Camptothecins in Cancer Therapy

Cancer Drug Discovery and Development

Beverly A. Teicher, Series Editor

Camptothecins in Cancer Therapy, edited by *Val R. Adams and Thomas G. Burke*, 2005

Combination Cancer Therapy: *Modulators and Potentiators*, edited by *Gary K. Schwartz*, 2005

Death Receptors in Cancer Therapy, edited by *Wafik S. El-Deiry*, 2005

Cancer Chemoprevention, Volume 2: *Strategies for Cancer Chemoprevention*, edited by *Gary J. Kelloff, Ernest T. Hawk, and Caroline C. Sigman*, 2005

Proteasome Inhibitors in Cancer Therapy, edited by *Julian Adams, 2004*

Nucleic Acid Therapeutics in Cancer, edited by *Alan M. Gewirtz, 2004*

Cancer Chemoprevention, Volume 1: *Promising Cancer Chemopreventive Agents*, edited by *Gary J. Kelloff, Ernest T. Hawk, and Caroline C. Sigman*, 2004

DNA Repair in Cancer Therapy, edited by *Lawrence C. Panasci and Moulay A. Alaoui-Jamali*, 2004

Hematopoietic Growth Factors in Oncology: *Basic Science and Clinical Therapeutics*, edited by *George Morstyn, MaryAnn Foote, and Graham J. Lieschke*, 2004

Handbook of Anticancer Pharmacokinetics and Pharmacodynamics, edited by *William D. Figg and Howard L. McLeod*, 2004

Anticancer Drug Development Guide: *Preclinical Screening, Clinical Trials, and Approval, Second Edition*, edited by *Beverly A. Teicher and Paul A. Andrews*, 2004

Handbook of Cancer Vaccines, edited by *Michael A. Morse, Timothy M. Clay, and Kim H. Lyerly*, 2004

Drug Delivery Systems in Cancer Therapy, edited by *Dennis M. Brown, 2003*

Oncogene-Directed Therapies, edited by *Janusz Rak*, 2003

Cell Cycle Inhibitors in Cancer Therapy: *Current Strategies*, edited by *Antonio Giordano and Kenneth J. Soprano*, 2003

Fluoropyrimidines in Cancer Therapy, edited by *Youcef M. Rustum*, 2003

Chemoradiation in Cancer Therapy, edited by *Hak Choy*, 2003

Targets for Cancer Chemotherapy: *Transcription Factors and Other Nuclear Proteins*, edited by *Nicholas B. La Thangue and Lan R. Bandara*, 2002

Tumor Targeting in Cancer Therapy, edited by *Michel Pagé*, 2002

Hormone Therapy in Breast and Prostate Cancer, edited by *V. Craig Jordan and Barrington J. A. Furr*, 2002

Tumor Models in Cancer Research, edited by *Beverly A. Teicher*, 2002

Tumor Suppressor Genes in Human Cancer, edited by *David E. Fisher*, 2001

Matrix Metalloproteinase Inhibitors in Cancer Therapy, edited by *Neil J. Clendeninn and Krzysztof Appelt*, 2001

Farnesyltransferase Inhibitors in Cancer, edited by *Saïd M. Sebti and Andrew D. Hamilton*, 2001

Platinum-Based Drugs in Cancer Therapy, edited by *Lloyd R. Kelland and Nicholas P. Farrell*, 2000

Signaling Networks and Cell Cycle Control: *The Molecular Basis of Cancer and Other Diseases*, edited by *J. Silvio Gutkind*, 1999

Apoptosis and Cancer Chemotherapy, edited by *John A. Hickman and Caroline Dive*, 1999

Antifolate Drugs in Cancer Therapy, edited by *Ann L. Jackman*, 1999

Antiangiogenic Agents in Cancer Therapy, edited by *Beverly A. Teicher*, 1999

Anticancer Drug Development Guide: *Preclinical Screening, Clinical Trials, and Approval*, edited by *Beverly A. Teicher*, 1997

Wolfgang Meyer, 04/2008

CAMPTOTHECINS IN CANCER THERAPY

Edited by

VAL R. ADAMS, PharmD

College of Pharmacy, University of Kentucky, Lexington, KY

and

THOMAS G. BURKE, PhD

Department of Pharmaceutical Sciences, College of Pharmacy and Lucille P. Markey Cancer Center, University of Kentucky; Tigen Pharmaceuticals Inc., Lexington, KY

HUMANA PRESS
TOTOWA, NEW JERSEY

999 Riverview Drive, Suite 208
Totowa, New Jersey 07512

www.humanapress.com

This publication is printed on acid-free paper. ∞
ANSI Z39.48-1984 (American National Standards Institute) Permanence of Paper for Printed Library Materials.

Production Editor: Wendy S. Kopf
Cover Design: Patricia F. Cleary
Cover Illustration: Figure 5 from Chapter 2, "Crystallographic Insight Into the Mechanism of Drug-Induced Topoisomerase I DNA Damage," by Alex B. Burgin, Jr., Michael D. Reese, Bart L. Staker, and Lance Stewart.

For additional copies, pricing for bulk purchases, and/or information about other Humana titles, contact Humana at the above address or at any of the following numbers: Tel.: 973-256-1699; Fax: 973-256-8341; E-mail: humana@humanapr.com or visit our Website at www.humanapress.com.

Printed in the United States of America. 10 9 8 7 6 5 4 3 2 1
eISBN 1-59259-866-8

Library of Congress Cataloging-in-Publication Data
Camptothecins in cancer therapy / edited by Thomas G. Burke and Val R. Adams.
p. ; cm. -- (Cancer drug discovery and development)
Includes bibliographical references and index.
ISBN 1-58829-027-1 (hardcover : alk. paper)
1. Camptothecin. 2. Cancer--Chemotherapy.
[DNLM: 1. Camptothecin--therapeutic use. 2. Neoplasms--drug therapy. 3. Antineoplastic Agents, Phytogenic--therapeutic use. 4. Camptothecin--analogs & derivatives. 5. Camptothecin--pharmacology. QV 269 C1989 2005] I. Burke, Thomas G., PhD. II. Adams, Val R. III. Series.
RC271.C35C345 2005
616.99'4061--dc22

2004013542

Dedication

I do not feel obliged to believe that the same God who has endowed us with sense, reason, and intellect has intended us to forgo their use.

Galileo Galilei

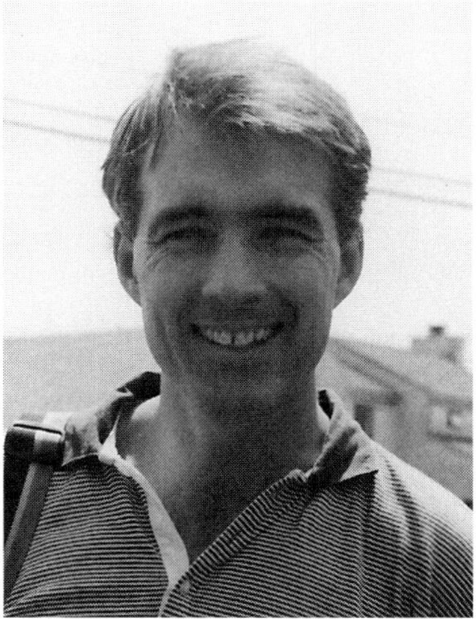

This book is lovingly dedicated to Dr. Thomas G. Burke, whose commitment to cancer research was exceeded only by his devotion to our marriage and our two young sons, Dylan and Aidan. In honor of his creative spirit and genuine enthusiasm for scientific inquiry, may this collection of articles serve both as a resource and as inspiration to researchers and clinicians alike.

Lori Latus

PREFACE

Clinical interest in the camptothecins continues to expand despite the fact that this class of agents has been studied for almost 50 years and two early generation members of the family have gained FDA approval. To date, the intensive research efforts carried have clearly validated the utility of this class of topoisomerase I inhibitor in the management of human cancer. The studies have also provided considerable insight into the shortcomings of the approved camptothecins and potential ways of improving upon the clinical performance of the family as a whole.

In the first part of *Camptothecins in Cancer Therapy* an up-to-date summary of what is known about the biochemistry, pharmacology, and chemistry of the camptothecins is presented. This section includes a discussion of the mechanism of topoisomerase I as well as a review of the means by which camptothecins poison this enzyme. The use of animal models in defining the anticancer potential of camptothecins and a discussion of camptothecin resistance is included. Chapters are also devoted to a review of new analog development, as well as drug delivery issues that are aimed at optimizing the anticancer activities of the camptothecins. In the third part of *Camptothecins in Cancer Therapy*, summaries are provided on each of the members of the camptothecin families that have been studied in the clinic. In addition, discussion of the potential use of camptothecins in a variety of different cancers has been included.

Camptothecins in Cancer Therapy aims to provide a thorough and up-to-date summary as well as define the central issues that will be the key focus areas in camptothecin research during the next 10 years.

Val R. Adams, ***PharmD***
Thomas G. Burke, ***PhD***

Contents

Contributors

Val R. Adams, PharmD • *Department of Pharmacy Practice and Science, College of Pharmacy, University of Kentucky, Lexington, KY*

Bradley D. Anderson, PhD • *Department of Pharmaceutical Sciences, College of Pharmacy, University of Kentucky, Lexington, KY*

Juana Barceló, PhD • *Laboratory of Molecular Pharmacology, Center for Cancer Research, National Center Institute, Bethesda, MD*

Aimee K. Bence, PhD • *Department of Pharmacy Practice and Science, College of Pharmacy, University of Kentucky, Lexington, KY*

Mary-Ann Bjornsti, PhD • *Department of Molecular Pharmacology, St. Jude Children's Research Hospital, Memphis, TN*

Alex B. Burgin, Jr., PhD • *deCODE Biostructures, Bainbridge Island, WA*

Thomas G. Burke, PhD (deceased) • *Department of Pharmaceutical Sciences, College of Pharmacy, and Experimental Therapeutics Program, Lucille P. Markey Cancer Center, University of Kentucky Medical Center, University of Kentucky, and Tigen Pharmaceuticals Inc., Lexington, KY*

Shyamal D. Desai, PhD • *Department of Pharmacology, UMDNJ–Robert Wood Johnson Medical School, Piscataway, NJ*

Michael D. Feese, PhD • *deCODE Biostructures, Bainbridge Island, WA*

Keith T. Flaherty, MD • *Division of Hematology/Oncology, Department of Medicine, University of Pennsylvania, Philadelphia, PA*

Henry S. Friedman, MD • *Brain Tumor Center, Duke University Medical Center, Durham, NC*

Takahisa Furuta, MD, PhD • *Laboratory of Molecular Pharmacology, Center for Cancer Research, National Cancer Institute, Bethesda, MD*

Jorge Gomez, MD • *Department of Thoracic Medicine, Memorial Sloan-Kettering Cancer Center, New York, NY*

Missak Haigentz, Jr., MD • *Department of Oncology, Montefiore Medical Center, Albert Einstein College of Medicine, Bronx, NY*

Sidney M. Hecht, PhD • *Departments of Chemistry and Biology, University of Virginia, Charlottesville, VA*

Hilary Hewes, MD • *Division of Hematology/Oncology, Cancer Research and Treatment Center, University of New Mexico, Albuquerque NM*

PETER J. HOUGHTON, PhD • *Department of Molecular Pharmacology, St. Jude Children's Research Hospital, Memphis, TN*

AARTI S. JUVEKAR, PhD • *Department of Molecular Pharmacology, St. Jude Children's Research Hospital, Memphis, TN and Cancer Research Institute, Parel, Bombay, India*

SCOTT H. KAUFMANN, MD, PhD • *Division of Hematology, Department of Internal Medicine and Department of Oncology, Mayo Clinic, Rochester, MN*

PANKAJ KUMAR, MD • *Department of Oncology, Montefiore Medical Center, Albert Einstein College of Medicine, Bronx, NY*

LORI J. LATUS, MD • *Tigen Pharmaceuticals Inc., Lexington, KY*

MARKOS LEGGAS, PhD • *Department of Pharmaceutical Sciences, College of Pharmacy, University of Kentucky, Lexington, KY*

ZHIYONG LIAO, PhD • *Laboratory of Molecular Pharmacology, Center for Cancer Research, National Cancer Institute, Bethesda, MD*

LEROY F. LIU, PhD • *Department of Pharmacology, UMDNJ–Robert Wood Johnson Medical School, Piscataway, NJ and Cancer Institute of New Jersey, New Brunswick, NJ*

BENJAMIN M. F. MOW, MD • *Department of Hematology/Oncology, National University Hospital, Singapore*

PETER J. O'DWYER, MD • *Division of Hematology–Oncology, Abramson Cancer Center, Department of Medicine, University of Pennsylvania, Philadelphia, PA*

ROMAN PEREZ-SOLER, MD • *Department of Oncology, Montefiore Medical Center, Albert Einstein College of Medicine, Bronx, NY*

YVES G. POMMIER, MD, PhD • *Laboratory of Molecular Pharmacology, Center for Cancer Research, National Cancer Institute, Bethesda, MD*

ZESHAAN A. RASHEED, MD, PhD • *Department of Pharmacology, Cancer Institute of New Jersey, New Brunswick, NJ*

LAURENT P. RIVORY, PhD • *Preclinical Development Team, Johnson and Johnson Research Pty. Ltd., Eveleigh, NSW, Australia*

ERIC K. ROWINSKY, MD • *Director of Clinical Research, Institute for Drug Development, Cancer Therapy and Research Center, University of Texas Health Science Center, San Antonio, TX*

ERIC H. RUBIN, MD • *Department of Pharmacology, Cancer Institute of New Jersey, New Brunswick, NJ*

JUDITH A. SMITH, PharmD • *Section of Gynecologic Medical Therapeutics, Division of Pharmacy and Division of Cancer Medicine, MD Anderson Cancer Center, University of Texas, Houston, TX*

Olivier Sordet, PhD • *Laboratory of Molecular Pharmacology, Center for Cancer Research, National Cancer Institute, Bethesda, MD*

Bart L. Staker, PhD • *deCODE Biostructures, Bainbridge Island, WA*

James P. Stevenson, MD • *Division of Hematology/Oncology, Department of Medicine, University of Pennsylvania, Philadelphia, PA*

Clinton F. Stewart, PharmD • *Department of Pharmaceutical Sciences, St. Jude Children's Research Hospital, Memphis, TN*

Lance Stewart, PhD • *deCODE Biostructures, Bainbridge Island, WA*

Haruyuki Takemura, MD, PhD • *Laboratory of Molecular Pharmacology, Center for Cancer Research, National Cancer Institute, Bethesda, MD*

Chris H. Takimoto, MD, PhD • *Division of Medical Oncology, Department of Medicine, University of Texas Health Science Center at San Antonio, and Institute for Drug Development, Cancer Therapy and Research Center, San Antonio, TX*

Joyce Thompson, MD • *Department of Hematology/Oncology, St. Jude Children's Research Hospital, Memphis, TN*

Christopher J. Twelves, MD • *Department of Medical Oncology, University of Glasgow, Glasgow, Scotland*

Robert C. A. M. van Waardenburg, PhD • *Department of Molecular Pharmacology, St. Jude Children's Research Hospital, Memphis, TN*

Claire Verschraegen, MD • *Division of Hematology/Oncology, Cancer Research and Treatment Center, University of New Mexico, Albuquerque NM*

Tian-Xiang Xiang, PhD • *Department of Pharmaceutical Sciences, College of Pharmacy, and Experimental Therapeutics Program, Lucille P. Markey Cancer Center, University of Kentucky, Lexington, KY*

I

Biochemistry, Pharmacology, and Chemistry

1 Mechanism of Action of Topoisomerase 1 Poisons

Leroy F. Liu, PhD,
and Shyamal D. Desai, PhD

CONTENTS

1. INTRODUCTION

DNA topoisomerases are important nuclear enzymes involved in many aspects of DNA metabolism, such as DNA replication, RNA transcription, chromosome condensation, and segregation *(1–5)*. They perform their topological transformation reactions on DNA via a concerted breakage/religation mechanism *(4,6–8)*. Because of their delicate act on DNA, topoisomerases can be double-edged swords. It is now well established that many xenobiotics, DNA lesions, and physiological stresses (e.g., oxidative stress, acidic pH stress, thiol stress) can interfere with the breakage/religation

Camptothecins in Cancer Therapy
Edited by: V. R. Adams and T. G. Burke © Humana Press Inc., Totowa, NJ

reactions of topoisomerases, resulting in topoisomerase-mediated DNA damage *(9–14)*. Among the five human DNA topoisomerases (hTOP1, hTOP2α, hTOP2β, hTOP3α, and hTOP3β), the first three have been identified to be molecular targets of anticancer drugs *(1,9,11,15–22)*.

DNA topoisomerase I was originally identified as the molecular target of the plant alkaloid camptothecin (CPT) *(8,15,23,24)*. CPT exhibits impressive antitumor activities against a broad spectrum of tumors in animal models *(25–27)*. Two CPT derivatives, irinotecan and topotecan, have been successfully developed in the clinic *(28–31)*, and second-generation CPTs such as silatecan and homocamptothecin appear quite promising in preclinical development *(32–39)*.

2. MECHANISM OF ACTION OF CAMPTOTHECIN

CPT specifically inhibits the relegation step of the TOP1 catalyzed cleavage/relegation reaction, resulting in the accumulation of a covalent reaction intermediate, often referred to as the cleavable or cleavage complex *(7,8,18)*. Insight into the structure of the TOP1 cleavable complex has been obtained from both biochemical and X-ray crystallographic studies *(40–43)*. These studies were performed using a self-poisoning DNA sequence (a TOP1 binding/cleavage hotspot sequence) derived from *Tetrahymena* recombinant (rDNA) *(43)*. This self-poisoning DNA sequence contains multiple A tracts located both upstream and downstream from the cleavage site. These A tracts are known to induce DNA bends *(44,45)*. Biochemical studies have demonstrated that TOP1 protects a 20-bp DNA region in which the cleavage position is centrally located *(42)*. A core of six bases (core element) located upstream of the cleavage site is of critical importance for TOP1 binding. The importance of this core element in TOP1 binding is also mirrored by the presence of a weak TOP1 cleavage consensus sequence located from +1 to –4 (+ and – refer to downstream and upstream positions from the site of cleavage, respectively). X-ray crystallographic studies of the cleavable complex formed between this self-poisoning DNA sequence and TOP1 have confirmed the essential interaction between TOP1 and the nucleotides located from +1 to –5. Both biochemical and X-ray crystallographic studies have demonstrated some weak interactions downstream from the site of DNA cleavage *(40,43,46)*.

Models explaining the molecular mechanism of TOP1 poisoning by CPT have been proposed. A base-flipping model was suggested based on the crystallographic structure of the TOP1-DNA cleavable complex and the results from the crosslinking studies using an alkylating CPT derivative *(41,47)*. In this model, CPT intercalates between the +1 and –1 bases, and the +1 base on the scissile strand is flipped out of the DNA helical stack *(41)*. Using computer modeling, a CPT pseudointercalation model has also been pro-

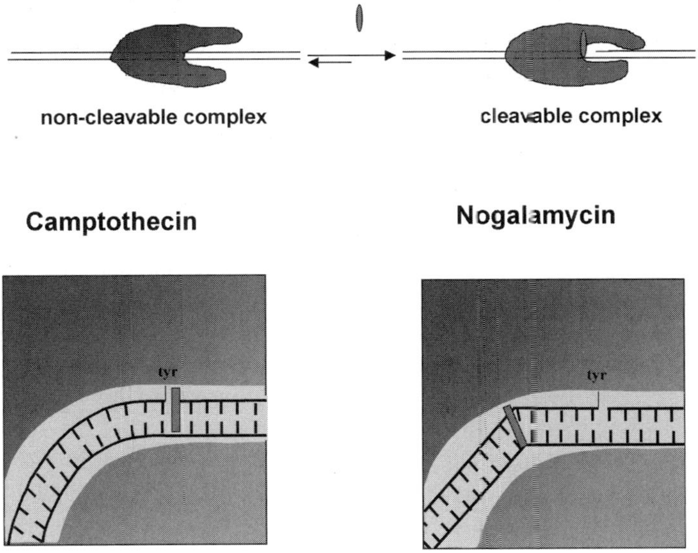

Fig. 1. Two proposed molecular mechanisms for topoisomerase (TOP1) poisoning by different TOP1 poisons. The intercalation model proposed for camptothecins is shown on the left; the DNA bending model proposed for nogalamycin is shown on the right.

posed, in which CPT is inserted between the +1 and –1 bases *(44)*. More recently based on other computer modeling studies, a CPT intercalation model in which CPT is completely intercalated between the +1 and –1 bases has been proposed *(49)* (Fig. 1). In this model, CPT is intercalated between the +1 and –1 bases, with the E-ring pointing into the minor groove and the A-ring directed toward the major groove *(49)*. These models highlight the importance of CPT binding to the site of DNA cleavage to interfere with the relegation step of the TOP1-catalyzed reaction. A recent study has solved the crystal structure of the TOP1 (topo70)-topotecan-DNA ternary complex at 2.1 Angstrom *(50)*. In this structure, topotecan is completely intercalated between +1 and –1 bases *(50)*.

3. NONCAMPTOTHECIN TOPOISOMERASE 1 POSIONS

In addition to CPT, a growing list of compounds (e.g., indolocarbazoles, nitidines, saintopin, intoplicine, fagaronine, bulgarein, morpholinyl doxorubicin, aclacinomycin A, indeno[1,2-c]isoquinolines, nogalamycin, actinomycin D, protoberberines, 2-phenylbenzimidazoles, dibenzo[*c,h*] cinnolines, terbenzimidazoles) has been identified to be TOP1 poisons *(51–61)*. Unlike CPT, the majority of these TOP1 poisons are DNA binders, suggesting that DNA binding may underlie the mechanism of TOP1 poisoning by at least some of these TOP1 poisons *(51,54,59,62,63)*. Studies on nogalamycin have provided some important clues to the role of DNA binding in the mechanism of TOP1 poisoning *(64)*. Nogalamycin is a strong DNA binder that exhibits both intercalative and minor groove-directed modes of interactions *(65–69)*. The minor groove-directed interaction of nogalamycin, as in the case of minor groove-binding Hoechst 33342, has been shown to be critical for TOP1 poisoning *(51)*. Studies of the interaction between nogalamycin and the TOP1-DNA complex have suggested that nogalamycin binds to a site that is three to six bases upstream of the site of TOP1-mediated DNA cleavage *(64)*. Neither the base-flipping model nor the intercalation models *(41,48,49)*, which requires that the drug bind between +1 and –1 bases, can explain the poisoning action of nogalamycin. Further studies have suggested that a nogalamycin-induced DNA bend located upstream of the cleavage site is responsible for enhanced TOP1 cleavage *(64)* (*see* Fig. 1). This DNA-bending model for TOP1 poisoning induced by nogalamycin is quite reminiscent of the DNA curvature model proposed for TOP1 poisoning by the self-poisoning sequence derived from *Tetrahymena* rDNA *(43)*. In fact, the nogalamycin-induced TOP1 cleavage hotspot shares a 10-bp identity (–2 to +8) with the self-poisoning sequence from *Tetrahymena* rDNA. In the case of the self-poisoning sequence, the presence of the DNA curvature has been suggested to be responsible for enhanced TOP1 binding and hence TOP1-mediated DNA cleavage. It seems plausible that nogalamycin may enhance TOP1 cleavage by a similar mechanism (i.e., enhanced TOP1 binding resulting from nogalamycin-induced DNA bend). Studies on nogalamycin have clearly implicated the importance of DNA structural perturbation on TOP1 poisoning.

4. DNA LESIONS AS TOPOISOMERASE 1 POISONS

The importance of DNA structural perturbation in the mechanism of TOP1 poisoning is also echoed by the observations that many DNA lesions (e.g., ultraviolet (UV) adducts, araC-substituted DNA, uracil-containing DNA, abasic sites, base mismatches, nicks and gaps, oxidized DNA, benzo[a]pyrene diol epoxide-DNA adducts) can poison TOP1 *(70–75)*. Many of these DNA lesions are known to either induce DNA bends or increase DNA flexibility *(76–84)*. Studies of 8-oxoguanine–containing DNA has also demonstrated that TOP1 poisoning is not caused by inhibition of relegation but rather, is a result of enhanced binding/cleavage *(75)*. Consequently, nogalamycin and some of these DNA lesions may share the same mechanism of TOP1 poisoning.

5. CELLULAR PROCESSING OF TOP1 CLEAVABLE COMPLEXES

The TOP1 cleavable complex, being a reversible protein-DNA covalent complex, represents a rather unique type of cellular lesion. So far, most studies have focused on its DNA damaging effect. Indeed, as with many other DNA damaging agents, CPT induces mutation/recombination, G2 cell cycle arrest, apoptotic cell death, elevation of *c-fos/c-jun* mRNAs, elevation of p53, phosphorylation of Chk1, and activation of nuclear factor κB *(85–97)*. Expression of most, if not all, of these DNA damaging effects of CPT requires ongoing DNA synthesis *(96–100)*. Inhibition of DNA synthesis with replication inhibitors can completely abrogate CPT cytotoxicity and other DNA-damaging effects *(99,101)*. A replication collision model has been proposed to explain the DNA-damaging effect of TOP1 cleavable complexes induced by CPT *(101)*. On collision between the replication fork, the reversible TOP1 cleavable complex is transformed into a potentially lethal double-strand DNA break *(98–101)*. Aspects of this replication model have been reproduced in a SV40 cell-free replication system *(102,103)* and confirmed by additional studies in mammalian cells *(104)*. Further support for the model comes from studies in yeast in which rad52 mutant yeast defective in double-strand break repair has been shown to be hypersensitive to CPT *(105–109)*.

In addition to the DNA replication machinery, the RNA transcription machinery also appears to process TOP1 cleavable complexes *(110)*. It has been demonstrated in an in vitro study that transcription can process TOP1-cleavable complexes into TOP1-linked DNA breaks on the template but not on the nontemplate DNA strand *(110)*. However, the role of transcription in CPT cytotoxicity is still unclear.

6. COVALENT MODIFICATION OF TOP1 CLEAVABLE COMPLEXES

In addition to the DNA damaging effects, TOP1 cleavable complexes induced by CPT have been shown to trigger other cellular responses, which appear to be unrelated to the DNA damage responses *(111–114)*. Two of these cellular responses, which occur immediately downstream from the TOP1-cleavable complexes have been described: the formation of ubiquitin-TOP1 conjugates and the formation of small ubiquitin-related modifier (SUMO-1)-TOP1 conjugates *(111–114)*. Although ubiquitin-TOP1 conjugates are destined for 26S proteasome-mediated degradation (TOP1 downregulation), the fate of SUMO-1-TOP1 conjugates is still unclear *(115–126)*. Although modification of TOP1 by ubiquitin and SUMO-1 occurs on TOP1-cleavable complexes, these cellular responses appear distinct from DNA damage responses. First, unlike the DNA damage response induced by CPT, the formation of ubiquitin-TOP1 and SUMO-1-TOP1 conjugates is unaffected by DNA replication inhibitors *(9,112,114)*. Second, ICRF-193, which is a catalytic inhibitor of TOP2 and does not induce TOP2-cleavable complexes *(111)*, can also induce the formation of ubiquitin/SUMO-1-TOP2 conjugates *(111,115)*. ICRF-193 is known to inhibit ATP hydrolysis and thereby trapping TOP2 in a protein clamp conformation *(127,128)*. Third, heat shock and other cellular stresses that damage proteins have been shown to induce ubiquitination and SUMOlation *(111,126,129–137)*, suggesting that ubiquitination and SUMOlation are protein stress responses. One attractive hypothesis is that ubiquitin/SUMO-1 conjugation to TOP1 is a direct result of the conformational change of TOP1 associated with the formation of TOP1-cleavable complexes.

7. UBIQUITIN/26S PROTEASOME-DEPENDENT DOWN-REGULATION OF TOP1

The role of ubiquitination of TOP1-cleavable complexes has been explored to some extent. As expected, ubiquitination of TOP1-cleavable complexes leads to 26S proteasome-mediated degradation of TOP1 (TOP1 down-regulation) *(114)*. It has been suggested that TOP1 down-regulation induced by CPT is an effective means to reduce the level of TOP1-cleavable complexes in cells *(114,138)*. Studies using a panel of breast and colorectal cancer cell lines have demonstrated that CPT-induced down-regulation exhibits a high degree of heterogeneity *(139–141)*. There was a general correlation between the extent of TOP1 downregulation and CPT resistance among these cancer cells. The breast cancer cell line ZR-75-1, being most sensitive to CPT, was completely defective in CPT-induced down-regulation of TOP1, whereas the BT474 breast cancer cell line, being least sensitive to CPT, exhibited effective CPT-induced down-regulation of TOP1 *(140,141)*. The 26S proteasome inhibitor MG132 was shown to inhibit CPT-induced downregulation of TOP1 in BT474 cells and concomitantly sensitized BT474 cells to CPT-induced apoptosis. By contrast, MG132 had little effect on CPT-induced apoptosis in ZR-75-1 cells *(141)*. These results suggest that CPT-induced down-regulation of TOP1 could be an important parameter for determining CPT sensitivity/resistance in tumor cells. The role of TOP1 down-regulation in CPT resistance is reasonable because removal of TOP1 by degradation is expected to reduce the cellular level of TOP1-cleavable complexes and hence resistance to CPT. However, it is also possible that TOP1 degradation is part of the repair mechanism for repairing TOP1 covalent complexes. Degradation of TOP1 may be necessary to reveal the hidden strand break for repair to occur.

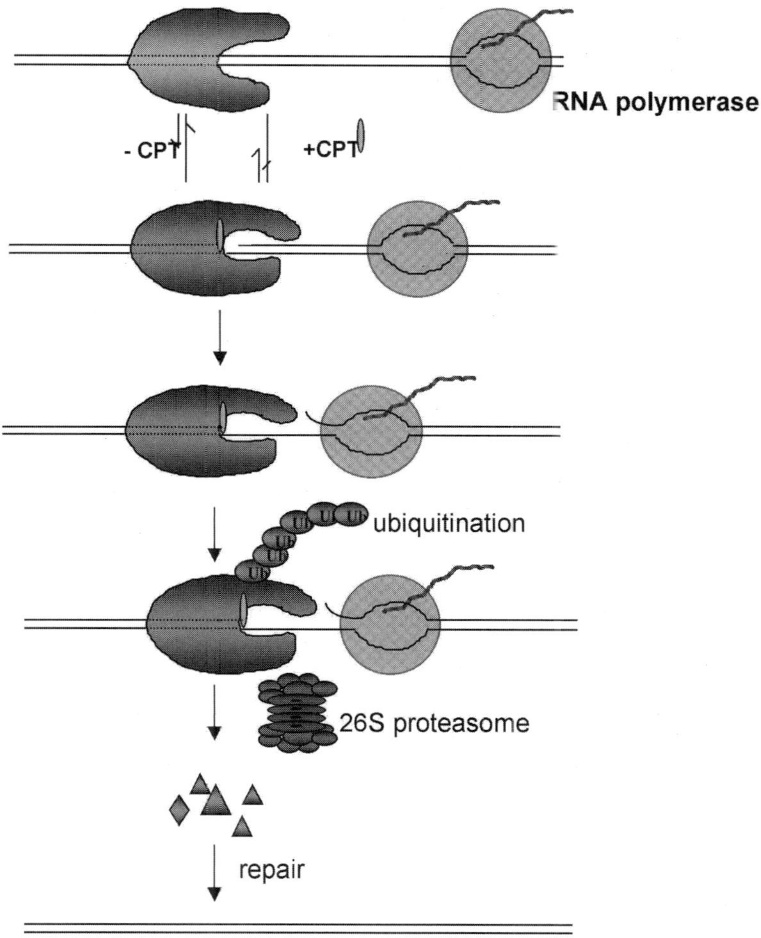

Fig. 2. A working model for camptothecin-induced down-regulation of topoisomerase 1.

Recent studies have demonstrated that transcription inhibitors such as DRB and α-amanitin inhibit CPT-induced TOP1 down-regulation, suggesting that transcription may be involved in this process. Further studies have suggested that transcription may be involved in the conversion of TOP1-cleavable complexes into irreversible TOP1-linked DNA breaks *(142)*. The working model for the role of transcription in CPT-induced down-regulation is shown in Fig. 2.

It has also been noted that CPT-induced TOP1 down-regulation is generally absent or reduced in tumor cells as compared with normal cells both in tissue culture models (141) and in patients *(143,144)*. Defect in CPT-induced down-regulation in tumor cells could contribute to the sensitivity of tumor cells to CPT. However, it is unclear why tumor cells are generally defective in CPT-induced down-regulation of TOP1. There is an inverse correlation between the extent of TOP1 down-regulation and the level of UCRP (ubiquitin cross-reactive protein) *(145–147)*. UCRP is the interferon-inducible protein ISG15 *(145–147)* and conjugates to substrate targets in a way similar but not identical to that of ubiquitin *(145–147)*. It remains to be determined if altered regulation of UCRP in tumor cells is responsible for defective TOP1 down-regulation.

8. SUMO-1 MODIFICATION OF TOP1 CLEAVABLE COMPLEXES

CPT induces rapid SUMO-1 conjugation to TOP1-cleavable complexes *(112,140)*. Both SUMO-1 and SUMO-2/3 have been demonstrated to conjugate to TOP1 in CPT-treated cells *(108)* (Yong M, Liu LF, unpublished results). Human SUMO-1 (also called UBL1, PIC1, GMP1, SMT3C, and sentrin in the literature) *(96,98,148–152)* is a ubiquitin-like protein. It shares an approximate 18% identity with ubiquitin *(124–126)*. Human SUMO-1 and its yeast homolog, Smt3p, also share a similar activation and conjugation pathway with ubiquitin, but employ distinct sets of E1 and E2 enzymes *(153–158)*. The E1 enzymes for activating human SUMO-1 and yeast Smt3p are the heterodimeric proteins, SAE1/SAE2 and Aos1p/Uba2p, respectively *(158,159)*. UBC9 is the only E2 identified for SUMO-1/Smt3p, whereas a dozen E2 enzymes have been identified for ubiquitin in yeast *(115–123)*. Recently, proteases that specifically activate SUMO-1/Smt3p precursors and cleave SUMO-1/Smt3p from their protein conjugates have been identified in yeast and mammalian cells *(122,124,162,163)*. Many proteins—such as RanGAP1, PML, IκBα, RAD51, RAD52, p53, and centromere proteins, which have diverse functions—have been shown to interact with UBC9/SUMO-1 or be covalently modified by SUMO-1 *(122,164–172)*. Except for RanGAP1 and perhaps a limited number of proteins, SUMO-1 appears to target nuclear proteins exclusively *(111,122,137,174)*. Although the function of SUMO-1 is still elusive, there are a few interesting observations that may shed light on the function of SUMO-1. First, PODs (PML oncogenic domains, also called nuclear bodies or ND10) *(175–177)* and the nuclear envelope appear to be the major sites of localization of SUMO-1 conjugates in the nucleus *(122,174)*. Second, SUMO-1 and ubiquitin appear to share the same conjugation sites on some target proteins (e.g., IκBα, MDM2) *(164,171)*. Third, SUMO has been shown to interact with the proteasome machinery *(179)*. This suggests that SUMO-conjugation to TOP1-cleavable complexes may be for the purpose of recruiting 26S proteasome machinery. As with TOP1, many substrates (e.g., IκBα, PML,

P53), which are conjugated to SUMO-1, are also conjugated to ubiquitin and are destroyed by 26S proteasome *(164,165,167,171)*. The role of sumoylation of TOP1-cleavable complexes is much less clear. However, sumoylation of TOP1 has been suggested to affect nucleolar delocalization in response to TOP1 inhibitors *(180,181)*. SUMO-1 conjugation to intact DNA topoisomerase I has also been shown to amplify cleavable complex formation on camptothecin treatment *(182)*.

The possibility that SUMOlation may be important for CPT cytotoxicity has been explored in yeast expressing human TOP1. It has been shown that partial inactivation of UBC9 leads to increased CPT sensitivity *(112)*. In addition, overexpression of Smt3p leads to an increase in CPT resistance *(112)*. These preliminary studies suggest that Smt3p/SUMO and UBC9 do affect CPT cytotoxicity *(112)*. However, whether the effect of Smt3p and UBC9 on CPT cytotoxicity is through their SUMOlation reaction on TOP1-cleavable complexes or through some other indirect events is unclear. Further studies are necessary to establish the role of SUMO-1-TOP1 conjugation in CPT sensitivity/resistance.

ACKNOWLEDGMENT

This work was supported by National Institute of Health grants CA39662 and CA077433.

REFERENCES

1. Liu LF. 1989 DNA topoisomerase poisons as antitumor drugs. Annu Rev Biochem 58:351–375.
2. Castano IB, Brzoska PM, Sadoff BU, Chen H, Christman MF. 1996 Mitotic chromosome condensation in the rDNA requires TRF4 and DNA topoisomerase I in Saccharomyces cerevisiae. Genes Dev 10:2564–2576.
3. Champoux JJ, Dulbecco R. 1972 An activity from mammalian cells that untwists superhelical DNA—a possible swivel for DNA replication (polyoma-ethidium bromide-mouse- embryo cells-dye binding assay). Proc Natl Acad Sci USA 69:143–146.
4. Wang JC. 1996 DNA topoisomerases. Annu Rev Biochem 65:635–692.
5. Zhang CX, Chen AD, Gettel NJ, Hsieh TS. 2000 Essential functions of DNA topoisomerase I in Drosophila melanogaster. Dev Biol 222:27–40.
6. Halligan BD, Davis JL, Edwards KA, Liu LF. 1982 Intra- and intermolecular strand transfer by HeLa DNA topoisomerase I. J Biol Chem 257:3995–4000.
7. Porter SE, Champoux JJ. 1989 The basis for camptothecin enhancement of DNA breakage by eukaryotic topoisomerase I. Nucleic Acids Res 17:8521–8532.
8. Hsiang YH, Hertzberg R, Hecht S, Liu LF. 1985 Camptothecin induces protein-linked DNA breaks via mammalian DNA topoisomerase I. J Biol Chem 260:14873–14878.
9. Li TK, Liu LF. 2001 Tumor cell death induced by topoisomerase-targeting drugs. Ann Rev Pharmacol Toxicol 41:53–77.

10. Li TK, Chen AY, Yu C, Mao Y, Wang H, Liu LF. 1999 Activation of topoisomerase II-mediated excision of chromosomal DNA loops during oxidative stress. Genes Dev 13:1553–1560.
11. Chen AY, Liu LF. 1994 DNA topoisomerases: essential enzymes and lethal targets. Annu Rev Pharmacol Toxicol 34:191–218
12. Kingma PS, Corbett AH, Burcham PC, Marnett LJ, Osheroff N. 1995 Abasic sites stimulate double-stranded DNA cleavage mediated by topoisomerase II. DNA lesions as endogenous topoisomerase II poisons. J Biol Chem 270:21441–21444.
13. Frydman B, Marton LJ, Sun JS, Neder K, Witiak DT, Liu AA, et al. 1997 Induction of DNA topoisomerase II-mediated DNA cleavage by beta-lapachone and related naphthoquinones. Cancer Res 57:620–627.
14. Vizan JL, Hernandez-Chico C, del CI, Moreno F. 1991 The peptide antibiotic microcin B17 induces double-strand cleavage of DNA mediated by E. coli DNA gyrase. EMBO J 10:467–476.
15. Hsiang YH, Liu LF. 1988 Identification of mammalian DNA topoisomerase I as an intracellular target of the anticancer drug camptothecin. Cancer Res 48:1722–1726.
16. Mao Y, Yu C, Hsieh TS, Nitiss JL, Liu AA, Wang H, et al. 1999 Mutations of human topoisomerase II alpha affecting multidrug resistance and sensitivity. Biochemistry 38:10793–10800.
17. Kupfer G, Bodley AL, Liu LF. 1987 Involvement of intracellular ATP in cytotoxicity of topoisomerase II-targetting antitumor drugs. NCI Monogr 4:37–40.
18. Nitiss JL, Wang JC. 1996 Mechanisms of cell killing by drugs that trap covalent complexes between DNA topoisomerases and DNA. Mol Pharmacol 50:1095–1102.
19. Goulaouic H, Roulon T, Flamand O, Grondard L, Lavelle F, Riou JF. 1999 Purification and characterization of human DNA topoisomerase IIIalpha. Nucleic Acids Res 27:2443–2450.
20. Seki T, Seki M, Onodera R, Katada T, Enomoto T. 1998 Cloning of cDNA encoding a novel mouse DNA topoisomerase III (Topo IIIbeta) possessing negatively supercoiled DNA relaxing activity, whose message is highly expressed in the testis. J Biol Chem 27:28553–28556.
21. Bennett RJ, Noirot-Gros MF, Wang JC. 2000 Interaction between yeast sgs1 helicase and DNA topoisomerase III. J Biol Chem 275:26898–26905.
22. Hanai R, Caron PR, Wang JC. 1996 Human TOP3: a single-copy gene encoding DNA topoisomerase III. Proc Natl Acad Sci USA 93:3653–3657.
23. Wall ME, Wani MC, Cook CE, Palmer KH, Mc Phail AT, Sim GM. 1966 Plant antitumor agents. I. The isolation and structure of camptothecin, a novel alkaloidal leukemia and tumor inhibitor from Camptotheca acuminata. J Am Chem Soc 88:3888–3890.
24. Wani MC, Wall ME. 1969 Plant antitumor agents. II. The structure of two new alkaloids from Camptotheca acuminata. J Org Chem 34:1364–1367.
25. Giovanella BC, Stehlin JS, Wall ME, Wani MC, Nicholas AW, Liu LF, et al. 1989 DNA topoisomerase I-targeted chemotherapy of human colon cancer in xenografts. Science 246:1046–1048.
26. Pantazis P, Early JA, Kozielski AJ, Mendoza JT, Hinz HR, Giovanella BC. 1993 Regression of human breast carcinoma tumors in immunodeficient mice treated with 9-nitrocamptothecin: differential response of nontumorigenic and tumorigenic human breast cells in vitro. Cancer Res 53:1577–1582.
27. Pantazis P, Kozielski AJ, Mendoza JT, Early JA, Hinz HR, Giovanella BC. 1993 Camptothecin derivatives induce regression of human ovarian carcinomas grown

in nude mice and distinguish between non-tumorigenic and tumorigenic cells in vitro. Int J Cancer 53:863–871.

28. Ogawa M. Novel anticancer drugs in Japan. 1999 J Cancer Res Clin Oncol 125: 134–140.
29. Rosen LS. 1998 Irinotecan in lymphoma, leukemia, and breast, pancreatic, ovarian, and small-cell lung cancers. Oncology (Huntingt) 12:103–109.
30. Chang AY. 1997 The potential role of topotecan in the treatment of advanced breast cancer. Semin Oncol 24:S20.
31. Davis PL, Shaiu WL, Scott GL, Iglehart JD, Hsieh TS, Marks JR. 1998 Complex response of breast epithelial cell lines to topoisomerase inhibitors. Anticancer Res 18:2919–2932
32. Bom D, Curran DP, Kruszewski S, Zimmer SG, Thompson SJ, Kohlhagen G, et al. 2000 The novel silatecan 7-tert-butyldimethylsilyl-10-hydroxycamptothecin displays high lipophilicity, improved human blood stability, and potent anticancer activity. J Med Chem 43:3970–3980.
33. Urasaki Y, Takebayashi Y, Pommier Y. 2000 Activity of a novel camptothecin analogue, homocamptothecin, in camptothecin-resistant cell lines with topoisomerase I alterations. Cancer Res 60:6577–6580.
34. Lavergne O, Harnett J, Rolland A, Lanco C, Lesueur-Ginot L, Demarquay D, et al. 1999 BN 80927: a novel homocamptothecin with inhibitory activities on both topoisomerase I and topoisomerase II. Bioorg Med Chem Lett 9:2599–2602.
35. Lesueur-Ginot L, Demarquay D, Kiss R, Kasprzyk PG, Dassonneville L, Bailly C, et al. 1999 Homocamptothecin, an E-ring modified camptothecin with enhanced lactone stability, retains topoisomerase I-targeted activity and antitumor properties. Cancer Res 59:2939–2943.
36. Philippart P, Harper L, Chaboteaux C, Decaestecker C, Bronckart Y, Gordover L, et al. 2000 Homocamptothecin, an E-ring-modified camptothecin, exerts more potent antiproliferative activity than other topoisomerase I inhibitors in human colon cancers obtained from surgery and maintained in vitro under histotypical culture conditions. Clin Cancer Res 6:1557–1562.
37. Lavergne O, Lesueur-Ginot L, Pla RF, Kasprzyk PG, Pommier J, Demarquay D, et al. 1998 Homocamptothecins: synthesis and antitumor activity of novel E-ring-modified camptothecin analogues. J Med Chem 41:5410–5419.
38. Demarquay D, Coulomb H, Huchet M, Lesueur-Ginot L, Camara J, Lavergne O, et al. 2000 The homocamptothecin, BN 80927, is a potent topoisomerase I poison and topoisomerase II catalytic inhibitor. Ann N Y Acad Sci 922:301–302.
39. Lavergne O, Demarquay D, Bailly C, Lanco C, Rolland A, Huchet M, et al. 2000 Topoisomerase I-mediated antiproliferative activity of enantiomerically pure fluorinated homocamptothecins. J Med Chem 43:2285–2289.
40. Stewart L, Redinbo MR, Qiu X, Hol WG, Champoux JJ. 1998 A model for the mechanism of human topoisomerase I. Science 279 1534–1541.
41. Redinbo MR, Stewart L, Kuhn P, Champoux JJ, Hol WG. 1998 Crystal structures of human topoisomerase I in covalent and noncovalent complexes with DNA. Science 279:1504–1513.
42. Stevnsner T, Mortensen UH, Westergaard O, Bonven BJ. 1989 Interactions between eukaryotic DNA topoisomerase I and a specific binding sequence. J Biol Chem 264:10110–10113.
43. Krogh S, Mortensen UH, Westergaard O, Bonven BJ. 1991 Eukaryotic topoisomerase I-DNA interaction is stabilized by helix curvature. Nucleic Acids Res 19:1235–1241.

44. Koo HS, Wu HM, Crothers DM. 1986 DNA bending at adenine thymine tracts. Nature 320:501–506.
45. Chan SS, Breslauer KJ, Austin RH, Hogan ME. 1993 Thermodynamics and premelting conformational changes of phased (dA)5 tracts. Biochemistry 32:11776–11784.
46. Christiansen K, Svejstrup AB, Andersen AH, Westergaard O. 1993 Eukaryotic topoisomerase I-mediated cleavage requires bipartite DNA interaction. Cleavage of DNA substrates containing strand interruptions implicates a role for topoisomerase I in illegitimate recombination. J Biol Chem 268:9690–9701.
47. Pommier Y, Kohlhagen G, Kohn KW, Leteurtre F, Wani MC, Wall ME. 1995 Interaction of an alkylating camptothecin derivative with a DNA base at topoisomerase I-DNA cleavage sites. Proc Natl Acad Sci USA 92:8861–8865.
48. Fan Y, Weinstein JN, Kohn KW, Shi LM, Pommier Y. 1998 Molecular modeling studies of the DNA-topoisomerase I ternary cleavable complex with camptothecin. J Med Chem 41:2216–2226.
49. Kerrigan JE, Pilch DS. 2001 A structural model for the ternary cleavable complex formed between human topoisomerase I, DNA and camptothecin. Biochemistry 40:9792–9798.
50. Staker BL, Hjerrild K, Feese MD, Behnke CA, Burgin AB, Stewart L. 2002 The mechanism of topoisomerase I poisoning by a camptothecin analog. Proc Nat Acad Sci USA 99:15387–15392.
51. Sim SP, Gatto B, Yu C, Liu AA, Li TK, Pilch DS, et al. 1997 Differential poisoning of topoisomerases by menogaril and nogalamycin dictated by the minor groove-binding nogalose sugar. Biochemistry 36:13285–13291.
52. Leteurtre F, Fujimori A, Tanizawa A, Chhabra A, Mazumder A, Kohlhagen G, et al. 1994 Saintopin, a dual inhibitor of DNA topoisomerases I and II, as a probe for drug-enzyme interactions. J Biol Chem 269:28702–28707.
53. Chen AY, Yu C, Bodley A, Peng LF, Liu LF. 1993 A new mammalian DNA topoisomerase I poison Hoechst 33342: cytotoxicity and drug resistance in human cell cultures. Cancer Res 53:1332–1337.
54. Chen AY, Yu C, Gatto B, Liu LF. 1993 DNA minor groove-binding ligands: a different class of mammalian DNA topoisomerase I inhibitors. Proc Natl Acad Sci USA 90:8131–8135.
55. Sun Q, Gatto B, Yu C, Liu A, Liu LF, LaVoie EJ. 1995 Synthesis and evaluation of terbenzimidazoles as topoisomerase I inhibitors. J Med Chem 38:3638–3644.
56. Kim JS, Gatto B, Yu C, Liu A, Liu LF, LaVoie EJ. 1996 Substituted 2,5'-Bi-1H-benzimidazoles: topoisomerase I inhibition and cytotoxicity. J Med Chem 39:992–998.
57. Kim JS, Sun Q, Gatto B, Yu C, Liu A, Liu LF, et al. 1996 Structure-activity relationships of benzimidazoles and related heterocycles as topoisomerase I poisons. Bioorg Med Chem 4:621–630.
58. Gatto B, Sanders MM, Yu C, Wu HY, Makhey D, LaVoie EJ, et al. 1996 Identification of topoisomerase I as the cytotoxic target of the protoberberine alkaloid coralyne. Cancer Res 56:2795–2800.
59. Xu Z, Li TK, Kim JS, LaVoie EJ, Breslauer KJ, Liu LF, et al. 1998 DNA minor groove binding-directed poisoning of human DNA topoisomerase I by terbenzimidazoles. Biochemistry 37:3558–3566.
60. Makhey D, Gatto B, Yu C, Liu A, Liu LF, LaVoie EJ. 1996 Coralyne and related compounds as mammalian topoisomerase I and topoisomerase II poisons. Bioorg Med Chem 4:781–791.

61. Li TK, Bathory E, LaVoie EJ, Srinivasan AR, Olson WK, Sauers RR, et al. 2000 Human topoisomerase I poisoning by protoberberines: potential roles for both drug-DNA and drug-enzyme interactions. Biochemistry 39:7107–7116.
62. Pilch DS, Xu Z, Sun Q, LaVoie EJ, Liu LF, Breslauer KJ. 1997 A terbenzimidazole that preferentially binds and conformationally alters structurally distinct DNA duplex domains: a potential mechanism for topoisomerase I poisoning. Proc Natl Acad Sci USA 94:13565–13570.
63. Pilch DS, Yu C, Makhey D, LaVoie EJ, Srinivasan AR, Olson WK, et al. 1997 Minor groove-directed and intercalative ligand-DNA interactions in the poisoning of human DNA topoisomerase I by protoberberine analogs. Biochemistry 36:12542–12553.
64. Sim SP, Pilch DS, Liu LF. 2000 Site-specific topoisomerase I-mediated DNA cleavage induced by nogalamycin: a potential role of ligand-induced DNA bending at a distal site. Biochemistry 39:9928–9934.
65. Li LH, Krueger WC. 1991 The biochemical pharmacology of nogalamycin and its derivatives. Pharmacol Ther 51:239–255.
66. Liaw YC, Gao YG, Robinson H, van der Marel GA, van Boom JH, Wang AH. 1989 Antitumor drug nogalamycin binds DNA in both grooves simultaneously: molecular structure of nogalamycin-DNA complex. Biochemistry 28:9913–9918.
67. Gao YG, Liaw YC, Robinson H, Wang AH. 1990 Binding of the antitumor drug nogalamycin and its derivatives to DNA: structural comparison. Biochemistry 29:10307–10316.
68. Searle MS, Hall JG, Denny WA, Wakelin LP. 1988 NMR studies of the interaction of the antibiotic nogalamycin with the hexadeoxyribonucleotide duplex d(5'-GCATGC)2. Biochemistry 27:4340–4349.
69. Zhang XL, Patel DJ. 1990 Solution structure of the nogalamycin-DNA complex. Biochemistry 29:9451–9466.
70. Pourquier P, Takebayashi Y, Urasaki Y, Gioffre C Kohlhagen G, Pommier Y. 2000 Induction of topoisomerase I cleavage complexes by 1-beta-D-arabinofuranosylcytosine (ara-C) in vitro and in ara-C-treated cells. Proc Natl Acad Sci USA 97:1885–1890.
71. Pommier Y, Kohlhagen G, Pourquier P, Sayer JM Kroth H, Jerina DM. 2000 Benzo[a]pyrene diol epoxide adducts in DNA are potent suppressors of a normal topoisomerase I cleavage site and powerful inducers of other topoisomerase I cleavages. Proc Natl Acad Sci USA 97:2040–2045.
72. Pourquier P, Ueng LM, Kohlhagen G, Mazumder A, Gupta M, Kohn KW, et al. 1997 Effects of uracil incorporation, DNA mismatches, and abasic sites on cleavage and relegation activities of mammalian topoisomerase I. J Biol Chem 272:7792–7796.
73. Pourquier P, Pilon AA, Kohlhagen G, Mazumder A, Sharma A, Pommier Y. 1997 Trapping of mammalian topoisomerase I and recombinations induced by damaged DNA containing nicks or gaps. Importance of DNA end phosphorylation and camptothecin effects. J Biol Chem 272:26441–26447.
74. Pourquier P, Bjornsti MA, Pommier Y. 1998 Induction of topoisomerase I cleavage complexes by the vinyl chloride adduct 1,N6-ethenoadenine. J Biol Chem 273:27245–27249.
75. Pourquier P, Ueng LM, Fertala J, Wang D, Park HJ, Essigmann JM, et al. 1999 Induction of reversible complexes between eukaryotic DNA topoisomerase I and DNA-containing oxidative base damages. 7,8-dihydro-8-oxoguanine and 5-hydroxycytosine. J Biol Chem 274:8516–8523.

76. Barsky D, Foloppe N, Ahmadia S, Wilson DM, MacKerell AD. 2000 New insights into the structure of abasic DNA from molecular dynamics simulations. Nucleic Acids Res 28:2613–2626.
77. Cline SD, Jones WR, Stone MP, Osheroff N. DNA abasic lesions in a different light: solution structure of an endogenous topoisomerase II poison. Biochemistry 1999;38:15500–15507.
78. Gmeiner WH, Skradis A, Pon RT, Liu J. 1999 Cytarabine-induced destabilization and bending of a model Okazaki fragment. Nucleosides Nucleotides. 18:1577–1578.
79. Hogan ME, Dattagupta N, Whitlock JP. 1981 Carcinogen-induced alteration of DNA structure. J Biol Chem 256:4504–4513.
80. Kahn JD, Yun E, Crothers DM. 1994 Detection of localized DNA flexibility. Nature 368:163–166.
81. Pietrasanta LI, Smith BL, MacLeod MC. 2000 A novel approach for analyzing the structure of DNA modified by Benzo[a]pyrene diol epoxide at single-molecule resolution. Chem Res Toxicol 13:351–355.
82. Roll C, Ketterle C, Faibis V, Fazakerley GV, Boulard Y. 1998 Conformations of nicked and gapped DNA structures by NMR and molecular dynamic simulations in water. Biochemistry 37:4059–4070.
83. Wang CI, Taylor JS. 1991 Site-specific effect of thymine dimer formation on dAn.dTn tract bending and its biological implications. Proc Natl Acad Sci USA 88:9072–9076.
84. Yamaguchi H, van Aalten DM, Pinak M, Furukawa A, Osman R. 1998 Essential dynamics of DNA containing a cis.syn cyclobutane thymine dimer lesion. Nucleic Acids Res 26:1939–1946.
85. Ribas G, Xamena N, Creus A, Marcos R. 1996 Sister-chromatid exchanges (SCE) induction by inhibitors of DNA topoisomerases in cultured human lymphocytes. Mutat Res 368:205–211.
86. Frei H, Wurgler FE. 1996 Induction of somatic mutation and recombination by four inhibitors of eukaryotic topoisomerases assayed in the wing spot test of Drosophila melanogaster. Mutagenesis 11: 315–325.
87. Pommier Y, Jenkins J, Kohlhagen G, Leteurtre F. 1995 DNA recombinase activity of eukaryotic DNA topoisomerase I; effects of camptothecin and other inhibitors. Mutat Res 337:135–145.
88. Huang TT, Wuerzberger-Davis SM, Seufzer BJ, Shumway SD, KuramaT, Boothman DA, et al. 2000 NF-kappaB activation by camptothecin. A linkage between nuclear DNA damage and cytoplasmic signaling events. J Biol Chem 275:9501–9509.
89. Nelson WG, Kastan MB. 1994 DNA strand breaks: the DNA template alterations that trigger p53-dependent DNA damage response pathways. Mol Cell Biol 14:1815–1823.
90. Piret B, Piette J. 1996 Topoisomerase poisons activate the transcription factor NF-kappaB in ACH-2 and CEM cells. Nucleic Acids Res 24:4242–4248.
91. Shao RG, Cao CX, Zhang H, Kohn KW, Wold MS, Pommier Y. 1999 Replication-mediated DNA damage by camptothecin induces phosphorylation of RPA by DNA-dependent protein kinase and dissociates RPA:DNA-PK complexes. EMBO J 18:1397–1406.
92. Wan S, Capasso H, Walworth NC. 1999 The topoisomerase I poison camptothecin generates a Chk1-dependent DNA damage checkpoint signal in fission yeast. Yeast 15:821–828.

93. Tolis C, Peters G, Ferreira CG, Pinedo HM, Giaccone G. 1999 Cell cycle disturbances and apoptosis induced by topotecan and gemcitabine on human lung cancer cell lines. Eur J Cancer 35:796–780.
94. Gradzka I, Skierski J, Szumiel I. 1998 DNA repair, cell cycle progression and cell death following camptothecin treatment in two murine lymphoma L5178Y sub-lines. Cell Biochem Funct 16:239–252.
95. Kaufmann WK, Kies PE. 1998 DNA signals for G2 checkpoint response in diploid human fibroblasts. Mutat Res. 400:153–167.
96. Maity A, Hwang A, Janss A, Phillips P, McKenna W G, Muschel RJ. 1996 Delayed cyclin B1 expression during the G2 arrest following DNA damage. Oncogene 13:1647–1657.
97. Goldwasser F, Shimizu T, Jackman J, Hoki Y, O'Connor PM, Kohn KW, et al. 1996 Correlations between S and G2 arrest and the cytotoxicity of camptothecin in human colon carcinoma cells. Cancer Res 56:4430–4437.
98. Tsao YP, D'Arpa P, Liu LF. 1992 The involvement of active DNA synthesis in camptothecin-induced G2 arrest: altered regulation of p34cdc2/cyclin B. Cancer Res 52:1823–1829.
99. D'Arpa P, Beardmore C, Liu LF. 1990 Involvement of nucleic acid synthesis in cell killing mechanisms of topoisomerase poisons. Cancer Res 50:6919–6924.
100. Zhang H, D'Arpa P, Liu LF. 1990 A model for tumor cell killing by topoisomerase poisons. Cancer Cells 2:23–27.
101. Hsiang YH, Lihou MG, Liu LF. 1989 Arrest of replication forks by drug-stabilized topoisomerase I-DNA cleavable complexes as a mechanism of cell killing by camptothecin. Cancer Res 49:5077–5082.
102. Yang L, Wold MS, Li JJ, Kelly TJ, Liu LF. 1987 Roles of DNA topoisomerases in simian virus 40 DNA replication in vitro. Proc Natl Acad Sci USA 84:950–954.
103. Tsao YP, D'Arpa P, Liu LF. 1993 Interaction between replication forks and topoisomerase I-DNA cleavable complexes: studies in cell free SV40 DNA replication system. Cancer Res 53:5908–5914.
104. Pourquier P, Jensen AD, Gong SS, Pommier Y, Rogler CE. 1999 Human DNA topoisomerase I-mediated cleavage and recombination of duck hepatitis B virus DNA in vitro. Nucleic Acid Res 27:1919–1925.
105. D'Arpa P, Liu LF. 1989 Topoisomerase-targeting antitumor drugs. Biochim Biophys Acta 989:163–177.
106. Eng WK, Faucette L, Johnson RK, Sternglanz R. 1988 Evidence that DNA topoisomerase I is necessary for the cytotoxic effects of camptothecin. Mol Pharmacol 34:755–760.
107. Nitiss J, Wang JC. 1988 DNA topoisomerase-targeting antitumor drugs. Proc Natl Acad Sci USA 85:7501–7505.
108. Nitiss JL, Rose A, Sykes KC, Harris J, Zhou J. 1996 Using yeast to understand drugs that target topoisomerase. Ann N Y Acad Sci 803:32–43.
109. Nitiss J, Wang JC. 1991 Yeast as a Genetic System in the Dissection of the Mechanism of Cell-Killing by Topoisomerase-Targeting Anticancer Drugs. In: DNA Topoisomerase in Cancer. Potmesil M, Kohn KW, eds. Oxford University Press, New York, 77–90.
110. Wu J, Liu LF. 1997 Processing of topoisomerase I cleavable complexes into DNA damage by transcription. Nucleic Acids Res 25:4181–4186.
111. Mao Y, Desai SD, Liu LF. 2000 SUMO-1 conjugation to human DNA topoisomerase II isozymes. J Biol Chem 275:26066–26073.

112. Mao Y, Sun M, Desai SD, Liu LF. 2000 SUMO-1 conjugation to topoisomerase I: A possible repair response to topoisomerase-mediated DNA damage. Proc Natl Acad Sci USA 97:4046–4051.
113. Duann P, Sun M, Lin CT, Zhang H, Liu LF. 1999 Plasmid linking umber change induced by topoisomerase I-mediated DNA damage. Nucleic Acids Res 27:2905–2911.
114. Desai SD, Liu LF, Vazquez-Abad D, D'Arpa P. 1997 Ubiquitin-dependent destruction of topoisomerase I is stimulated by the antitumor drug camptothecin. J Biol Chem 272: 24159–24164.
115. Mao Y, Desai SD, Ting CY, Hwang J, Liu LF. 2001 26 S proteasome-mediated degradation of topoisomerase II cleavable complexes. J Biol Chem 276:40652–40658.
116. Hochstrasser M. 2000 Biochemistry. All in the ubiquitin family. Science 289: 563–564.
117. Hochstrasser M. 1996 Ubiquitin-dependent protein degradation. Annu Rev Genet 30:405–439.
118. Hochstrasser M. 1992 Ubiquitin and intracellular protein degradation. Curr Opin Cell Biol 4:1024–1031.
119. Haas AL, Siepmann TJ. 1997 Pathways of ubiquitin conjugation. FASEB J 11:1257–68.
120. Pickart CM. 1997 Targeting of substrates to the 26S proteasome. FASEB J 11:1055–1066.
121. Hershko A, Ciechanover A, Varshavsky A. 2000 The ubiquitin system. Nat Med 6:1073–1081.
122. Melchior F. 2000 Sumo nonclassical ubiquitin. Annu Rev Cell Dev Biol 16: 591–626.
123. Schwienhorst I, Johnson ES, Dohmen RJ. 2000 SUMO conjugation and deconjugation. Mol Gen Genet 263:771–786.
124. Yeh ET, Gong L, Kamitani T. 2000 Ubiquitin-like proteins: new wines in new bottles. Gene 248:1–14.
125. Kretz-Remy C, Tanguay RM. 1999 SUMO/sentrin: protein modifiers regulating important cellular functions. Biochem Cell Biol 77:299–309.
126. Saitoh H, Pu RT, Dasso M. 1997 SUMO-1: wrestling with a new ubiquitin-related modifier. Trends Biochem Sci 22:374–376.
127. Roca J, Ishida R, Berger JM, Andoh T, Wang JC. 1994 Antitumor bisdioxopiperazines inhibit yeast DNA topoisomerase II by trapping the enzyme in the form of a closed protein clamp. Proc Natl Acad Sci USA 91:1781–1785.
128. Hamatake M, Andoh T, Ishida R. 1997 Effects of ICRF-193, a catalytic inhibitor of DNA topoisomerase II, on sister chromatid exchange. Anticancer Drugs 8:637–642.
129. Pirkkala L, Alastalo TP, Zuo X, Benjamin IJ, Sistonen L. 2000 Disruption of heat shock factor 1 reveals an essential role in the ubiquitin proteolytic pathway. Mol Cell Biol 20:2670–2675.
130. Wyttenbach A, Carmichael J, Swartz J, Furlong RA, Narain Y, Rankin J, et al. 2000 Effects of heat shock, heat shock protein 40 (HDJ-2), and proteasome inhibition on protein aggregation in cellular models of Huntington's disease. Proc Natl Acad Sci USA 97:2898–2903.
131. Kaye FJ, Modi S, Ivanovska I, Koonin EV, Thress K, Kubo A, et al. 2000 A family of ubiquitin-like proteins binds the ATPase domain of Hsp70-like Stch. FEBS Lett 467:348–355.

132. Luders J, Demand J, Hohfeld J. 2000 The ubiquitin-related BAG-1 provides a link between the molecular chaperones Hsc70/Hsp70 and the proteasome. J Biol Chem 275:4613–4617.
133. Tongaonkar P, Beck K, Shinde UP, Madura K. 1999 Characterization of a temperature-sensitive mutant of a ubiquitin-conjugating enzyme and its use as a heat-inducible degradation signal. Anal. Biochem 272:263–269.
134. Sharp FR, Massa SM, Swanson RA. 1999 Heat-shock protein protection. Trends Neurosci 22:97–99.
135. Kim D, Kim SH, Li GC. 1999 Proteasome inhibitors MG132 and lactacystin hyperphosphorylate HSF1 and induce hsp70 and hsp27 expression. Biochem Biophys Res Commun 254:264–268.
136. Mathew A, Mathur SK, Morimoto RI. 1998 Heat shock response and protein degradation: regulation of HSF2 by the ubiquitin-proteasome pathway. Mol Cell Biol 18:5091–5098.
137. Saitoh H, Hinchey J. 2000 Functional heterogeneity of small ubiquitin-related protein modifiers SUMO-1 versus SUMO-2/3. J Biol Chem 275:6252–6258.
138. Murren JR, Beidler DR, Cheng YC. 1996 Camptothecin resistance related to drug-induced down-regulation of topoisomerase I and to steps occurring after the formation of protein-linked DNA breaks. Ann N Y Acad Sci 803:74–92.
139. Liu LF, Desai SD, Li TK, Mao Y, Sun M, Sim SP. 2000 Mechanism of action of camptothecin. Ann N Y Acad Sci 922:1–10.
140. Desai SD, Mao Y, Sun M, Li TK, Wu J, Liu LF. 2000 Ubiquitin, SUMO-1 and UCRP in camptothecin sensitivity and resistance. Ann N Y Acad Sci 922:306–308.
141. Desai SD, Li TK, Rodriguez-Bauman A, Rubin E, Liu LF. 2001 Ubiquitin/26S proteasome-mediated degradation of topoisomerase I as a resistance mechanism to camptothecin in tumor cells. Cancer Res 61:5926–5932.
142. Desai SD, Zhang H, Rodriguez-Bauman A, Yang JM, Wu X, Gounder MK, et al. 2003 Transcription-dependent degradation of topoisomerase I-DNA covalent complexes. Mol Cell Biol 23:2341–2350.
143. Eder JP, Rubin E, Stone R, Bryant M, Xi G-X, Supko J, et al. 1996 Trials of 9-amino-20(S)-camptothecin in Boston. Ann N Y Acad Sci 803:247–255.
144. Rubin E, Wood V, Bharati A, Trites D, Lynch C, Hurwitz S, et al. 1995 A phase I and pharmacokinetic study of a new camptothecin derivative, 9-aminocamptothecin. Clin Cancer Res 1:269–276.
145. Narasimhan J, Potter JL, Haas AL. 1996 Conjugation of the 15-kDa interferon-induced ubiquitin homolog is distinct from that of ubiquitin. J Biol Chem 271:324–330.
146. Haas AL, Ahrens P, Bright PM, Ankel H. 1987 Interferon induces a 15-kilodalton protein exhibiting marked homology to ubiquitin. J Biol Chem 262:11315–11323.
147. Loeb KR, Haas AL. 1992 The interferon-inducible 15-kDa ubiquitin homolog conjugates to intracellular proteins. J Biol Chem 267:7806–7813.
148. Shen Z, Pardington-Purtymun PE, Comeaux JC, Moyzis RK, Chen DJ. 1996 Associations of UBE2I with RAD52, UBL1, p53, and RAD51 proteins in a yeast two-hybrid system. Genomics 37:183–186.
149. Boddy MN, Howe K, Etkin LD, Solomon E, Freemont PS. 1996 PIC1, a novel ubiquitin-like protein which interacts with the PML component of a multiprotein complex that is disrupted in acute promyelocytic leukaemia. Oncogene 13:971–982.
150. Okura T, Gong L, Kamitani T, Wada T, Okura I, Wei CF, et al. 1996 Protection against Fas/APO-1- and tumor necrosis factor-mediated cell death by a novel protein, sentrin. J Immunol 157:4277–4281.

151. Matunis MJ, Coutavas E, Blobel G. 1996 A novel ubiquitin-like modification modulates the partitioning of the Ran-GTPase-activating protein RanGAP1 between the cytosol and the nuclear pore complex. J Cell Biol 135:1457–1470.
152. Lapenta V, Chiurazzi P, van der Spek P, Pizzuti A, Hanaoka F, Brahe C. 1997 SMT3A, a human homologue of the S. cerevisiae SMT3 gene, maps to chromosome 21qter and defines a novel gene family. Genomics 40:362–366.
153. Gong L, Li B, Millas S, Yeh ET. 1999 Molecular cloning and characterization of human AOS1 and UBA2, components of the sentrin-activating enzyme complex. FEBS Lett 448:185–189.
154. Okuma T, Honda R, Ichikawa G, Tsumagari N, Yasuda H. 1999 In vitro SUMO-1 modification requires two enzymatic steps, E1 and E2. Biochem Biophys Res Commun 254:693–698.
155. Schwarz SE, Matuschewski K, Liakopoulos D, Scheffner M, Jentsch S. 1998 The ubiquitin-like proteins SMT3 and SUMO-1 are conjugated by the UBC9 E2 enzyme. Proc Natl Acad Sci USA 95:560–564.
156. Desterro JM, Thomson J, Hay RT. 1997 Ubch9 conjugates SUMO but not ubiquitin. FEBS Lett 417:297–300.
157. Johnson ES, Blobel G. 1997 Ubc9p is the conjugating enzyme for the ubiquitin-like protein Smt3p. J Biol Chem 272:26799–26802.
158. Johnson ES, Schwienhorst I, Dohmen RJ, Blobel G. 1997 The ubiquitin-like protein Smt3p is activated for conjugation to other proteins by an Aos1p/Uba2p heterodimer. EMBO J 16:5509–5519.
159. Desterro JM, Rodriguez MS, Kemp GD, Hay RT. 1999 Identification of the enzyme required for activation of the small ubiquitin-like protein SUMO-1. J Biol Chem 274:10618–10624.
160. Desterro JM, Thomson J, Hay RT. 1997 Ubch9 conjugates SUMO but not ubiquitin. FEBS Lett 417:297–300.
161. Johnson ES, Blobel G. 1997 Ubc9p is the conjugating enzyme for the biquitin-like protein Smt3p. J Biol Chem 272:26799–26802.
162. Li SJ, Hochstrasser M. 2000 The yeast ULP2 (SMT4) gene encodes a novel protease specific for the ubiquitin-like Smt3 protein. Mol Cell Biol 20:2367–2377.
163. Li SJ, Hochstrasser M. 1999 A new protease required for cell-cycle progression in yeast. Nature 398:246–151.
164. Buschmann T, Fuchs SY, Lee CG, Pan ZQ, Ronai Z. 2000 SUMO-1 modification of Mdm2 prevents its self-ubiquitination and increases Mdm2 ability to ubiquitinate p53. Cell 101:753–762.
165. Muller S, Berger M, Lehembre F, Seeler JS, Haupt Y, Dejean A. 2000 c-Jun and p53 activity is modulated by SUMO-1 modification. J Biol Chem 275:13321–13329.
166. Zhong S, Muller S, Ronchetti S, Freemont PS, Dejean A, Pandolfi PP. 2000 Role of SUMO-1-modified PML in nuclear body formation. Blood 95:2748–2752.
167. Gostissa M, Hengstermann A, Fogal V, Sandy P, Schwarz SE, Scheffner M, et al. 1999 Activation of p53 by conjugation to the ubiquitin-like protein SUMO-1. EMBO J 18:6462–6471.
168. Rodriguez MS, Desterro JM, Lain S, Midgley CA, Lane DP, Hay RT. 1999 SUMO-1 modification activates the transcriptional response of p53. EMBO J 18:6455–6461.
169. Sternsdorf T, Puccetti E, Jensen K, Hoelzer D, Will H, Ottmann OG, et al. 1999 PIC-1/SUMO-1-modified PML-retinoic acid receptor alpha mediates arsenic trioxide-induced apoptosis in acute promyelocytic leukemia. Mol Cell Biol 19:5170–5178.

170. Muller S, Dejean A. 1999 Viral immediate-early proteins abrogate the modification by SUMO-1 of PML and Sp100 proteins, correlating with nuclear body disruption. J Virol 73:5137–5143.
171. Desterro JM, Rodriguez MS, Hay RT. 1998 SUMO-1 modification of IkappaBalpha inhibits NF-kappaB activation. Mol Cell 2:233–239.
172. Saitoh H, Sparrow DB, Shiomi T, Pu RT, Nishimoto T, Mohun TJ, et al. 1998 Ubc9p and the conjugation of SUMO-1 to RanGAP1 and RanBP2. Curr Biol 8:121–124.
173. Matunis MJ, Wu, J, Blobel G. 1998 SUMO-1 modification and its role in targeting the Ran GTPase-activating protein, RanGAP1 to the nuclear pore complex. J Cell Biol 140:499–509.
174. Kamitani T, Nguyen HP, Yeh ET. 1997 Preferential modification of nuclear proteins by a novel ubiquitin-like molecule. J Biol Chem 272:14001–14004.
175. Cho Y, Lee I, Maul GG, Yu E. 1998 A novel nuclear substructure, ND10: distribution in normal and neoplastic human tissues. Int J Mol Med 1:717–724.
176. Maul GG. 1998 Nuclear domain 10, the site of DNA virus transcription and replication. Bioessays 20:660–667.
177. Sternsdorf T, Grotzinger T, Jensen K, Will H. 1997 Nuclear dots: actors on many stages. Immunobiology 198:307–331.
178. Buschmann T, Fuchs SY, Lee CG, Pan ZQ, Ronai Z. 2000 SUMO-1 modification of Mdm2 prevents its self-ubiquitination and increases Mdm2 ability to ubiquitinate p53. Cell 101:753–762.
179. Lallemand-Breitenbach V, Zhu J, Puvion F, Koken M, Honore N, Doubeikovsky A, et al. 2001 Role of promyelocytic leukemia (PML) sumolation in nuclear body formation, 11S proteasome recruitment, and As(2)O(3)-induced PML or PML/retinoic acid receptor alpha degradation. J Exp Med 193:1361–1372.
180. Rallabhandi P, Hashimoto K, Mo YY, Beck WT, Moitra PK, D'Arpa P. 2002 Sumoylation of topoisomerase I is involved in its partitioning between nucleoli and nucleoplasm and its clearing from nucleoli in response to camptothecin. J Biol Chem 277:40020–40026.
181. Mao YY, Yu Y, Shen Z, Beck WT. 2002 Nucleolar delocalization of human topoisomerase I in response to topotecan correlates with sumoylation of the protein. J Biol Chem 277:2958–2964.
182. Horie K, Tomida A, Sugimoto Y, Yasugi T, Yoshikawa H, Taketani Y, et al. 2002 SUMO-1 conjugation to intact DNA topoisomerase I amplifies cleavable complex formation induced by camptothecin. Oncogene 21:7913–7922.

2 Crystallographic Insight Into the Mechanism of Drug-Induced Topoisomerase I DNA Damage

Alex B. Burgin, Jr., PhD,
Michael D. Feese, PhD,
Bart L. Staker, PhD,
and Lance Stewart, PhD

CONTENTS

1. BACKGROUND

Topoisomerase I (TOP-I) is an essential eukaryotic enzyme that acts to remove supercoils generated during transcription and DNA replication *(1)*. Because of the size of the eukaryotic chromosome, removal of these supercoils can only be accomplished locally by introducing breaks into the DNA helix. Being a type 1 enzyme, TOP-I mediates DNA relaxation by creating a transient, single-strand break in one strand of the DNA duplex. This tran-

Camptothecins in Cancer Therapy
Edited by: V. R. Adams and T. G. Burke © Humana Press Inc., Totowa, NJ

sient nicking allows the broken strand to rotate around its intact complement, effectively removing local supercoils. Strand nicking results from the transesterification of an active-site tyrosine (Tyr723 in the human TOP-I) at a DNA phosphodiester bond forming a 3'-phosphotyrosine covalent enzyme–DNA complex. The covalent intermediate is reversed when the released 5'-OH of the broken strand reattacks the phosphotyrosine intermediate in a second transesterification reaction *(1)*. The rate of relegation is normally much faster than is the rate of cleavage *(2)*. This ensures that the steady state concentration of the covalent 3'-phosphotyrosyl TOP-I–DNA complex is extremely low. Several DNA lesions and drugs, however, have been shown to stabilize the covalent 3'-phosphotyrosyl intermediate *(3)*. For example, camptothecin (CPT) is a natural product that was originally discovered because of its antitumor activity *(4)* and was later demonstrated to promote the accumulation of TOP-I-DNA adducts in vitro and in vivo *(5,6)*. It is generally believed that CPTs act to convert TOP-I into a DNA-damaging agent by binding the covalent 3'-phosphotyrosyl intermediate and, specifically, blocking DNA relegation *(7,8)*. Topo I is the sole intramolecular target of CPT and the cytotoxic effects of CPT poisoning are S-phase-specific *(9)*. Both in vitro and in vivo data support the idea that during DNA replication, the replication complex can collide with the "trapped" TOP-I-DNA complex, resulting in a double-strand break and subsequent apoptotic cell death *(10)*. Presumably, these compounds have anticancer activity because rapidly dividing cells (e.g., cancer cells) enter S-phase more frequently than do normal cells.

2. THE TERNARY TOP-I–DNA–DRUG COMPLEX

It has been extremely difficult to study the mechanism of CPT activity because the drug acts as an uncompetitive inhibitor and binds only to the transient enzyme-substrate complex *(7,11)*. There is no reported equilibrium binding constant for any TOP-I poison. To overcome this fundamental problem, we have used DNA substrates containing a 5'-bridging phosphorothioate linkage to covalently trap the enzyme-substrate complex *(12)*. TOP-I-mediated cleavage of these substrates generates a 5'-sulfhydryl, instead of a 5'-hydroxyl, which is inert in subsequent ligation reactions. These substrates have allowed the crystallization of human TOP-I covalently joined to duplex DNA in the absence (3.2 Å) and presence (2.1 Å) of topotecan, a clinically approved CPT analog (Hycamtin®) *(13)*.

A comparative analysis of these structures demonstrates that topotecan intercalates at the site of DNA cleavage, forming base-stacking interactions with both the –1 (upstream) and +1 (downstream) base pairs. The planar five-membered ring system of topotecan mimics a DNA base pair in the DNA duplex and occupies the same space as the +1 base pair in the structure without drug bound (Figs. 1,2). The intercalation binding site is created by conformational changes at the phosphodiester bond between the +1 and –

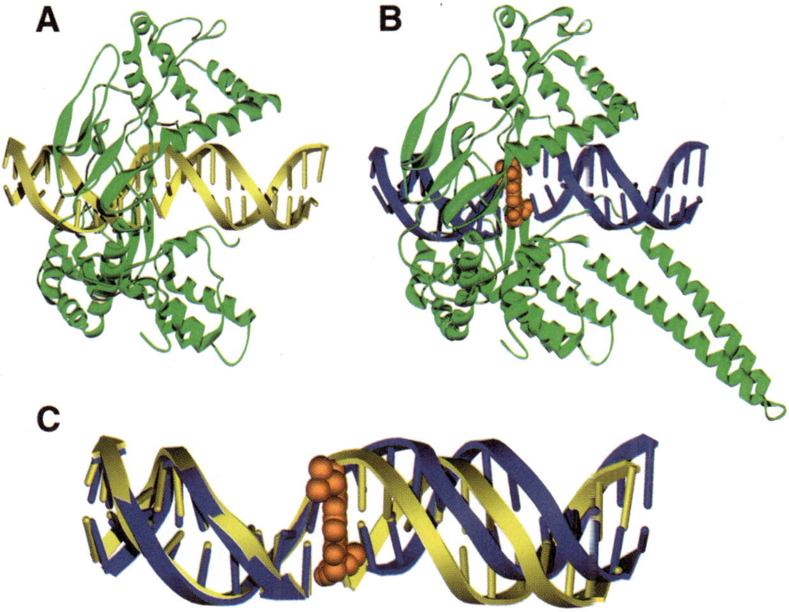

Fig. 1. Model of topoisomerase I (TOP-I)–DNA complex without **(A)** and with bound topotecan **(B)** is diagrammed with protein (green), DNA unbound (**A**: yellow), DNA-topotecan bound (**B**: blue), and topotecan (orange, CPK representation). A comparison of the topotecan ternary complex structure to the non-topotecan structure reveals minor differences in the overall C-α backbone trace with an RMSD = 1.33 Å, excluding C-terminal linker residues Gln633-Gln697, which were not visible in the electron density of the non–drug-bound protein. The 2.1 Å drug-bound structure represents the most complete TOP-I structure reported to date, providing visible electron density from Gln201 to the COOH-terminal Phe765. The specific activity and sensitivity to camptothecin of topo70 is indistinguishable from that of the full-length native human TOP-I *(34,35)*. Previously reported crystal structures of human TOP-I include the inactive Tyr723Phe versions of topo70 and topo58/6.3 (a reconstituted linkerless enzyme) in noncovalent complex with DNA, and topo58/6.3 in covalent complex with DNA *(29,36)*. Each of these structures contained unresolvable portions of the protein in the connector region (Pro635–Phe640). Moreover, the reconstituted enzyme has altered kinetics and is not sensitive to camptothecin in a plasmid relaxation assay *(35)*. Hence, the structures reported here are the first structures of a fully active human TOP-I in covalent complex with DNA in the absence and presence of bound drug. **(C)** Comparison of the 22mer duplex oligonucleotides of the drug-bound (blue) and nondrug-bound (yellow). Topotecan (orange, CPK) binds to the enzyme-substrate complex by intercalating in the DNA. Intercalation is accommodated by unwinding of the DNA and translation downstream of the cleavage site. The binding pocket is stabilized primarily by contacts between the enzyme and DNA substrate. A detailed analysis of the contacts between the ternary complex of TOP-I and DNA reveals a total of 36 direct protein-DNA contacts and 6 additional water-mediated protein-DNA contacts.

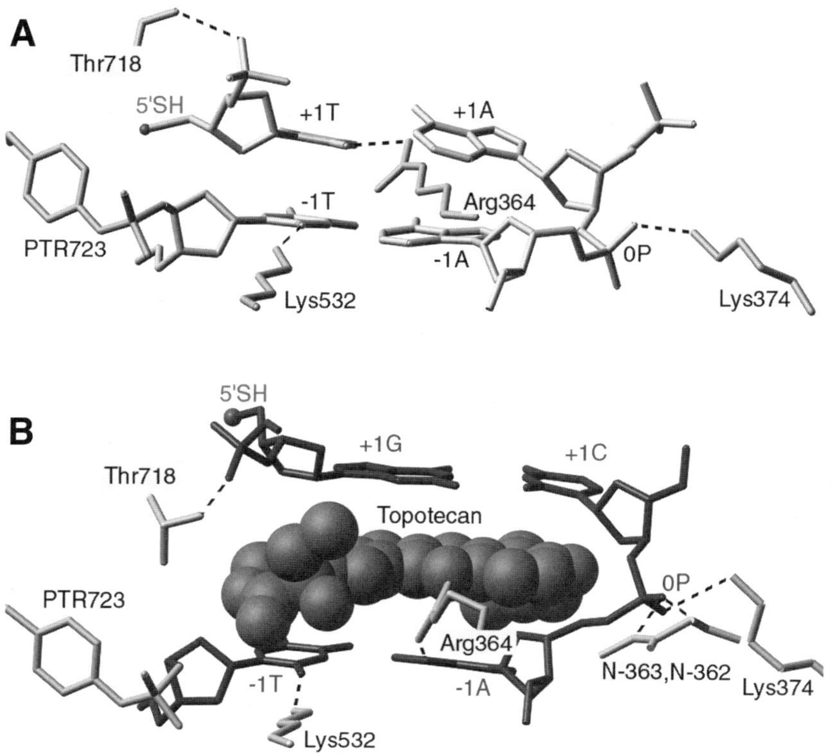

Fig. 2. Topotecan binding pocket. **(A)** Molecular diagram showing the nondrug-bound topoisomerase I–DNA complex. The +1 and –1 bases of the duplex DNA are shown making four contacts to the surrounding protein to stabilize the protein-DNA complex. **(B)** Topotecan (CPK) intercalates between the +1 and –1 bases of the duplex DNA (stick). Six protein contacts stabilize the open form of the DNA. Topo70 residues, whose mutation leads to drug resistance, are highlighted with gray boxes. 5'SH of the +1 G is indicated and the covalent phosphotyrosine attachment to DNA is shown between PTR723 and the –1 T of the cleaved strand. Mobile phosphodiester of the intact DNA strand is labeled 0P.

1 base pairs of the uncleaved strand (0P). This conformational change in the DNA requires only a minimal change within the protein (Fig. 1). The intercalation pocket, however, is stabilized by several protein-DNA interactions (Fig. 2). The hydroxyl of Thr718 makes a hydrogen bond contact with the nonbridging phosphodiester oxygen of guanosine at position +1 of the cleaved strand (+1G). Arg364 makes a hydrogen bond contact with N3 of adenosine at position –1 of the uncleaved strand (–1A). Lys532 makes a hydrogen bond with the oxygen of thymidine at position –1 (–1T). Lys374 and the main chain nitrogens of 362 and 363 make hydrogen bond contacts

with the nonbridging phosphodiester of the uncleaved strand (0P). Consistent with the observed drug-binding mode, mutations at position Arg364 *(14)* would be expected to destabilize the topotecan binding site and are known to result in camptothecin resistance. Lys532 acts as the general acid during strand cleavage *(15)*, and mutations could not result in camptothecin resistance because these mutations produce an inactive enzyme. Interestingly, substitution of alanine for threonine at position 718 stabilizes the enzyme-DNA complex even in the absence of camptothecin *(16)*.

The intercalation binding mode explains how CPTs specifically block DNA relegation, because the binding/intercalation results in a 3.4 Å shift of the downstream duplex and displaces the reactive 5'-OH of the cleaved strand 10 Å away from the phosphotyrosine (Fig. 2). For a relegation event to occur, the topotecan molecule must be released from the nicked DNA and diffuse out of the complex. The results also explain why CPTs bind the enzyme-substrate complex, but do not bind the enzyme or substrate alone; the topotecan-binding pocket is located within the DNA substrate, but this binding site can only form after TOP-I-mediated cleavage. Approximately 380 $Å^2$ of the total 626 $Å^2$ solvent-accessible portion of topotecan, or 61% of the drug surface, is covered by base stacking interactions with DNA. An additional 27% of the solvent-accessible region of topotecan is covered by protein side chains; the remaining 11% is solvent accessible. The single direct-protein contact mediated by Asp533 that hydrogen bonds to the 20(S) hydroxyl represents only 5% of the total solvent accessible surface of topotecan.

The E-ring is known to be in equilibrium between the closed lactone form and a hydrolyzed open carboxylate form *(4)* (Fig. 3A). It is therefore not surprising that difference Fourier maps of the ternary TOP-I–DNA-topotecan structure demonstrate the presence of both the open and closed E-ring conformers of topotecan (Fig. 3B). An unrestrained full matrix refinement of occupancy factors *(17)* (with all positional and thermal parameters fixed) for the closed lactone and open carboxylate versions of topotecan converge to an occupancy of 63% (standard uncertainty 7%) closed lactone and 37% (standard uncertainty 7%) open carboxylate conformers.

It is not possible to determine the relative affinities of open (carboxylate) versus closed (lactone) forms of topotecan based on a crystal structure; however, the model demonstrates that both conformers can bind within the same intercalation pocket (Fig. 3C) and presumably inhibit relegation. There may be differences in the binding affinities of the lactone and carboxylate forms; however, it is unlikely that this difference would be apparent in the crystals because the crystallizations were performed at extremely high topotecan concentrations (0.1 m*M*). This concentration is probably well above the K_D of both the lactone and the carboxylate, therefore both would be expected to bind. In addition, it is not possible to determine if there

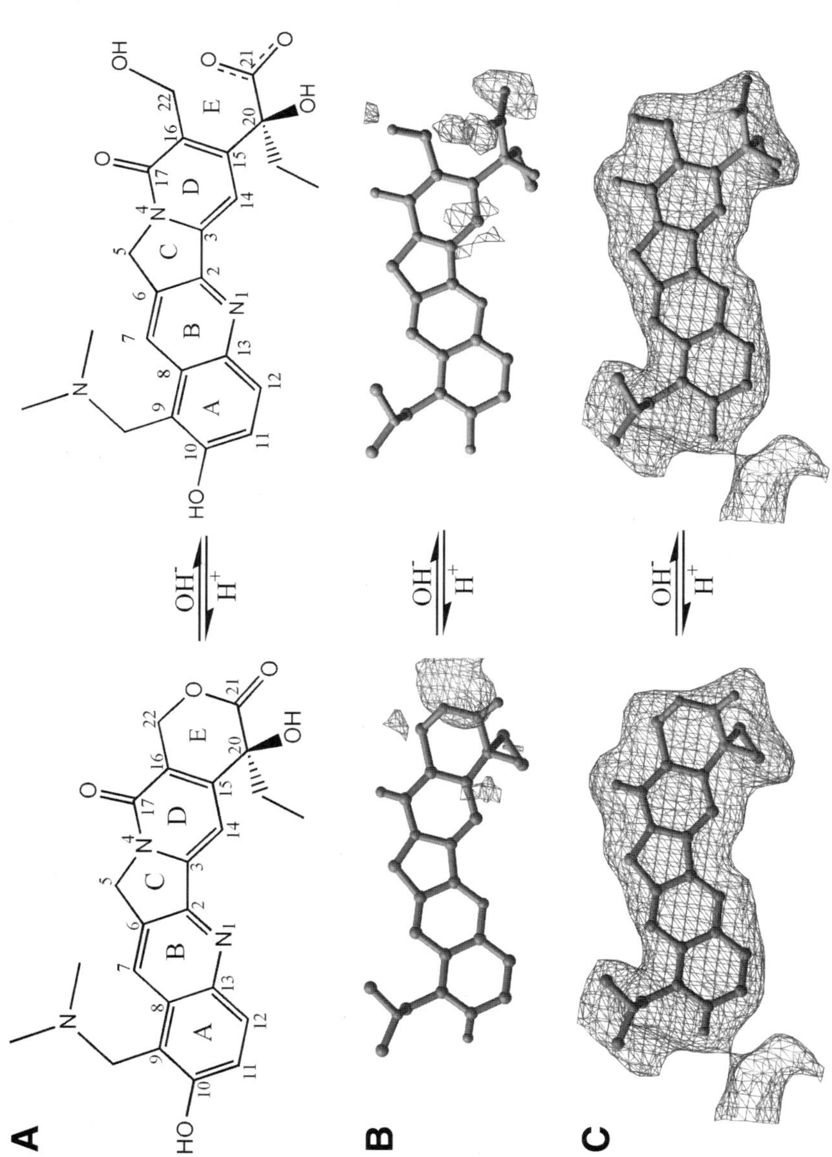
A
B
C

is preferential binding of the carboxylate or lactone forms because it is not possible to determine the true equilibrium ratio within the micro-environment of the active site.

3. DRUG INTERACTIONS

Stacking interactions with the +1 and –1 base pairs are one the primary forces stabilizing topotecan in the ternary complex. This feature may explain the preference for a G:C base pair at the +1 position of sites stabilized by camptothecins and may also explain why modifications that disrupt the planar ring system eliminate drug binding. There are relatively few hydrogen bonds stabilizing the drug (Fig. 4). Two water-mediated hydrogen bonds assist in coordinating topotecan: the oxygen of the D-ring pyridone makes a water mediated contact to Asn722, and the C-21 oxygen of the E-ring is bridged by a water molecule to the phosphotyrosine (Tyr723). In the carboxylate model, the 22-hydroxyl is 2.7 Å from the R-group of Asn722, and the 21-carboxylate oxygen is 2.8 Å from Lys532, a known catalytic residue *(15)*. The 20(S)-hydroxyl can still coordinate Asp533, and can make an additional hydrogen bond contact (3.1 Å) to the ε-nitrogen of Arg364 (Fig. 4). Consistent with the proposed structural model, mutations at residues Asp533, Arg364, and Asn722 would be expected to destabilize the bound drug and enzymes with mutations at these positions are resistant to camptothecin *(14,18,19)*.

The observed Asp533:20-(OH) interaction is the only hydrogen bond contact made in both the lactone and carboxylate models and emphasizes the importance of the 20-(OH) for CPT activity. Many studies demonstrate

---

Fig. 3. *(opposite page)* Topotecan electron density. **(A)** Topotecan with reversible hydrolysis of the base-labile E-ring from the closed lactone conformation to the open carboxylate form is diagrammed. **(B)** Left panel: 3.0 σ $|F_o|–|F_c|$ electron density map calculated with the lactone form of topotecan (100% closed E-ring) is diagrammed. Negative electron density (indicated by contours) is seen in the vicinity of the lactone oxygen, and positive (indicated by contours) electron density peaks are located nearby. **(B)** Right panel: 3.0 σ $|F_o|–|F_c|$ electron density calculated with the carboxylate form of topotecan (100% open E-ring) is diagrammed. Negative electron density (contoured) surrounds the terminal hydroxyl and carboxylic acid moieties, whereas a positive (contoured) electron density peak is in the location of what would be the lactone oxygen in the closed E-ring conformation. **(C)** 3.0 σ $|F_o|–|F_c|$ omit map of electron density for topotecan is illustrated. The electron density map reveals that both the lactone (left panel) and carboxylate (right panel) forms of the E-ring are present in the crystal structure. The E-ring of topotecan is oriented toward the phosphotyrosine. The c-9-dimethyl-amine group of topotecan projects into the major groove of the B-form DNA duplex. The c-20-ethylene group of the E-ring faces into the minor groove.

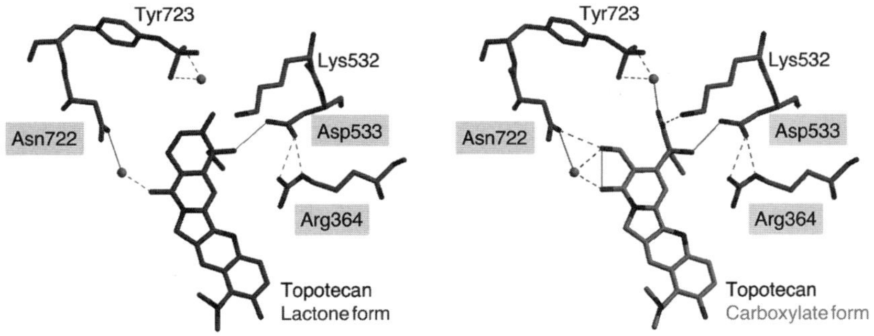

Fig. 4. Mode of topotecan binding. Topotecan interactions with protein side chains for the lactone (panel A) and carboxylate (panel B) forms of the drug. Hydrogen bonds (predicted by contact distance and geometry of the refined atomic positions) are shown as solid lines. Contacts less than 3.0 Å between polar atoms are shown as dashed lines. Labels for residues that, if mutated, produce a camptothecin resistant enzyme are highlighted in gray boxes. The oxygen atoms of water molecules are depicted as spheres. The left and right panels are oriented as a stereo pair so that a pseudostereo overlap of the lactone and carboxylate forms of topotecan can be achieved.

the importance of the 20-(OH) for CPT activity. For example, the 20(R) stereoisomer of CPT is inactive *(20,21)*. This is explained by the crystal structures that predict that the 20(R) ethyl group would sterically clash with the side chains of Asp533 and Lys532 (Fig. 5), and that the 20(R)-OH would also not be able to hydrogen bond with Asp533. Hertzberg et al. reported that if 20(S)-OH is substituted for hydrogen or acetate, no covalent complex accumulated in vitro *(22)*. The acetate modification would sterically clash with Asp533 and both modifications would eliminate the observed hydrogen bond contact. Similar observations were made by Wang et al., who have shown that conversion of the 20(S)-OH to 20(S/R)-H eliminates the accumulation of TOP-I–DNA covalent complex in vitro *(23)*. The difficulty in interpreting these data is that the 20-H modification would also be expected to prevent or minimize E-ring opening. These modifications would therefore be expected to simultaneously eliminate the 20-hydroxyl:Asp533, the 21-keto:Lys532, and the 22-hydroxyl:Asn722 hydrogen bond interactions of the carboxylate form of topotecan. Fortunately, Wang et al. have also synthesized analogs in which the 20-hydroxyl was replaced with chlorine or bromine. The advantage of these substrates is that they would be expected to eliminate the 20-hydroxyl:Asp533 interaction; however, these analogs should still allow E-ring opening and therefore should still allow the 21-keto:Lys532 and the 22-hydroxyl:Asn722 hydrogen bond interactions. Indeed, the 20-Cl and 20-Br have intermediate effects on in vitro stabilization of the covalent complex *(23)*, and provide circumstantial evidence that E-ring opening is important for CPT binding and activity.

It is widely believed that the closed lactone E-ring is essential for inhibition of TOP-I *(24)*, and several analogs have been synthesized that stabilize the lactone form. For example, homocamptothecin is a seven-member E-ring analog that has in vitro and in vivo activity *(25)*. This analog still contains an appropriately positioned 20-(OH) group, and the slightly larger ring can still fit within the intercalation binding pocket. This E-ring modification results in a slower rate of hydrolysis (formation of carboxylate); however, the equilibrium is actually shifted in favor of formation of the carboxylate over the lactone *(26)*. In addition, conversion of the E-ring lactone to a lactam prevents E-ring opening and simultaneously destroys in vitro activity of the drug *(22)*. In light of the structural model, these results suggest that opening of the E-ring is actually necessary for activity. There is experimental evidence for E-ring opening on formation of the ternary protein–DNA–drug complex *(27)*; in vitro activity *(21)* and in vivo activity *(28)* of the carboxylate form have been previously reported.

The structures also provide an explanation for the observed structure-activity relationships that improve in vivo efficacy. For example, previous functional analyses have demonstrated that a large number of modifications can be placed at positions 7, 9, and 10 of CPT *(24)*, and in some cases these modifications can increase in vivo activity. The structural model demonstrates that these positions face into the major groove of the DNA and modifications that improve solubility or stability would not sterically interfere with drug binding (Fig. 5).

4. POISON EFFECTS ON DNA RELAXATION

TOP-I has been proposed to relax DNA via a mechanism of "controlled rotation" in which the DNA duplex located downstream of the cleavage site rotates around the phosphodiester bond (0P) between the +1 and –1 base pairs of the uncleaved strand, effectively passing the unbroken strand through the single-strand break with each complete rotation event *(29)*. The rotation event is thought to occur in a controlled manner because the simplified models for the trajectory of the DNA during rotation predict that the rotating DNA, located downstream of the cleavage site, will experience transient electrostatic interactions with positively charged regions of the TOP-I enzyme that are in close proximity to the downstream DNA *(29)*. The protein encircles the DNA, and the linker (residues Gln633 to Gln697) and nose cone (residues Thr303 to Glu337) domains of TOP-I contain a variety of positively charged residues that are likely to contact the DNA during rotation. Within the framework of the controlled rotation model for DNA relaxation, intercalative camptothecin binding would not necessarily be expected

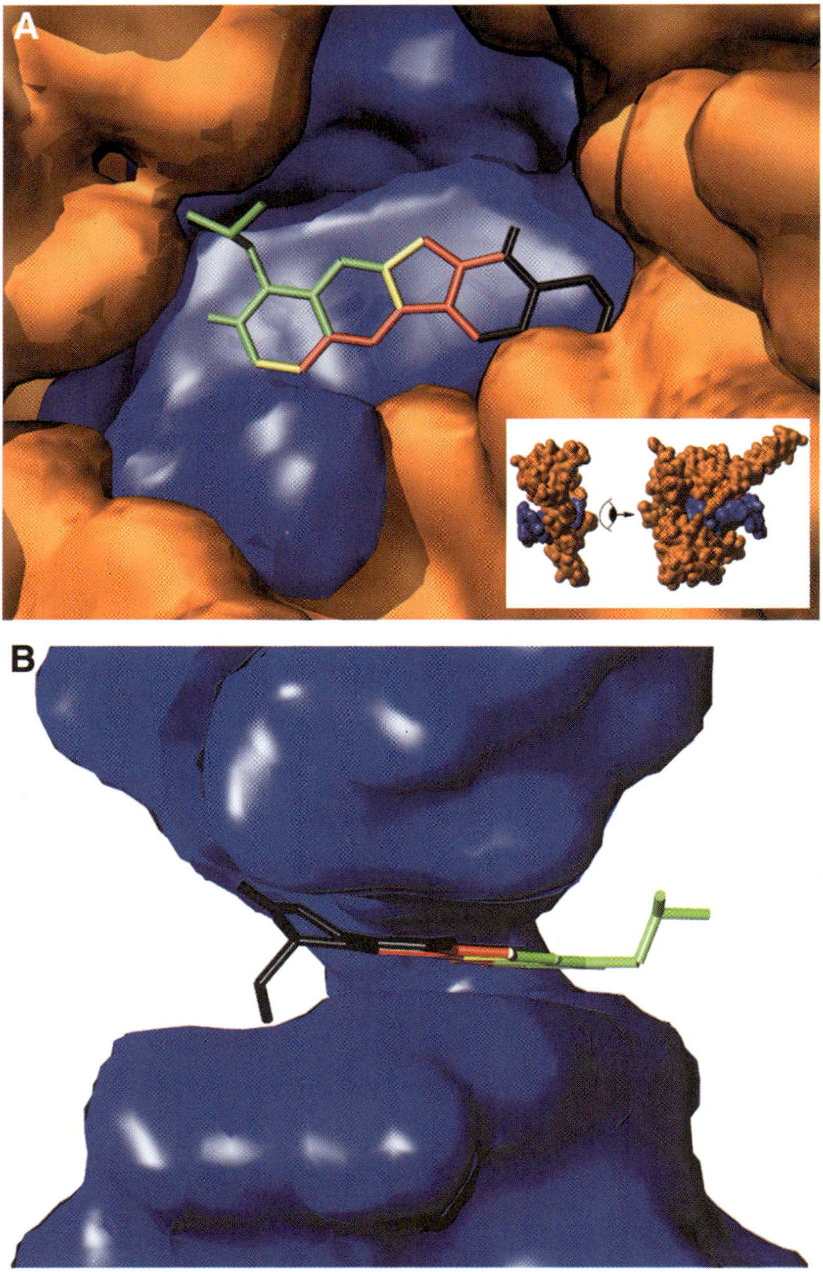
A
B

to have any affect on the speed with which DNA is relaxed. In fact, one might predict that, by inhibiting relegation, TOP-I poisons might be expected to enhance the rate of supercoil release. On the contrary however, it has been shown that TOP-I poisons such as camptothecin actually inhibit the rotation/relaxation process in vitro *(30)*.

It is also known that the inhibitory effects of camptothecin on DNA relaxation can only be observed with relatively high micromolar inhibitor concentrations, as compared with the much lower nanomolar concentrations of CPT needed to observe stabilization of the covalent complex in a typical detergent-mediated DNA breakage assay *(31,32)*. This observation is often interpreted as being a nonspecific inhibitory effect of large concentrations of inhibitor molecules binding nonspecifically to TOP-I. However, our structural observations suggest an alternative explanation, wherein the intercalative binding of inhibitor to the TOP-I–DNA covalent complex places constraints on DNA rotation that would otherwise not be present. That large concentrations of inhibitor are required to observe an inhibitory effect on plasmid relaxation is actually anticipated because the plasmid molecules (approximately 1–2 Kb supercoiled circles) used in the assay can be fully relaxed by a single TOP-I molecule, and there are thousands of possible TOP-I binding sites on a plasmid. As such, for an inhibitory effect on relaxation to be observed, a substantial proportion of all TOP-I–DNA

Fig. 5. *(opposite page)* Model of topotecan binding pocket. **(A)** Molecular surface diagram of both the protein (orange) and DNA (blue) of the topotecan binding pocket. The protein–DNA complex has been separated to show a view of the topotecan binding pocket (*see* inset). The convex surface of the topotecan faces into a pocket within the protein–DNA complex. The bonds of the topotecan molecule have been color-coded to represent the structure activity relationship (SAR) of chemical derivatives of the camptothecin scaffold. Bonds that are absolutely essential, such as the E-ring, and D-ring pyridole are colored black. Bonds in which additive moieties decrease inhibitory activity are colored red. Bonds in which additive moieties have a mixed effect on inhibitory activity (sometimes increasing, sometimes decreasing) are colored yellow. Bonds in which additive moieties can increase inhibitory activity are colored green. Although position 5 of the camptothecin scaffold is positioned toward the open pocket, substituents at this position do not increase inhibitory activity. It is likely that this is due to the sp3 stereochemistry at this position. Rather than planar extensions, as at sp2 positions 7 and 9, substituents at position 5 would project up or down into the surrounding DNA and thus disrupt the base stacking interactions that topotecan makes with both upstream and downstream DNA, shown in **(B)**. Molecular surface of DNA shown with protein removed. Topotecan intercalates the cleaved DNA and is tightly sandwiched between the upstream and downstream base pairs.

binding events would have to be rendered ineffective before a significant effect on relaxation could be observed. It logically follows that large concentrations of inhibitors will be required to observe an effect on plasmid relaxation.

Thus it has been a mystery how camptothecins stabilize the nicked complex but prevent DNA relaxation, because nicked DNA should be able to rotate and allow DNA relaxation *(30)*. To explain how intercalative binding of a TOP-I could inhibit both relaxation and relegation, one could invoke the idea that the rotating DNA may somehow clash with the bound poison. Alternatively, the intercalative binding of TOP-I poison may place constraints on rotatable bonds within the phosphodiester backbone of the uncleaved strand within the vicinity of drug binding. Indeed, a comparison of the unbound and CPT-bound structures shows that topotecan displaces the critical 0P phosphodiester bond and results in several interactions that could inhibit rotation (Fig. 6). In the drug-bound structure, Phe361 is positioned closely underneath the +1 phosphodiester and would be expected to sterically hinder rotation at 0P. Phe361Ser mutants are resistant to camptothecin poisoning of DNA relaxation *(14)*. In addition, drug binding and displacement of the +1 phosphodiester bond causes the nonbridging oxygens to form hydrogen bonds with the main chain nitrogens of residues Gly363 and Arg364. A hydrogen bond contact to Lys374 is present in both structures. The tight positioning of 0P against the peptide backbone of the protein effectively restrains three (α, β, γ) of the five potentially rotatable backbone bonds *(33)*. This tight packing arrangement would be expected to prevent the downstream DNA from rotating about 0P. This packing arrangement would not eliminate all possible DNA rotation; for example, rotation could still occur at the +2 (or +3, and so on) phosphodiester. However, additional base-pair hydrogen bond interactions would have to be broken to allow this rotation. Alternatively, rotation could still occur at +1 because two rotatable bonds are not hindered. However, in both cases, the trajectory of the rotating DNA would be significantly altered, and this would require significant conformational flexibility that is not likely to be present in the protein.

It is also important to note that the DNA must unwind or open through conformational changes at 0P to create the topotecan binding site. This suggests that the partially unwound DNA conformation observed in the ternary complex may represent a conformational intermediate that normally forms during the unpoisoned catalytic reaction. For example, the open conformation may be the first step of DNA relaxation; after DNA cleavage, conformational changes at 0P would break the stacking interactions between the +1 base pair and the –1 base pair and could facilitate unwinding. It is important to note that this opening is clearly stabilized by several protein–DNA interactions (Fig. 6).

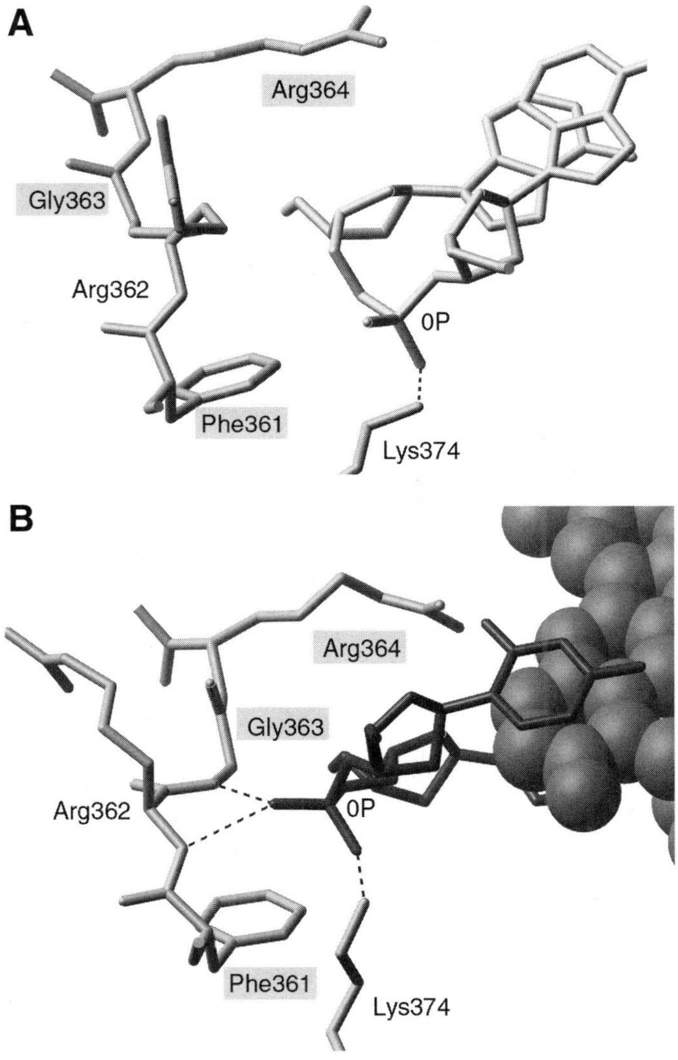

Fig. 6. Topotecan inhibits DNA relaxation. **(A)** Molecular diagram showing the nondrug-bound topoisomerase I–DNA complex. The +1 and –1 bases of the intact DNA strand are shown making a contact to Lys374 of the surrounding protein. **(B)** Topotecan (CPK) intercalates between the +1 and –1 bases of the duplex DNA (stick). Three protein contacts stabilize the open form of the intact DNA strand. Topo70 residues, whose mutation leads to drug resistance, are highlighted with gray boxes. Mobile phosphodiester of the intact DNA strand is labeled 0P.

5. CONCLUSIONS

In conclusion, the 2.1 Å structure of topotecan bound to the TOP-I–DNA covalent complex solves a 40-year mystery of how the camptothecins bind to their molecular target. The structures explain why the drugs only bind the enzyme-substrate complex and specifically block both DNA relegation and relaxation. The drug binds to the complex by intercalating between DNA bases of both strands at the enzyme-induced nick and makes specific hydrogen bond contacts with both the DNA and the enzyme. The ternary structure demonstrates that topotecan is tightly wedged against the protein and phosphodiester backbone that could prevent DNA rotation. Close examination of the ternary complex also indicates that the bound drug exists in both the closed lactone and open carboxylate forms. This result is important because it has been generally agreed that the E-ring open carboxylate form is inactive in vivo. This result demonstrates that the E-ring is in equilibrium between lactone and carboxylate forms when bound to the TOP-I–DNA complex and raises the possibility that both forms can poison the reaction.

Acknowledgments

The authors would like to thank G. Ireton, E. Wallace, and D. Connor for their technical assistance, H. Kim for intellectual support and review of this manuscript, S. Wasserman at Com-CAT, Advanced Photon Source, and Argonne National Laboratory, for assistance in data collection, as well as L. Berman and the staff of X25 at the National Synchrotron Light Source, Brookhaven National Laboratory, for assistance in data collection and helpful support. This work was supported by National Cancer Institute Grants R43 CA82964 and R43 CA79439, NIGMS Grant GM58598, and the Pacific West Cancer Fund. PDB accession numbers are 1K4T for the ternary topo70-DNA-Topotecan complex, and 1K4S for the binary topo70-DNA complex (patents pending).

REFERENCES

1. Champoux JJ. DNA 2001 Topoisomerases: structure, function, and mechanism. Ann Rev Biochem 70:369–413.
2. Stivers JT, Shuman S, Mildvan AS. 1994 Vaccinia DNA topoisomerase I: single-turnover and steady-state kinetic analysis of the DNA strand cleavage and ligation reactions. Biochemistry 33:327–329.
3. Pourquier P, Pommier Y. 2001 Topoisomerase I-mediated DNA damage. Adv Cancer Res 80:189–216.
4. Wall ME, et al. The isolation and structure of camptothecin, a novel alkaloidal leukemia and tumor inhibitor from *Camptotheca acuminata*. J Am Chem Soc 1966;88:3888–3890.
5. Hsiang YH, Hertzberg, R, Hecht S, Liu LF. 1985 Camptothecin induces protein-linked DNA breaks via mammalian DNA topoisomerase I. J Biol Chem 260:14873–14878.

6. Nitiss JL, Wang JC. 1988 DNA topoisomerase-targeting antitumor drugs can be studied in yeast. Proc Natl Acad Sci USA 85:7501–7505.
7. Hertzberg RP, Caranfa MJ, Hecht SM. 1989 On the mechanism of topoisomerase I inhibition by camptothecin: evidence for binding to an enzyme-DNA complex. Biochemistry 28:4629–4638.
8. Chen AY, Liu LF. 1994 DNA topoisomerases: essential enzymes and lethal targets. Rev Pharmacol Toxicol 34:191–218.
9. Bjornsti MA, Benedetti P, Viglianti GA, Wang JC. 1989 Expression of human DNA topoisomerase I in yeast cells lacing yeast DNA topoisomerase I: restoration of sensitivity of the cells to the antitumor drug camptothecin. Cancer Res 49:6318–6323.
10. Li TK, Liu LF. 2001 Tumor cell death induced by topoisomerase-targeting drugs. Annu Rev Pharmacol Toxicol 41:53–77.
11. Horwitz SB, Chang CK, Grollman AP. 1971 On the mechanism of topoisomerase I inhibition by camptothecin: evidence for binding to an enzyme-DNA complex. Biochemistry 7:632–644.
12. Burgin AB Jr, Huizenga BN, Nash HA. 1995 A novel suicide substrate for DNA topoisomerases and site-specific recombinases. Nucleic Acids Res 23:2973–2979.
13. Staker BL, Hjerrild K, Feese MD, Behnke CA, Burgin AB, Stewart L. 2002 The mechanism of topoisomerase I poisoning by a camptothecin analog. Proc Natl Acad Sci 99:15387–15392.
14. Li XG, Haluska P Jr, Hsiang YH, et al. 1997 Involvement of amino acids 361 to 364 of human topoisomerase I in camptothecin resistance and enzyme catalysis. Biochem Pharmacol 53:1019–1027.
15. Krogh BO, Shuman S 2000. Catalytic mechanism of DNA topoisomerase IB. Mol Cell 5:1035–1041.
16. Fiorani P, Amatruda JF, Silvestri A, Butler RH, Bjornsti MA, Benedetti P. 1999 Domain interactions affecting human DNA topoisomerase I catalysis and camptothecin sensitivity. Mol Pharm 56:1105–1115.
17. Sheldrick GM. SHELXL-97. University of Göttingen, 1997.
18. Tamura H, Kohchi C, Yamada R, et al. 1991 Molecular cloning of a cDNA of a camptothecin-resistant human DNA topoisomerase I and identification of mutation sites. Nucleic Acids Res 19:69–75.
19. Fertala J, Vance JR, Pourquier P, Pommier Y, Bjornsti M-A. 2000 Substitutions of Ans-726 in the active site of yeast DNA topoisomerase I define novel mechanisms of stabilizing the covalent enzyme-DNA intermediate. J Biol Chem 275:15246–15253.
20. Jaxel C, Kohn KW, Wani MC, Wall ME, Pommier Y. 1989 Structure-activity study of the actions of camptothecin derivatives on mammalian topoisomerase I: evidence for a specific receptor site and a relation to antitumor activity. Cancer Res 49:1465–1469.
21. Hsiang YH, Liu LF, Wall ME, et al. 1989 DNA topoisomerase I-mediated DNA cleavage and cytotoxicity of camptothecin analogues. Cancer Res 49:4385–4389.
22. Hertzberg RP, Caranfa MJ, Holden KG, et al. 1989 Modification of the hydroxy lactone ring of camptothecin: inhibition of mammalian topoisomerase I and biological activity. J Med Chem 32:715–720.
23. Wang X, Zhou X, Hecht SM. 1999 Role of the 20-hydroxyl group in camptothecin binding by the topoisomerase I-DNA binary complex. Biochemistry 38:4374–4381.

24. Kehrer DFS, Soepenberg O, Loows WJ, Verweij J, Sparreboom A. 2001 Modulation of camptothecin analogs in the treatment of cancer: a review. Anti-Cancer Drugs 12:89–105.
25. Lesuer-Ginot L, Demarquay D, Kiss R, et al. 1999 Homocamptothecin, an E-ring modified camptothecin with enhanced lactone stability, retains topoisomerase I-targeted activity and antitumor properties. Cancer Res 59:2939–2943.
26. Chauvier D, Chourpa I, Bigg DC, Manfait M. 2000 Kinetics of in vitro hydrolysis of homocamptothecins as measured by fluorescence. Ann N Y Acad Sci 922: 314–316.
27. Chourpa I, Riou JF, Millot J, Pommier Y, Manfait M. 1998 Modulation in kinetics of lactone ring hydrolysis of camptothecins upon interaction with topoisomerase I cleavage sites on DNA. Biochemistry 37:7284–7291.
28. Giovanella BC, Stehlin JS, Wall ME, et al. 1989 DNA topoisomerase I—targeted chemotherapy of human colon cancer in xenografts. Science 246:1046–8.
29. Stewart L, Redinbo MR, Qiu X, Hol WG J, Champoux JJ. 1998 A model for the mechanism of human topoisomerase I. Science 279:1534–1541.
30. Champoux JJ. 2000 Structure-based analysis of the effects of camptothecin on activities of human topoisomerase I. Ann N Y Acad Sci 922:56–64.
31. Fiorani P, Hann CL, Benedetti P, Bjornsti MA. 2001 Drug-induced stabilization of covalent DNA topoisomerase I-DNA intermediates. DNA cleavage assays. Methods Mol Biol 95:291–301.
32. Shen LL. 2001 DNA-unwinding test using eukaryotic DNA topoisomerase I. Methods Mol Biol 95:149–160.
33. Saenger W.1983 Principles of Nucleic Acid Structure. In: Advanced Texts in Chemistry. Cantor C, ed. Springer-Verlag, New York, pp. 13–15.
34. Stewart L, Ireton GC, Parker LH, Madden KR, Champoux JJ. 1996 Biochemical and biophysical analyses of recombinant forms of human topoisomerase I. J Biol Chem 271:7593–7601.
35. Stewart L, Ireton GC, Champoux JJ. 1999 A functional linker in human topoisomerase I is required for maximum sensitivity to camptothecin in a DNA relaxation assay. J Biol Chem 274:32950–32960.
36. Redinbo MR, Stewart L, Kuhn P, Champoux JJ, Hol WGJ. 1998 Crystal structures of human topoisomerase I in covalent and noncovalent complexes with DNA. Science 279:1504–1513.

3 Inhibitors of Topoisomerase I Function

Sidney M. Hecht, PhD

CONTENTS

1. INTRODUCTION

As noted elsewhere in this book, the locus of action of camptothecin (CPT) *(1)* (Fig. 1) as an antitumor agent involves the noncovalent binding of this agent to the covalent binary complex formed between topoisomerase I (TOP-I) and DNA (Fig. 2) *(1)*. Although the equilibrium between free enzyme and the enzyme-DNA binary complex normally lies far toward free enzyme and DNA, in the presence of CPT, the equilibrium is rapidly displaced toward ternary complex *(2)*. At this level, the action of CPT on TOP-I function is entirely analogous to those of several agents that inhibit the function of topoisomerase II, including 4-(9-acridinylamino)-*N*-(methanesulfonyl)-*m*-anisidine (m-AMSA), etoposide, and teniposide *(3)*.

The persistence of the ternary complex during DNA replication would be expected to result in the introduction of DNA lesions, and these have been postulated to form the biochemical basis for the killing of cells treated with CPT *(4,5)*.

Camptothecins in Cancer Therapy
Edited by: V. R. Adams and T. G. Burke © Humana Press Inc., Totowa, NJ

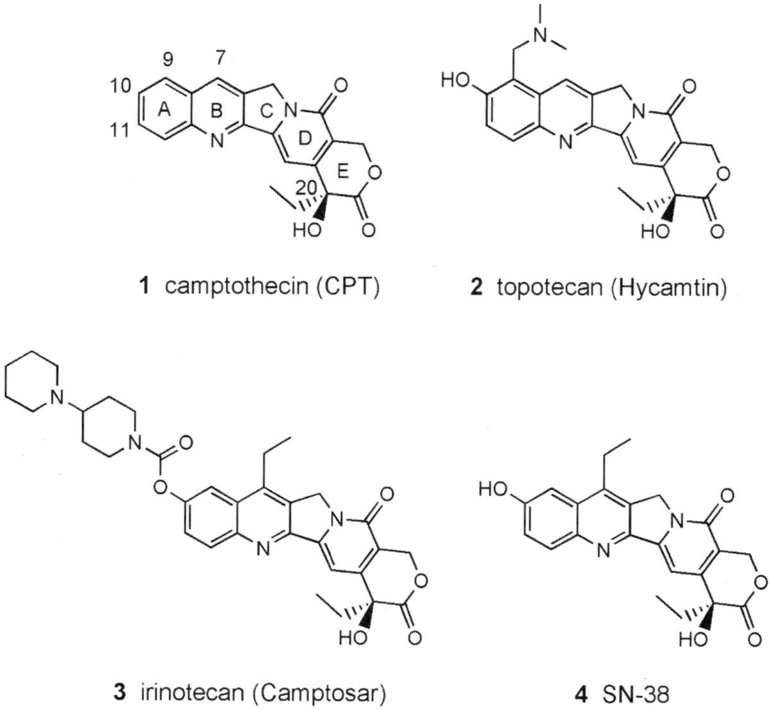

Fig. 1. Chemical structures of camptothecin (**1**) and two clinically used congeners (**2**and **3**). Compound **3** is a prodrug of **4**.

As shown in Fig. 1, subsequent to the identification of the locus of action of CPT (**1**), two camptothecin analogs have undergone clinical development and are marketed as antitumor agents. Hycamtin (topotecan) (**2**) is a more water-soluble analogue of CPT marketed by GlaxoSmithKline for the treatment of ovarian cancer and small-cell lung cancer. Camptosar (irinotecan) (**3**), a prodrug of SN-38 (**4**), is marketed by Pfizer; it is effective in the treatment of colorectal cancer and non–small-cell lung cancer.

Although numerous chemical strategies can be envisioned for the modification of the CPTs to produce more effective antitumor agents, other approaches can also be envisioned. These include other structural classes of TOP-I inhibitors, some of which may function in a different fashion than the CPTs. It has also become increasingly clear that TOP-I participates in cellular processes other than simple alteration of the linking number of DNA; targeting of these TOP-I–linked functions may also provide access to novel agents.

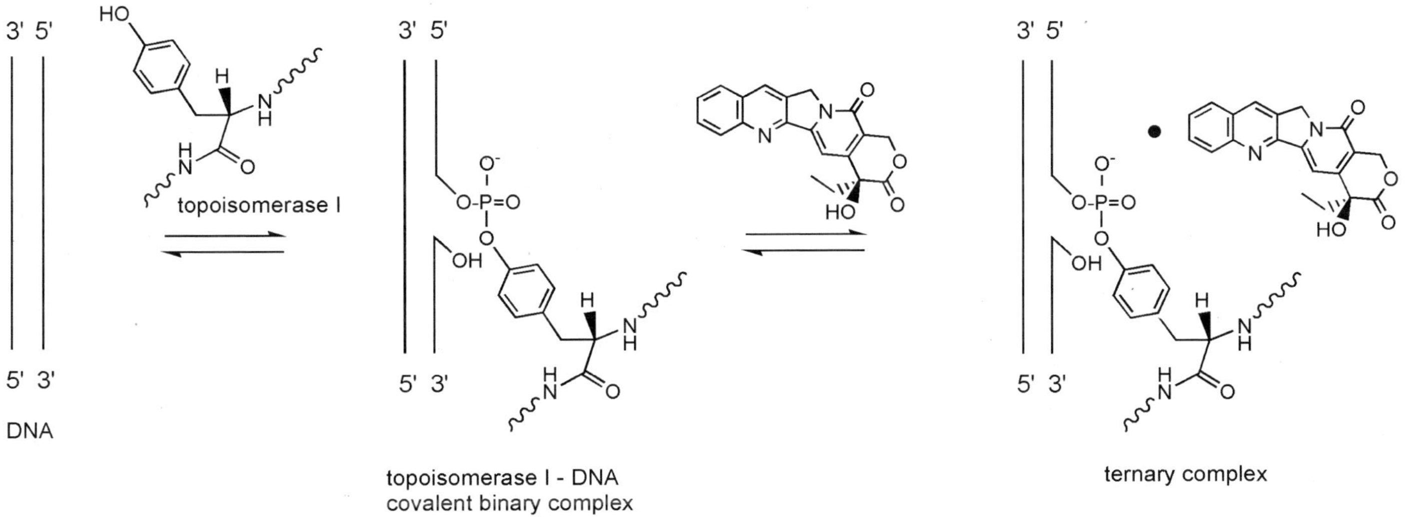

Fig. 2. Effect of CPT on the reversible nicking of DNA by TOP-I.

2. AGENTS THAT TARGET THE TOP-I–DNA COVALENT BINARY COMPLEX

2.1. CPT Analogs

The structure-activity relationships for the CPTs have been studied extensively *(6,7)*. From the perspective of identifying new derivatives having improved properties, it may be noted that the **7**, **9**, and **10** positions (Figs. 3 and 4) are quite tolerant of substitution, and that 11- and 12-substituted derivatives have also been reported. It seems clear that a 20-hydroxyl group having the *S*-configuration is also important, because 20-deoxy CPT is inactive as a TOP-I inhibitor *(6,8)*, although a recent study with 20-chloro, bromo, and amino derivatives has indicated that other functions may substitute for the OH group at this position *(8)*.

Analogs of CPT that have been studied in phase I–II clinical trials or preclinically include the water-soluble derivative DX-8951f (**5**) and the lipophilic derivative BNP1350 (**6**), 9-amino CPT (**7**), and CPT alkyl esters exemplified by **8** (Fig. 3) *(9)*. In addition to the usual pharmacokinetic issues that can be addressed through the use of derivatives such as **5–8**, the camptothecins have an additional property that has been the focus of considerable attention.

As shown in Fig. 4, CPT undergoes a pH-sensitive hydrolysis/lactonization of ring E (i.e., the reversible interconversion of hydroxy acid **9** and the lactone form of CPT [**1**]). This property was first noted by Wall and was used for the formulation of the otherwise insoluble CPT lactone *(10)*. It was later shown in a cell-free system that **9** does not inhibit TOP-I function (Fig. 2) *(6,11)*, suggesting that the formulation of CPT lactone as hydroxy acid **9** could have contributed to the failure of CPT itself in early clinical trials.

The consequences of the hydrolysis/lactonization process for CPT analogs that have greater water solubility than CPT itself would seem logically to be minimal, because the equilibrium should be rapid on a therapeutic time scale; indeed the spontaneous conversion of a ring E-opened carboxamide **10** to **1** (Fig. 4) *(12)* underscores the considerable facility of the lactonization. Nonetheless, it has been shown that individual CPT derivatives differ in their lactone-hydroxy acid ratios after lipid bilayer partitioning and argued that this may affect their properties sufficiently to alter their activities as antitumor agents *(13)*. The finding that the ring-opened form of CPT analogs can bind to serum proteins with greater efficiencies than the respective lactones adds to the complexity of the analysis *(14,15)*.

Although alteration of ring E of CPT has generally resulted in a loss of cytotoxic potential *(12)*, there is one important recent exception—namely homocamptothecin (**11**) (Fig. 5) and its derivatives *(16)*. These compounds induce DNA cleavage in the presence of TOP-I and stabilize the covalent

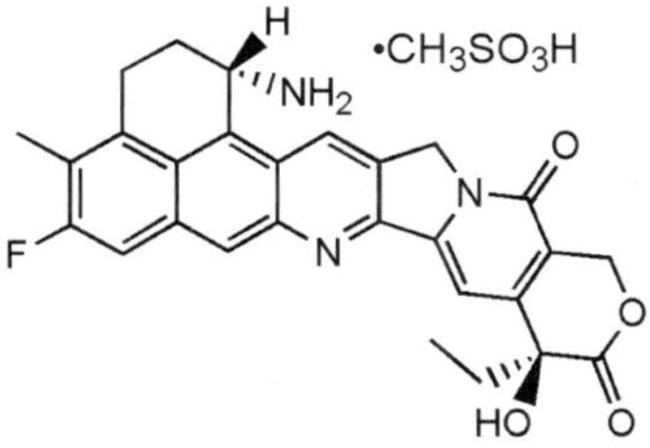

5 DX-8951f

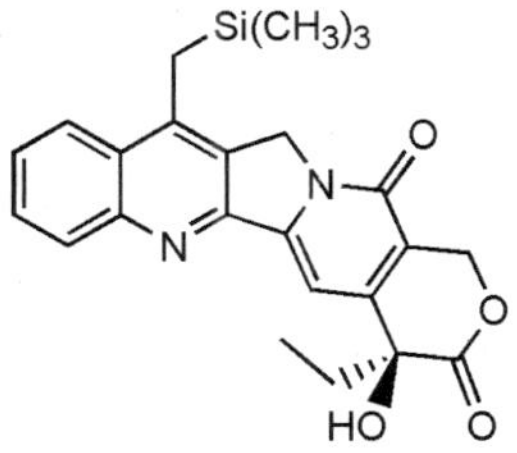

6 BNP1350

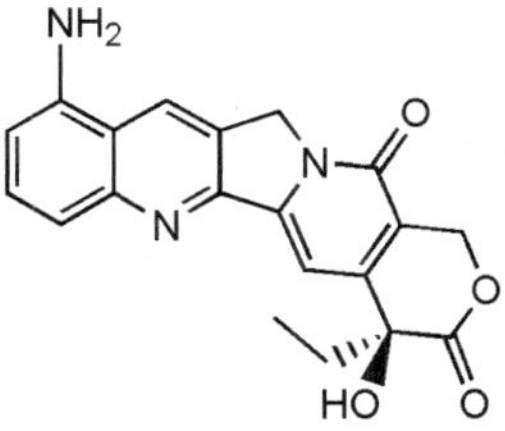

7 9-aminoCPT

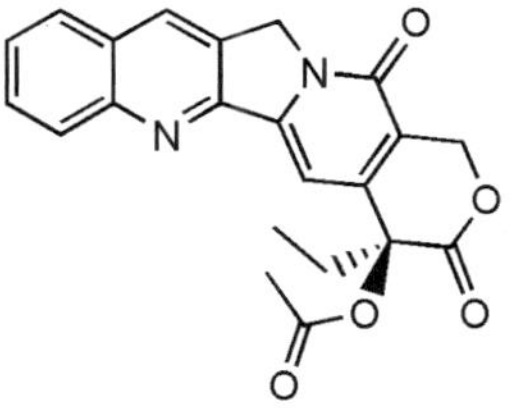

8

Fig. 3. Structural analogs of camptothecin.

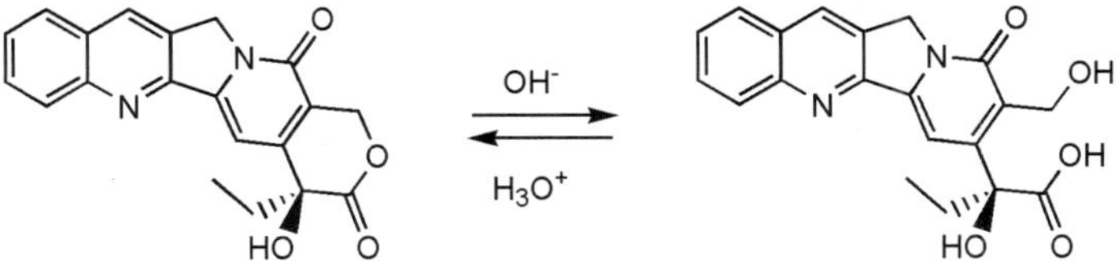

1 CPT, lactone form

9 CPT hydroxy acid

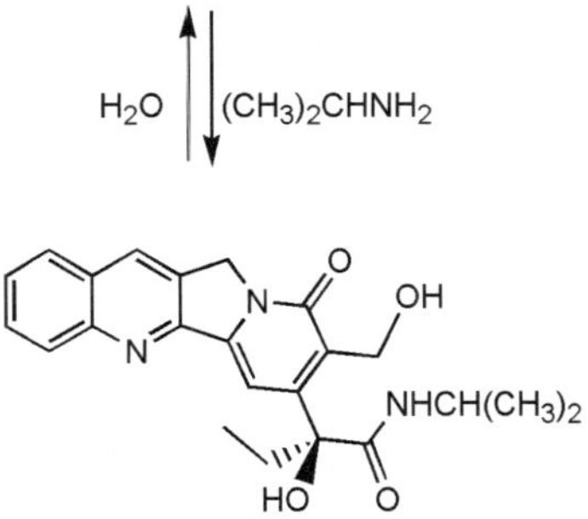

10

Fig. 4. Transformations of ring E in camptothecin.

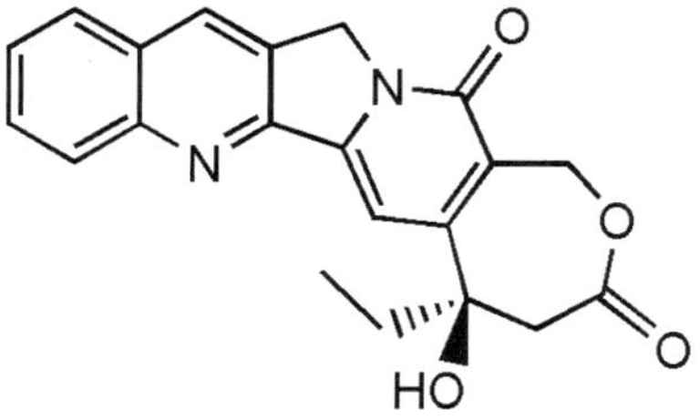

11 homocamptothecin

Fig. 5. Structure of homocamptothecin (**11**).

binary complex formed between the enzyme and DNA. The lactone (E-) ring does not undergo solvolysis readily, and ring opening is not readily reversed under physiological conditions. It is not clear to what extent the absence of reversible ring opening may contribute to the antitumor activity of the homocamptothecins, but derivatives have been prepared that exhibit strong antiproliferative activity *(17,18)*.

There is an important characteristic of TOP-I inhibition at the level of binary complex stabilization that probably contributes to the ability of such inhibitors to function as antineoplastic agents. Although the effects of simple enzyme inhibitors can often be overcome in a cellular context by overexpression of the targeted enzyme, overexpression of TOP-I actually renders cells hypersensitive to CPT *(19–21)*, presumably by increasing the number of associated DNA lesions. Because TOP-I is an essential enzyme in humans, it is also not possible to avoid inhibition by CPT via dramatic lowering of intracellular TOP-I levels. Accordingly, resistance to CPT is often characterized by alteration of TOP-I structure *(22,23)*.

2.2. Other Nitrogen Heterocycles

In addition to the camptothecins, several other classes of nitrogen heterocycles have been found to promote the cleavage of DNA by TOP-I, with concomitant stabilization of the formed enzyme-DNA covalent binary complex. These have included the benzophenanthridine alkaloids nitidine (**12**) and fagaronine (**13**) *(24)*, protoberberine-type alkaloids such as coralyne (**14**) and dihydrocoralyne (**15**), and a number of indolocarbazole derivatives, exemplified by **16** and **17** *(25)* (Fig. 6).

It is interesting that a number of compounds within these structural series had been identified as antineoplastic agents before their identification as TOP-I inhibitors. These include the benzophenanthridine alkaloids *(26)*, more than 80 of which have been characterized from natural sources, in addition to those prepared by chemical synthesis *(26–28)*.

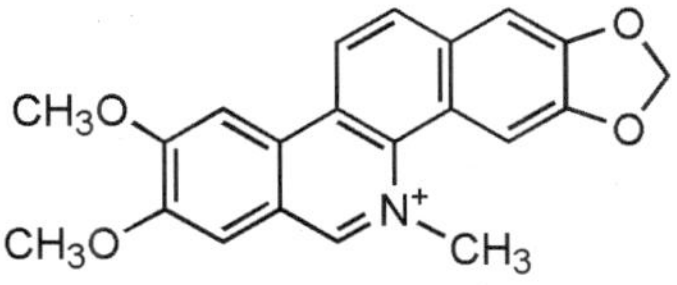

12 nitidine

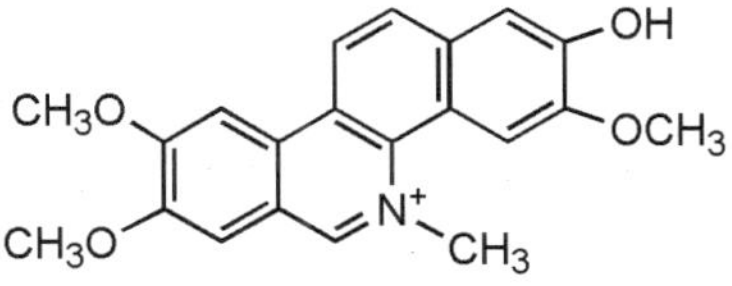

13 fagaronine

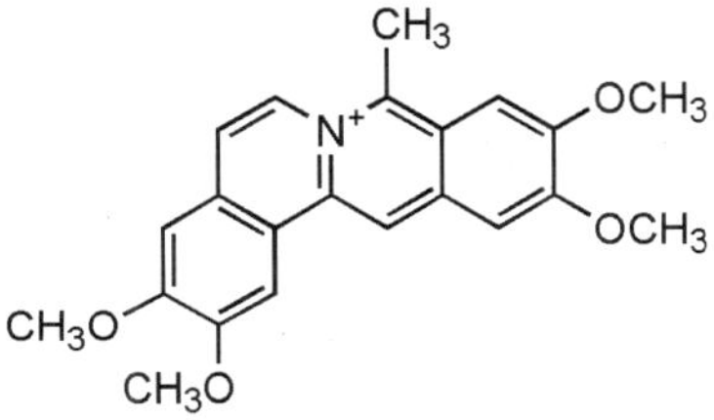

14 coralyne

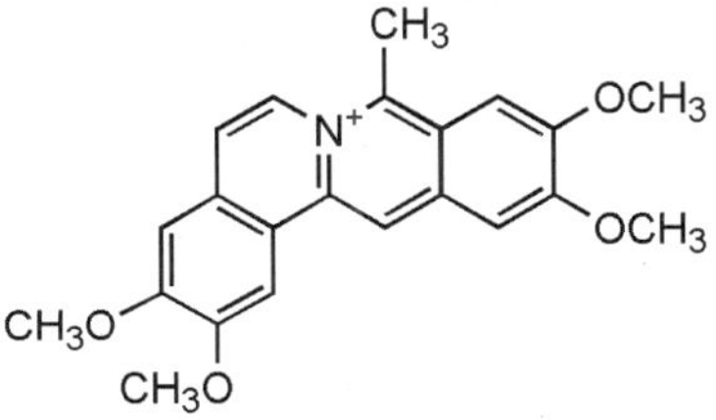

15 dihydrocoralyne

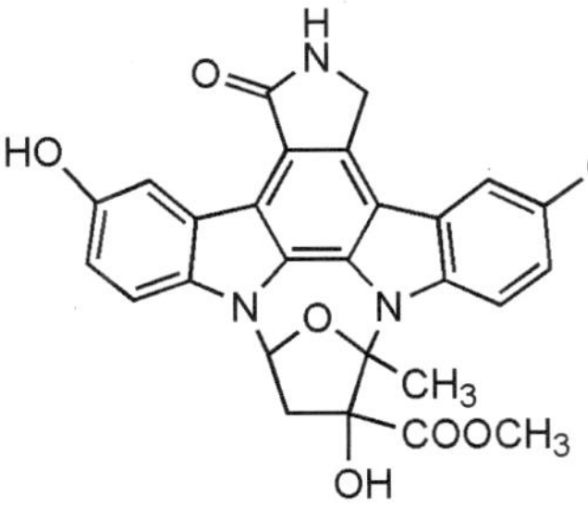

16

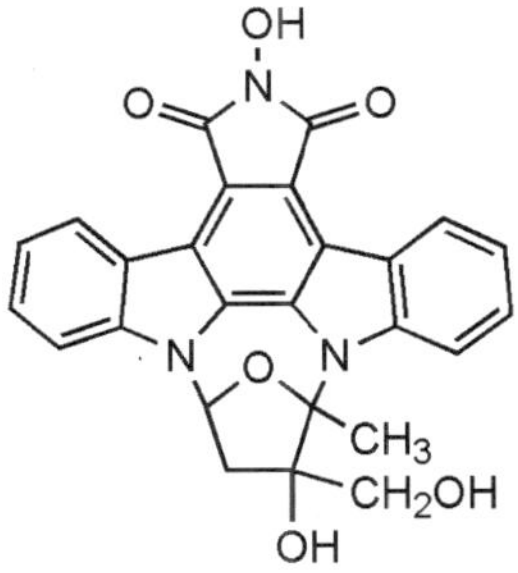

17

Fig. 6. Nitrogen heterocycles that inhibit TOP-I in analogy with camptothecin.

One issue that is of concern for compounds of the type discussed here is the extent to which the antineoplastic activity reported actually reflects inhibition of TOP-I function. For example, in addition to stabilizing the TOP-I–DNA covalent binary complex, nitidine (**12**) and fagaronine (**13**) also bind directly to DNA *(24)*. This is illustrated for fagaronine in Fig. 7, which shows the concentration-dependent effects of **13** on covalent binary complex formation. Although fagaronine promoted the formation of enzyme-DNA covalent binary complex in a concentration-dependent fashion, at higher concentrations (4.9–78 μ*M*) the compound also altered the mobility of DNA on an agarose gel via direct binding to DNA. Nitidine and fagaronine also inhibited DNA and RNA polymerases *(29)* and reverse transcriptases *(29–31)*, although only at rather high concentrations. Nonetheless, it is encour-

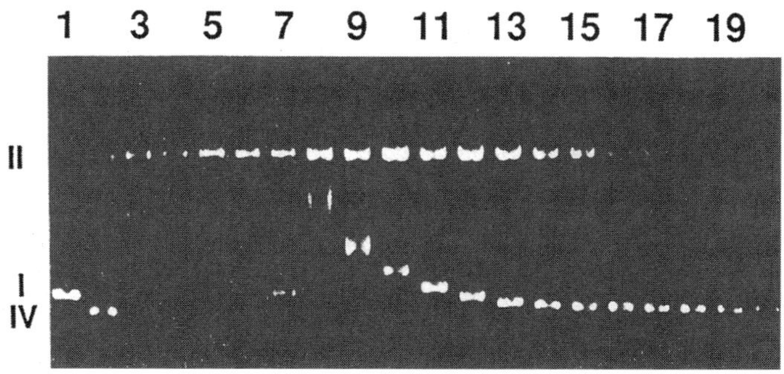

Fig. 7. Analysis of the effects of fagaronine (**13**) on TOP-I–DNA complex formation. *Lane 1*, supercoiled pSP64 plasmid DNA; *lane 2*, supercoiled DNA + calf thymus TOP-I; *lanes 3–20*, supercoiled DNA + topoisomerase I + 2500, 1250, 625, 312, 156, 78, 39, 19.5, 9.8, 4.9, 2.4, 1.2, 0.6, 0.3, 0.15, 0.075, 0.037, and 0.018 μ*M* fagaronine, respectively. Reprinted with permission from Chem Res Toxicol 1993;6:813–818. Copyright 1993 American Chemical Society.

aging that only those benzophenanthridine alkaloids found to stabilize the covalent binary complex formed from TOP-I and DNA in vitro had been identified in earlier studies as agents having antitumor activity in experimental animal models.

3. OTHER THERAPEUTIC STRATEGIES INVOLVING TOP-I

Although the focus of activity in developing inhibitors of TOP-I function has involved compounds that stabilize the enzyme-DNA covalent binary complex, other strategies for enzyme inhibition can be readily envisioned. For example, the overall mechanism of DNA relaxation by TOP-I involves initial DNA binding, nicking of one strand of the DNA backbone by TOP-I, and then strand passage (in a processive or distributive fashion *[32]*) to effect DNA relaxation. Resealing of the nick then affords free TOP-I and relaxed DNA (Fig. 2). Any of the individual processes leading to DNA relaxation (i.e., DNA binding, nicking, strand passage) should be amenable to inhibition. Additionally, it should be possible to target free TOP-I.

There are examples of compounds that exhibit some of the foregoing properties. Corilagin and chebulagic acid both exhibited strong inhibition of TOP-I-mediated DNA relaxation, although neither stabilized the enzyme-DNA covalent binary complex. Chebulagic acid was also approximately 10- to 50-fold more potent than CPT at inhibiting DNA relaxation. Additionally, chebulagic acid was also >800-fold more potent than CPT in inhibiting the nicking of DNA by TOP-I *(33)*.

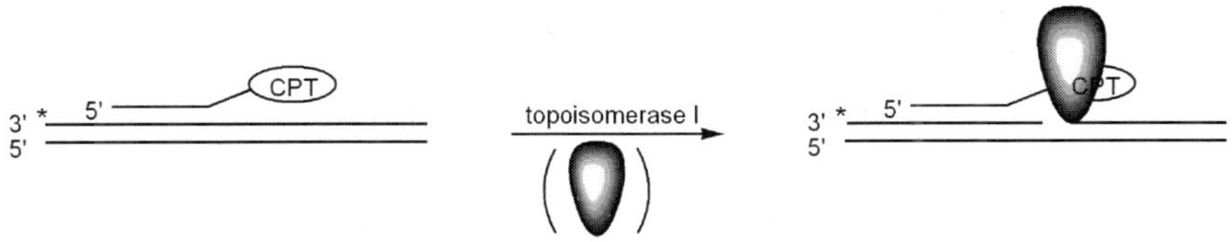

Fig. 8. Targeting and cleavage of a camptothecin-DNA conjugate by TOP-I.

Another strategy has been reported recently by Matteucci et al. *(34)*, who appended CPT covalently to a DNA oligonucleotide. When hybridized to a larger DNA target having a sequence complementary to the sequence in the probe oligonucleotide, the formed duplex promoted TOP-I-mediated cleavage of the DNA target in a sequence-selective fashion (Fig. 8).

4. DATA THAT MAY ENABLE THE DESIGN OF IMPROVED TOP-I INHIBITORS

4.1. Chemical Modification of TOP-I by Electrophilic CPTs

In 1990, Hertzberg et al. demonstrated that bromoacetamido CPTs **18** and **19** (Fig. 9) effected covalent modification of TOP-I in the enzyme-DNA binary complex in a time-dependent fashion after binding to the same site normally occupied by CPT *(35)*. Although the identity of the amino acid residue that was alkylated has never been reported, this experiment was important in establishing the nature of the matrix in proximity to position 10 of CPT within the formed ternary complex with the enzyme and its DNA substrate. More generally, the experiment also established the feasibility of using electrophilic CPT derivatives to map the orientation of CPT at the interface of the formed protein-nucleic acid binary complex.

A conceptually analogous experiment was later described by Pommier et al. *(36)* involving CPT derivative **20**. This compound, which contains an electrophilic chlorine at position 7 of the CPT system, was found to alkylate N-3 of guanosine in the +1 position of the scissile strand of the DNA substrate. On the basis of this finding and a number of observations that had been made in biochemical experiments, Fan et al. *(37)* proposed a model for the binding site of CPT within the enzyme-DNA binary complex (Fig. 10). Both the alkylation of G+1 by CPT **20** and stabilization of the covalent binary complex by CPT is most efficient at 5'-TG-3' cleavage sites, which allow putative stacking of CPT to the G residue at the terminus of the cleaved oligonucleotide to orient CPT within the ternary complex. Additional key amino acid residues putatively involved in the binding of CPT include Asn 722 (Fig. 10). A more recent computational model has also been proposed by Kerrigan and Pilch *(38)*. This model also posits the intercala-

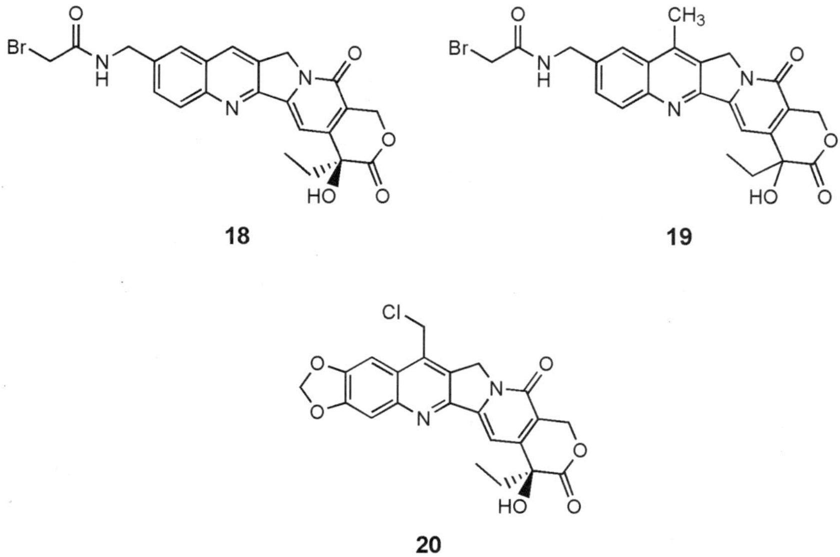

Fig. 9. Electrophilic analogues of camptothecin used to map the inhibitor binding pocket within the TOP-I–DNA covalent binary complex.

tion of the bound CPT and makes predictions about the preferred mode of orientation of the bound CPT within the enzyme-DNA ternary complex.

4.2. X-Ray Crystallographic Analysis of Human DNA TOP-I

Recently, Hol and Champoux have reported the crystal structures of reconstituted and truncated human TOP-I in both noncovalent and covalent complexes with DNA oligonucleotide substrates *(39)*. None of the complexes contained bound CPT, but analysis of the structures nonetheless permitted these workers to propose a CPT binding model for the covalent binary complex. This model, shown in Fig. 10, was substantially different than the model proposed by Fan et al. *(37)*. As illustrated, key CPT binding interactions were posited for Arg364 and Asp533, both of which were envisioned to form H-bonding interactions with ring E.

4.3. Use of CPT Binding Models to Guide Hypothesis Testing

Although the CPT binding models outlined in Fig. 10 differ in most respects, both involve the participation of the 20-OH group of CPT as a H-bond donor to amino acid residues within the binding pocket of the enzyme-DNA binary complex. This seemed entirely sensible given the reports *(6,8)* that 20-deoxy CPT (**21**) lacks antitumor activity and cannot

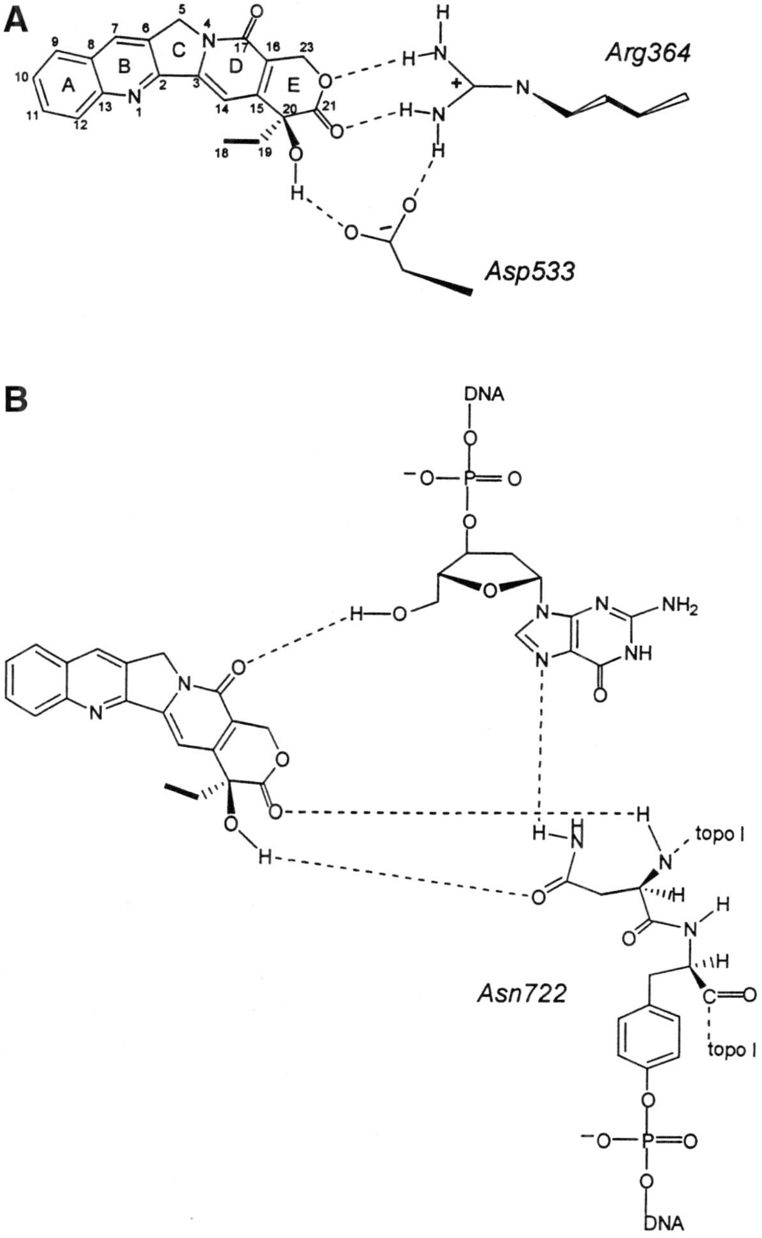

Fig. 10. Models of the binding of camptothecin to the covalent binary complex based on biochemical (**B**) and X-ray crystallographic (**A**) studies. Reprinted with permission from Biochemistry 1999;38:4374–4381. Copyright 1999 American Chemical Society.

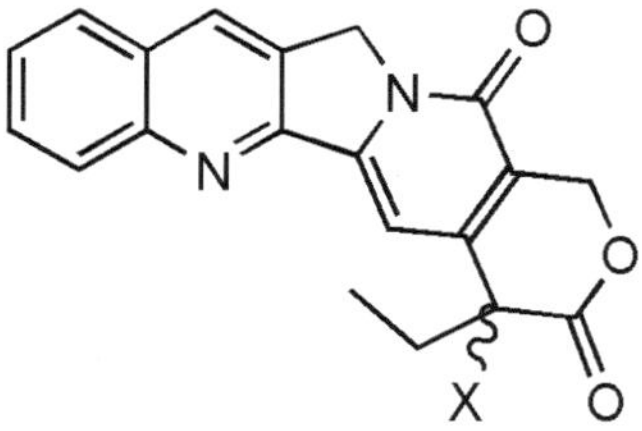

21 X = H
22 X = Cl
23 X = Br
24 X = NH_2

Fig. 11. Camptothecin analogues modified at position 20.

stabilize the covalent enzyme-DNA binary complex. Wang et al. *(8)* tested the importance of the 20 OH group in a series of experiments involving CPT (**1**), 20-deoxy CPT (**21**) and CPT derivatives bearing substituents other than an OH group at position 20. These included 20-chloro CPT (**22**), 20-bromo CPT (**23**) and 20-amino CPT (**24**), all of which were essentially racemic at position 20 (Fig. 11). Compounds **1** and **21–24** were tested for their abilities to stabilize the covalent binary complex between human TOP-I and the DNA oligonucleotide duplex whose scissile strand had the sequence 5'-GGCGCG GAGACTTGGAGAAATTTGGCGCGG; cleavage occurred at the $T_{13}G_{14}$ sequence *(8)*.

As summarized in Table 1, 20 deoxy CPT failed to stabilize the covalent binary complex to a significant extent, but 20-chloro CPT (**22**), 20-bromo CPT (**23**) and 20-amino CPT (**24**) exhibited reasonable binary complex stabilization, especially considering that each was racemic at C-20 and the 20*R* isomer of CPT has been reported *(11)* to be inactive.

To assess the ability of **21–24** to mediate cytotoxicity as a consequence of stabilization of the binary complex, Wang et al. *(8)* tested these analogs in a yeast strain lacking the homologous TOP-I but harboring a plasmid that contained human TOP-I under the control of an inducible promotor. As shown in Table 2, CPT **21** was not cytotoxic at any tested concentration, whereas **22–24** were all reasonably cytotoxic. Because halo CPT derivatives **22** and **23** lack a H-bond donor at C-20, it seems clear that the models represented in Fig. 10 likely require some revision. Perhaps the heteroatoms attached to C-20 in compounds **1**, **22**, **23**, and **24** actually function as H-bond acceptors, assuming that all of these agents interact with the enzyme-DNA binary complex in the same fashion.

Table 1
Stabilization of a TOP-I–DNA Oligonucleotide Complex by CPT Analogs

	% Ternary complex		
CPT analog	*50 μM CPT*	*20 μM CPT*	*5 μM CPT*
1	82	78	71
21	5	3	2
22	26	29	7
23	33	24	7
24	34	21	12

Table 2
TOP-I-Dependent Cytotoxicity of CPT Analogs

CPT analog	IC_{50} (μM)
1	0.2
21	—[a]
22	2.1
23	6.7
24	47

[a] No cytotoxicity observed up to 100 m*M* concentration.

4.4. Modified TOP-I

Bjornsti and coworkers have made numerous point mutants of TOP-I, some of which exhibit substantially modified properties *(40)*. One example is the substitution of amino acids at position 722 in the human enzyme, which normally contains Asn. These mutant enzymes exhibited a range of properties in mediating the reversible cleavage of DNA and in supporting cell viability *(40)*. For example, the introduction of serine, leucine, asparagine, or alanine at this position afforded enzymes that were resistant to CPT. That specific amino acid changes in TOP-I can affect CPT binding suggests that key substitutions may be of great utility in defining the nature of the binding of CPT and other inhibitors to the covalent enzyme-DNA binary complex.

A further refinement of this approach is suggested by the work of Hecht, Schultz, and others in introducing structurally modified amino acids into specific sites in proteins *(41–48)*. Clearly, the substitution of numerous analogues of amino acids found to be essential for CPT binding can potentially provide a detailed picture of the nature of inhibitor binding to the covalent enzyme-DNA binary complex.

5. BIOCHEMICAL PROCESSES PUTATIVELY LINKED TO TOP-I

5.1. Nonhomologous Recombination

Nonhomologous, or illegitimate, recombination refers to processes by which chromosomal rearrangements occur in DNA regions having little or no sequence homology. Although this phenomenon is quite common and is thought to be linked to cancer and genetic diseases *(49)*, the underlying molecular mechanisms are not clear. However, it certainly is clear that any such rearrangement must involve the formation and ultimate joining of DNA ends. Enzymes such as topoisomerases that catalyze DNA cleavage and ligation reactions must, therefore, be regarded as candidates for mediating such transformations. Topoisomerases I are particularly good candidates because site-specific recombinases exhibit TOP-I activity *(50,51)*, and TOP-I can subserve certain recombinase functions *(52)*. Further, in a study of chromosomal excision of SV40, which is believed to involve illegitimate recombination, Bullock et al. *(53,54)* found that the excision crossover points were in proximity to DNA sequences that are preferred cleavage sites for eukaryotic TOP-I. Given the deep-seated chromosomal rearrangements that are sometimes associated with carcinogenesis, the apparent involvement of TOP-I in illegitimate recombination may provide a potential new target for antitumor therapy.

Henningfeld and Hecht *(55)* modeled three types of transformations that may occur during illegitimate recombination using branched, nicked, and gapped substrates. The transformations involved in the use of nicked and gapped DNA oligonucleotide substrates are shown in Fig. 12. Also illustrated in this figure is TOP-I-mediated ligation of the nicked substrate. As shown in Fig. 12, ligation could occur across one- or three-nucleotide gaps produced by the enzyme and was influenced by the complementarity of the nucleotide at the 5′-end of the acceptor oligonucleotide to the nucleotide downstream from the cleavage site on the nonscissile strand.

The model duplexes were subsequently used to test the inhibitory properties of CPT analogues, most of which had been shown to stabilize the covalent TOP-I–DNA binary complex formed from B-DNA duplexes *(8,56)*. Although many of the CPT analogues were inhibitory in all of the assay systems, some showed a substantial variation in potency from one system to another. This is illustrated in Table 3 for the five CPT derivatives characterized in Table 1 *(8)*. The transformations studied were those outlined in Fig. 12, namely the ligation of nicked and gapped substrates. As shown in Table 3, the rank order of potencies of analogs **21–24** in inhibiting the ligation of the nicked DNA were not dissimilar to their potencies in stabilizing the covalent binary complex formed from B-form DNA

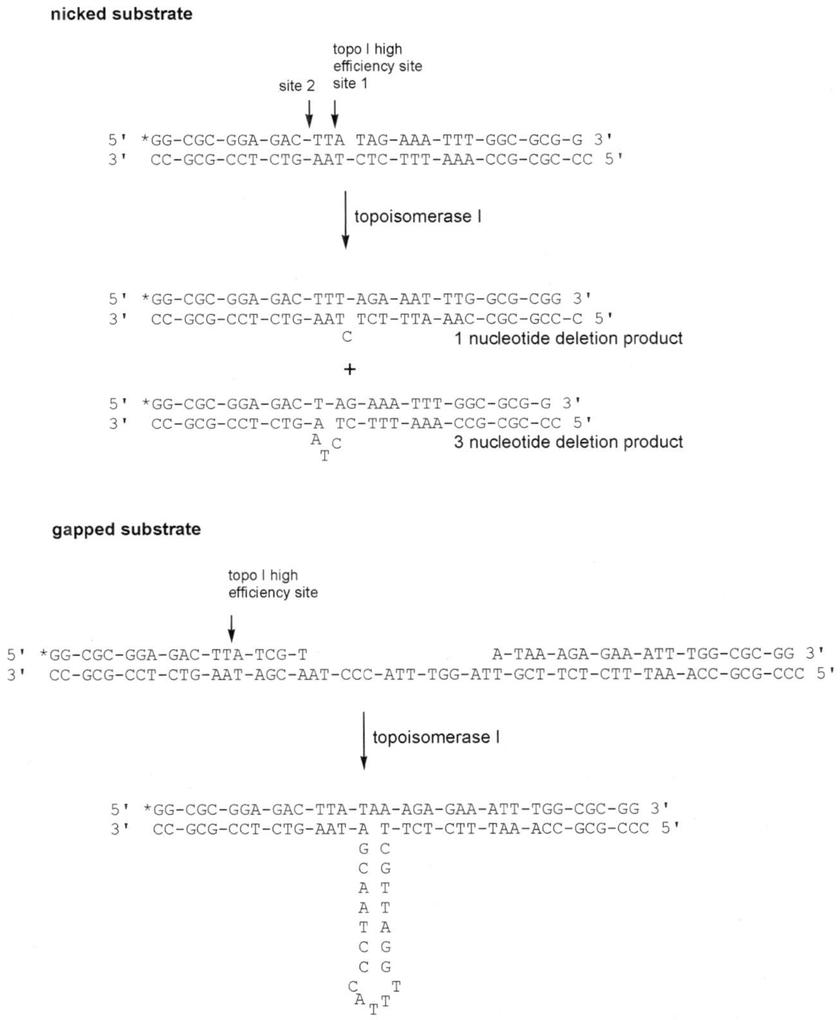

Fig. 12. **(A)** Models of illegitimate recombination using nicked and gapped DNA oligonucleotide substrates. **(B)** TOP-I–mediated ligation of a nicked substrate.

(Tables 1 and 3). However, ligation of inhibition of the gapped DNA substituted was effected only by CPT itself and by 20-deoxy CPT (**21**), the latter of which failed to inhibit any of the other ligation reactions. Thus it seems clear that differential inhibition of individual TOP-I-mediated transformations should be possible.

Table 3
Inhibition of the TOP-I-Mediated Ligation of Nicked and Gapped DNA Oligonucleotides by CPTs

	Extent of inhibition ligation (%)	
CPT analog[a]	*Nicked substrate*[b]	*Gapped substrate*
1	62	47
21	5	13
22	21	0
23	37	0
24	32	0

[a]50 μ*M* concentration.
[b]Inhibition of ligation after cleavage at site 2.

5.2. SR Protein Phosphorylation

Recently, Tazi and coworkers have documented the ability of TOP-I to mediate the phosphorylation of SR proteins (i.e. proteins containing arginine-serine repeats). Prominent among these are splicing factors that contain ribonucleoprotein consensus sequences. These proteins are phosphorylated exclusively on serine and appear to be excellent candidates for regulation of gene expression because they have the wherewithal to control (alternative) splicing of key structural genes *(57–60)*. It has been reported that CPT can inhibit the phosphorylation of SR proteins by TOP-I, and it seems plausible that protein phosphorylation may be an important component of the expression of antitumor activity by CPT.

An intriguing report by Labourier et al. *(61)* describes the stabilization of the TOP-II–DNA binary complex and inhibition of TOP-I SR protein kinase activity by an indolocarbazole. Although several indolocarbazoles have been shown to stabilize the TOP-I–DNA binary complex *(25,62,63)*, the finding of a second inhibitory locus for a compound of this type is intriguing. The contribution of inhibition of these two loci to the development of cytotoxicity is clearly of great interest and may suggest a general strategy for developing TOPI inhibitors having enhanced efficacy as antitumor agents.

5.3. Contribution of TRF Genes to the Expression of Cytotoxicity by TOP-I Inhibitors

In yeast there is a family of genes denoted *TRF* (DNA topoisomerase-related function), the protein products of which seem to have a function related to TOP-I function. For example, although *TRF* and *TOP-I* single deletion mutants are viable, the double mutants are inviable. Further, it has been found that a *TRF4* mutant is hypersensitive to CPT. Because the *TRF* genes are known to be required for proper nuclear segregation, it seems likely that this family of proteins augments TOP-I function at the level of chromatin (i.e., the actual in vivo locus of TOP-I inhibitors such as the camptothecins). There are *TRF* homologues in widely divergent species (e.g., *Drosophila*, *C. elegans*, oat, humans) suggesting a high level of evolutionary conservation.

Recently, Christman and coworkers have identified the product of *TRF4* as a novel DNA polymerase *(64)*, now denoted polymerase σ *(65)*. Although no inhibitor of this enzyme has been reported, it will be of great interest to learn whether a specific inhibitor of polymerase σ is capable of potentiating the cytotoxicity of DNA TOP-I inhibitors. Clearly, such a finding could provide an important new strategy for enhancing the utility of TOP-I inhibitors as antitumor agents.

ACKNOWLEDGMENTS

The work described in this chapter from the Hecht laboratory was supported by NIH Research Grant CA78415, awarded by the National Cancer Institute.

REFERENCES

1. Hsiang YH, Hertzberg R, Hecht SM, Liu LF. 1985 Camptothecin induces protein-linked DNA breaks via mammalian DNA topoisomerase I. J Biol Chem 260:14873–14878.
2. Hertzberg RP, Caranfa MJ, Hecht SM. 1989 On the mechanism of topoisomerase I inhibition by camptothecin: evidence for binding to an enzyme-DNA complex. Biochemistry 28:4629–4638.
3. Liu LF. 1989 DNA topoisomerase poisons as antitumor drugs. Annu Rev Biochem 58:351–375.
4. Hsiang Y, Lihour MG, Liu LF. 1989 Arrest of replication forks by drug-stabilized topoisomerase I-DNA cleavable complexes as a mechanism of cell killing by camptothecin. Cancer Res 49:5077–5082.
5. Liu LF. 1990 Anticancer drugs that convert DNA topoisomerases into DNA damaging agents. In: DNA Topology and Its Biological Effects. Cozzarelli NR, Wang JC, eds. Cold Spring Harbor Laboratory, New York, 371–389.
6. Hertzberg RP, Caranfa MJ, Holden KG, et al. 1989 Modification of the hydroxy lactone ring of camptothecin: inhibition of mammalian topoisomerase I and biological activity. J Med Chem 32:715–720.
7. Kingsbury WD, Boehm JC, Jakas DR, et al. 1991 Synthesis of water-soluble (aminoalkyl)camptothecin analogues: inhibition of topoisomerase I antitumor activity. J Med Chem 34:98–107.
8. Wang X, Zhou X, Hecht SM. 1999 Role of the 20-hydroxyl group in camptothecin binding by the topoisomerase I-DNA binary complex. Biochemistry 38:4374–4381.
9. Liehr JG, Giovanella BC, Verschraegen CF, eds. 2000 The camptothecins. Unfolding their anticancer potential. Vol. 922. Annals New York Academy Sciences, New York.

10. Wani MC, Ronman PE, Lindley JT, Wall ME. 1980 Plant antitumor agents. 18. Synthesis and biological activity of camptothecin analogues. J Med Chem 23: 554–560.
11. Jaxel C, Kohn KW, Wani MC, Wall ME, Pommier Y. 1989 Structure-activity study of the actions of camptothecin derivatives on mammalian topoisomerase I: evidence for a specific receptor site and a relation to antitumor activity. Cancer Res 49:1465–1469.
12. Adamovics JA, Hutchinson CR. 1979 Prodrug analogues of the antitumor alkaloid camptothecin. J Med Chem 22:310–314.
13. Burke TG, Mishra AK, Wani MC, Wall ME. 1993 Lipid bilayer partitioning and stability of camptothecin drugs. Biochemistry 32:5352–5364.
14. Mi Z, Burke TG. 1994 Differential interactions of camptothecin lactone and carboxylate forms with human blood components. Biochemistry 33:10325–10336.
15. Mi Z, Malak H, Burke TG. 1995 Reduced albumin binding promotes the stability and activity of topotecan in human blood. Biochemistry 34:13722–13728.
16. Lavergne O, Demarquay D, Kasprzyk PG, Bigg DCH. 2000 Homocamptothecins E-ring modified CPT analogues. In: The camptothecins. Unfolding their anticancer potential. Vol. 922. Liehr JG, Giovanella BC, Verschraegen CF, eds. Annals New York Academy Sciences, New York, 100–111.
17. Lavergne O, Lesueur-Ginot L, Pla Rodas F, Bigg DCH. 1997 BN 80245: an E-ring modified camptothecin with potent antiproliferative and topoisomerase I inhibitory activities. Bioorg Med Chem Lett 7:2235–2238.
18. Lavergne O, Lesueur-Ginot F, Pla Rodas F, et al. 1998 Homocamptothecins: synthesis and antitumor activity of novel E-ring-modified camptothecin analogues. J Med Chem 41:5410–5419.
19. Nitiss JL, Wang JC. 1988 DNA topoisomerase-targeting antitumor drugs can be studied in yeast. Proc Natl Acad Sci USA 85:7501–7505.
20. Eng WK, Faucette L, Johnson RK, Sternglanz R. 1988 Evidence that DNA topoisomerase I is necessary for the cytotoxic effects of camptothecin. Mol Pharmacol 34:755–760.
21. Bjornsti MA, Benedetti P, Viglianti GA. 1989 Expression of human DNA topoisomerase I in yeast cells lacking yeast DNA topoisomerase I: restoration of sensitivity of the cells to the antitumor drug camptothecin. Cancer Res 49:6318–6323.
22. Gupta RS, Gupta R, Eng B, et al. 1988 Camptothecin-resistant mutants of Chinese hamster ovary cells containing a resistant form of topoisomerase I. Cancer Res 48:6404–6410.
23. Kjeldsen E, Bonven BJ, Andoh T, et al. 1988 Characterization of a camptothecin-resistant human DNA topoisomerase I. J Biol Chem 263:3912–3916.
24. Wang LK, Johnson RK, Hecht SM. 1993 Inhibition of topoisomerase I function by nitidine and fagaronine. Chem Res Toxicol 6:813–818.
25. Yamashita Y, Fujii N, Murakata C, Ashizawa T, Okabe M, Nakano H. 1992 Induction of mammalian DNA topoisomerase I mediated DNA cleavage by antitumor indolocarbazole derivatives. Biochemistry 31:12069–12075.
26. Suffness M, Cordell GA. 1985 Antitumor alkaloids. In: The Alkaloids. Vol. XXV. Brossi A, ed. Academic Press, Florida, 178–188.
27. Phillips SD, Castle RN. 1981 A review of the chemistry of the antitumor benzo[c]phenanthridine alkaloids nitidine and fagaronine and of the related antitumor alkaloid coralyne. J Heterocycl Chem 18:223–232.
28. Cushman M, Mohan P, Smith ECR. 1984 Synthesis and biological activity of structural analogues of the anticancer benzophenanthridine alkaloid nitidine chloride. J Med Chem 27:544–547.

29. Sethi VS. 1976 Inhibition of mammalian and oncornavirus nucleic acid polymerase activities by alkoxybenzophenanthridine alkaloids. Cancer Res 36:2390–2395.
30. Sethi ML. 1979 Inhibition of reverse transcriptase activity by benzophenanthridine alkaloids. J Nat Prod 42:187–196.
31. Tan GT, Miller JF, Kinghorn AD, Hughes SH, Pezzuto JM. 1992 HIV-1 and HIV-2 reverse transcriptases: a comparative study of sensitivity to inhibition by selected natural products. Biochem Biophys Res Commun 185:370–378.
32. Stivers JT, Harris TK, Mildvan AS. 1997 Vaccinia DNA topoisomerase I: evidence supporting a free rotation mechanism for DNA supercoil relaxation. Biochemistry 36:5212–5222.
33. Berry DE, MacKenzie L, Shultis EA, Chan JA, Hecht SM. 1992 Naturally occurring inhibitors of topoisomerase I-mediated DNA relaxation. J Org Chem 57:420–422.
34. Matteucci M, Lin KY, Huang T, et al. 1997 Sequence-specific targeting of duplex DNA using a camptothecin-triple helix forming oligonucleotide conjugate and topoisomerase I. J Am Chem Soc 119:6939–6940.
35. Hertzberg RP, Busby RW, Caranfa MJ, et al. 1990 Irreversible trapping of the DNA-topoisomerase I covalent complex. J Biol Chem 265:19287–19295.
36. Pommier Y, Kohlhagen G, Kohn KW, Leteurtre F, Wani MC, Wall ME. 1995 Interaction of an alkylating camptothecin derivative with a DNA base at topoisomerase I-DNA cleavage sites. Proc Natl Acad Sci USA 92:8861–8865.
37. Fan Y, Weinstein JN, Kohn KW, Shi LM, Pommier Y. 1998 Molecular modeling studies of the DNA-topoisomerase I ternary cleavable complex with camptothecin. J Med Chem 41:2216–2226.
38. Kerrigan JE, Pilch DS. 2001 A structural model for the ternary cleavable complex formed between human topoisomerase I, DNA, and camptothecin. Biochemistry 40:9792–9798.
39. Redinbo MR, Stewart L, Kuhn P, Champoux JJ, Hol WG. 1998 Crystal structures of human topoisomerase I in covalent and noncovalent complexes with DNA. Science 279:1504–1513.
40. Fiorani P, Bjornsti MA. 2000 Mechanisms of DNA topoisomerase I-induced cell killing in the yeast. In: The camptothecins. Unfolding their anticancer potential. Vol. 922. Liehr JG, Giovanella BC, Verschraegen CF, eds. New York Academy of Sciences, New York, 65–75.
41. Cornish VW, Kaplan MI, Veenstra DL, Kollman PA, Schultz PG. 1994 Stabilizing and destabilizing effects of placing β-branched amino acids in protein α-helices. Biochemistry 33:12202–12031.
42. Thorson JS, Chapman E, Schultz PG. 1995 Analysis of hydrogen bonding strengths in proteins using unnatural amino acids. J Am Chem Soc 117:9361–9362.
43. Sonar S, Liu XM, Lee CP, et al. 1995 Site-directed isotope labeling and FT-IR spectroscopy: the Tyr 185/Pro peptide bond of bacteriorhodopsin is perturbed during the primary photoreaction. J Am Chem Soc 117:11614–11615.
44. Hohsaka T, Ashizuka S, Murakami H, Sisido M. 1996 Incorporation of nonnatural amino acids into streptavidin through in vitro frame-shift suppression. J Am Chem Soc 118:9778–9779.
45. Mamaev SV, Laikhter AL, Arslan T, Hecht SM. 1996 Firefly luciferase: alteration of the color of emitted light resulting from substitutions at position 286. J Am Chem Soc 118:7243–7244.
46. Karginov VA, Mamaev SV, An H, et al. 1997 Probing the role of an active site aspartic acid in dihydrofolate reductase. J Am Chem Soc 119:8166–8176.

47. Steward LE, Collins CS, Gilmore MA, Carlson JE, Ross JBA, Chamberlin AR. 1997 In vitro site-specific incorporation of fluorescent probes into β-galactosidase. J Am Chem Soc 119:6–11.
48. England PM, Lester HA, Davidson N, Dougherty DA. 1997 Photochemical proteolysis applied to ion channels in vivo. Proc Natl Acad Sci USA 94:11025–11030.
49. Schimke RT, Sherwood SW, Hill AB, Johnston RN. 1986 Overreplication and recombination of DNA in higher eukaryotes: potential consequences and biological implications. Proc Natl Acad Sci USA 83:2157–2161.
50. Landy A. 1989 Dynamic, structural, and regulatory aspects of lambda site-specific recombination. Annu Rev Biochem 58:913–949.
51. Ikeda H. 1990 DNA topoisomerase-mediated illegitimate recombination. In: DNA Topology and Its Biological Effects. Cozzarelli NR, Wang JC, eds. Cold Spring Harbor Laboratory Press, New York, 341–359.
52. Shuman S. 1991 Recombination mediated by vaccinia virus DNA topoisomerase I in *Escherichia coli* is sequence specific. Proc Natl Acad Sci USA 88:10104–10108.
53. Bullock PW, Forrester W, Botchan M. 1984 DNA sequence studies of simian virus 40 chromosomal excision and integration in rat cells. J Mol Biol 174:55–84.
54. Bullock P, Champoux JJ, Botchan M. 1985 Association of crossover points with topoisomerase I cleavage sites: a model for nonhomologous recombination. Science 230:954–958.
55. Henningfeld KA, Hecht SM. 1995 Topoisomerase I-mediated illegitimate recombination with duplex DNA substrates containing branches, nicks and gaps. Biochemistry 34:6120–6129.
56. Wang X, Wang LK, Kingsbury WD, Johnson RK, Hecht SM. 1998 Differential effects of camptothecin derivatives on topoisomerase I-mediated DNA structure modification. Biochemistry 37:9399–9408.
57. Rossi F, Labourier E, Forné T, et al. 1996 Specific phosphorylation of SR proteins by mammalian DNA topoisomerase I. Nature 381:80–82.
58. Tazi J, Rossi F, Labourier E, Gallouzi I, Brunel C, Antoine E. 1997 DNA topoisomerase I: customs officer at the border between DNA and RNA worlds? J Mol Med 75:786–800.
59. Labourier E, Rossi F, Gallouzi I, Allemand E, Divita G, Tazi J. 1998 Interaction between the N-terminal domain of human DNA topoisomerase I and the arginine-serine domain of its substrate determines phosphorylation of SF2/ASF splicing factor. Nucleic Acids Res 26:2955–2962.
60. Rossi F, Labourier F, Gallouzi I, et al. 1998 The C-terminal domain but not the tyrosine 723 of human DNA topoisomerase I active site contributes to kinase activity. Nucleic Acids Res 26:2963–2970.
61. Labourier E, Riou JF, Prudhomme M, Carrasco C, Bailly C, Tazi J. 1999 Poisoning of topoisomerase I by an antitumor indolocarbazole drug: stabilization of topoisomerase I-DNA covalent complexes and specific inhibition of the protein kinase activity. Cancer Res 59:52–55.
62. Anizon F, Belin L, Moreau P, et al. 1997 Syntheses and biological activity (topoisomerases inhibition antitumoral and antimicrobial properties) of rebeccamycin analogues bearing modified sugar moieties and substituted on the imide nitrogen with a methyl group. J Med Chem 40:3456–3465.
63. Bailly C, Riou JF, Colson P, Houssier C, Rodrigues-Pereira E, Prudhomme M. 1997 DNA cleavage by topoisomerase I in the presence of indolocarbazole derivatives of rebeccamycin. Biochemistry 36:3917–3929.

64. Wang Z, Castaño IB, De Las Peñas A, Adams, C, Christman MF. 2000 Pol Kappa, a DNA polymerase required for sister chromatid cohesion. Science 289:774–779.
65. Carson D, Christman MF.2001 Evidence that replication fork components catalyze the establishment of sister chromatid cohesion. Proc Natl Acad Sci USA 98:8270–8275.

4 Cytotoxic Mechanisms of Topoisomerase 1 Inhibitors

Yves G. Pommier, MD, PhD,
Juana Barceló, PhD,
Takahisa Furuta, MD, PhD,
Haruyuki Takemura, MD, PhD,
Olivier Sordet, PhD,
and ZhiYong Liao, PhD

CONTENTS

Camptothecins in Cancer Therapy
Edited by: V. R. Adams and T. G. Burke © Humana Press Inc., Totowa, NJ

1. INTRODUCTION

Topoisomerase 1 (Top1) is a validated target for cancer chemotherapy *(1–3)* because of its identification as the sole target of camptothecin (CPT) *(4)*. The sodium salt of CPT was found to be clinically active, but its use was discontinued in the 1970s because of severe side effects and lack of understanding of the drug's mechanism of action *(5)*. The finding in 1985 that CPT specifically poisons Top1 has generated great interest to find water-soluble, more efficacious, and less toxic analogs of CPT.

Top1 inhibitors exemplify classical anticancer agents that have been discovered by screening the antiproliferative activity of extracts from natural products. Although Top1 is clearly the primary cellular target of CPTs, it is less well understood why CPTs selectively kill tumor cells. Indeed, Top1 is essential and present in all cells, including tumor and normal cells, which indicates that the selectivity of CPTs and Top1 inhibitors must arise from molecular mechanisms/determinants of cellular response that are specifically altered in tumors.

This chapter is an update of our previous reviews *(2,3,6)*. First, we give an update on the clinical development of novel Top1 inhibitors and on the DNA-damaging lesions that poison Top1. Next, we present a common molecular model for the poisoning of Top1–DNA complexes, which we will refer to as the 5'-end misalignment model. The third and final part of this review focuses on the multiple molecular pathways implicated in the repair of Top1–mediated DNA damage and in the cell death signaling. These pathways can be referred to as "secondary targets" because their alterations probably contribute to the tumor selectivity of Top1 poisons and because they can potentially be targeted to enhance the cellular activity of Top1 poisons.

2. NOVEL TOP1 INHIBITORS

Discovery of Top1 inhibitors is facilitated by the availability of a variety of biochemical and cellular assays. Indeed, Top1 can be expressed as a biochemically active recombinant protein *(7)*, and several crystal structures of Top1 bound to a DNA substrate have been reported recently *(8–12)*. Thus our understanding of Top1's molecular structure and mechanisms of action provides insights into the physiological functions of Top1, and have facilitated the screening and rational design of non-CPT Top1 inhibitors.

Yeast and mouse cells deficient for Top1 can be used to assess the selectivity of Top1 inhibitors. In these cellular systems, the hallmark of Top1 poisons is lack of drug activity *(13,14)*. A panel of cell lines with point mutations that confer resistance to CPTs can be used to test cross-resistance between CPT and non-CPT poisons *(3,15,16)*. Analysis of the drug sensitivity for the corresponding recombinant Top1 enzymes can also be used to assess the binding site of the new inhibitors in comparison with CPTs *(16,17)*.

In this first section, we review briefly the most recently developed CPT derivatives and the non-CPT Top1 poisons. More detailed reviews of the non-CPT Top1 inhibitors can be found elsewhere *(18–20)*. We will also (*see* Section 4.4.) stress the point that Top1 can be poisoned by agents that damage DNA. This type of Top1 poisoning probably occurs frequently under physiological conditions, which gives a biological relevance to the repair mechanisms for Top1 cleavage complexes.

2.1. CPTs

The US Food and Drug Administration has approved two water-soluble CPT derivatives recently: Topotecan (Hycamtin®, Glaxo SmithKline) as a second-line chemotherapy for ovarian cancers and for the treatment of small-cell lung cancer, and CPT-11 (Irinotecan, Camptosar®, Yakult Honsha KK) for colon cancers *(21)*. The derivatized positions 7, 9, and 10 for these CPT derivatives are indicated in Fig. 1. Several other CPT derivatives are in clinical trials: 9-nitrocamptothecin (9-NC) (SuperGen) *(22)*, exatecan mesylate (DX-8951f) *(23)*, Afeletecan® (Bayer AG), CKD-602 (Chong Kun Dang Pharmaceutical Corp.), DRF-1042 (Dr. Reddys Research Foundation), PEG-camptothecin (Prothecan®) (Enzon Inc.), MAG-camptothecin (PNU-166148) (Pharmacia), ST1481 (Sigma-Tau Healthsci SpA), Homa-copolymer-camptothecin (University of London), and Karenitecin® (BioNumerik Pharmaceuticals) *(21)*.

Recently, CPT analogs bearing a seven-member E-ring (Fig. 1) have been generated chemically and found to retain potent Top1 inhibition both in biochemical systems with purified Top1 and in cells *(15,24–26)*. These derivatives have been synthesized and studied by the Beaufour Ipsen group and named homocamptothecins (Fig. 1). The presence of an additional methylene group stabilizes the E-ring and limits the conversion to the carboxylate. Conversely, the inactive carboxylate of homocamptothecin cannot be converted to the lactone after the E-ring has been opened *(25)*. The binding of these compounds in the Top1–DNA complex is probably very similar to (but possibly better than) the binding of CPTs, based on the recent finding that mutations that confer resistance to CPTs also confer cross-resistance to homocamptothecin *(15)*. However, because of its greater potency, homocamptothecin remains more active in CPT-resistant cells *(15)*. The difluorohomocamptothecin derivative BN-80915 (diflomotecan) (Fig. 1), which is more potent than SN-38, the active metabolite of CPT-11 (Fig. 1), and produces more stable cleavage complexes in cells *(27)*, has been selected for clinical trials.

The CPT derivatives presently in the clinic have two major limitations: (1) at physiological pH, the labile α-hydroxylactone function, which is essential for CPT activity *(28)* is in equilibrium with its inactive (carboxylate) form that is bound to serum albumin *(29)* (Fig. 1); and (2) the CPT-trapped cleavage complexes reverse within minutes after drug removal, which imposes long or repeated infusions for cancer treatment.

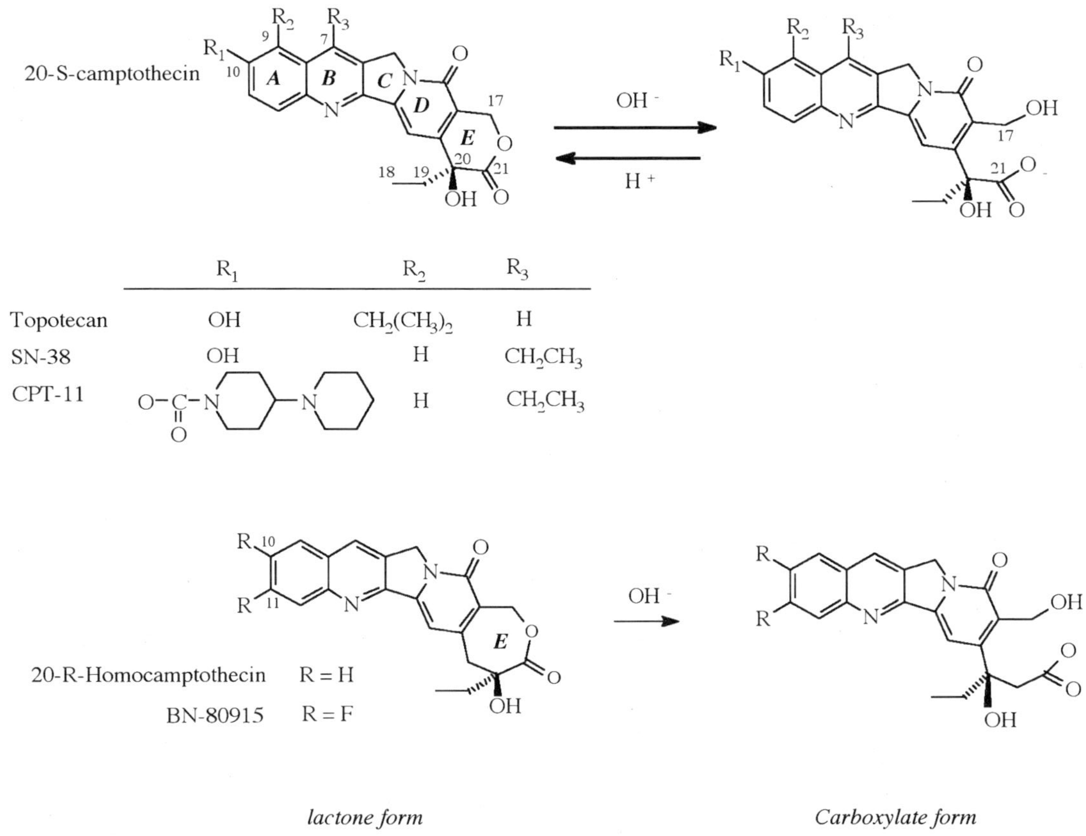

Fig. 1. Camptothecin (CPT) derivatives used in the clinic. SN-38 is the active metabolite of CPT-11.

2.2. Non-CPT Top1 Poisons: Polyheterocyclic Aromatic Inhibitors

The indolocarbazoles represent the most advanced class of non-CPT derivatives in terms of chemotype, clinical development, and structure-activity *(19,20,30)*. Among the numerous Top1 inhibitor indolocarbazole derivatives, NB-506 and J-107088 (Fig. 2) have recently been selected for clinical trials. As with CPTs, indolocarbazoles prevent the religation of a subset of Top1 cleavage complexes. The DNA sequence selectivity of these cleavages is globally different from the pattern of cleavage sites induced by CPTs *(16,31,32)*. Furthermore, by contrast to CPTs, indolocar-bazole Top1 poisons generally can bind to DNA by intercalation *(33)*.

A second class of non-CPT polyheterocyclic aromatic inhibitors is the indenoisoquinolines. The synthesis of the indenoisoquinoline NSC-314622 (Fig. 2) was first reported in 1978 *(34)*. Consecutively, a series of indenoisoquinolines were synthesized and found to possess significant anticancer activity *(35,36)*. However, little was known about their anticancer mechanism until recently, when a statistical analysis of cytotoxicity results obtained with the National Cancer Institute in vitro Anticancer Drug Discovery Screen of 60 cell lines revealed that NSC-314622 is a Top1 inhibitor *(37)*. The patterns of DNA breaks produced in the presence of camptothecins and NSC-314622 are different. Because of their novel structure, several dozens of indenoisoquinolines have been synthesized and tested for Top1 inhibition and for antiproliferative activity in the National Cancer Institute cell screen over the past 3 years *(38–40)*. Generally, the indenoisoquinoline derivatives that inhibit Top1 are cytotoxic in the National Cancer Institute cell lines *(38–40)*. Antitumor activity is also observed for some of these compounds in animal models *(40)*. Indenoisoquinolines are in preclinical development, and efforts are focused on testing the antitumor activity of selected indenoisoquinolines (i.e., compound MJ-III-65 shown in Fig. 2) in animal models and on obtaining cocrystal structure of indenoiso quinolines in the Top1–DNA complex.

Other polyheterocyclic Top1 poisons include nitidine, coralyne, berberine, and benzo[*a*]acridine derivatives (Fig. 2). These compounds share a common heterocyclic ring system, and generally bind to DNA by intercalation. Although some of them exhibit antiproliferative activity, to the best of our knowledge, they are not in clinical development; for further details *see* ref. *20*.

2.3. Non-CPT Top1 Poisons: Benzimidazoles and Minor Groove Ligands

The *bis*-benzimidazole dyes Hoechst 33342 (Ho-33342) and parent compound Hoechst 33258 (Ho-33258, NSC-32291, pibenzimol) (Fig. 3) represent a structurally unique class of Top1 poisons. Ho-33342 is commonly

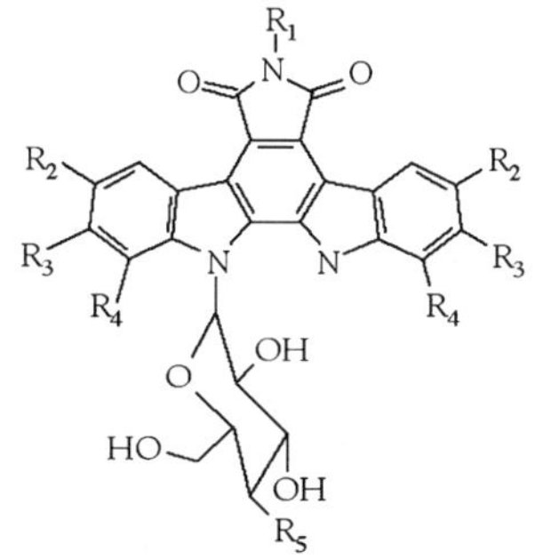

Indolocarbazoles

Compounds	R1	R2	R3	R4	R5
NB-506	NHCHO	H	H	OH	OH
J-107088	$NH(CH_2OH)_2$	H	OH	H	OH
BMS0250749	H	F	H	H	F

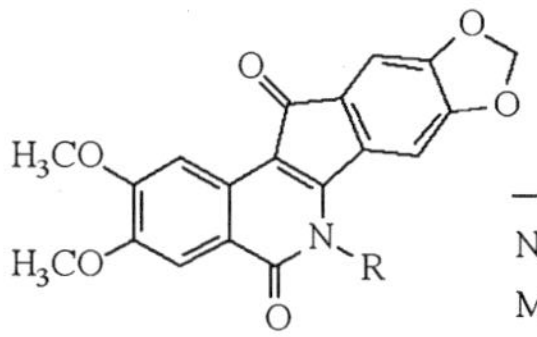

Indenoisoquinolines

	R
NSC-314622	CH_3
MJ-III-65	$(CH_2)_3NH(CH_2)_2OH$

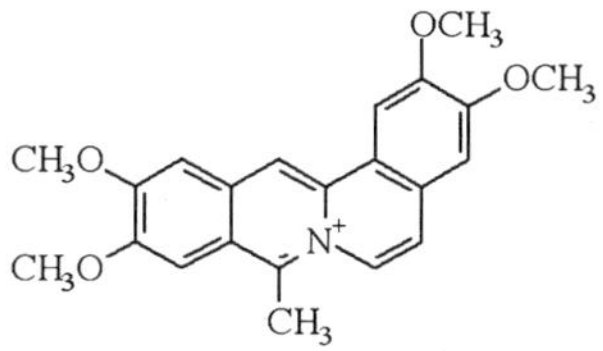

Coralyne

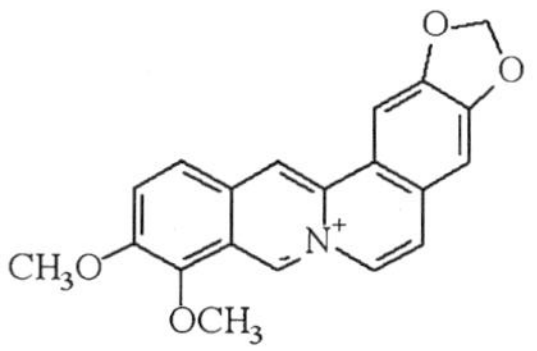

Berberine

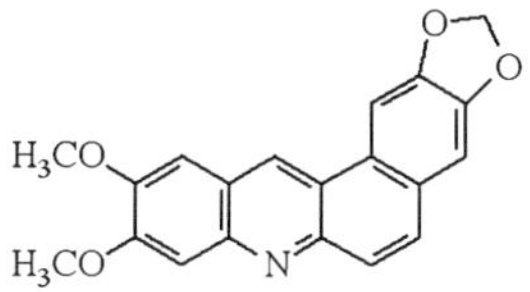

Benzo[a]acridine

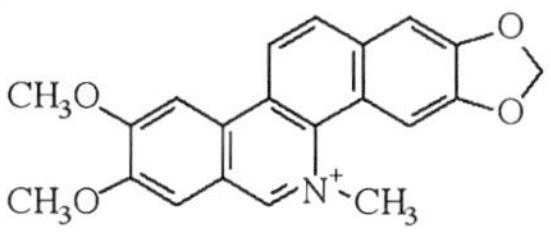

Nitidine

Fig. 2. Noncamptothecin polycyclic TOP-I poisons.

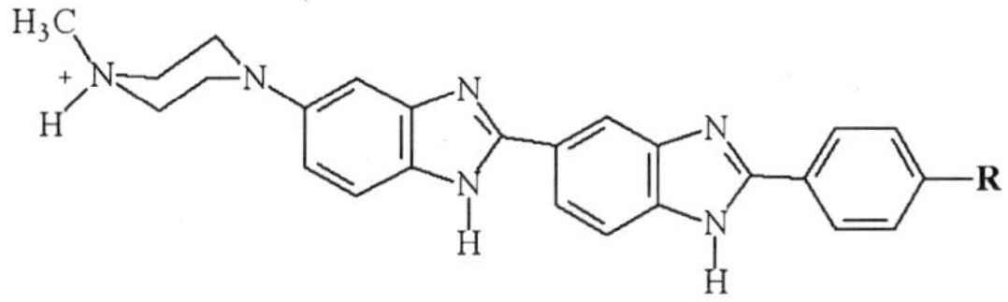

Hoechst 33258 R = OH (Pibenzimol)
Hoechst 33342 R = OCH_2CH_3

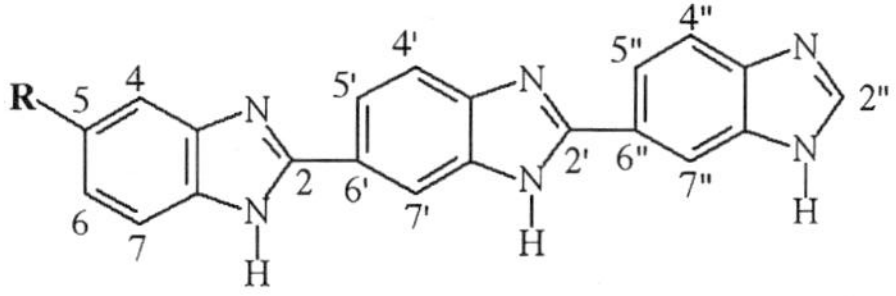

TB R = H
5PTB R = Phenyl } **Terbenzimidazoles**

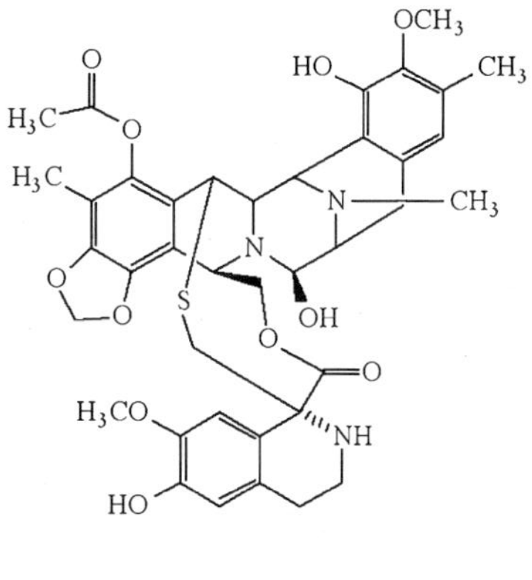

Ecteinascidin 743

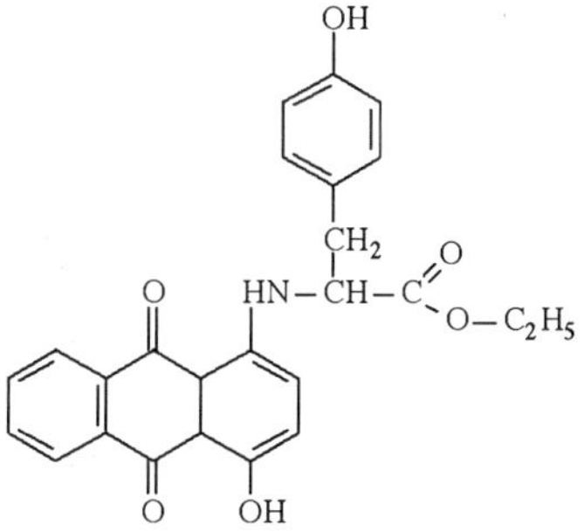

NU/ICRF 505

Fig. 3. Noncamptothecin minor groove binding TOP-I poisons.

used for histochemical staining and flow cytometry analysis of DNA content. Ho-33342 and 33258 reversibly trap Top1 cleavage complexes with a different sequence selectivity than CPT *(41)*. They both bind to AT-rich sequences, causing widening of the DNA minor groove *(42)*. However, minor groove binding is not sufficient for Top1 trapping because Distamycin, Berenil, and netropsin do not poison Top1 *(41)*. Ho-33258 is two orders of magnitude less cytotoxic than Ho33342 because of its low membrane permeability. Ho-33342 also disrupts TATA box-binding protein/TATA box element binding *(43)*, suggesting that it targets other cellular pathways besides Top1. A limitation of Ho-33342 as an anticancer drug is that it is not effective against tumor cell lines overexpressing MDR1 *(44)*.

In recent years, the Liu and Lavoie group has synthesized and investigated a series of benzimidazoles *(45)*, bibenzemidazoles *(46)*, and terbenzimidazole derivatives *(47,48)*. Recent studies focused on modifications of the 5- or 2"-positions of terbenzimidazoles (Fig. 3). A number of 5-substituted terbenzimidazoles can poison Top1 in biochemical assays. 5-phenylterbenzimidazole (Fig. 3) is the most effective in cell culture assays *(47,48)*. Studies with poly(dA)·poly(dT) duplex DNA suggest that 5-phenylterbenzimidazole binds to DNA both by intercalation and in the minor groove *(47)*.

Ecteinascidin 743 (Et-743, NSC-648766) is a potent antitumor agent from the Caribbean tunicate ("sea squirt") *Ecteinascidia turbinata*. Et-743 is in phase II and III clinical trials, with remarkable activity in soft-tissue sarcomas and solid tumors, including ovarian carcinoma *(49,50)*. Et-743 binds tightly in the DNA minor groove, where it alkylates guanine-N2 in a sequence-selective manner, preferentially binding guanines that are followed by a guanine or cytosine *(51)*. The bond between Et-743 and DNA is reversible on DNA denaturation *(51)* and even spontaneously *(52)*, which sets Et-743 apart from the DNA alkylating agents presently used in cancer chemotherapy. Top1 was identified as a cellular target of Et-743 during a systematic search of nuclear proteins that bind to Et-743–DNA adducts *(53)*. Biochemical and cellular studies demonstrate that Et-743 can trap Top1–DNA cleavage complexes in vitro and in cancer cells *(53,54)*. The distribution of the drug-induced Top1 sites is different for Et-743 and CPT *(53)*. A derivative of Et-743, phthalascidin (Pt-650), was also found to poison Top1 cleavage complexes in vitro and in cells *(54)*. However, Top1 is probably not the primary cellular target of Et-743 because the drug remains active in yeast with a deletion in the Top1 gene *(55)* and in mammalian cells deficient for Top1 *(56)*. Furthermore, Top1 inhibition is only detectable at micromolar concentrations that exceed pharmacologically active concentrations *(57,58)*. Recent studies revealed that Et-743 acts by a novel mechanism of action: poisoning of transcription-coupled nucleotide excision repair *(59)*.

Another recently identified DNA minor groove binding Top1 poisons is NU/ICRF 505, a tyrosine conjugate of anthraquinone modified at the C-terminus of the amino acid as an ethyl ester *(60)*. Molecular modeling of the drug interaction with the DNA sequence d(CGTACG) suggests that the amino acid occupies the DNA minor groove *(60)*. Cellular pharmacology of NU/ICRF 505 shows G1 arrest in cells overexpressing Top1 and induction of apoptosis *(61)*. Clinical development of NU/ICRF 505 has recently been abandoned because of variable metabolism results in both mouse and human plasma *(19)*.

2.4. Non-CPT Top1 Poisons: DNA Damaging Agents

Chemotherapeutic agents that target and damage DNA can also trap Top1; for a comprehensive review *see* ref. *62*. Using oligonucleotides with defined modifications, we found that incorporation of the nucleoside analogs, 5-fluorouracile and gemcitabine (2'-difluorocytosine) immediately downstream from a Top1 cleavage complex prevent the Top1–mediated DNA religation *(14,63)*. Chemotherapeutic alkylating agents have also been shown to trap Top1, which contributes to the cytotoxicity of the MNNG *(64)*. Oxidative lesions such as 8-oxoguanine and 5-hydroxycytosine also enhance Top1 cleavage complexes *(65)*. The contribution of Top1 poisoning to the antiproliferative activity of these drugs is suggested by the resistance of Top1-deficient cells to these drugs *(14,64)*.

Besides chemotherapeutic agents, Top1 can be trapped by naturally occurring endogenous and carcinogenic DNA lesions, ranging from UV-induced thymine dimers *(66,67)*, oxidative base lesions *(65)*, base mismatches and abasic sites *(68)*, DNA strand breaks *(69)*, the carcinogenic adducts, N6-ethenoadenine *(70)*, and benzo[*a*]pyrene diol epoxide adducts *(71–73)*; *see* ref. *62* for a review. It is not known how frequently such Top1 cleavage complexes form. However, the fact that all cells expressing a type IB topoisomerase express tyrosyl-DNA phosphodiesterase (Tdp1; *see* Section 5.1.), suggest selective pressure for removing Top1 cleavage complexes, and therefore for the natural occurrence of these complexes.

3. MOLECULAR MODEL FOR TOP1 INHIBITION: MISALIGNMENT OFTHE 5'-HYDROXYL END OF THE CLEAVED DNA

3.1. Binding of CPTs and Polycyclic/Heterocyclic Poisons to the Top1–DNA Complex

CPT and its derivatives are noncompetitive inhibitors of Top1. They inhibit the enzyme by binding in a ternary complex with Top1 and the cleaved DNA *(28,74)*. Consequently, they uncouple the enzyme DNA nicking-closing reaction by preventing the DNA religation ("closing") step.

This unique mode of action represents a paradigm for the concept that it is possible to interfere with two macromolecules (i.e., Top1 and DNA) by stabilizing their interaction. This concept is important because one of the present objectives in drug development is to interfere with macromolecule interactions. Thus it is conceivable to look for agents that act by preventing the dissociation of the two macromolecules rather than by inhibiting their binding, which might be more difficult because of a required competitively high drug binding constant.

Not all the Top1 cleavage complexes are equally trapped by CPTs, and trapping is most effective at DNA sequences with a T at the 3'-end of the scissile DNA strand (position –1 in Fig. 4, which corresponds to the DNA end covalently linked to Top1) and a G at the 5'-end of the broken DNA (position +1 in Fig. 4). This DNA sequence-dependence led to the hypothesis that CPT forms a ternary complex with Top1 and the DNA by binding at the enzyme-DNA interface at the DNA break site *(75)*. This hypothesis was further strengthened by the finding that a derivative of CPT with an alkylating group at position 7 can form an adduct with the +1 guanine (at the N3 position) in the presence of active Top1 *(76)*.

It is accepted that CPT or its derivatives stabilize Top1 cleavage complexes by forming a ternary complex including: Top1+DNA+drug. In the proposed models (discussed by Stewart in Chapter 15), CPT intercalates/stacks at the enzyme-DNA interface between the bases that flank the cleavage site in the cleaved DNA generated by Top1 *(8,28,75–78)* (Fig. 4B) and prevents DNA religation by keeping the 5'-end of the broken DNA out of alignment with the Top1-DNA phosphotyrosyl bond that needs to be attacked by the 5'-hydroxyl of the broken DNA during religation (Fig. 4A).

Recently, experiments with intercalating ligands demonstrated position-specific trapping of Top1 cleavage complexes by polycyclic hydrocarbons (benzo[*a*]pyrene diol epoxide adducts) intercalated between the bases that flank the Top1 cleavage site or that are immediately downstream from the cleavage site *(72,73)*. A unifying model is that the polycyclic aromatics (CPTs, indolocarbazoles, indenoisoquinolines, coralyne, berberine, and nitidine derivatives) bind to a common site in the Top1–DNA complex by stacking (intercalating) either on the 5'-side or the 3'-side of the base pair immediately downstream (position +1 in Fig. 4B) from the Top1 cleavage site *(78)*. The differences in DNA cleavage patterns (i.e., differential intensity of cleavage at any given site) between compounds might be due to specific interactions between particular drugs and the bases flanking the Top1 cleavage site *(78)*.

A potential exception to this model has been proposed for nogalamycin *(79)*, which traps Top1 cleavage complexes by intercalating upstream from the Top1 cleavage complex. In this case, drug binding was proposed to induce a local bent downstream from the Top1 cleavage, which interferes

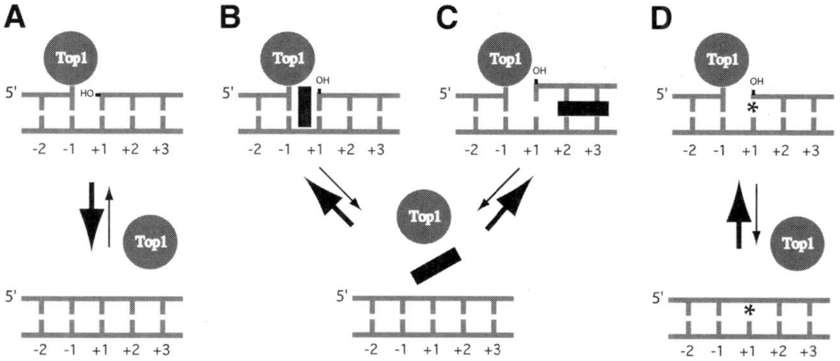

Fig. 4. Proposed molecular interactions between TOP-I poisons and TOP-I–DNA complexes leading to misalignment of the DNA 5'-terminus at the cleavage site. **(A)** Under normal conditions, cleavage complexes are readily reversible by nucleophilic attack from the 5'-hydroxyl end generated by TOP-I–mediated DNA cleavage (*see* Fig. 6B). **(B)** Binding of camptothecin and intercalators (black rectangle) at the enzyme-DNA interface trap TOP-I cleavage complexes by altering the +1 base position. (Note that intercalation between the +1 and +2 base pairs can also trap TOP-I cleavage complexes *[72]*). The resulting cleavage complexes can only reverse when the drug dissociates from the TOP-I–DNA complex. **(C)** Minor groove ligands (black rectangle) widen the minor groove, which displaces the 5'-DNA terminus. **(D)** Base modifications induced by endogenous, carcinogenic, or chemotherapeutic lesions (oxidative lesions, abasic sites, mismatches, and adducts) can also misalign the 5'-DNA terminus and trap TOP-I cleavage complexes independently of chemotherapy.

with DNA religation. Thus nogalamycin bound to a Top1–DNA complex may act similarly to minor groove ligands (*see* Section 3.2.).

3.2. Molecular Model for Top1 Poisoning by DNA Minor Groove Ligands

Experiments with oligonucleotides containing a single benzo[*a*]pyrene diol epoxide dG adducts at specific positions have shed some light on the spatial relationship between minor groove ligand binding sites and Top1 cleavage (Fig. 4C). These experiments demonstrated that Top1 was trapped when ligands are bound in the minor groove downstream from the Top1 cleavage site between positions +2 and +3 *(71)*. By contrast, Top1 was prevented from cleaving the DNA if the minor groove ligand covered the +1 or the –1 base pair *(71)*. In such a case, Top1 cleavage was observed a few bases upstream from minor groove ligand, which is consistent with trapping of Top1 when the minor groove ligand is downstream from the potential Top1 cleavage. Blockade of Top1 cleavage by minor groove ligands at the

+1 position is also consistent with the crystal structure of Top1 showing close contacts between the enzyme and the DNA minor groove at this position *(8)*. Thus we propose that minor groove binding drugs (such as benzimidazoles and Et-743) poison Top1 by binding immediately downstream (3') from the cleaved DNA strand without contacting the +1 base pair (Fig. 4C). Minor groove binding downstream from the cleavage site would alter the structure of the DNA downstream from (on the 3'-side of) the cleavage site resulting in a misalignment of the 5'-hydroxyl DNA terminus to be relegated by Top1.

3.3. Top1 Poisoning by Nucleotide Modifications

Base modifications at specific sites demonstrated that Top1 trapping occurs when the +1 base is altered; *see* ref. *62* for a review. This probably results in structural modifications of the broken end downstream from the Top1 cleavage site (Fig. 4D).

3.4. General Model for Top1 Poisoning: "5'-Terminus Misalignment"

Together, the molecular observation presented previously leads to a relatively simple and general mechanism for trapping Top1 cleavage complexes: presence of a ligand that either intercalates or binds to the minor groove, or presence of DNA modifications that result in a misalignment of the 5'-hydroxyl DNA terminus, interfere with the religation of Top1 cleavage complexes. As indicated at the beginning of this section, the inhibitors act in a noncompetitive manner by preventing the dissociation of Top1–DNA complex.

By contrast, DNA modifications upstream from the Top1 cleavage complex (positions –1, –2, and upstream) generally prevent DNA cleavage *(62,71–73)*, which is consistent with the structure of Top1–DNA complexes showing that the enzyme major contacts are immediately upstream of the site of cleavage *(8,12)*.

4. CELLULAR LESIONS INDUCED BY TOP1 CLEAVAGE COMPLEXES

4.1. DNA Damage Resulting From Top1 Cleavage Complexes

Top1 cleavage complexes are normally readily reversible. Early experiments also demonstrated that short exposures (less than 60 minutes in cell culture) to CPT are relatively noncytotoxic *(80–82)*. These observations are consistent with a time-dependent conversion of Top1 cleavage complexes into DNA lesions by cellular metabolism. Figure 5 shows how reversible Top1 cleavage complexes can be converted into DNA damage (irreversible

Top1 covalent complexes). Collisions between transcription and replication complexes are shown in panels A and B, respectively. These lesions and the cellular consequences of transcription and replication inhibition will be discussed in Section 4.2.

Panels C–F (Fig. 5) show the genesis of irreversible Top1 cleavage complexes (commonly referred to as "suicide complexes") by preexisting DNA lesions (strand breaks in panels C and D; base lesions in panel E); for review *see* ref. *62*. The probability for forming such lesions is enhanced by treatment with Top1 poisons because the drugs enhance the frequency of Top1 cleavage complexes. Thus the higher the drug concentration, the greater the probability that cleavage complexes might form in the vicinity of a preexisting DNA lesion. This might explain the synergism between CPTs and ionizing radiations *(83)*. Also, at high CPT concentrations, it is plausible that two Top1 cleavage complexes might form on opposite strands, close enough for melting of the duplex and generation of a double-strand break (Fig. 5F).

4.2. Replication vs Transcription

The Top1–linked DNA breaks resulting from the collision between DNA and RNA polymerases with the Top1 cleavage complex on the DNA template strand are represented in Fig. 5A,B. In most cancer cells in tissue culture *(81,84,85)* and in yeast *(86)*, cytotoxicity appears primarily related to replication-mediated DNA lesions. However, the protective effect of aphidicolin is generally limited to the lowest (submicromolar) doses of CPT *(82)*. Replication-independent cytotoxicity can be observed at micromolar CPT concentrations *(87–89)*. This may be related to the observed fundamental differences at the gene expression level between the molecular mechanisms of reversible G2 cell-cycle delay after mild DNA damage induced by CPT and permanent G2 arrest after more extensive DNA damage *(90)*. Replication-independent cytotoxicity seems to be cell type–specific. The XRCC1 mutant Chinese hamster ovary (CHO) EM9 cells (*see* Section 5.3.) are hypersensitive to CPT even when DNA replication is blocked *(91)*.

4.3. Replication Inhibition by Top1 Poisons

CPT treatment produces a rapid and persistent inhibition of DNA synthesis *(80,81,92)*. The rapid inhibition of DNA synthesis is primarily the result of replication fork collisions (Fig. 5B), as demonstrated in replicating SV40 DNA *(93,94)* and recently in human cells *(95)*. Interestingly, it appears that the leading strand DNA synthesis proceeds up to the 5'-end of the Top1 cleaved DNA, and this process has been referred to as "replication run-off" *(95)*. Furthermore, this 5'-terminus is rapidly phosphorylated in vivo, possibly by polynucleotide kinase phosphatase (*see* Fig. 5B and 6). DNA synthesis inhibition might also be related to inhibition of thymidine kinase *(96)*.

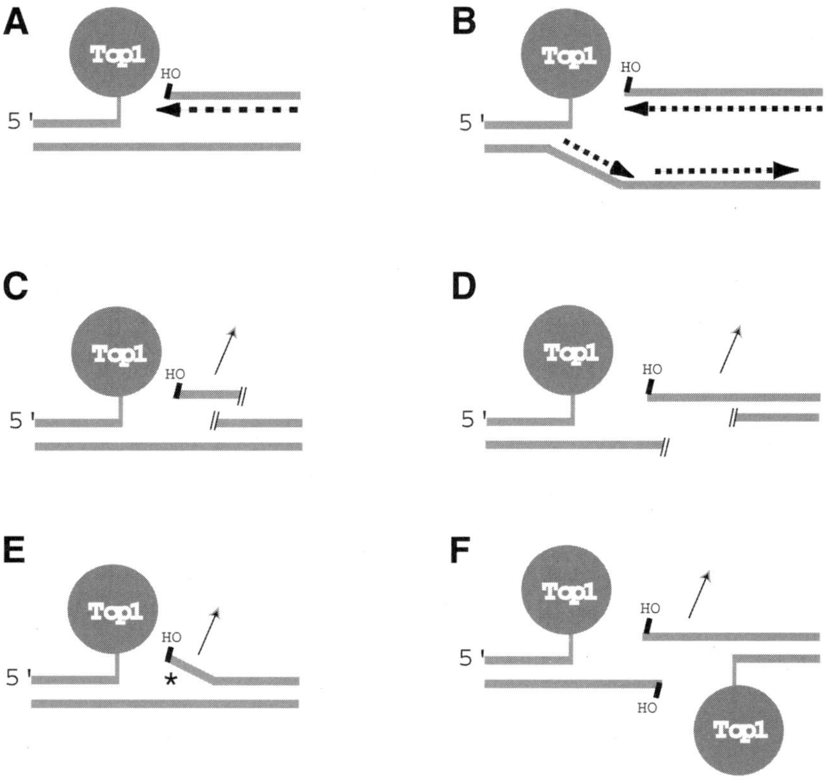

Fig. 5. Conversion of reversible TOP-I cleavage complexes into DNA damage. DNA single-strand breaks are shown on the left (panels **A,C,E**) and DNA double-strand breaks on the right (panels **B,D,F**). **(A)** Transcription complex collision can generate a DNA single-strand break in which the 5'-hydroxyl end is misaligned and is prevented from TOP-I–mediated relegation. The RNA is shown as a dashed arrow. **(B)** Replication fork collision generates a DNA double-strand break on the leading strand and a single-stranded segment on the lagging strand. The leading strand is shown as a dashed arrow pointing left. Okasaki fragments are shown as dashed arrows pointing right. The 5'-hydroxyl end has been found to be phosphorylated in camptothecin-treated cells *(95)*, possibly by PNKP (*see* Fig. 6). **(C)** TOP-I cleavage complexes in DNA containing a preexisting single-strand break on the scissile strand in the proximity of the TOP-I site can result in dissociation of the small DNA segment (small arrow pointing up) and generation of a single-stranded segment on the non-scissile strand (the double lines with *A* and *A'* represent the corresponding ends of the broken DNA). **(D)** A TOP-I cleavage complex opposite to a preexisting single-strand break in the proximity of the TOP-I site can result in dissociation of the DNA duplex downstream from the TOP-I cleavage (small arrow pointing up) and generation of a DNA double-strand break (the double lines represent the ends of the broken DNA). **(E)** Base lesions (for instance an abasic site at position +1

The observed persistent inhibition of DNA synthesis (for up to 8 hours) after CPT removal *(92)* is probably the result of activation of an S-phase checkpoint *(92)*. This S-phase checkpoint probably is due primarily to a delayed firing of the late replicons. Checkpoint activation would prevent cells from entering mitosis with damaged DNA and provide additional time for DNA repair. Furthermore, replication fork arrest would prevent the generation of new collisions. Inhibition of the S-phase checkpoint by the 7-hydroxystaurosporine (UCN-01), a cell-cycle checkpoint abrogator, produces a marked synergistic cell killing *(97)*. This observation is potentially important for cancer chemotherapy because UCN-01 is presently in clinical trials and because the synergism is more pronounced in cells with defective p53 *(97)*. Thus it is attractive to propose clinical trials associating CPT derivatives and UCN-01.

4.4. Transcriptional Effects of Top1 Poisons

Early pharmacological studies showed that CPT is a potent inhibitor of transcription for both nucleolar and nucleoplasmic RNA *(80,98–100)*. This effect is primarily the result of transcription elongation blocks from drug-trapped Top1 cleavage complexes (Fig. 5A) *(101–104)*. CPT treatment produces an accumulation of abortive transcripts in the 5'-end of the genes by premature termination of growing RNA chains *(103,105)*. The response to Top1 inhibition was also found to be context-dependent *(106)* and to cause, in certain genes, the transcription complex to stall in the midst of transcription units *(107)*. In agreement with these observations, in vitro assays demonstrated that transcription complexes could convert CPT-stabilized Top1–cleavable complexes into irreversible strand breaks by the elongation of the RNA polymerase on the template strand (*see* Fig. 5A) *(88,108)*.

Studies of the effect of CPT on the transcription from the dihydrofolate reductase (*DHFR*) gene in CHO cells showed that CPT stimulated RNA synthesis from promoter-proximal sequences, whereas transcription from promoter-distal sequences was reduced *(105)*. CPT appeared to stimulate initiation while inhibiting elongation of the RNA polymerase II transcribed *DHFR* gene *(105)*. A recent study demonstrated that transcription inhibition by CPT is not uniform *(107)*. For instance, CPT caused a strong holdback

---

(Fig 5 continued) or +2; *see* Fig. 4D) can generate an irreversible DNA single-strand break. **(F)** At high camptothecin concentrations, two TOP-I cleavage complexes may form near each other and after melting of the duplex (arrow pointing up), generate in a DNA double-strand break. In general irreversible TOP-I cleavage complexes are referred to as "suicide complexes." (For further details on lesions shown in panels **C-E**, *see [62]*).

of the endogenous c-*myc* gene at the P2 promoter while having minimal effect on an episomal c-*myc* gene or on the basal expression of the *Hsp70* and *Gadph* genes *(107)*. CPT provoked no alteration of transcription complexes at most of the rRNA promoters and transcription by RNA polymerase III of 7*SK RNA* was fully resistant to CPT. By contrast, CPT treatment enhanced expression of *c-fos* mRNA *(107)*. Thus the transcriptional effects of CPT are gene- and cell type-dependent. Transcription inhibition has been shown to recover rapidly after CPT treatment *(100,105)*. Interestingly, Cockayne syndrome cells, which are deficient in transcription recovery after DNA damage and in transcription-coupled nucleotide excision repair, show CPT hypersensitivity *(109)*. This hypersensitivity suggests that RNA transcription inhibition and recovery are potential cellular determinants of drug response.

The pleiotropic effects of Top1 poisons on transcription probably are a result of the fact that Top1 affects transcription in more than one way. Besides producing physical blocks for RNA elongation by RNA polymerase, Top1 cleavage complexes can activate a cellular transcriptional stress response. CPT treatment produces an elevation of transcription factors including *p53 (110)*, *AP1* (*c-fos* and *c-Jun*) *(111,112)*, and NF-κB *(113,114)*. Using microarray analysis, we recently found that many genes are rapidly upregulated following *(90)* and during CPT treatment in p53-dependent and -independent manners *(115)*.

Inhibition of transcription by Top1 poisons could also be exerted by inhibition of the enzyme's catalytic activity rather than by a direct collision of RNA polymerase with cleavage complexes. Inhibition of Top1–mediated DNA relaxation could block RNA polymerase progression by producing an accumulation of positive supercoils upstream from the polymerase in transcribing chromatin domains *(107,116)* and by compacting chromatin in specific gene domains *(107,117)*. The transcriptional effects of CPTs could also be related to two other functions of Top1 that are independent of its DNA nicking-closing activity. First, Top1 is known to regulate transcription initiation by binding to TATA binding proteins and by repressing basal transcription and enhancing transcription activation *(118–120)*. However, to our knowledge, there is no published information on the effect of CPT on this activity. Second, Top1 may activate RNA splicing by acting as a specific kinase for RNA splicing factors from the SR family such as SF2/ASF *(121–123)*, and by binding to RNA splicing factors PSF/p54 *(124)*. CPT has been found to block this Top1 SR kinase activity in vitro *(121)*.

5. REPAIR OF TOP1 COVALENT COMPLEXES

The various lesions resulting from the conversion of reversible Top1 cleavage complexes into DNA damage (Fig. 5) are sometimes referred to as "suicide complexes" or "dead-end covalent complexes" to denote their irreversibility. They exhibit the unique characteristic of having a covalently linked Top1 molecule at the 3'-end of a DNA break. These lesions also frequently include a double-strand break at the other end of the broken DNA (Fig. 5), which prevents the relegation of the 5'-DNA terminus. In the case of the transcription-mediated Top1 suicide complexes (Fig. 5A), the double-strand break corresponds to a DNA–RNA hydride, and it is not known whether the RNA extends to the end of the template DNA. In the case of the replication-mediated suicide complexes on the leading strand for DNA synthesis (Fig. 5B), the double-strand break corresponds to a DNA duplex made of the template and the newly synthesized leading DNA strands (*see* Section 4.4.). In the case of Top1 suicide complexes resulting from cleavage complexes in nicked DNA (Fig. 5C,D) or from neighboring cleavage complexes on opposite strands of the DNA duplex (Fig. 5F), a staggered DNA double-strand break is formed.

The repair/removal of the Top1-DNA adduct at the 3'-end of the suicide complex is effected by a specific pathway centered around a recently discovered enzyme, Tdp1 enzyme.

5.1. Implication of Tdp1 in 3'-End Processing of the Top1 Covalent Complexes

The isolation of the gene encoding Tdp1, a protein that hydrolyzes the covalent bond between Top1 and DNA, was recently described *(125)*. The biochemical activity of this enzyme is to catalyze the cleavage of the chemical bond that joins the active site tyrosine of Top1 to the 3' end of DNA *(126)* (Fig. 6). The result is a clean hydrolysis of the tyrosyl-DNA phosphodiester linkage, thereby liberating a DNA terminated with a 3' phosphate (Fig. 6C). Tdp1 belongs to the phospholipase D superfamily *(127)*, which includes enzymes implicated in phospholipid metabolisms that catalyze phosphoryl transfer reactions. The HKD motif *(128)* has been implicated in Tdp1's catalytic mechanism *(127)*. Tdp1 is ubiquitous and highly conserved in eukaryotes. The 1.69 Å crystal structure of Tdp1 consists of a monomer composed of two similar domains that are related by a pseudo-2-fold axis of symmetry. The catalytic site of each domain contains conserved histidine, lysine, and asparagine residues *(129)*. Specificity of Tdp1 for processing 3'- but not 5'-tyrosyl-DNA complexes, suggests that Tdp1 belongs to a pathway specific for the repair of Top1-DNA adducts.

To this point no inhibitors of Tdp1 have been identified, and there are no reports of Tdp1 mutations in mammalian cells. Screening through chemically mutagenized yeast revealed one single mutation-derived mutant strain that possessed very low Tdp1 activity. This mutant strain failed to show enhanced sensitivity to CPT. However, when disruption of the Tdp1 gene was combined with disruption of the Rad9 gene in the same strain, CPT sensitivity was increased by a factor of 12 *(125)*. Exposure to other DNA

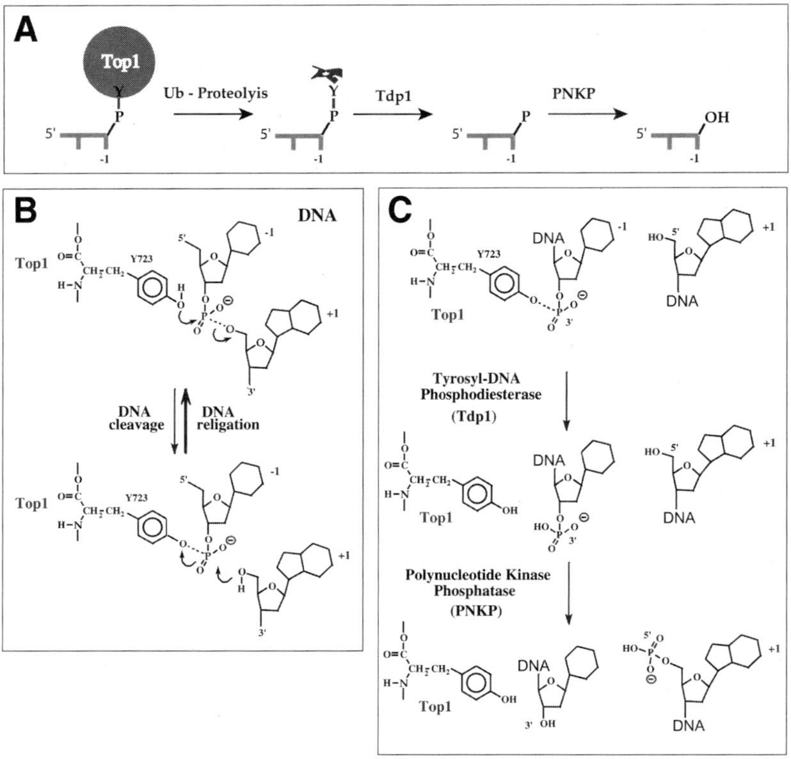

Fig. 6. Proposed model for 3'-end repair of TOP-I cleavage complexes by Tdp1 and PNKP. **(A)** Schematic representation of the consecutive steps required for 3'-end processing. First, TOP-I must be proteolyzed (probably by the 26S proteasome after ubiquitination). Tdp1 can then remove the remaining TOP-I peptide fragment bound to the 3'-DNA terminus and generate a DNA end bearing a 3'-phosphate. Finally polynucleotide kinase phosphatase (PNKP) can hydrolyze the 3'-phosphate and generate a 3'-hydroxyl ribose end. **(B)** The normal nicking (cleavage)/closing (religation) reactions catalyzed by TOP-I are SN2 reactions that require alignment of the attacking nucleophiles: tyrosyl hydroxyl group for cleavage and 5'-hydroxyl ribose for religation. **(C)** Tdp1 hydrolyzes specifically the tyrosyl-phosphodiester bond. PNKP can process both DNA termini: it can dephosphorylate the 3'-DNA terminus and phosphorylate the 5'-DNA terminus. Such termini are substrates for DNA polymerases and ligases.

damaging agents such as methyl methane sulfonate did not show an increased hypersensitivity of these mutant cells lines, and inactivation of the Top1 gene in the same cells increased their survival by a factor of 1000. Overexpression of religation-defective mutants of Top1 in low Tdp1 expressing yeast strains had a similar effect to CPT. These data suggest high specificity of Tdp1 activity for Top1 catalysis-derived Tyrosyl-DNA covalent complexes *(125)*. They also demonstrate that, at least in yeast, additional pathways besides Tdp1 are implicated for the repair of Top1 covalent complexes. It is tempting to speculate that Tdp1 is primarily required when the G2 checkpoint is deficient as in the case of the yeast *RAD9* mutant, and that these alternative pathways are Rad9-dependent (and possibly operate in G2-arrested cells by recombination) (*see* Section 6.4.).

A model of the possible repair pathways of Top1-induced DNA damage should take into account recent findings related to Tdp1 biochemical activity. Both the structure of the DNA segment bound to Top1 *(125,130)* and the length of the Top1 polypeptide chain determine Tdp1 biochemical activity in vitro *(130)*. Optimum Tdp1 substrates include: (1) a DNA segment consisting of at least a few nucleotides *(130)*, consistent with the presence of a potential DNA binding groove in the Tdp1 structure *(129)*, (2) an exposed phosphotyrosyl bond at the Top1-DNA junction (a tyrosyl group linked to the 3'-end of a nick is a poor substrate *[125]*), suggesting that Tdp1 activity would be optimum after the 5'-end of the broken DNA has been either digested or displaced to render the 3'-phosphotyrosyl bond accessible to Tdp1, and (3) a short Top1 polypeptide segment, because the effectiveness of Tdp1 decreases as the length of Top1 polypeptide chain is extended *(130)*. It is therefore likely that Top1 probably needs to be proteolyzed at least partially for efficient Tdp1 activity *(126,130)* (Fig. 6). As discussed in Section 6.1., such a degradation in association with Top1 ubiquitination has been observed after CPT treatment *(131,132)*.

Because Tdp1 generates a 3'-phosphate end, this phosphate needs to be removed because neither DNA polymerases nor ligases can process this end unless it bears a 3'-hydroxyl. Although Tdp1 is the only known enzyme to remove tyrosine from complexes in which the amino acid is linked to the 3'-end of DNA fragments, the multifunctional apurinic endonucleases appear well suited for the removal of the resulting 3' phosphate substrates. Other enzymes believed to be involved in the repair of the 3' phosphate lesions, and specifically those introduced in the process of repair of Top1–induced DNA lesions in yeast are Tpp1 *(133)* and polynucleotide kinase phosphatase (PNKP) *(134)*. PNKP is a plausible candidate for such an activity in human cells (*see* Section 5.3.).

5.2. Repair of Replication-Mediated DNA Double-Strand Breaks

The repair mechanisms for these lesions implicates known elements of the DNA double-strand break repair pathways including the Ku/DNA-PK complex *(92)*, ATM *(135,136)* (*see* Section 6.3.), and Rad52 *(13,137)* (a well-established homologous recombination factor). Indirect evidence for

PNKP activity is supported by the observation that the 5'-end of the replication-mediated DNA double-strand breaks are rapidly phosphorylated in CPT-treated cells *(95)* (*see* Fig. 5B).

Figure 7 shows two possible pathways for replication fork repair and restart after collision with Top1 cleavage complexes. The pathway shown on the left (panel A) is initiated by the regression of the blocked replication fork. This reaction is commonly referred to as replication fork regression *(138,139)*. This regression associated with annealing of the newly replicated leading and lagging strands and formation of a DNA cruciform (four-stranded junction), commonly referred to as a "chickenfoot" because of the morphology of the resulting structure *(139)* (Fig. 7A). The molecular mechanisms driving this reverse movement are not well characterized. They might involve protein complexes that stabilize DNA strand exchange and annealing (duplex formation) such as Rad51, the eukaryotic equivalent of the bacterial RecA protein that forms nucleoprotein filaments and promotes exchange/annealing between homologous DNA sequences *(138,140)*. Positive supercoiling ahead of the blocked replication fork, which would force branch migration, has also been invoked *(138)*. After the DNA downstream from the Top1 cleavage complex has been reannealed, it is conceivable that the Top1 cleavage complex could reverse without intervention of repair enzymes because the 5'-hydroxyl end of the DNA can be aligned with the Top1–DNA phosphotyrosyl bond. It is also possible that Tdp1 could remove the Top1 and that the resulting gap is repaired by the BER (base excision repair) pathway (*see* Section 5.3.). After the repair/removal of the Top1 cleavage complex, the fork would restart by unwinding the cruciform. This unwinding is believed to be carried out by the RecQ helicases: BLM (Bloom) and WRN (Werner), which are very effective in vitro for unwinding cruciforms structures. In the absence of these helicases, "chickenfoot" structures would need to be resolved by recombination, which might explain the high frequency of sister chromatid exchanges in Bloom syndrome cells; for recent review, *see* ref. *141*.

The second pathway shown on the right in Fig. 7B speculates that the first step consists in the removal of the Top1 cleavage complex, possibly by Tdp1 and gap repair (*see* section 5.3 and Fig. 8), which would result in the ligation of the template strand for leading strand synthesis with a newly synthesized Okasaki fragment. The second step would be a strand invasion/exchange probably involving Rad51, which would result in the formation of a Holliday junction. After resolution, the recombined DNA segment could be used to restart the replication fork. Analysis of such pathways is challenging and it is likely that additional mechanisms exist for the repair of the broken replication forks in mammalian cells. Implication of the Rad51 recombination pathway in the repair of Top1-mediated DNA damage is suggested by the hypersensitivity of Rad51-deficient cells to CPT *(142–144)*.

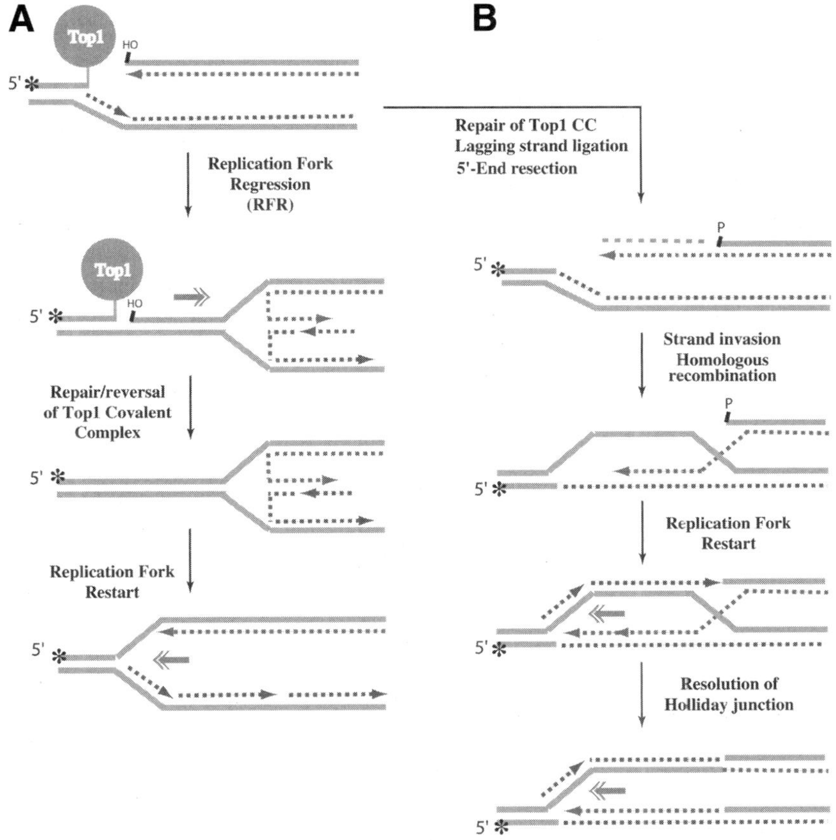

Fig. 7. Hypothetical pathways for repairing or resolving replication fork damage produced by TOP-I cleavage complex collision. **(A)** Replication fork regression (RFR) is a branch migration reaction associated with annealing of the two newly replicated strand to each other forming a "chickenfoot" *(138,139)*. RFR allows the reversal (or repair) of the TOP-I cleavage complex. Replication restart is assumed to require the activity of RecQ helicases (Bloom and Werner syndrome helicases). **(B)** Example of homologous recombination leading to the resolution and restart of the collapsed replication fork after collision with a TOP-I cleavage complex.

5.3. Possible Role of the XRCC1/Poly(ADP-Ribose-Polymerase/PNKP/ β -Polymerase/Ligase III Complex

Several observations implicate the XRCC1/poly(ADP-ribose)polymerase (PARP)/β-polymerase/ligase III complex in the cellular response to and repair of Top1 cleavage complexes. Regarding the implication of PARP, the observations are as follows: (1) PARP activity is increased in CPT-

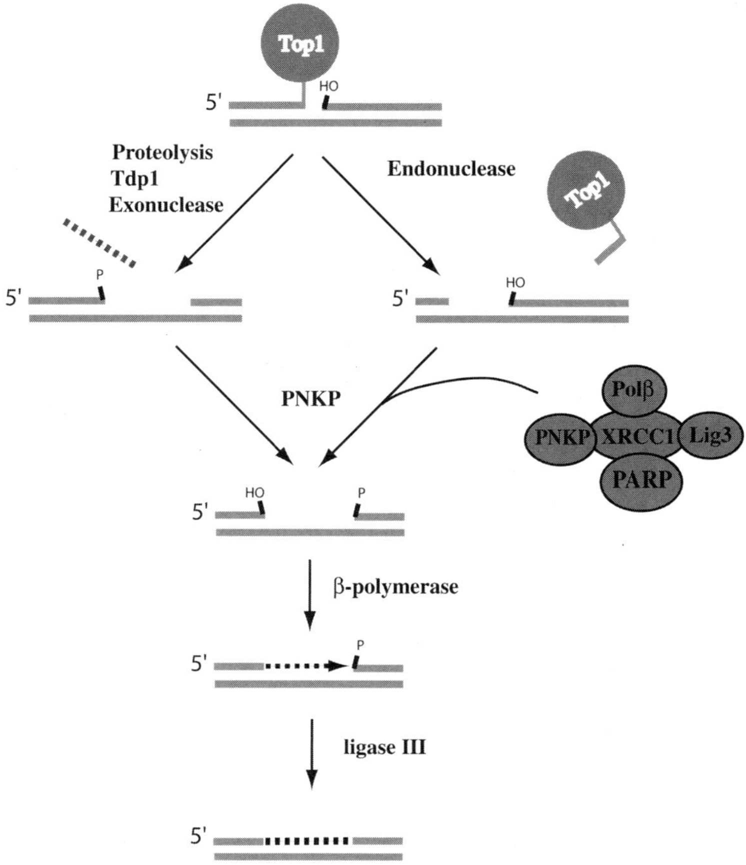

Fig. 8. Hypothetical pathways involving the base excision repair (BER) pathway. Topoisomerase-I cleavage complexes can be processed either by the Tdp1 pathway followed by exonuclease processing of the DNA ends (left) or by a hypothetical endonuclease (right). The resulting gap is processed by the PNKP (polynucleotide kinase phosphatase), which produces 3'-hydroxyl and 5'-phosphate ends. PNKP is shown at right in a multiprotein complex with XRCC1 (which serves as a scaffolding protein), poly(ADP-ribose)polymerase (PARP), β-polymerase (Polβ), and ligase III (Lig3). β-polymerase extends the 3'-hydroxyl end and fill the gap. Ligase III completes gap repair by ligating the DNA ends.

treated cells *(145)*, (2) CPT hypersensitivity was reported in mutant cells lines, derived from the Chinese hamster V79 cell line, deficient in PARP or its activity *(146,147)* (Table 1), (3) we recently observed hypersensitivity to CPT, expressed as reduced survival, and slow repair of Top1–induced DNA lesions in PARP knock-out mouse fibroblasts (Barceló et al., unpublished),

Table 1
Genetic Alterations Sensitizing Cell to Topoisomerase 1 Poisons

Genes	*Functions*	*Reference*
ATM	Protein kinase from the P13K family Implicated in DSB response	*135,176–178*
NBS1	Scaffolding protein forming a complex with Mre11 and Rad50 *MRN complex) DSB repair and recombination pathways	*202,203*
DNA-PKcs	Protein kinase from the PI3K family Implicated in DSB response	*92*
ATR	Protein kinase from the PI3K family Implicated in replication stress response	*222*
WRN	Replication helicase from the RecQ family	*237–239*
BLM	Replication helicase from the recQ family	*240*
XRCC2	One of the seven members ot the Rad51 family Implicated in DNA strand exchange/homologous recombination	*142,143*
Ead51C	One of the seven members of the Rad51 family Implicated in DNA strand exchange/homologous recombination	*144*
XRCC1	BER	*91,143,151*
PARP	BER	*146,147*
CSA/CSB	TCR/BER	*109*
γ-H2AX	Corehistone Phosphorylated in response to DSB	*248*
p53/p21	Apoptosis	*250,265*
Bcl-2	Apoptosis	*266*

ATM, ataxia telangiectasia mutant; ATR, ataxia telangiectasia and Rad3 homolog; BER, base excision repair; BLM, bloom syndrome; CSA/CSB, Cockayne syndrome complementation groups A and B; DNA-PKcs, DNA-dependent protein kinase catalytic subunit; DSB, DNA double-strand breaks; NER, nucleotide excision repair; PARP, poly(ADP-ribose) polymerase; PI3K, phosphatidyl inositol 3 kinase; TCR, transcription-coupled repair.

(4) increased PARP-1 levels have been observed in a CPT-resistant cell-line *(148)* and, (5) pharmacological inhibitors of PARP such as 3-aminobenzamide *(149)* or the novel inhibitor NU1025 *(150)* sensitize cells to CPTs.

The implication of XRCC1 stems from the following observations: (1) the CHO XRCC1-mutant EM9 cells are hypersensitive to CPT *(91,143)* and (2) some CPT-resistant cell lines show increased XRCC1 levels, and the increased resistance to CPT acquired by XRCC1 transfection can be reversed by treatment with 3-aminobenzamide *(151)*.

XRCC1, PARP, β-polymerase, ligase III ,and PNKP form a multiprotein complex with specific activity for BER *(152,153)* (Fig. 8). PARP is a relatively abundant nuclear protein with a zinc finger motif used as a nick-sensor that binds to double- and single-stranded DNA breaks. These breaks could be the direct result of ionizing radiations or result from enzymatic excision of a DNA lesion repaired by the BER pathway (reviewed in refs. *154* and *155*). Binding of PARP-1 to nicked DNA catalyzes the transfer by this protein of successive units of the ADP-ribose moiety of nicotinamide adenine dinucleotide as a substrate, which results in transient covalent binding of large, negatively charged poly(ADP-ribose) polymers to macromolecular acceptors, including PARP itself *(154,155)*. This modification alters the structure and function of the protein acceptors and marks the beginning of the DNA repair process. Top1 is one of the poly(ADP-ribose) acceptors and is inhibited by poly(ADP-ribosylation) *(156–158)*. However, it has also been reported that association of PARP and Top1 may activate Top1 *(159)*.

XRCC1 has no enzymatic activity and probably functions as a scaffolding factor by bringing together the enzymes required for BER, including human PNKP *(152)*. Figure 8 proposes a hypothetical scheme in which PNKP acts after removal of the Top1–DNA complex to prepare the DNA ends for β-polymerase and ligase III action. PARP's nick sensor function could implicate this protein in a damage survey mechanism that involves the recruitment of XRCC1 and associated proteins to the sites of CPT-induced DNA damage. The absence of PARP-1 may hinder XRCC1 access, which could explain that nuclear extracts from PARP- and XRCC1-deficient cells exhibit slow repair activity by Tdp1, PNKP, and β-polymerase, on substrates mimicking CPT-induced DNA damage (Barceló and Pommier, unpublished).

6. MOLECULAR PATHWAYS IMPLICATED IN THE CELLULAR RESPONSES TO TOP1 CLEAVAGE COMPLEXES: DETERMINANTS OF RESPONSE AND RESISTANCE WITH POTENTIAL CLINICAL RELEVANCE

Cellular responses to Top1 poisons determine cell survival and therefore tumor response and host toxicity. Efficient repair (*see* Section 5.) is probably coupled with checkpoint activation to stop cell cycle. Cell-cycle arrest would have two beneficial consequences: (1) it would give time to the repair machinery for removing the lesions before the generation of unviable or mutated cells after mitosis and (2) it would prevent further replication- and transcription-dependent DNA damage. Cell-cycle checkpoints activated by Top1 poisons include the S-phase and the G2 checkpoints *(97)*, but also activation of the p53/p21 pathways in response to replication-mediated DNA damage *(110)*. Cell-cycle checkpoints are probably also connected to the apoptosis machinery, and it is likely that in the presence of extensive DNA damage, the same DNA damage sensors and checkpoints that stop cell-cycle progression and promote DNA repair activate apoptosis. Thus an exciting and challenging new area of research is the elucidation of the relationships between sensor proteins, checkpoints, DNA repair, and apoptosis. Integration of these pathways should enable us to understand the cellular determinants of cellular response to Top1 poisons. The next section focuses on some cellular pathways and responses known to be elicited by Top1 poisons.

6.1. Ubiquitination, Sumoylation, and Proteolysis of Top1

CPT treatment reduces the intracellular content of Top1 in peripheral blood mononuclear cells and in tissue culture cells *(131,132,160)*. This reduction has been reported to be DNA replication–independent because it is not affected by aphidicolin *(161)*. It is, however, abolished by inhibitors of the 26S proteasome, and ubiquitin–Top1 conjugates have been detected in cells treated with CPT, suggesting that CPT induces ubiquitin/26S-proteasome–dependent degradation of Top1, a phenomenon referred to as Top1 downregulation *(132)*. Ubiquitination can be schematically divided in three steps: (1) activation: ubiquitin becomes linked to the ubiquitin-activating enzyme (E1), (2) transfer: ubiquitin is transferred to a conjugating enzyme (E2), and (3) ligation: a ubiquitin-ligating enzyme (E3) connects ubiquitin to its target protein *(162)*. The subcellular localization for Top1 ubiquitination and its subsequent degradation seems to be nuclear *(160)*, which is consistent with the nuclear localization of a fraction of the 26S proteasome.

Top1 degradation may serve two roles: (1) confer cellular tolerance to further CPT treatment and (2) take part in a repair pathway of Top1–mediated DNA damage before Tdp1 action (*see* Section 5.1. and Fig. 6). Top1 degradation appears to be primarily a cellular response to transcription block rather than replication-mediated DNA lesions *(161)* and to be specific for hyperphosphorylated forms of Top1, which are associated with transcription *(163)*. These observations suggest that the collisions between RNA polymerase complexes and Top1 cleavage complexes (*see* Fig. 5A) trigger Top1 ubiquitination and subsequent degradation by the 26S proteasome.

Interestingly, Top1 degradation is cell-type-specific and attenuated in transformed cells, suggesting that oncogenic transformation is associated with the resistance of cells to CPT-induced Top1 degradation *(164)*. Studies performed with patient samples consistently demonstrate that normal peripheral blood cells downregulate Top1 *(165)*, whereas Top1 protein levels remain unchanged in leukemic cells *(166)*. Top1 downregulation has been found to be correlated with CPT resistance in various cell lines in culture, and prevention of Top1 degradation by the 26S proteasome inhibitor MG132 sensitizes the cells to CPT-induced apoptotic cell death *(164)*. Theses observations could, at least in part, explain the synergy observed between CPT and the phase II trial proteasome inhibitor PS-341 *(167)* (for review see ref. *168*).

CPT or its clinically derivative, topotecan, induce also small ubiquitin-like modifier (SUMO)-1 (also SUMO-2/3) conjugation to Top1 *(161,169)*. This process (named SUMOylation) takes place early in response to CPT and appears to be very transient. Human SUMO-1, also named UBL1 *(170)*, PIC1 *(171)*, GMP1 *(172)*, SMTC3 *(173)*, and sentrin *(174)* is a 15-kDa protein with 18% sequence similarity to ubiquitin. SUMOylation mimics the classical ubiquitination pathway. The first step is activation of SUMO; the second is transfer of SUMO to the conjugation enzyme; and the last step, ligation of SUMO to its target protein. SUMOylation employs a distinct set of E1 and E2 enzymes. UBC9 is the only E2 enzyme identified for SUMO-1, whereas a dozen of E2 enzymes have been identified for ubiquitin in yeast. In addition, no E3-type ligases specific for the sumoylation pathway have been identified (for review *see* ref. *175*).

Top1 SUMOylation shares some characteristics with ubiquitination. Both reactions are dependent on the formation of Top1 cleavage complexes and are independent of DNA replication *(132,161)*. However, they differ in the following ways: (1) SUMOylation is independent of transcription *(161)*, (2) SUMOylation appears to be specific for dephosphorylated Top1, (3) SUMOylation is effective in both normal and tumor cells *(161)*, and (4) SUMOylation has not been linked to protein degradation. The role of SUMO-1 Top1 conjugation is still not clear. It may competitively inhibit Top1 ubiquitination and degradation because the same lysine residues are used for both ubiquination and SUMOylation. By tagging of Top1, SUMOylation may modulate the Top1 cellular location, function, or activity *(169)*. The importance of SUMO conjugation to Top1 in CPT cytotoxicity is not known, and it is not clear whether the increased sensitivity of yeast defective in UBC9 to CPT is directly related to Top1 or to downstream cellular response pathways *(161)*.

6.2. The ATM-Mre11/Rad50/NBS1 Double-Strand Break Repair Pathways

Theataxia telangiectasia modified (ATM) gene product is a central component of the S-phase checkpoint pathway (Fig. 9) as AT cells fail to arrest DNA replication in the presence of DNA damage ("radioresistant DNA synthesis" phenotype). The mechanism of ATM activation after DNA damage is not yet understood. More specifically, it is not clear whether ATM can be directly activated by the double-stranded ends of broken DNA or by some sensor proteins that bind to the DNA ends. Various studies have established that AT cells are hypersensitive to CPT *(135,176)* (Table 1). Similarly,

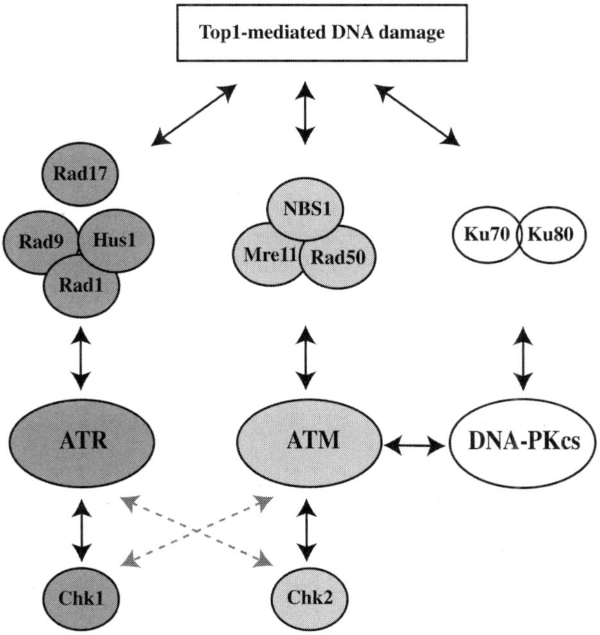

Fig. 9. Simplified representation of the cell cycle checkpoint pathways implicated in DNA damage response to TOP-I poisoning. Each pathway is shown with its DNA sensors (9.1.1 heterotrimer at left, MRN heterotrimer in the middle, and Ku heterodimer at right), its primary kinase (ATM, ATR, and DNA-PKcs), and two effectors (Chk1 and Chk2). Activation of Chk1 and Chk2 by direct phosphorylation are believed to be selective for ATR and ATM, respectively.

deficiencies in the ATM ortholog in Chinese hamster cells enhance their sensitivity to CPT *(177,178)*.

ATM is a protein kinase from the phosphatidyl inositol 3 kinase (PI3 kinase) family whose substrates include several proteins implicated in DNA repair and cell-cycle checkpoints: p53 *(179–181)*, Chk2 *(182)*, Nbs1 *(183–186)*, BRCA1 *(187)*, and 53BP1 *(188)*. Checkpoint proteins, including Nbs1, Mre11, BRCA1, and 53BP1 colocalize in nuclear foci after ionizing irradiation *(189)* and cooperate in the ionizing radiation-induced S-phase checkpoint *(190)*. AT cells are also deficient in activating NF-κB after CPT treatment *(191)*, suggesting that multiple pathways downstream from ATM are implicated in the cellular response to CPT.

Mutations of the NBS1 gene (mutated in Nijmegen breakage syndrome) result in an AT-related phenotype with radioresistant DNA synthesis *(192)*. The NBS1 gene product functions as a heterotrimer with the Mre11 and Rad50 gene products. This trimeric complex is commonly referred to as the

MRN complex *(193)* (Fig. 9), which forms foci at double-strand break sites *(192)*, probably in association with other proteins including mismatch repair factors (MSH2, MSH6, MLH1), BRCA1, the Bloom (BLM) protein, the DNA replication factor C (RFC) and ATM *(194,195)*. These large protein complexes have been named BASC (BRCA1-associated genome surveillance complexes) *(195,196)*.

The MRN complex is also a nuclease and could play a direct role in processing the DNA ends for repair/recombination reactions *(197,198)*. The link between the MRN complex and the S-phase checkpoint pathway was recently strengthened by the finding that an AT-like disorder (including radioresistant DNA synthesis) is caused by mutations in the Mre11 gene *(199)*. Because the DNA binding of the Mre11 complex does not require ATM *(185,200)*, it seems plausible that binding of the MRN complex to DSBs activates and possibly recruits ATM. ATM then phosphorylates NBS1 *(183–186)* and activates the S-phase checkpoint *(183,201)*. These observations suggest the existence of a regulatory loop between the MRN complex, the ATM kinase, and the S-phase checkpoint.

Both AT *(135,176)* and NBS cells *(202,203)* are hypersensitive to CPT (Table 1), indicating the importance of the MRN-ATM pathway for cellular response to CPT. Furthermore, CPT treatment induces phosphorylation of NBS1 and BRCA1 *(204)*.

6.3. The Ku/DNA-PK Double-Strand Repair Pathway

CPT-induced replication-mediated double-strand breaks were recently found to induce phosphorylation of the middle-size subunits of the human single-strand DNA binding protein (RPA2) by DNA-dependent protein kinase (DNA-PK) *(92)*. Like ATM, the catalytic subunit of DNA-PK (DNA-PKcs) belongs to the PI3 kinase family. DNA-PKcs functions with the heterodimer of Ku proteins (Ku70/80), which bind to the ends of the double-strand breaks and activate the kinase activity of DNA-PKcs. DNA-PKcs-deficient (MO-59-J) cells are hypersensitive to CPT (see Table 1) and defective in DNA synthesis inhibition following CPT treatment *(92)*, suggesting that DNA-PK might regulate the S-phase checkpoint and that RPA2 may be one of the effectors in this pathway. Although the exact roles of RPA2 phosphorylation remain to be elucidated, RPA2 is essential for stabilizing single-stranded DNA during replication and repair. An intriguing observation is that the cell cycle checkpoint abrogator UCN-01 inhibits RPA2 phosphorylation by acting in cells upstream from DNA-PK *(92)*. Based on the recent findings that UCN-01 inhibits both Chk1 *(205,206)* and Chk2, it is possible that "cross-talks" exist between the Chk1/Chk2 and DNA-PK pathways. Furthermore, "cross-talk" probably exist between the ATM and DNA-PK pathways since ATM can be directly activated by DNA-PK *(208)*.

6.4. The 9.1.1 and ATR Pathways: Implication in the S-Phase Checkpoint Induced by Top1 Poisons

In fission yeast, a group of six checkpoint proteins, Hus1, Rad1, Rad3, Rad9, Rad17, and Rad26, are required to block entry into mitosis when DNA replication is inhibited or in the presence of damaged DNA (for review *see* refs. *209* and *210*). Human homologs of these checkpoint regulators have been identified, indicating the conservation of the DNA integrity/checkpoint pathways from yeast to humans.

These factors form multiprotein complexes. The Hus1 protein interacts with Rad1 and Rad9 *(211–213)*. In human cells, this "9.1.1" complex *(214)* interacts with hRad17 *(215)* and PCNA (the proliferating cell nuclear antigen) *(216)*. hRad17 is homologous to RFC1 (the largest subunit of the pentameric replication factor C) and Hus1, Rad1 and Rad9 are homologous to PCNA *(216)*, suggesting mechanistic similarities between the 9.1.1/Rad17 pathway and components of the normal replicative DNA polymerase complex *(216)*. Rad17 would be the clamp loader (equivalent of RFC) and the 9.1.1 complex the sliding clamp for DNA polymerase (~ PCNA) *(217)*. It is therefore assumed that Rad17 and the 9.1.1 complex act as sensors for DNA damage and that Rad17 loads the 9.1.1 complex onto damaged DNA at arrested replication forks *(210)*.

Recent observations suggest that the 9.1.1 complex is implicated in the cellular response to CPT-induced DNA damage. In CPT-treated cells, hHus1 and hRad1 become hyperphosphorylated, and hRad9 becomes firmly anchored to nuclear components in association with hHus1 and the hyperphos phorylated form of hRad1 *(218)*. Hus1 is an essential gene whose inactivation results in genomic instability and massive apoptosis in mice *(219)*. p21 inactivation is required for cell viability, and *Hus1-/-p21-/-* cells display a unique sensitivity to hydroxyurea and UV, but only slightly increased sensitivity to ionizing radiation *(219)*.

ATR (Ataxia Telangiectasia and Rad 3-related) is also believed to function in this S-phase checkpoint pathway probably in connection with the 9.1.1 complex (for review *see* ref. *210*). ATR is with ATM and DNA-PK, a member of the PI3 kinase family. ATR binds to and is activated by damaged DNA and phosphorylates similar substrates as ATM. ATR function in close physical and functional association with ATRIP (the ATR Interacting Protein, which is the homolog of the yeast checkpoint gene Rad26) *(220)*. Although the three PI3 kinase pathways (ATM, ATR, DNA-PK) exhibit some degree of redundancy, it is presently believed that the ATM and DNA-PK pathways are primarily activated by DNA double-strand breaks (induced for instance by ionizing radiation) whereas the ATR pathway is activated by replication-mediated DNA damage and damaged replication forks (as in the case of UV, hydroxyurea, and Top1 poisons). The ATM and

ATR pathways are also believed to have some differential specificity with respect to their effector substrates: ATM preferentially activates Chk2, whereas ATR preferentially activates Chk1 *(210)*. Recent studies demonstrate that in ATR-kinase dominant-negative cells (ATR-kinase dead; ATR/kd) *(221)*, phosphorylation of Chk1 in response to Top1 poisons is not observed, and both S- and G2 checkpoints are abrogated *(222)*. Furthermore, these ATR-deficient cells are hypersensitive to topotecan *(222)* (Table 1), which implicates ATR in the cellular response and S-phase checkpoint activation in cells treated with Top1 poisons.

The ATR and 9.1.1 pathways are probably connected because in fission yeast, Rad1, Hus1, and Rad9 are essential for Chk1 activation *(223–225)*, and in human cells, the ATR-associated protein (ATRIP) is required for phosphorylation of hRad17 in response to DNA damage *(220)*.

6.5. The RecQ Pathway: Bloom and Werner Syndrome Pathways

The RecQ pathway has recently been proposed to be important for: (1) unwinding replicating DNA *(226)* possibly in association with Top3 *(227)*, (2) faithful chromosome segregation during anaphase *(228)*, (3) for meiotic recombinations in association with Top3 *(229)*, (4) for resolving stalled replication forks *(230)*, and (5) for restarting replication forks after their collapse *(231,232)* (Fig. 7).

The pathway is highly conserved. It is named after the E. Coli homolog, RecQ. In budding yeast, a sole gene encodes the RecQ homolog, SGS1 (slow growth suppressor 1), whose mutant allele was identified as a suppressor of the slow growth phenotype of Top3 mutants *(229)*. The SGS1 mutants show hyper-recombination and defects in chromosome segregation *(233)*. Sgs1 interacts with both Top2 and Top3 *(233–235)*. In humans, BLM and WRN (genes defective in Bloom and Werner syndrome, respectively) are two homologs of SGS1. Although BLM, WRN and SGS1 are similar in length, and *sgs1* mutant can be partially rescued by BLM and WRN *(236)*, these three gene products share little homology outside their helicase domain *(234)*. Also, by contrast to BLM cells, WRN cells do not show increased sister chromatin exchanges.

Both WRN *(237–239)*, and BLM *(240)* knockout cells are hypersensitive to CPT (Table 1). Further implication of WRN in Top1 poisoning was recently published *(241)*. WRN was found to form distinct nuclear foci in response to CPT and other DNA damaging agents, including etoposide, 4-nitroquinolin-N- oxide and bleomycin. Aphidicolin inhibited CPT-induced WRN foci strongly but not bleomycin-induced foci, indicating that WRN forms foci at replication-mediated DNA double-strand breaks. These WRN foci were colocalized with RPA foci almost entirely and with Rad51 foci partially, implicating cooperative functions of these proteins in response to

DNA damage. WRN foci partially colocalized with sites of 5-bromo-2'-deoxy-uridine incorporation, suggesting that WRN form nuclear foci in response to aberrant DNA structures, including DNA double-strand breaks and stalled replication forks and that WRN takes part in the homologous recombination repair and in the processing of stalled replication forks *(241)* (*see* Fig. 7).

As for the other pathways, it is likely that cross-talks exist between the RecQ and the ATR/ATM pathways. BLM was recently shown to be phosphorylated by ATR and to be required for correct relocalization of MRN complexes in the presence of stalled replication forks *(242)*. WRN binds to Ku70/80, which stimulates its exonuclease activity *(243,244)*. Taken together, these observations suggest that, when replication is impaired by CPT-induced DNA damage, WRN prevents the illegitimate recombination and promotes DNA-repair by non-homologous end joining (NHEJ) by the Ku/DNA-PK pathway *(240)*.

6.6. The Chromatin Remodeling Pathways (CSA/CSB/γ-H2AX)

Evidence for chromatin changes and histone modifications in DNA repair is emerging. CPT induces chromatin structural reorganization, which involves disassembly of a group of nucleosomes without loss of histone, resulting in DNA relaxation *(117,245)*.

Cockayne syndrome B (CSB) recombinant protein has been shown to act as a chromatin remodeling factor *(246)*. It is also known that Cockayne syndrome cells are hypersensitive to CPT (Table 1) and accumulate abnormally high levels of double strand breaks (DSBs) in nascent DNA *(109)*.

Recent studies demonstrated that one of the histones, histone H2AX is rapidly phosphorylated in response to DNA double-strand breaks *(247)*. Phosphorylated H2AX is referred to γ-H2AX. This phosphorylation could alter chromatin structure to allow access and action for DNA repair factors. γ-H2AX may also function in checkpoint function in association with other proteins that colocalize in nuclear foci, such as the MRN complex, BRCA1, and BLM *(247)*. Studies from our group indicates that γ-H2AX is formed in cells treated with CPT, and that H2AX mutation that prevents the formation of γ-H2AX increase the cellular sensitivity to CPT *(248)*. Because the kinases that induce γ-H2AX formation are related to the PI3 kinases, γ-H2AX formation might link the ATM, ATR, and DNA-PK pathways in mammalian cells.

53BP1 also forms nuclear foci within 1 hour after CPT treatment *(188)*. 53BP1 was identified as a p53-binding protein in yeast two-hybrid systems. It contains a tandem of BRCT motifs in its C-terminus, and its function has not yet been elucidated. 53BP1 is rapidly phosphorylated by ATM (although may be not exclusively) after ionizing radiations and colocalizes with γ-H2AX *(188)*, suggesting that 53BP1 is implicated in DNA strand break repair and possibly checkpoints.

6.7. Other Pathways: p53 and Fanconi Anemia Pathways

Although p53 levels are induced following CPT treatment, p53 deficiencies in tumor cells in culture do not translate in hypersensitivity to CPT *(249)*. However, transfection of E6 papilloma virus ubiquitin ligase, which degrades p53 increase the CPT sensitivity both in colon and breast human carcinoma cells *(250)*. p53 elevation is replication-dependent *(110)*, which is consistent with a DNA damage response. By contrast to ionizing radiation, p53 elevation is preserved in AT cells treated with CPT or the top2 inhibitor, etoposide *(251)*, indicating that p53 elevation in response to CPT is independent of ATM. Because of the diversity of the p53 responses, which can either induce apoptosis or cell cycle arrest or enhance DNA repair, the outcome of p53 deficiencies is probably dependent upon the cellular context.

The sensitivity of Fanconi anemia cells to CPT is controversial. Saito and coworkers found that Fanconi anemia cells are hypersensitive to CPT, whereas their Top1 gene is normal *(252)*. By contrast, two independent studies found no difference in sensitivity to CPT *(253,254)*. This apparent discrepancy might be result of the fact that Fanconi anemia cells have eight complementation groups and that the cell lines used in the previously cited studies belonged to different complementation groups *(255)*.

7. APOPTOTIC RESPONSE TO TOP1 POISONING: BALANCE BETWEEN CELL DEATH AND SURVIVAL

As with other DNA damaging agents, Top1 poisons are efficient inducers of apoptosis. This effect is both cell type– and dose-dependent, suggesting that the same types of lesions can activate different pathways. In this section, we will focus on the potential connections between Top1–mediated DNA damage and the apoptotic pathway. A working hypothesis is that the same sensors that are implicated in cell-cycle checkpoint response initiate the apoptotic cascade. Rad9, a member of the 9.1.1 complex (*see* Section 6.4.), has recently been shown to bind to and block the activity of the antiapoptotic proteins Bcl-2 and Bcl-xL *(256,257)*. Several observations suggest that the nonreceptor tyrosine kinase c-abl could be one of the upstream signals that control the differential activity of Rad9 (checkpoint or apoptosis): (1) c-abl is activated in response to DNA damage *(258)*, and the Ku/DNA-PK complex *(208,259)* and the ATM gene product *(260,261)* have been implicated in its activation and (2) c-abl phosphorylates Rad9 and increases its ability to interact with Bcl-xL *(262)*. In addition, the finding that c-abl also phosphorylates the Rad51 protein and modulates its activity has supported a role for c-abl in coordinating DNA repair with the induction of apoptosis *(263,264)*. Whether apoptosis induced by Top1 poisons is also, at least in part, dependent for c-abl activation and implicates some of the cell cycle checkpoint proteins remains to be determined.

REFERENCES

1. Li TK, Liu LF. 2001 Tumor cell death induced by topoisomerase-targeting drugs. Annu Rev Pharmacol Toxicol 41:53–77.
2. Pommier Y, Pourquier P, Fan Y, Strumberg D. 1998 Mechanism of action of eukaryotic DNA topoisomerase I and drugs targeted to the enzyme. Biochim Biophys Acta 1400:83–105.
3. Pommier Y, Pourquier P, Urasaki Y, Wu J, Laco G. 1999 Topoisomerase I inhibitors: selectivity and cellular resistance. Drug Resistance Update 2:307–318.
4. Hsiang YH, Hertzberg R, Hecht S, Liu LF. 1985 Camptothecin induces protein-linked DNA breaks via mammalian DNA topoisomerase I. J Biol Chem 260:14873–14878.
5. Wall ME, Wani MC. 1995 Camptothecin and taxol: discovery to clinic—thirteenth Bruce F. Cain Memorial Award lecture. Cancer Res 55:753–760.
6. Gupta M, Fujimori A, Pommier Y. 1995 Eukaryotic DNA topoisomerases I. Biochim Biophys Acta 1262:1–14.
7. Pourquier P, Kohlhagen G, Ueng L-M, Pommier Y. 1999 Topoisomerase I and II activity assays. In: Methods in molecular medicine: cytototoxic drug resistance mechanisms. Vol. 28. Brown R, and Böger-Brown, U, eds. Humana Press, New Jersey, 95–110.
8. Redinbo MR, Stewart L, Kuhn P, Champoux JJ, Hol WG. 1998 Crystal structure of human topoisomerase I in covalent and noncovalent complexes with DNA. Science 279:1504–1513.
9. Redinbo MR, Champoux JJ, Hol WG. 1999 Structural insights into the function of type IB topoisomerases. Curr Opin Struct Biol 9:29–36.
10. Redinbo MR, Stewart L, Champoux JJ, Hol WG. 1999 Structural flexibility in human topoisomerase I revealed in multiple non-isomorphous crystal structures. J Mol Biol 292:685–696.
11. Redinbo MR, Champoux JJ, Hol WG. 2000 Novel insights into catalytic mechanism from a crystal structure of human topoisomerase I in complex with DNA. Biochemistry 39:6832–40.
12. Stewart L, Redinbo MR, Qiu X, Hol WG, Champoux JJ. 1998 A model for the mechanism of human topoisomerase I. Science 279:1534–1541.
13. Nitiss J, Wang JC. 1988 DNA topoisomerase-targeting antitumor drugs can be studied in yeast. Proc Natl Acad Sci USA 85:7501–7505.
14. Pourquier P, Takebayashi Y, Urasaki Y, Gioffre C, Kohlhagen G, Pommier Y. 2000 Induction of topoisomerase I cleavage complexes by 1-β-D-arabinofuranosylcytosine (Ara-C) in vitro and in ara-C-treated cells. Proc Natl Acad Sci USA 97:1885–1890.
15. Urasaki Y, Takebayashi Y, Pommier Y. 2000 Activity of a novel camptothecin analogue, homocamptothecin, in camptothecin-resistant cell lines with topoisomerase I alterations. Cancer Res 60:6577–6580.
16. Urasaki Y, Laco G, Takebayashi Y, Bailly C, Kohlhagen G, Pommier Y. 2001 Use of camptothecin-resistant mammalian cell lines to evaluate the role of topoisomerase I in the antiproliferative activity of the indolocarbazole, NB-506, and its topoisomerase I binding site. Cancer Res 61:504–508.
17. Woo MH, Vance JR, Marcos AR, Bailly C, Bjornsti MA. 2002 Active site mutations in DNA topoisomerase I distinguish the cytotoxic activities of camptothecin and the indolocarbazole, rebeccamycin. J Biol Chem 277:3813–3822.
18. Pommier Y. 1998 Diversity of DNA topoisomerases I and inhibitors. Biochimie 80:255–270.

19. Long BH, Balasubramanian BN. 2000 Non-camptothecin topoisomerase I active compounds as potential anticancer agents. Exp Opin Ther Patents 10:655–686.
20. Meng L-H, Liao Z-H, Pommier Y. 2003 Non-camptothecin DNA topoisomerase I inhibitors in cancer chemotherapy. Curr Topics Med Chem 3:305–320.
21. Garcia-Carbonero R, Supko JG. 2002 Current perspectives on the clinical experience, pharmacology, and continued development of the camptothecins. Clin Cancer Res 8:641–661.
22. Konstadoulakis MM, Antonakis PT, Tsibloulis BG, et al. 2001 A phase II study of 9-nitrocamptothecin in patients with advanced pancreatic adenocarcinoma. Cancer Chemother Pharmacol 48:417–420.
23. Verschraegen CF, Levenback C, Vincent M, et al. 2000 Phase II study of intravenous DX-8951f in patients with advanced ovarian, tubal, or peritoneal cancer refractory to platinum, taxane, and topotecan. Ann N Y Acad Sci 922:349–351.
24. Lavergne O, Lesueur-Ginot L, Pla Rodas F, et al. 1998 Homocamptothecins: synthesis and antitumor activity of novel E-ring- modified camptothecin analogs. J Med Chem 41:5410–5419.
25. Lesueur-Ginot L, Demarquay D, Kiss R, et al. 1999 Homocamptothecin, an E-ring modified camptothecin with enhanced lactone stability, retains topoisomerase I-targeted activity and antitumor properties. Cancer Res 59:2939–2943.
26. Philippart P, Harper L, Chaboteaux C, et al. 2000 Homocamptothecin, an E-ring-modified camptothecin, exerts more potent antiproliferative activity than other topoisomerase I inhibitors in human colon cancers obtained from surgery and maintained in vitro under histotypical culture conditions. Clin Cancer Res 6:1557–1562.
27. Larsen AK, Gilbert C, Chyzak G, et al. 2001 Unusual potency of BN 80915, a novel fluorinated E-ring modified camptothecin, toward human colon carcinoma cells. Cancer Res 61:2961–2967.
28. Jaxel C, Kohn KW, Wani MC, Wall ME, Pommier Y. 1989 Structure-activity study of the actions of camptothecin derivatives on mammalian topoisomerase I: evidence for a specific receptor site and a relation to antitumor activity. Cancer Res 49:1465–1469.
29. Burke TG, Mi Z. 1994. The structural basis of camptothecin interactions with human serum albumin: impact on drug stability. J Med Chem 37:40–46.
30. Prudhomme M. 2000 Recent developments of rebeccamycin analogs as topoisomerase I inhibitors and antitumor agents. Curr Med Chem 7:1189–1212.
31. Bailly C, Riou J-F, Colson P, Houssier C, Rodriguez-Pereira E, Prudhomme M. 1997 DNA cleavage by topoisomerase I in the presence of indolocarbazole derivatives of rebeccamycin. Biochemistry 36:3917–3929.
32. Fukasawa K, Komatani H, Hara Y, et al. 1998 Sequence-selective DNA cleavage by a topoisomerase I poison, NB-506. Int J Cancer 75:145–150.
33. Ren J, Bailly C, Chaires JB. 2000 NB-506, an indolocarbazole topoisomerase I inhibitor, binds preferentially to triplex DNA. FEBS Lett 470:355–359.
34. Cushman M, Cheng L. 1978 Total synthesis of nitidine chloride. J Org Chem 43:286–288.
35. Cushman M, Mohan P, Smith EC. 1984 Synthesis and biological activity of structural analogs of the anticancer benzophenanthridine alkaloid nitidine chloride. J Med Chem 27:544–547.
36. Cushman M, Mohan P. 1985 Synthesis and antitumor activity of structural analogs of the anticancer benzophenanthridine alkaloid fagaronine chloride. J Med Chem 28:1031–1036.

37. Kohlhagen G, Paull K, Cushman M, Nagafufuji P, Pommier Y. 1998 Protein-linked DNA strand breaks induced by NSC 314622, a non-camptothecin topoisomerase I poison. Mol Pharmacol 54:50–58.
38. Cushman M, Jayaraman M, Vroman JA, et al. 2000 Synthesis of new Indeno[1,2-c]isoquinolines: cytotoxic non-camptothecin topoisomerase I inhibitors. J Med Chem 43:3688–98.
39. Strumberg D, Pommier Y, Paull K, Jayaraman M, Nagafuji P, Cushman M. 1999 Synthesis of cytotoxic indenoisoquinoline topoisomerase I poisons. J Med Chem 42:446–457.
40. Jayaraman M, Fox BM, Hollingshead M, Kohlhagen G, Pommier Y, Cushman M. 2002. Synthesis of new dihydroindeno[1,2-c]isoquinoline and indenoisoquinolinium chloride topoisomerase I inhibitors having high in vivo anticancer activity in the hollow fiber animal model. J Med Chem 45:242–249.
41. Chen AY, Yu C, Gatto B, Liu LF. 1993 DNA minor groove-binding ligands: a different class of mammalian topoisomerase I inhibitors. Proc Natl Acad Sci USA 90:8131–8135.
42. Beerman TA, McHugh MM, Sigmund R, Lown JW, Rao KE, Bathini Y. 1992 Effects of analogs of the DNA minor groove binder Hoechst 33258 on topoisomerase II and I mediated activities. Biochim Biophys Acta 1131:53–61.
43. Zhang X, Kiechle F. 2001 Hoechst 33342-induced apoptosis is associated with decreased immunoreactive topoisomerase I and topoisomerase I-DNA complex formation. Ann Clin Lab Sci 31:187–198.
44. Chen AY, Yu C, Bodley A, Peng LF, Liu LF. 1993 A new mammalian DNA topoisomerase I poison Hoechst 33342: cytotoxicity and drug resistance in human cell cultures. Cancer Res 53:1332–1337.
45. Kim JS, Sun Q, Gatto B, et al. 1996 Structure-activity relationships of benzimidazoles and related heterocycles as topoisomerase I poisons. Bioorg Med Chem 4:621–630.
46. Jin S, Kim JS, Sim SP, et al. 2000 Heterocyclic bibenzimidazole derivatives as topoisomerase I inhibitors. Bioorg Med Chem Lett 10:719–723.
47. Pilch DS, Xu Z, Sun Q, LaVoie EJ, Liu LF, Breslauer KJ. 1997 A terbenzimidazole that preferentially binds and conformationally alters structurally distinct DNA duplex domains: a potential mechanism for topoisomerase I poisoning. Proc Natl Acad Sci USA 94:13565–13570.
48. Rangarajan M, Kim JS, Jin S, et al. 2000 2"-Substituted 5-phenylterbenzimidazoles as topoisomerase I poisons. Bioorg Med Chem 8:1371–1382.
49. Aune G, Furuta T, Pommier Y. 2002 Ecteinascidin 743: a novel anticancer drug with a unique mechanism of action. Anticancer Drugs 13:545–555.
50. Verschraegen CF, Glover K. 2001 ET-743 (PharmaMar/NCI/Ortho Biotech). Curr Opin Investig Drugs 2:1631–1638.
51. Pommier Y, Kohlhagen G, Bailly C, Waring M, Mazumder A, Kohn KW. 1996 DNA sequence- and structure-selective alkylation of guanine N2 in the DNA minor groove by ecteinascidin 743, a potent antitumor compound from the Caribbean tunicate *Ecteinascidia Turbinata*. Biochemistry 35:13303–13309.
52. Zewail-Foote M, Hurley LH. 2001 Differential rates of reversibility of ecteinascidin 743-DNA covalent adducts from different sequences lead to migration to favored bonding sites. J Am Chem Soc 123:6485–6495.
53. Takebayashi Y, Pourquier P, Yoshida A, Kohlhagen G, Pommier Y. 1999 Poisoning of human DNA topoisomerase I by ecteinascidin 743, an anticancer drug that selectively alkylates DNA in the minor groove. Proc Natl Acad Sci USA 96:7196–7201.

54. Martinez EJ, Owa T, Schreiber SL, Corey EJ. 1999 Phthalascidin, a synthetic antitumor agent with potency and mode of action comparable to ecteinascidin 743. Proc Natl Acad Sci USA 96:3496–3501.
55. Damia G, Silvestri S, Carrassa L, et al. 2001 Unique pattern of ET-743 activity in different cellular systems with defined deficiencies in DNA-repair pathways. Int J Cancer 92:583–588.
56. Takebayashi Y, Goldwasser F, Urasaki Y, Kohlhagen G, Pommier Y. 2001 Ecteinascidin 743 induces protein-linked DNA breaks in human colon carcinoma HCT116 cells and is cytotoxic independently of topoisomerase I expression. Clin Cancer Res 7:185–191.
57. Ryan DP, Supko JG, Eder PP, et al. 2001 Phase I and pharmacokinetic study of ecteinascidin 743 administered as a 72-hour continuous intravenous infusion in patients with sold malignancies. Clin Cancer Res 7:231–242.
58. Taamma A, Misset JL, Riofrio M, et al. 2001 Phase I and pharmacokinetic study of ecteinascidin-743, a new marine compound, administered as a 24-hour continuous infusion in patients with solid tumors. J Clin Oncol 19:1256–1265.
59. Takebayashi Y, Pourquier P, Zimonjic DB, et al. 2001 Antiproliferative activity of ecteinascidin 743 is dependent upon transcription-coupled nucleotide-excision repair. Nat Med 7:961–966.
60. Cummings J, Macpherson JS, Meikle I, Smyth JF. 1996 Development of anthracenyl-amino acid conjugates as topoisomerase I and II inhibitors that circumvent drug resistance. Biochem Pharmacol 52:979–990.
61. Macpherson JS, Cummings J, Meikle I, Miller EP, Smyth JF. 1997 Cell cycle effects of the novel topoisomerase I inhibitor NU/ICRF 505 in a panel of Chinese hamster ovary cell lines. Eur J Cancer. 33:280–283.
62. Pourquier P, Pommier Y. 2001 Topoisomerase I-mediated DNA damage. Adv Cancer Res 80:189–216.
63. Pourquier P, Gioffre C, Kohlhagen G, et al. 2002 Gemcitabine (2',2'-difluoro-2'-deoxycytidine), an antimetabolite that poisons topoisomerase I. Clin Cancer Res 8:2499–2504.
64. Pourquier P, Waltman JL, Urasaki Y, et al. 2001 Topoisomerase I-mediated cytotoxicity of *N*-methyl-*N*'-nitro-*N*-nitrosoguanidine: trapping of topoisomerase I by the O^6-methylguanine. Cancer Res 61:53–58.
65. Pourquier P, Ueng L-M, Fertala J, et al. 1999 Induction of reversible complexes between eukaryotic DNA topoisomerase I and DNA-containing oxidative base damages. J Biol Chem 274:8516–8523.
66. Lanza A, Tornatelli S, Rodolfo C, Scanavini MC, Pedrini AM. 1996 Human DNA topoisomerase I-mediated cleavages stimulated by ultraviolet light-induced DNA damage. J Biol Chem 271:6978–6986.
67. Subramanian D, Rosenstein BS, Muller MT. 1998 Ultraviolet-induced DNA damage stimulates topoisomerase I-DNA complex formation in vivo: possible relationship with DNA repair. Cancer Res 58:976–984.
68. Pourquier P, Ueng L-M, Kohlhagen G, et al. 1997 Effects of uracil incorporation, DNA mismatches, and abasic sites on cleavage and religation activities of mammalian topoisomerase I. J Biol Chem 272:7792–7796.
69. Pourquier P, Pilon A, Kohlhagen G, Mazumder A, Sharma A, Pommier Y. 1997 Trapping of mammalian topoisomerase I and recombinations induced by damaged DNA containing nicks or gaps: importance of DNA end phosphorylation and camptothecin effects. J Biol Chem 272:26441–26447.

70. Pourquier P, Bjornsti M-A, Pommier Y. 1998 Induction of topoisomerase I cleavage complexes by the vinyl chloride adduct, 1,*N*6-ethenoadenine. J Biol Chem 273:27245–27249.
71. Pommier Y, Kohlhagen G, Pourquier P, Sayer JM, Kroth H, Jerina DM. 2000 Benzo[*a*]pyrene epoxide adducts in DNA are potent inhibitors of a normal topoisomerase I cleavage site and powerful inducers of other topoisomerase I cleavages. Proc Natl Acad Sci USA 97:2040–2045.
72. Pommier Y, Kohlhagen G, Laco GS, Sayer JM, Kroth H, Jerina DM. 2000 Position-specific trapping of topoisomerase I-DNA cleavage complexes by the intercalated benzo[a]pyrene diol epoxide adducts at the 6-amino group of adenine. Proc Natl Acad Sci USA 97:10739–10744.
73. Pommier Y, Kohlhagen G, Laco GS, Kroth H, Sayer JM, Jerina DM. 2002 Different effects on human topoisomerase I by minor groove and intercalated deoxyguanosine adducts derived from two polycyclic aromatic hydrocarbon diol epoxides at or near a normal cleavage site. J Biol Chem 277:13666–13672.
74. Hertzberg RP, Caranfa MJ, Hecht SM. 1989 On the mechanism of topoisomerase I inhibition by camptothecin: Evidence for binding to an enzyme-DNA complex. Biochemistry 28:4629–4638.
75. Jaxel C, Capranico G, Kerrigan D, Kohn KW, Pommier Y. 1991 Effect of local DNA sequence on topoisomerase I cleavage in the presence or absence of camptothecin. J Biol Chem 266:20418–20423.
76. Pommier Y, Kohlhagen G, Kohn F, Leteurtre F, Wani MC, Wall ME. 1995 Interaction of an alkylating camptothecin derivative with a DNA base at topoisomerase I-DNA cleavage sites. Proc Natl Acad Sci USA 92:8861–8865.
77. Kerrigan JE, Pilch DS. 2001 A structural model for the ternary cleavable complex formed between human topoisomerase I, DNA, and camptothecin. Biochemistry 40:9792–9798.
78. Laco G, Collins JR, Luke BT, et al. 2002 Human topoisomerase I inhibition: docking camptothecin and derivatives into a structure-based active site model. Biochemistry 41:1428–1435.
79. Sim SP, Pilch DS, Liu LF. 2000 Site-specific topoisomerase I-mediated DNA cleavage induced by nogalamycin: a potential role of ligand-induced DNA bending at a distal site. Biochemistry 39:9928–9934.
80. Horwitz SB, Chang CK, Grollman AP. 1971 Studies on camptothecin. I. Effects of nucleic acid and protein synthesis. Mol Pharmacol 7:632–644.
81. Holm C, Covey JM, Kerrigan D, Pommier Y. 1989 Differential requirement of DNA replication for the cytotoxicity of DNA topoisomerase I and II inhibitors in Chinese hamster DC3F cells. Cancer Res 49:6365–6368.
82. O'Connor PM, Nieves-Neira W, Kerrigan D, et al. 1991 S-Phase population analysis does not correlate with the cytotoxicity of camptothecin and 10,11-methylenedioxycamptothecin in human colon carcinoma HT-29 cells. Cancer Commun 3:233–240.
83. Mattern MR, Hofmann GA, McCabe FL, Johnson RK. 1991 Synergic cell killing by ionizing radiation and topoisomerase I inhibitor topotecan (SK&F 10864). Cancer Res 51:5813–5816.
84. Hsiang Y-H, Lihou MG, Liu LF. 1989 Arrest of DNA replication by drug-stabilized topoisomerase I-DNA cleavable complexes as a mechanism of cell killing by camptothecin. Cancer Res 49:5077–5082.

85. Goldwasser F, Shimizu T, Jackman J, et al. 1996 Correlations between S- and G2-phase arrest and cytotoxicity of camptothecin in human colon carcinoma cells. Cancer Res 56:4430–4437.
86. Nitiss JL, Wang JC. 1996 Mechanisms of cell killing by drugs that trap covalent complexes between DNA topoisomerases and DNA. Mol Pharmacol 50:1095–1102.
87. Morris EJ, Geller HM. 1996 Induction of neuronal apoptosis by camptothecin, an inhibitor of DNA topoisomerase-I: evidence for cell cycle-independent toxicity. J Cell Biol 134:757–770.
88. Wu J, Liu LF. 1997 Processing of topoisomerase I cleavable complexes into DNA damage by transcription. Nucleic Acids Res 25:4181–4186.
89. Borovitskaya AE, D'Arpa P. 1998 Replication-dependent and -independent camptothecin cytotoxicity of seven human colon tumor cell lines. Oncol Res 10:271–276.
90. Zhou Y, Gwadry FG, Reinhold WC, et al. 2002 Transcriptional regulation of mitotic genes by camptothecin-induced DNA damage: microarray analysis of dose- and time-dependent effects. Cancer Res 62:1688–1695.
91. Barrows LR, Holden JA, Anderson M, D'Arpa P. 1998 The CHO XRCC1 mutant, EM9, deficient in DNA ligase III activity, exhibits hypersensitivity to camptothecin independent of DNA replication. Mutat Res 408:103–110.
92. Shao R-G, Cao C-X, Zhang H, Kohn KW, Wold MS, Pommier Y. 1999 Replication-mediated DNA damage by camptothecin induces phosphorylation of RPA by DNA-dependent protein kinase and dissociates RPA: DNA-PK complexes. EMBO J 18:1397–1406.
93. Snapka RM. 1986 Topoisomerase inhibitors can selectively interfere with different stages of simian virus 40 DNA replication. Mol Cell Biol 6:4221–4227.
94. Tsao YP, Russo A, Nyamusa G, Silber R, Liu LF 1993. Interaction between replication forks and topoisomerase I-DNA cleavable complexes: studies in a cell-free SV40 DNA replication system. Cancer Res 53:5908–5914.
95. Strumberg D, Pilon AA, Smith M, Hickey R, Malkas L, Pommier Y. 2000 Conversion of topoisomerase I cleavage complexes on the leading strand of ribosomal DNA into 5′-phosphorylated DNA double-strand breaks by replication runoff. Mol Cell Biol 20:3977–3987.
96. Voeller DM, Grem JL, Pommier Y, Paull K, Allegra CJ. 2000 Identification and proposed mechanism of action of thymidine kinase inhibition associated with cellular exposure to camptothecin analogs. Cancer Chemother Pharmacol 45:409–416.
97. Shao R-G, Cao C-X, Shimizu T, O'Connor P, Kohn KW, Pommier Y. 1997 Abrogation of an S-phase checkpoint and potentiation of camptothecin cytotoxicity by 7-hydroxystaurosporine (UCN-01) in human cancer cell lines, possibly influenced by p53. Cancer Res 57:4029–4035.
98. Kessel D. 1971 Effects of camptothecin on RNA synthesis in leukemia cells. Biochim Biophys Acta 246:225–232.
99. Wu RS, Kumar A, Warner JR. 1971 Ribosome formation is blocked by camptothecin, a reversible inhibitor of RNA synthesis. Proc Natl Acad Sci USA 68: 3009–3014.
100. Kann HE Jr, Kohn KW. 1972 Effects of deoxyribonucleic acid-reactive drugs on ribonucleic acid synthesis in leukemia L1210 cells. Mol Pharmacol 8:551–560.
101. Gilmour DS, Elgin SC. 1987 Localization of specific topoisomerase I interactions within the transcribed region of active heat shock genes by using the inhibitor camptothecin. Mol Cell Biol 7:141–148.

102. Rowe TC, Couto E, Kroll DJ. 1987 Camptothecin inhibits hsp 70 heat-shock transcription and induces DNA strand breaks in hsp 70 genes in Drosophila. NCI Monogr 4:49–53.
103. Zhang H, Wang JC, Liu LF. 1988 Involvement of DNA topoisomerase I in transcription of human ribosomal RNA genes. Proc Natl Acad Sci USA 85:1060–1064.
104. Stewart AF, Herrera RE, Nordheim A. 1990 Rapid induction of c-fos transcription reveals quantitive linkage of RNA polymerase II and DNA topoisomerase I enzyme activities. Cell 60:141–146.
105. Ljungman M, Hanawalt PC. 1996 The anti-cancer drug camptothecin inhibits elongation but stimulates initiation of RNA polymerase II transcription. Carcinogenesis 17:31–35.
106. Muscarella DE, Rachlinski MK, Sotiriadis J, Bloom SE. 1998 Contribution of gene-specific lesions, DNA-replication-associated damage, and subsequent transcriptional inhibition in topoisomerase inhibitor-mediated apoptosis in lymphoma cells. Exp Cell Res 238:155–167.
107. Collins I, Weber A, Levens D. 2001 Transcriptional consequences of topoisomerase inhibition. Mol Cell Biol 21:8437–8451.
108. Bendixen C, Thomsen B, Alsner J, Westergaard O. 1990 Camptothecin-stabilized topoisomerase I-DNA adducts cause premature termination of transcription. Biochemistry 29:5613–5619.
109. Squires S, Ryan AJ, Strutt HL, Johnson RT. 1993 Hypersensitivity of Cockayne's syndrome cells to camptothecins is associated with the generation of abnormally high levels of double strand breaks in nascent DNA. Cancer Res 53:2012–2019.
110. Nelson WG, Kastan MB. 1994 DNA strand breaks: the DNA template alterations that trigger p53-dependent DNA damage response pathways. Mol Cell Biol 14:1815–1823.
111. Kharbanda S, Rubin E, Gunji H, et al. 1991 Camptothecin and its derivatives induce expression of the c-jun protooncogene in human myeloid leukemia cells. Cancer Res 51:6636–6642.
112. Zhao H, Jin S, Fan F, Fan W, Tong T, Zhan Q. 2000 Activation of the transcription factor Oct-1 in response to DNA damage. Cancer Res 60:6276–6280.
113. Piret B, Piette J. 1996 Topoisomerase poisons activate the transcription factor NF-kappaB in ACH-2 and CEM cells. Nucleic Acids Res 24:4242–4248.
114. Huang TT, Wuerzberger-Davis SM, Seufzer BJ, et al. 2000 NF-kappa B Activation by camptothecin. A linkage between nuclear DNA damage and cytoplasmic signaling events. J Biol Chem 275:9501–9509.
115. Daoud SS, Munson PJ, Reinhold WC, et al. 2002 A new approach (GEM) for design, analysis, and visualization of gene expression experiments in molecular pharmacology: application to p53- and topotecan-dependence studies. Proc Am Assoc Cancer Res 43:1085.
116. Wang JC. 1996 DNA topoisomerases. Annu Rev Biochem. 65:635–692.
117. Duann P, Sun M, C-T L, Zhang H, Liu LF. 1999 Plasmid linking number change induced by topoisomerase I-mediated DNA damage. Nucleic Acids Res 27: 2905–2911.
118. Merino A, Madden KR, Lane WS, Champoux JJ, Reinberg D. 1993 DNA topoisomerase I is involved in both repression and activation of transcription. Nature 365:227–232.
119. Kretzschmar M, Meisterernst M, Roeder RG. 1993 Identification of human DNA topoisomerase I as a cofactor for activator-dependent transcription by RNA polymerase II. Proc Natl Acad Sci USA 90:11508–11512.

120. Shykind BM, Kim J, Stewart L, Champoux JJ, Sharp PA. 1997 Topoisomerase I enhances TFIID-TFIIA complex assembly during activation of transcription. Genes Develop 11:397–407.
121. Rossi F, Labourier E, Forne T, et al. 1996 Specific phosphorylation of SR proteins by mammalian DNA topoisomerase I. Nature 381:80–82.
122. Rossi E, Labourier E, Gallouzi I-E, et al. 1998 The C-terminal domain but not the tyrosine 723 of human DNA topoisomerase I active site contributes to kinase activity. Nucleic Acids Res 26:2963–2970.
123. Labourier E, Rossi F, Gallouzi I-E, Allemand E, Divita G, Tazi J. 1998 Interaction between the N-terminal domain of human DNA topoisomerase I and the arginine-serine domain of its substrate determines phosphorylation of SF2/ASF splicing factor. Nucleic Acids Res 26:2955–2962.
124. Straub T, Grue P, Uhse A, et al. 1998 The RNA-splicing factor PSF/p54 controls DNA-topoisomerase I activity by a direct interaction. J Biol Chem 273:26261–26264.
125. Pouliot JJ, Yao KC, Robertson CA, Nash HA. 1999 Yeast gene for a Tyr-DNA phosphodiesterase that repairs topo I covalent complexes. Science 286:552–555.
126. Yang S-W, Burgin AB, Huizenga BN, Robertson CA, Yao KC, Nash HA. 1996 A eukaryotic enzyme that can disjoin dead-end covalent complexes between DNA and type I topoisomerases. Proc Natl Acad Sci USA 93:11534–11539.
127. Interthal H, Pouliot JJ, Champoux JJ. 2001 The tyrosyl-DNA phosphodiesterase Tdp1 is a member of the phospholipase D superfamily. Proc Natl Acad Sci USA 98:12009–12014.
128. Stuckey JA, Dixon JE. 1999 Crystal structure of a phospholipase D family member. Nat Struct Biol 6:278–284.
129. Davies DR, Interthal H, Champoux JJ, Hol WG. 2002 The crystal structure of human tyrosyl-DNA phosphodiesterase, Tdp1. Structure (Camb) 10:237–248.
130. Debethune L, Kohlhagen G, Grandas A, Pommier Y. 2002 Processing of nucleopeptides mimicking the topoisomerase I-DNA covalent complex by tyrosyl-DNA phosphodiesterase. Nucleic Acids Res 30:1198–1204.
131. Beidler DR, Cheng Y-C. 1995 Camptothecin induction of a time- and concentration-dependent decrease of topoisomerase I and its implication in camptothecin activity. Mol Pharmacol 47:907–914.
132. Desai SD, Liu LF, Vazquez-Abad D, D'Arpa P. 1997 Ubiquitin-dependent destruction of topoisomerase I is stimulated by the antitumor drug camptothecin. J Biol Chem 272:24159–24164.
133. Vance JR, Wilson TE. 2001 Uncoupling of 3′-phosphatase and 5′-kinase functions in budding yeast. Characterization of Saccharomyces cerevisiae DNA 3′-phosphatase (TPP1). J Biol Chem 276:15073–15081.
134. Meijer M, Karimi-Busheri F, Huang TY, Weinfeld M, Young D. 2002 Pnk1, a DNA kinase/phosphatase required for normal response to DNA damage by gamma-radiation or camptothecin in Schizosaccharomyces pombe. J Biol Chem 277:4050–4055.
135. Smith PJ, Makinson TA, Watson JV. 1989 Enhanced sensitivity to camptothecin in ataxia telangiectasia cells and its relationship with the expression of DNA topoisomerase I. Int J Radiat Biol 55:217–231.
136. Shiloh Y. 2003 ATM and related protein kinases: safeguarding genome integrity. Nat Rev Cancer 3:155–168.
137. Eng WK, Faucette L, Johnson RK, Sternglanz R. 1988 Evidence that DNA topoisomerase I is necessary for the cytotoxic effects of camptothecin. Mol Pharmacol 34:755–760.

138. Michel B, Flores MJ, Viguera E, Grompone G, Seigneur M, Bidnenko V. 2001 Rescue of arrested replication forks by homologous recombination. Proc Natl Acad Sci USA 98:8181–8188.
139. Klein HL, Kreuzer KN. 2002 Replication, recombination, and repair: going for the gold. Mol Cell 9:471–480.
140. Baumann P, West SC. 1998 Role of the human RAD51 protein in homologous recombination and double- stranded-break repair. Trends Biochem Sci 23:247–251.
141. Gaymes TJ, North PS, Brady N, Hickson ID, Mufti GJ, Rassool FV. 2002 Increased error-prone non homologous DNA end-joining—a proposed mechanism of chromosomal instability in Bloom's syndrome. Oncogene 21:2525–2533.
142. Thacker J, Ganesh AN. 1990 DNA-break repair, radioresistance of DNA synthesis, and camptothecin sensitivity in the radiation-sensitive irs mutants: comparisons to ataxia-telangiectasia cells. Mutat Res 235:49–58.
143. Caldecott K, Jeggo P. 1991 Cross-sensitivity of gamma-ray-sensitive hamster mutants to cross- linking agents. Mutat Res 255:111–121.
144. Godthelp BC, Wiegant WW, van Duijn-Goedhart A, et al. 2002 Mammalian Rad51C contributes to DNA cross-link resistance, sister chromatid cohesion and genomic stability. Nucleic Acids Res 30:2172–2182.
145. Simbulan-Rosenthal CM, Rosenthal DS, Iyer S, Boulares AH, Smulson ME. 1998 Transient poly(ADP-ribosyl)ation of nuclear proteins and role of poly(ADP-ribose) polymerase in the early stages of apoptosis. J Biol Chem 273:13703–13712.
146. Chatterjee S, Cheng M-F, Trivedi D, Petzold SJ, Berger NA. 1989 Camptothecin hypersensitivity in poly(adenosine diphosphate-ribose) polymerase-deficient cell lines. Cancer Commun 1:389–394.
147. Chatterjee S, Hirschler NV, Petzold SJ, Berger SJ, Berger NA. 1989 Mutant cells defective in poly(ADP-ribose) synthesis due to stable alterations in enzyme activity or substrate availability. Exp Cell Res 184:1–15.
148. Staron K, Kowalska-Loth B, Nieznanski K, Szumiel I. 1996 Phosphorylation of topoisomerase I in L5178Y-S cells is associated with poly(ADP-ribose) metabolism. Carcinogenesis 17:383–387.
149. Mattern MR, Mong SM, Bartus HF, Mirabelli CK, Crooke ST, Johnson RK. 1987 Relationship between the intracellular effects of camptothecin and the inhibition of DNA topoisomerase I in cultured L1210 cells. Cancer Res 47:1793–1798.
150. Bowman KJ, Newell DR, Calvert AH, Curtin NJ. 2001 Differential effects of the poly (ADP-ribose) polymerase (PARP) inhibitor NU1025 on topoisomerase I and II inhibitor cytotoxicity in L1210 cells in vitro. Br J Cancer 84:106–112.
151. Park SY, Lam W, Cheng YC. 2002 X-ray repair cross-complementing gene I protein plays an important role in camptothecin resistance. Cancer Res 62:459–465.
152. Whitehouse CJ, Taylor RM, Thistlethwaite A, et al. 2001 XRCC1 stimulates human polynucleotide kinase activity at damaged DNA termini and accelerates DNA single-strand breaks. Cell 104:107–117.
153. Thompson LH, West MG. 2000 XRCC1 keeps DNA from getting stranded. Mutat Res 459:1–18.
154. de Murcia G, Menissier de Murcia J. 1994 Poly(ADP-ribose) polymerase: a molecular nick-sensor. Trends Biochem Sci 19:172–176.
155. D'Amours D, Desnoyers S, D'Silva I, Poirier GG. 1999 Poly(ADP-ribosyl)ation reactions in the regulation of nuclear functions. Biochem J 342:249–268.
156. Kasid UN, Halligan B, Liu LF, Dritschilo A, Smulson M. 1989 Poly(ADP-ribose)-mediated post-translational modification of chromatin-associated human topoisomerase I. Inhibitory effects on catalytic activity. J Biol Chem 264:18687–18692.

157. Ferro AM, Olivera BM. 1984 Poly(ADP-ribosylation) of DNA topoisomerase I from calf thymus. J Biol Chem 259:547–554.
158. Smith HM, Grosovsky AJ. 1999 PolyADP-ribose-mediated regulation of p53 complexed with topoisomerase I following ionizing radiation. Carcinogenesis 20:1439–1444.
159. Bauer PI, Buki KG, Comstock JA, Kun E. 2000 Activation of topoisomerase I by poly [ADP-ribose] polymerase. Int J Mol Med 5:533–540.
160. Fu Q, Kim SW, Chen HX, Grill S, Cheng YC. 1999 Degradation of topoisomerase I induced by topoisomerase I inhibitors is dependent on inhibitor structure but independent of cell death. Mol Pharmacol 55:677–683.
161. Mao Y, Sun M, Desai SD, Liu LF. 2000 SUMO-1 conjugation to topoisomerase I: A possible repair response to topoisomerase-mediated DNA damage. Proc Natl Acad Sci USA 97:4046–4051.
162. Almond JB, Cohen GM. 2002 The proteasome: a novel target for cancer chemotherapy. Leukemia 16:433–443.
163. D'Arpa P, Liu LF. 1995 Cell cycle-specific and transcription-related phosphorylation of mammalian topoisomerase I. Exp Cell Res 217:125–131.
164. Desai SD, Li TK, Rodriguez-Bauman A, Rubin EH, Liu LF. 2001 Ubiquitin/26S proteasome-mediated degradation of topoisomerase I as a resistance mechanism to camptothecin in tumor cells. Cancer Res 61:5926–5932.
165. Rubin E, Wood V, Bharti A, et al. 1995 A phase I and pharmacokinetic study of a new camptothecin derivative, 9- aminocamptothecin. Clin Cancer Res 1:269–276.
166. Saleem A, Edwards TK, Rasheed Z, Rubin EH. 2000 Mechanisms of resistance to camptothecins. Ann N Y Acad Sci 922:46–55.
167. Cusack JC Jr, Liu R, Houston M, Abendroth K, Elliott PJ, Adams J, Baldwin AS Jr. 2001 Enhanced chemosensitivity to CPT-11 with proteasome inhibitor PS-341:implications for systemic nuclear factor-kappaB inhibition. Cancer Res 61:3535–3540.
168. Adams J. 2002 Development of the proteasome inhibitor PS-341. Oncologist 7: 9–16.
169. Mo Y-Y, Yu Y, Shen Z, Beck WT. 2002 Nucleolar delocalization of human topoisomerase I in response to topotecan correlates with sumoylation of the protein. J Biol Chem 277:2958–2964.
170. Shen Z, Pardington-Purtymun PE, Comeaux JC, Moyzis RK, Chen DJ. 1996 UBL1, a human ubiquitin-like protein associating with human RAD51/RAD52 proteins. Genomics 36:271–279.
171. Boddy MN, Howe K, Etkin LD, Solomon E, Freemont PS. 1996 PIC 1, a novel ubiquitin-like protein which interacts with the PML component of a multiprotein complex that is disrupted in acute promyelocytic leukaemia. Oncogene 13:971–982.
172. Matunis MJ, Coutavas E, Blobel G. 1996 A novel ubiquitin-like modification modulates the partitioning of the Ran-GTPase-activating protein RanGAP1 between the cytosol and the nuclear pore complex. J Cell Biol 135:1457–1470.
173. Lapenta V, Chiurazzi P, van der Spek P, Pizzuti A, Hanaoka F, Brahe C. 1997 SMT3A, a human homologue of the S. cerevisiae SMT3 gene, maps to chromosome 21qter and defines a novel gene family. Genomics 40:362–366.
174. Okura T, Gong L, Kamitani T, et al. 1996 Protection against Fas/APO-1- and tumor necrosis factor-mediated cell death by a novel protein, sentrin. J Immunol 157:4277–4281.
175. Wilson VG, Rangasamy D. 2001 Intracellular targeting of proteins by sumoylation. Exp Cell Res 271:57–65.

176. Johnson RT, Gotoh E, Mullinger AM, Ryan AJ, Shiloh Y, Squires S. 1999 Targeting double-strand breaks to replicating DNA identifies a subpathway of DSB repair that is defective in Ataxia-Telangiectasia cells. Biochem Biophys Res Comm 261:317–325.
177. Jones NJ, Ellard S, Waters R, Parry EM. 1993 Cellular and chromosomal hypersensitivity to DNA crosslinking agents and topoisomerase inhibitors in the radiosensitive Chinese hamster irs mutants: phenotypic similarities to ataxia telangiectasia and Fanconi's anaemia cells. Carcinogenesis 14:2487–2494.
178. Johnson MA, Bryant PE, Jones NJ. 2000 Isolation of camptothecin-sensitive Chinese hamster cell mutants: phenotypic heterogeneity within the ataxia telangiectasia-like XRCC8 (irs2) complementation group. Mutagenesis 15:367–374.
179. Banin S, Moyal L, Shieh, S-Y, et al. 1998 Enhanced phosphorylation of p53 by ATM in response to DNA damage. Science 281:1674–1677.
180. Canman CE, Lim DS, Cimprich KA, et al. 1998 Activation of the ATM kinase by ionizing radiation and phosphorylation of p53. Science 281:1677–1679.
181. Khanna KK, Keating KE, Kozlov S, et al. 1998 ATM associates with and phosphorylates p53: mapping the region of interaction. Nat Genet 20:398–400.
182. Matsuoka S, Huang M, Elledge SJ. 1998 Linkage of ATM to cell cycle regulation by the Chk2 protein kinase. Science 282:893–897.
183. Lim DS, Kim ST, Xu B, et al. 2000 ATM phosphorylates p95/nbs1 in an S-phase checkpoint pathway. Nature 404:613–617.
184. Zhao S, Weng YC, Yuan SS, et al. 2000 Functional link between ataxia-telangiectasia and Nijmegen breakage syndrome gene products. Nature 405:473–477.
185. Gatei M, Young D, Cerosaletti KM, et al. 2000 ATM-dependent phosphorylation of nibrin in response to radiation exposure. Nat Genet 25:115–119.
186. Wu X, Ranganathan V, Weisman DS, et al. 2000 ATM phosphorylation of Nijmegen breakage syndrome protein is required in a DNA damage response. Nature 405:477–482.
187. Cortez D, Wang Y, Qin J, Elledge SJ. 1999 Requirement of ATM-dependent phosphorylation of brca1 in the DNA damage response to double-strand breaks. Science 286:1162–1166.
188. Rappold I, Iwabuchi K, Date T, Chen J. 2001 Tumor suppressor p53 binding protein 1 (53BP1) is involved in DNA damage-signaling pathways. J Cell Biol 153:613–620.
189. Wu X, Petrini JH, Heine WF, Weaver DT, Livingston DM, Chen J. 2000 Independence of R/M/N focus formation and the presence of intact BRCA1. Science 289:11.
190. Xu B, Kim S, Kastan MB. 2001 Involvement of Brca1 in S-phase and G(2)-phase checkpoints after ionizing irradiation. Mol Cell Biol 21:3445–3450.
191. Piret B, Schoonbroodt S, Piette J. 1999 The ATM protein is required for sustained activation of NF-kappaB following DNA damage. Oncogene 18:2261–2271.
192. Petrini JH. 2000 The Mre11 complex and ATM: collaborating to navigate S phase. Curr Opin Cell Biol 12:293–296.
193. Hopfner KP, Putnam CD, Tainer JA. 2002 DNA double-strand break repair from head to tail. Curr Opin Struct Biol 12:115–122.
194. Zhong Q, Chen CF, Li S, et al. 1999 Association of BRCA1 with the hRad50-hMre11-p95 complex and the DNA damage response. Science 285:747–750.
195. Wang Y, Cortez D, Yazdi P, Neff N, Elledge SJ, Qin J. 2000 BASC, a super complex of BRCA1-associated proteins involved in the recognition and repair of aberrant DNA structures. Genes Dev 14:927–939.

196. Furaki M, Liu JM. 2001 Chromosomal breakage syndromes and the BRCAL genome surveilance complex. Trends Mol Med 7:560–562.
197. Paull TT, Gellert M. 1998 The 3′ to 5′ exonuclease activity of Mre11 facilitates repair of DNA double-strand breaks. Mol Cell 1:969–979.
198. Paull TT, Rogakou EP, Yamazaki V, Kirchgessner CU, Gellert M, Bonner WM. 2000 A critical role for histone H2AX in recruitment of repair factors to nuclear foci after DNA damage. Curr Biol 10:886–895.
199. Stewart GS, Maser RS, Stankovic T, et al. 1999 The DNA double-strand break repair gene hMRE11 is mutated in individuals with an ataxia-telangiectasia-like disorder. Cell 99:577–587.
200. Mirzoeva OK, Petrini JH. 2001 DNA damage-dependent nuclear dynamics of the mre11 complex. Mol Cell Biol 21:281–288.
201. Dong Z, Zhong Q, Chen PL. 1999 The Nijmegen breakage syndrome protein is essential for Mre11 phosphorylation upon DNA damage. J Biol Chem 274: 19513–19516.
202. Johnson MA, Jones NJ. 1999 The isolation and genetic analysis of V79-derived etoposide sensitive Chinese hamster cell mutants: two new complementation groups of etoposide sensitive mutants. Mutation Res 435:271–282.
203. Kraakman-van der Zwet M, Overkamp WJ, Friedl AA, et al. 1999 Immortalization and characterization of Nijmegen Breakage syndrome fibroblasts. Mutat Res 434:17–27.
204. Wu J, Yin MB, Hapke G, Toth K, Rustum YM. 2002 Induction of biphasic DNA double strand breaks and activation of multiple repair protein complexes by DNA topoisomerase I drug 7-ethyl- 10-hydroxy-camptothecin. Mol Pharmacol 61:742–748.
205. Busby EC, Leistritz DF, Abraham RT, Karnitz LM, Sarkaria JN. 2000 The radiosensitizing agent 7-hydroxystaurosporine (UCN-01) inhibits the DNA damage checkpoint kinase hChk1. Cancer Res 60:2108–2112.
206. Graves PR, Yu L, Schwarz JK, et al. 2000 The Chk1 protein kinase and the Cdc25C regulatory pathways are targets of the anticancer agent UCN-01. J Biol Chem 275:5600–5605.
207. Yu Q, La Rose JH, Zhang H, Takemura H, Kohn KW, Pommier Y. 2002 UCN-01 inhibits p53 up-regulation and abrogates γ-radiation-induced G(2)-M checkpoint independently of p53 by targeting both of the checkpoint kinases, Chk2 and Chk1. Cancer Res 62:5743–5748.
208. Kharbanda S, Pandey P, Jin S, et al. 1997 Functional interaction between DNA-PK and c-Abl in response to DNA damage. Nature 386:732–735.
209. Zhou BB, Elledge SJ. 2000 The DNA damage response: putting checkpoints in perspective. Nature 408:433–439.
210. Caspari T, Carr AM 2002. Checkpoints: how to flag up double-strand breaks. Curr Biol 12:R105–R107.
211. Caspari T, Dahlen M, Kanter-Smoler G, et al. 2000 Characterization of Schizosaccharomyces pombe Hus1: a PCNA-related protein that associates with Rad1 and Rad9. Mol Cell Biol 20:1254–1262.
212. Kondo T, Matsumoto K, Sugimoto K. 1999 Role of a complex containing rad17, mec3, and ddc1 in the yeast DNA damage checkpoint pathway. Mol Cell Biol 19:1136–1143.
213. Kostrub CF, al-Khodairy F, Ghazizadeh H, Carr AM, Enoch T. 1997 Molecular analysis of hus1+, a fission yeast gene required for S-M and DNA damage checkpoints. Mol Gen Genet 254:389–399.

214. Volkmer E, Karnitz LM. 1999 Human homologs of Schizosaccharomyces pombe rad1, hus1, and rad9 form a DNA damage-responsive protein complex. J Biol Chem 274:567–570.
215. Rauen M, Burtelow MA, Dufault VM, Karnitz LM. 2000 The human checkpoint protein hRad17 interacts with the PCNA-like proteins hRad1, hHus1, and hRad9. J Biol Chem 275:29767–39771.
216. Komatsu K, Miyashita T, Hang H, et al. 2000 Human homologue of S. *pombe* Rad9 interacts with BCL-2/BCL-XL and promotes apoptosis. Nat Cell Biol 2:1–6.
217. Venclovas C, Thelen MP. 2000 Structure-based predictions of rad1, rad9, hus1 and rad17 participation in sliding clamp and clamp-loading complexes. Nucleic Acids Res 28:2481–2493.
218. Burtelow MA, Kaufmann SH, Karnitz LM. 2000 Retention of the human Rad9 checkpoint complex in extraction-resistant nuclear complexes after DNA damage. J Biol Chem 275:26343–26348.
219. Weiss RS, Enoch T, Leder P. 2000 Inactivation of mouse Hus1 results in genomic instability and impaired responses to genotoxic stress. Genes Dev 14:1886–1898.
220. Cortez D, Guntuku S, Qin J, Elledge SJ. 2001 ATR and ATRIP: partners in checkpoint signaling. Science 294:1713–1716.
221. Cliby WA, Roberts CJ, Cimprich KA, et al. 1998 Overexpression of a kinase-inactive ATR protein causes sensitivity to DNA-damaging agents and defects in cell cycle checkpoints. Embo J 17:159–169.
222. Cliby WA, Lewis KA, Lilly KK, Kaufmann SH. 2002 S phase and G2 arrests induced by topoisomerase I poisons are dependent on ATR kinase function. J Biol Chem 277:1599–1606.
223. Walworth N, Bernards R. 1996 *Rad*-dependent responses of the *Chk1*-encoded protein kinase at the DNA damage checkpoint. Science 271:353–356.
224. Walworth NC. 1998 Rad9 comes of age. Science. 281:185–186.
225. Brondello JM, Boddy MN, Furnari B, Russell P. 1999 Basis for the checkpoint signal specificity that regulates chk1 and cds1 protein kinases. Mol Cell Biol 19:4262–4269.
226. Liao S, Graham J, Yan H. 2000 The function of xenopus Bloom's syndrome protein homolog (xBLM) in DNA replication. Genes Dev 14:2570–2575.
227. Chakraverty RK, Kearsey JM, Oakley TJ, et al. 2001 Topoisomerase III acts upstream of Rad53p in the S-phase DNA damage checkpoint. Mol Cell Biol 21:7150–7162.
228. Goodwin A, Wang SW, Toda T, Norbury C, Hickson ID. 1999 Topoisomerase III is essential for accurate nuclear division in Schizosaccharomyces pombe. Nucleic Acids Res 27:4050–4058.
229. Gangloff S, de Massy B, Arthur L, Rothstein R, Fabre F. 1999 The essential role of yeast topoisomerase III in meiosis depends on recombination. Embo J 18: 1701–1711.
230. Yankiwski V, Marciniak RA, Guarente L, Neff NF 2000. Nuclear structure in normal and Bloom syndrome cells. Proc Natl Acad Sci USA 97:5214–5219.
231. Kamath-Loeb AS, Johansson E, Burgers PM, Loeb LA. 2000 Functional interaction between the werner syndrome protein and DNA polymerase delta. Proc Natl Acad Sci USA 97:4603–4608.
232. Rothstein R, Michel B, Gangloff S. 2000 Replication fork pausing and recombination or "gimme a break." Genes Develop 14:1–10.
233. Watt PM, Louis EJ, Borts RH, Hickson ID. 1995 Sgs1: a eukaryotic homolog of E. coli RecQ that interacts with topoisomerase II in vivo and is required for faithful chromosome segregation. Cell 81:253–260.

234. Gangloff S, MacDonald JP, Bendixen C, Arthur L, Rothstein R. 1994 The yeast type 1 topoisomerase top3 interacts with sgs1, a DNA helicase homolog: a potential eukaryotic reverse gyrase. Mol Cell Biol 14:8391–8398.
235. Lu J, Mullen JR, Brill SJ, Kleff, S, Romeo AM, Sternglanz R. 1996 Human homologues of yeast helicase. Nature 383:678–679.
236. Yamagata K, Kato J, Shimamoto A, Goto M, Furuichi Y, Ikeda H. 1998 Bloom's and Werner's syndrome genes suppress hyperrecombination in yeast sgs1 mutant: Implication for genomic instability in human diseases. Proc Natl Acad Sci USA 95:8733–8738.
237. Lebel M, Leder P. 1998 A deletion within the murine Werner syndrome helicase induces sensitivity to inhibitors of topoisomerase and loss of proliferative capacity. Proc Natl Acad Sci USA 95:13097–13102.
238. Poot M, Gollahon KA, Rabinovitch PS. 1999 Werner syndrome lymphoblastoid cells are sensitive to camptothecin- induced apoptosis in S-phase. Hum Genet 104:10–14.
239. Pichierri P, Franchitto A, Mosesso P, Palitti F. 2000 Werner's syndrome cell lines are hypersensitive to camptothecin-induced chromosomal damage. Mutat Res 456:45–57.
240. Imamura O, Fujita K, Itoh C, Takeda S, Furuichi Y, Matsumoto T. 2002 Werner and Bloom helicases are involved in DNA repair in a complementary fashion. Oncogene 21:954–963.
241. Sakamoto S, Nishikawa K, Heo SJ, Goto M, Furuichi Y, Shimamoto A. 2001 Werner helicase relocates into nuclear foci in response to DNA damaging agents and co-localizes with RPA and Rad51. Genes Cells 6:421–430.
242. Franchitto A, Pichierri P. 2002 Bloom's syndrome protein is required for correct relocalization of RAD50/MRE11/NBS1 complex after replication fork arrest. J Cell Biol 157:19–30.
243. Li B, Comai L. 2000 Functional interaction between Ku and the Werner syndrome protein in DNA end processing. J Biol Chem 275:39800.
244. Brosh RM Jr, Bohr VA. 2002 Roles of the Werner syndrome protein in pathways required for maintenance of genome stability. Exp Gerontol 37:491–506.
245. Sun M, Duann P, Lin CT, Zhang H, Liu LF. 2000 Rapid chromatin reorganization induced by topoisomerase I-mediated DNA damage. Ann N Y Acad Sci 922: 340–342.
246. Citterio E, Van Den Boom V, Schnitzler G, et al. 2000 ATP-Dependent chromatin remodeling by the cockayne syndrome B DNA repair-transcription-coupling factor. Mol Cell Biol 20:7643–7653.
247. Redon C, Pilch D, Rogakou E, Sedelnikova O, Newrock K, Bonner W. 2002 Histone H2A variants H2AX and H2AZ. Curr Opin Genet Dev 12:162–169.
248. Furuta T, Takemura H, Liao ZY, et al. 2003 Phosphorylation of histone H2AX and activation of Mre11, Rad50, and Nbs1 in response to replication-dependent DNA double-strand breaks induced by mammalian DNA topoisomerase 1 cleavage complexes. J Biol Chem 278:20303–20312.
249. Slichenmyer WJ, Nelson WG, Slebos RJ, Kastan MB. 1993 Loss of a *p53*-associated G1 checkpoint does not increase cell survival following DNA damage. Cancer Res 53:4164–4168.
250. Gupta M, Fan S, Zhan Q, Kohn KW, O'Connor PM, Pommier Y. 1997 Inactivation of p53 increases the cytotoxicity of camptothecin in human colon HCT116 and breast MCF-7 cancer cells. Clin Cancer Res 3:1653–1660.

251. Canman CE, Wolff AC, Chen C-H, Fornace AJ, Kastan MB. 1994 The p53-dependent cell cycle checkpoint pathway and ataxia-telangiectasia. Cancer Res 54:5054–5058.
252. Saito H, Grompe M, Neeley TL, Jakobs PM, Moses RE. 1994 Fanconi anemia cells have a normal gene structure for topoisomerase I. Hum Genet 93:583–586.
253. Poot M, Hoehn H. 1993 DNA topoisomerases and the DNA lesion in human genetic instability syndromes. Toxicol Lett 67:297–308.
254. Rosselli F, Duchaud E, Averbeck D, Moustacchi E. 1994 Comparison of the effects of DNA topoisomerase inhibitors on lymphoblasts from normal and Fanconi anemia donors. Mutation Res 325:137–144.
255. Taniguchi T, Dandrea AD. 2002 Molecular pathogenesis of fanconi anemia. Int J Hematol 75:123–128.
256. Komatsu K, Miyashita T, Hang H, et al. 2000 Human homologue of S. pombe Rad9 interacts with BCL-2/BCL-xL and promotes apoptosis. Nat Cell Biol 2:1–6.
257. Komatsu K, Hopkins KM, Lieberman HB, Wang H. 2000 Schizosaccharomyces pombe Rad9 contains a BH3-like region and interacts with the anti-apoptotic protein Bcl-2. FEBS Lett 481:122–126.
258. Kharbanda S, Ren R, Pandey P, et al. 1995 Activation of the c-Abl tyrosine kinase in the stress response to DNA-damaging agents. Nature 376:785–788.
259. Jin S, Kharbanda S, Mayer B, Kufe D, Weaver DT. 1997 Binding of Ku and c-Abl at the kinase homology region of DNA-dependent protein kinase catalytic subunit. J Biol Chem 272:24763–24766.
260. Baskaran R, Wood LD, Whitaker LL, et al. 1997 Ataxia telangiectasia mutant protein activates c-Abl tyrosine kinase in response to ionizing radiation. Nature 387:516–519.
261. Shafman T, Khanna KK, Kedar P, et al. 1997 Interaction between ATM protein and c-Abl in response to DNA damage. Nature 387:520–523.
262. Yoshida K, Komatsu K, Wang HG, Kufe D. 2002 c-Abl tyrosine kinase regulates the human Rad9 checkpoint protein in response to DNA damage. Mol Cell Biol 22:3292–3300.
263. Chen G, Yuan SS, Liu W, et al. 1999 Radiation-induced assembly of Rad51 and Rad52 recombination complex requires ATM and c-Abl. J Biol Chem 274: 12748–12752.
264. Yuan ZM, Huang Y, Ishiko T, et al. 1998 Regulation of Rad51 function by c-Abl in response to DNA damage. J Biol Chem 273:3799–3802.
265. Han Z, Wei W, Dunaway S, et al. 2002 Role of p21 in apoptosis and senescence of human colon cancer cells treated with camptothecin. J Biol Chem 277:17154–17160.
266. Walton MI, Whysong D, O'Connor PM, Hockenbery D, Korsmeyer SJ, Kohn KW. 1993 Constitutive expression of human Bcl-2 modulates nitrogen mustard and camptothecin induced apoptosis. Cancer Res 53:1853–1861.

5 Biochemical and Genetic Analyses of DNA Topoisomerase 1-Mediated DNA Damage

Robert C. A. M. van Waardenburg, PhD
and Mary-Ann Bjornsti, PhD

CONTENTS

1. INTRODUCTION

Eukaryotic DNA topoisomerase 1 (Top1) is a highly conserved enzyme that catalyzes changes in the linkage of DNA strands (reviewed in refs.*1–3*). Such changes in DNA topology are important during cellular processes involving DNA, including DNA replication, recombination, transcription, and chromosome condensation *(1–3)*. The monomeric Top1 enzyme, encoded by the *Top1* gene, binds to duplex DNA and catalyzes the transient cleavage and relegation of a single DNA strand. This is achieved by the nucleophilic attack of the active site tyrosine on a DNA phosphodiester bond to generate a phosphotyrosyl linkage between the enzyme and the 3'-end of the nicked DNA. The formation of this enzyme-linked nick allows for the rotation of the noncovalently held DNA end around phosphodiester bonds in the nonscissile strand to effect changes in DNA linking number. In

Camptothecins in Cancer Therapy
Edited by: V. R. Adams and T. G. Burke © Humana Press Inc., Totowa, NJ

a second transesterification reaction, the 5'OH DNA end attacks the phosphotyrosyl bond to restore the phosphodiester backbone bond and liberate the enzyme. The formation of a covalent Top1p-DNA complex is the hallmark of topoisomerase-catalyzed reactions and acts to conserve the energy of the cleaved DNA bond such that the concerted nicking and relegation of DNA stands does not require an exogenous energy source, such as adenosine triphosphate (ATP). The type IB enzymes, such as eukaryotic Top1, are distinct from type IA and type II enzymes in the formation of a 3'-phosphotyrosyl bond. Recent structural insights suggest mechanistic similarities between type IB enzymes and tyrosine recombinases, such as Cre and Int, which also form a covalent linkage with a 3'-phosphoryl DNA end *(4,5)*.

2. TOP1 POISONS

Several cancer chemotherapeutics interfere with the catalytic cycle of DNA Top1 and reversibly stabilize the covalent Top1-DNA intermediate (reviewed in refs. *6–8*). Camptothecin (CPT) is a plant alkaloid identified in a screen for natural products with antitumor activity initiated by the National Cancer Institute in the 1960s *(9)*. Subsequent studies determined that the cytotoxic activity of this novel agent derived from its ability to reversibly inhibit the resolution of the covalent Top1–DNA complex. Although the levels of ternary CPT–Top1–DNA complexes are relatively constant throughout the cell cycle, at pharmacologically achievable drug concentrations, CPT-induced toxicity is highly S-phase–dependent *(10)*. Numerous studies indicate irreversible DNA lesions are formed after the collision of advancing replication forks with these drug-enzyme–DNA complexes leading to cell cycle arrest and ultimately cell death *(6,7,10)*.

The camptothecin analogs, topotecan and the pro-drug CPT-11 (irinotecan), have significant activity against adult and pediatric solid tumors (reviewed in *[9,11,12]*). Additional analogs, DX 8951f, DRF-1042, and several liposomal formulations, are in Phase I/II trials. In addition, there has been considerable interest in the development of structurally distinct Top1 poisons as chemotherapeutic agents. For example, indolocarbazole derivatives, such as NB-506 *(13)*, are being evaluated in clinical trials, whereas other compounds, such as triazachrysenes *(14)*, are the subjects of preclinical investigation. Although Top1 has emerged as an important cellular target for drug development, significant questions remain concerning the cytotoxic mechanism of novel Top1 poisons and whether the enzyme constitutes the cellular target of these agents. As detailed in the following section, the use of model systems and isogenic cell lines have provided compelling data supporting Top1 as the relevant cellular target of the CPTs *(7,8,15,16)*. Recent studies also indicate the cytotoxic activity of the indolocarbazole derivative, rebeccamycin R-3, is a direct consequence of Top1 poisoning and requires Top1 transesterification catalytic activity *(17)*. This is in contrast to another indolocarbazole, NB-506, which appears to have cytotoxic activities in addition to Top1 poisoning *(18)*. Whether this is a consequence of specific alterations in indolocarbazole substituents or interactions with Top1–DNA complexes has yet to be resolved. Nevertheless, these studies highlight the utility of model systems in clarifying the mechanism of drug action.

3. YEAST AS A MODEL SYSTEM

In *Drosophila* and mouse models, the *TOP1* gene is essential during early embryonic development *(19,20)*. Consequently, it has not been possible to develop isogenic, untransformed cell lines that are homozygous $TOP1^{+/+}$ or $TOP1^{-/-}$ to investigate the cytotoxic mechanism of drugs that target Top1. In contrast, the *TOP1* gene is nonessential in the budding yeast *Saccharomyces cerevisiae (21)*.Yeast cells deleted for *TOP1* (*top1*Δ) are viable because of the presence of other cellular functions that compensate for the loss of Top1 activity *(22)*. For example, DNA topoisomerase II can maintain the viability of *top1*Δ yeast cells *(21)*. However, because this type II enzyme is not sensitive to CPT, the use of isogenic *TOP1* and *top1*? strains have been used to demonstrate the selective cytotoxicity of this Top1 poison *(23–25)*.

The yeast system has been extensively used to investigate complex biological processes that have proven intractable in higher eukaryotes (for reviews *see* refs. *15,26–32*). The well-developed genetics and extensive literature regarding specific gene functions provide a rich resource for investigations of drug action at the cellular level. For example, mitotically stable plasmids are available that can be stably maintained in low (ARS/CEN vectors) or high copy number (2 µm-based vectors) *(33,34)*. These shuttle vectors contain selectable markers to ensure their continued maintenance in yeast cells and sequences necessary for amplification in bacteria. This is complemented by a series of well-characterized constitutive or inducible promoters for gene expression. The yeast *TOP1* promoter (termed Sc) is a relatively weak promoter expressed constitutively throughout the cell cycle, whereas pGPD is a strong constitutive promoter. In contrast, the pGAL1 promoter is repressed in media containing dextrose, but induced to express at high levels in the presence of galactose.

Another advantage of yeast derives from the relatively high frequency of homologous recombination, in comparison with other eukaryotic cell systems *(35)*. This coupled with extensively annotated, public genome sequence database (such as the *Saccharomyces* Genome Database [SGD] and the YPD *[36,37]*), allows for polymerase chain reaction–based, one-step gene disruptions or DNA insertions to any site within the genome.

The derivation of heterothallic haploid strains of opposite mating type also simplifies the construction of isogenic haploid strains with which to investigate the phenotypic consequences of genetic alterations and identify cellular processes that modulate drug sensitivity. After sporulation of diploid cells, the meiotic haploid products can be dissected, recovered, and screened for the appropriate combination of genetic markers *(38)*. Thus it is possible to screen mutagenized yeast cells for a specific phenotype (such as CPT resistance), backcross the individual mutant strains to define single-gene defects, and isolate the corresponding wild-type allele by complementation of the mutant phenotype after transformation with a plasmid-based genomic DNA library *(15,39–41)*. The scarcity and limited size of introns within the yeast genome allows for the direct isolation of complementary gene sequences from DNA libraries where the entire genome is equally represented, rather than relying on cDNA libraries that are skewed toward expressed gene sequences.

*top1*Δ yeast cells are resistant to CPT. However, the introduction of plasmid-encoded yeast *TOP1* or human *TOP1* cDNA sequences was sufficient to restore cell sensitivity to CPT *(23–25)*. Moreover, drug-induced cytotoxicity required the expression of a catalytically active enzyme, because mutation of the active site tyrosine to phenylalanine abrogated enzyme catalysis and CPT sensitivity *(42)*. These data established Top1 as the cellular target of CPT and its analogs and further indicate that cell killing results from the conversion of a nonessential enzyme into cellular poison via the stabilization of the covalent Top1–DNA intermediate.

A potential drawback of this system is the relative impermeability of yeast cells to a wide range of drugs, in part because of the expression of transporter families such as the ATP binding cassette (ABC) transporters and major facilitator superfamily of transporters *(43,44)*. Yeast cell permeability to select agents can be enhanced by deletion of the *ERG6* gene, which alters lipid membrane composition, and, consequently, drug uptake/efflux or by deletion of the Pdr1p and Pdr3p transcriptional regulators of the pleiotropic drug resistance pathway that includes ABC transporters *(41,45,46)*. An alternative approach is to overexpress Top1, at levels tolerated by repair proficient yeast strains, to increase the intracellular concentration of the drug target *(42,47)*. A third option is to use repair defective strains, with the implicit assumption that the specific repair pathway deleted plays a critical role in protecting cells from drug-induced DNA lesions *(25)*. In the event that the cytotoxic mechanism of a given agent is unknown, a survey of isogenic strains defective in specific repair pathways may provide important mechanistic insights into drug action. One example is the enhanced sensitivity of *rad52*Δ strains to CPT *(23,25)*. Although Top1 is the cellular target of CPT, homologous recombination is clearly required for the repair of DNA lesion(s) induced by Top1 poisoning. Similar results have recently been obtained with the indolocarbazole, rebeccamycin R-3 *(17)*.

As detailed in the following section, the yeast system can also be exploited to investigate the effects of specific amino acid substitutions on Top1 catalysis and drug sensitivity and to define the cellular processes that function in the formation, recognition, and repair of DNA damage induced by Top1 poisons.

4. *top1* MUTANTS

The crystal structures of a catalytically active 70-kDa fragment of human DNA Top1 in noncovalent and covalent complexes with DNA have been reported *(48–50)*. Similar to other topoisomerases, the type IB enzyme forms a protein clamp that completely circumscribes the duplex DNA substrate. Opposing "lip" domains interact with each other and the DNA to effect clamp closure. The tight packing of DNA within these structures suggests dramatic domainal movements are necessary to effect DNA binding and possibly to allow strand rotation after DNA cleavage. Indeed, this question has recently been addressed in studies in which different lip domain residues were substituted by cysteines to induce the formation of a disulfide crosslink to lock the Top1 protein clamp *(51,52)*, with distinct effects on DNA rotation. Because the crosslinks were formed at different positions within the Top1-clamp, it appears that rather subtle changes in protein architecture can have profoundly distinct effects on enzyme catalysis. However, expression of the catalytically inactive Top1Y723F-clamp sufficed to induce cell death in yeast strains engineered to express elevated levels of oxidized glutathione *(52)*. This suggests a novel mechanism of Top1 poisoning reminiscent of ICRF-187 poisoning of DNA topoisomerase II *(53,54)*.

The core domains that constitute the clamp and comprise the active site of the enzyme are highly conserved at the amino acid level between yeast and human Top1 *(1–3)*. The N-terminal domains, for which no structural information is available, are quite divergent in sequence, yet exhibit a similar content of basic residues. In both cases, the N-terminal domain is dispensable for catalytic activity *(55,56)*, although recent studies suggest N-terminal residues modulate DNA binding and may suppress enzyme-mediated DNA strand transfers *(57,58)*. The linker regions that connect the protein clamp with the active site tyrosine domain also exhibit significant differences in length and sequence, yet are predicted to form two extended alpha helices.

Amino acid substitutions known to affect Top1 sensitivity to CPT are mostly clustered along one face of the enzyme that makes contact with the DNA *(48,49)*. The structure of the enzyme-DNA intermediate complexed with the CPT analog topotecan was recently reported *(59)*. The structure confirms an intercalative mode of drug binding with additional contacts formed with specific enzyme residues or mediated through water molecules. Within the active site of the enzyme, remarkably few residues make direct contacts with the DNA. However, these structures highlight the dramatic alterations in linker domain flexibility that accompanies drug binding *(60)*. This is consistent with recent studies of a human Top1 mutant in which alterations in linker domain flexibility reduced enzyme sensitivity to CPT *(61)*.

As *top1*Δ yeast strains are viable and CPT resistant, the effects of specific amino acid substitutions on enzyme catalysis, cell viability, and drug sensitivity can be assessed in the absence of endogenous wild-type Top1. Although Top1 mutations have been identified in yeast and in mammalian cell lines selected for CPT resistance (for example, *see* refs. *18,42,47,61–71)*, Top1 mutations have not emerged as a mechanism of CPT resistance in clinical samples. Nevertheless, the analysis of Top1 mutant activities has provided important information regarding enzyme mechanism and how interfering with Top1 catalysis can induce cytotoxic lesions.

In our studies, some of which are summarized in Table 1, specific residues in yeast or human Top1 were mutated in p*GAL1*-promoted vectors, and the vectors were transformed into repair proficient *top1*Δ strains *(17,42,47, 66,67,69,72)*. Individual transformants were grown in dextrose-containing media (to suppress p*GAL1* expression) and then induced to express the mutant *top1* allele with galactose. Using this approach, we have defined several mutations around the active site tyrosine in yeast and human Top1 that abolish the catalytic activity of the enzyme (yeast Top1Y727F, human Top1Y723F) or that render the enzyme CPT resistant without demonstrable changes in enzyme specific activity (yeast and human Top1vac, yeast Top1N726S, human Top1N722S proteins). The Asn722 to Ser substitution was previously selected in a drug-treated human cell line *(71)*. Additional mutations produce alterations in enzyme activity and CPT sensitivity, such as the yeast Top1N726D and TopN726L mutant enzymes. More surprising was the identification of single amino acid substitutions that alter the stability of the covalent enzyme-DNA intermediate and are able to induce cell lethality in the absence of CPT *(66,69,72)*. These include yeast Top1T722A, yeast Top1N726H, and yeast Top1N726D. Analogous substitutions of the conserved Thr718 and Asn722 residues in human Top1 produce similar alterations in enzyme catalysis *(17,67)*.

One remarkable aspect of this work is the finding that single residue changes can have such dramatic and diverse effects on Top1 enzymology, DNA binding, and drug sensitivity. For example, substituents of the conserved Asn residue immediately N-terminal to the active site Tyr produce distinct mechanism of Top1 poisoning that result from specific alterations in the DNA cleavage-relegation equilibrium. Relative to wild-type Top1, the Top1N726H mutant enzyme exhibits an enhanced rate of DNA cleavage in assays using suicide DNA substrates, with little change in specific activity *(69)*. In contrast, the introduction of an Asp residue at this position (in

Table 1
DNA Topoisomerase 1 Mutants

TOP1 allele	*Active site residues*	*Camptothecin sensitivity*	*Cell viability*	*Reference*
TOP1	Thr Ser Lys Ile Asn **Tyr**$_{727yeast}$ Leu $_{723human}$			*24,39, 42,72a*
top1T-A	Ala	**S**	**Lethal**	*66,67,72*
top1vac	ArgAla	**CPT^R**	—	*42,47,72a*
top1N-H	His	**S**	**Lethal**	*17,69*
top1N-S	Ser	**CPT^R**	—	*17,69,72a*
top1Y-F	Phe	**CPT^R**	—	*42,69,72a*
top1N726D	Asp	**CPT^R**	**Lethal**	*17,69*
top1N726L	Leu	**CPT^R**	—	*42,72a*

Wild-type and mutant *top1* alleles are listed on the left. The wild-type Top1 sequence is shown at the top, with the single or double amino acid changes listed below the wild-type residue. The active site of yeast Top1 is Tyr727 and human Top1 is Tyr 723. in the case of mutations engineered into yeast and human Top1, the specific residue numbers are deleted in the allele designation. Alterations in Top1N726Dp andTop1N726L mutant enzyme activity and cell viability are described for yeast *top1* mutants only. Enzyme sensitivity to camptothecin (CPT) was assesses in DNA cleavage assays with purified proteins. S indicates comparable levels of CPT-stabilizes enzyme-DNA complexes to that obtained with the respective wild-type enzyme, whereas CPT^R indicates diminished mutant *top1*-DNA complex formation. Mutant enzyme-induced cell lethality in the absence of CPT was assayed in *top1Δ* cells transformed with an ARS/CEN vector expressing the indicates yeast or human *top1* allele from the pGAL promoter in galactose-containing media. Viability was scored by the number of cells forming colonies. —, no effect on cell number.

Top1N726D) reduces the affinity of the enzyme for DNA. On formation of the covalent complex, the defect in DNA binding becomes localized to the noncovalently held 5' end of the cleaved DNA *(69)*, which adversely affects DNA relegation. Both of these alterations in enzyme catalysis are distinct from the action of CPT, which specifically inhibits DNA relegation with no detectable effects on DNA binding. A similar mechanism of Top1 poisoning is also evident in the Top1T722A mutant enzyme, where substitution of Ala for the conserved Th722 residue appears to mimic CPT by reducing the rate of DNA relegation, without affecting DNA binding or cleavage in vitro *(66,72)* (Colley WC, van der Merwe M, Vance JR, Burgin A, Bjornsti MA, unpublished results).

Because each of these "self-poisoning" Top1 mutant enzymes appears to directly or indirectly increase the stability of the covalent complex, the prediction would be that they also induce similar DNA lesions as CPT during S-phase and have similar effects on cell cycle progression, checkpoint activation, and cell death. Indeed, overexpression of either yeast Top1T722A or the analogous human mutant, Top1T718Ap, in *top1Δ* yeast cells induces a terminal phenotype indistinguishable from CPT-treated cells expressing wild-type Top1 *(67,72)*. Low levels of Top1T722A expression also induces hyperrecombination among the tandemly repeated rDNA sequences, as do sublethal concentrations of CPT *(72)*. Ectopic expression of yeast Top1T722A in COS cells also induces apoptosis, consistent with the cytotoxic mechanism of CPT *(73)*. Thus the in vivo and biochemical characterizations of Top1T722A activity indicate this mutant enzyme acts as a CPT mimetic.

The Top1N726H and Top1N726D mutant enzymes also induce similar terminal phenotypes in yeast *(69)*; however, isogenic mutant yeast strains that exhibit enhanced sensitivity to CPT and Top1T722A do not necessarily exhibit similar responses to Top1N726H (Colley WC, van der Merwe M, Bjornsti M-A, unpublished results). These data suggest that distinct alterations in Top1 catalysis may induce different patterns of DNA lesions and, consequently, cellular responses. Additional support for this model comes from more recent experiments with the double Top1T722A,N726H mutant enzyme. Here, the combination of the two mutations in a single enzyme potentiates the cytotoxic activity of the mutant protein to yield greater than additive cell kill (Colley WC, van der Merwe M, Bjornsti M-A, unpublished results). These data further suggest that both mechanisms of Top1 poisoning can occur in the context of a single molecule, which raises the intriguing possibility that structurally diverse Top1 poisons can be used in combination therapy to achieve enhanced antitumor activity.

These mutants also provide valuable reagents with which to investigate structural aspects of drug-enzyme interactions, particularly with regard to non-CPT Top1p poisons. For example, although the mutant enzymes summarized in Table 1 exhibit varying levels of sensitivity and resistance to CPT, they all exhibit enhanced covalent complex stability in the presence of the rebeccamycin indolocarbazole, R-3, in DNA cleavage assays *(17)*. In particular, the yeast Top1N726S mutant enzyme, which is resistant to CPT in DNA cleavage assays and in yeast cells, is hypersensitive to rebeccamycin R-3, both in vitro and in vivo. These data suggest that structural features of the Top1 active site necessary for effective CPT binding are distinct from those required for the productive interaction of rebeccamycin R-3. Whether this translates into enhanced antitumor activity when both agents are used in combination therapy has yet to be determined.

5. CELLULAR RESPONSES TO TOP1 POISONS

Numerous studies have established that Top1 poisoning by CPTs is required for the cytotoxic action of this class of chemotherapeutics. However, other factors can modulate cellular responses to Top1 poisons by affecting the levels of CPT-induced DNA damage, the recognition or repair of Top1-DNA lesions, or cell cycle progression in the presence of such DNA damage *(6–8,10,41)*. For example, homologous recombination appears to be required for the effective repair of Top1–DNA lesions, as yeast strains defective for the recombinational repair of DNA breaks, because of the deletion of the *RAD52* gene, are hypersensitive to CPT *(23–25)*. DNA damage checkpoints also modulate cell survival after Top1 poisoning, because yeast cells deleted for the *RAD9* DNA damage checkpoint exhibit enhanced cell killing in response to CPT (in the presence of wild-type Top1) or expression of the self-poisoning Top1T722A mutant enzyme *(46,67,72)*. Yet, in contrast to rather extensive investigations of drug effects on Top1 catalysis, considerably less is known about the specific cellular processes involved in the formation and repair of drug-induced Top1–DNA lesions.

Because the phenotypic consequences of CPT action are faithfully reiterated in yeast, we have developed several genetic screens to identify gene products, other than Top1, that influence cell sensitivity to CPT *(15)*. Initially, *top1Δ* cells expressing wild-type *TOP1* from a plasmid-borne *GAL1* promoter were mutagenized and screened for CPT resistance on galactose-containing media *(39)*. To eliminate vector-based *top1* mutants and trivial mutations affecting *GAL1* promoter function, the resistant colonies were cured of the original vector and rescreened for CPT resistance with a plasmid that constitutively expresses *TOP1*. This approach identified several dominant mutations that mapped to the *PDR1* gene, which encodes a transcription factor that regulates the expression of a large family of ABC transporters in the pleiotropic drug resistance network *(45)*. These membrane- spanning proteins can transport a wide variety of small molecules through plasma membranes, and their increased expression has been linked with cellular drug resistance *(43,44)*. Subsequent genetic analyses of the *PDR1* dominant mutants revealed that the greater than 1000-fold resistance to CPT resulted primarily from the increased expression of the Snq2 transporter *(45)*. Even at physiological levels, this transporter conferred some protection against CPT-induced lethality. However, because ABC transporters are rather promiscuous in terms of substrate specificity, overexpression of the closely related Pdr5 transporter also induced a CPT-resistant phenotype *(45)*.

At the time of these studies, ABC transporters had not been shown to play a significant role in human cell resistance to CPTs. Consequently, we posited that similar, as yet unidentified ABC transporters would affect CPT analog efflux from human cells *(45)*. This prediction was borne out by the identification of a new ABC transporter, BCRP, in ovarian cell lines selected for resistance to topotecan or mitoxantrone and in multidrug-resistant MCF-7/AdrVp cells *(74,75)*. BCRP is a half transporter, similar to the *Drosophila* white and brown transporters and the yeast Snq2 and Pdr5 transporters, that effectively effluxes the CPT analogs, TPT, and CPT-11 *(16,75,76)*.

Although mechanisms of drug uptake and efflux are important, these initial yeast screens failed to reveal downstream events occurring after stabilization of the covalent complex. Moreover, upregulation of drug efflux pathways would obfuscate the analysis of any alterations in these processes. To circumvent issues of drug transport, a genetic screen was designed to identify conditional mutants that exhibit enhanced sensitivity to the self-poisoning Top1T722A mutant enzyme at the nonpermissive temperature of 35°C *(8,40)*. Constitutive low levels of this mutant enzyme mimicked sublethal doses of CPT. In repair-proficient, checkpoint-competent yeast strains, sufficient DNA damage was induced to elicit a hyperrecombination phenotype with little effect on overall cell survival *(8,40)*. In contrast, yeast cells defective for homologous recombination (*rad52Δ* strains) or the *RAD9* DNA damage checkpoint (*rad9Δ* strains) were unable to tolerate even low levels of the Top1T722A enzyme.

Using this approach, yeast mutants were isolated that exhibited temperature sensitive lethality in the presence of Top1T722A. Further characterization of these *tah* mutants (for *top1T722A* hypersensitive) identified nine *TAH* genes that normally function to protect cells from Top1–induced DNA damage *(8,40)*. The *tah* mutants were viable at 26°C, yet exhibited a greater than 3-log drop in cell viability at 35°C in the presence of Top1T722Ap. Isogenic *tah* mutant strains also demonstrated similar patterns of temperature sensitivity to CPT, when expressing wild-type Top1, and to DNA replication inhibition by hydroxyurea, in the absence of Top1. The *tah* mutants exhibited varying levels of sensitivity to other DNA damaging agents such as methylmethane sulfonate (MMS) and ultraviolet light. Nevertheless, the pattern of *tah* mutant hypersensitivity to Top1T722A, CPT and hydroxyurea at 35°C and the terminal phenotypes observed under these conditions were consistent with S-phase induced lethality.

Complementation of the *tah* mutant phenotypes with a single-copy vector-based yeast genomic DNA library identified the wild-type *TAH* alleles. Despite a common cytotoxic response to CPT or the self-poisoning Top1T722A mutant enzyme, the *TAH* genes represent an extremely diverse group of cellular processes *(8,40)*. These include DNA replication (*TAH11*, *CDC45*, *DPB11*), ubiquitin-mediated proteolysis (*DOA4*), Smt3 (SUMO)-conjugation (*UBC9*), transcription (*TAF47*), cortical actin organization (*SLA1*, *SLA2*), and a gene of unknown function (*TAH18*). Although the mechanism by which each of these gene products protects cells from Top1–induced DNA damage is the subject of ongoing experimentation, the results of several studies have begun to reveal the involvement of common pathways.

Cdc45 is required for initiation of chromosomal DNA replication and functions to recruit DNA polymerase α *(77,78)*. Dpb11 also has an essential function in DNA replication *(79)*. It physically interacts with DNA polymerase ε and is required for the S-phase checkpoint. The *cdc45-10* and *dpb11-10* mutant alleles identified in the *tah* screen retain sufficient function to remain viable at 35°C in the absence of DNA damage, yet, both single mutants exhibit a slight delay in early S-phase that corresponds with a transient accumulation of Okazaki-sized DNA fragments *(40)*. In contrast, the double *cdc45-10, dpb11-10* mutant is inviable at 35°C, even in the absence of a DNA damaging agent *(40)*. This synthetic lethal phenotype indicates the proteins share a common essential function. The persistent accumulation of Okazaki-sized DNA fragments in the double mutant and the rapid drop in cell viability that accompanies cell-cycle transit through S-phase suggests a defect in processive DNA synthesis. In the presence of Top1T722A, the accumulation of Okazaki fragments behind the replication fork may preclude the effective repair of DNA lesions produced by the collision of the advancing replication fork with the Top1T722A-DNA complexes. A similar cytotoxic mechanism would apply to CPT–Top1–DNA complexes. In both cases, the stability of the replication fork and the integrity of the newly replicated strands may be required for the effective repair of the Top1p-DNA lesions (*see* ref. *80* for discussion of repair and DNA synthesis).

More recent studies with two additional *tah* mutant strains, *doa4-10*, and *sla1-10*, indicate a synthetic lethal interaction of these mutants at the nonpermissive temperature in the absence of Top1 poisoning *(81)*. The nonessential *DOA4* gene encodes a C-terminal ubiquitin hydrolase that associates with the 26S proteasome and recycles ubiquitin from proteins targeted for proteolytic degradation *(82,83)*. Although Doa4 is not required for cell viability, the resultant decrease in free ubiquitin pools induces a wide range of conditional phenotypes. *SLA1* is also not essential for cell viability, yet plays an important role in the reorganization of cortical actin patches during the cell cycle *(84)*. Results obtained with single and double *doa4-10/sla1-10* mutants reveal a genetic interaction between the organization of the actin cytoskeleton, ubiquitin-mediated proteolysis, and cellular responses to Top1 poisons. In particular, the actin cytoskeletal defects in *doa4-10* or *sla1-10* cells arrested in late S-phase, in response to Top1–DNA lesions, render the cells extremely fragile and prone to cell lysis *(81)*. This is also evident in the double *doa4-10, sla1-10* mutants at high temperature in the absence of DNA damage. In the case of *doa4-10*, a specific defect in *RAD9* DNA damage checkpoint responses also appear to contribute to the enhanced sensitivity of these cells to Top1-T722A.

The characterization of extragenic mutations that complement *doa4-10* mutant cell sensitivity to Top1T722A-induced DNA damage will define the specific cellular functions that are altered by the loss of Doa4 function and that normally protect cells from Top1 poisons. Similar genetic analyses of extragenic suppressors of other *tah* mutant are also under way. A complementary approach is to identify gene products that complement specific *tah* mutant phenotypes when overexpressed from a high-copy vector. The characterization of these high-copy suppressors, in conjunction with the related analysis of extragenic mutations that also restore *tah* mutant cell resistance to Top1 poisons, will continue to define the pathways required for the recognition and repair of the DNA lesions induced by CPT. The function of related human *TAH* genes in modulating untransformed and transformed cell sensitivity to CPT analogs is also being addressed using siRNA technology. These combined approaches will determine the extent to which mechanisms of CPT-induced cytotoxicity are conserved from yeast to human.

Additional efforts are under way to investigate the novel mechanism of human Top1Y723F–clamp-induced lethality *(52)*. The lack of an S-phase terminal phenotype suggests the formation of replication-independent cytotoxic lesions, which may also be exploited in the development of non-camptothecin Top1 poisons.

ACKNOWLEDGMENTS

This work has been supported, in part, by National Institute of Health grants CA58755 and CA23099 project 2 (to M-AB), CA21675 Cancer center grant, and ALSAC. We wish to thank our friend and collaborator, Piero Benedetti, and present and past members of the Bjornsti lab for their contributions to this work. In particular, we thank William C. Colley, Paola Fiorani, Hervé Jacquiau, Cynthia Lancaster, Nabil Matmati, Komaraiah Palle, Changxian Shen, Marie van der Merwe, and Michael Woo for helpful discussions and Alice Gibson, Hong Guo, Andrew Larkin, and Padma Thimmaiah for their expert technical assistance.

REFERENCES

1. Champoux JJ. 2001 DNA topoisomerases: structure, function, and mechanism. Annu Rev Biochem 70:369–413.
2. Keck JL, Berger JM. 1999 Enzymes that push DNA around. Nat Struct Biol 6: 900–902.
3. Wang JC. 2002 Cellular roles of DNA topoisomerases: a molecular perspective. Nat Rev Mol Cell Biol 3:430–440.
4. Woodfield G, Cheng C, Shuman S, Burgin AB. 2000 Vaccinia topoisomerase and Cre recombinase catalyze direct ligation of activated DNA substrates containing a 3'-para-nitrophenyl phosphate ester. Nucleic Acids Res 28:3323–3331.
5. Krogh BO, Shuman S. 2000 Catalytic mechanism of DNA topoisomerase IB. Mol Cell 5:1035–1041.

6. Li TK, Liu LF. 2001 Tumor cell death induced by topoisomerase-targeting drugs. Annu Rev Pharmacol Toxicol 41:53–77.
7. Kohn K, Pommier Y. 2000 Molecular and biological determinants of the cytotoxic actions of camptothecins. Perspective for the development of new topoisomerase I inhibitors. Ann NY Acad Sci 922:11–26.
8. Fiorani P, Bjornsti M-A. 2000 Mechanisms of DNA topoisomerase I-induced cell killing in the yeast *Saccharomyces cerevisiae*. Ann N Y Acad Sci 922:65–75.
9. Arbuck SG, Takimoto CH. 1998 An overview of topoisomerase I-targeting agents. Semin Hematol 35:3–12.
10. Kaufmann SH. 1998 Cell death induced by topoisomerase-targeted drugs: more questions than answers. BBA 1400:195–212.
11. Rodriguez-Galindo C, Radomski K, Stewart CF, Furman W, Santana VM, Houghton PJ. 2000 Clinical use of topoisomerase I inhibitors in anticancer treatment. Med Pediatr Oncol 35:385–402.
12. Pizzolato JF, Saltz LB. 2003 The camptothecins. Lancet 361:2235–2242.
13. Bailly C. 2000 Topoisomerase I poisons and suppressors as anticancer drugs. Curr Med Chem 7:39–58.
14. Ruchelman AL, Singh SK, Wu X, et al. 2002 Diaza- and triazachrysenes: potent topoisomerase-targeting agents with exceptional antitumor activity against the human tumor xenograft, MDA-MB-435. Bioorg Med Chem Lett 12:3333–3336.
15. Bjornsti M-A. 2002 Cancer therapeutics in yeast. Cancer Cell 2:267–273.
16. Benedetti P, Benchokroun Y, Houghton PJ, Bjornsti M-A. 1998 Analysis of camptothecin resistance in yeast: relevance to cancer. Drug Res Updates 1:176–183.
17. Woo MH, Vance JR, Marcos AR, Bailly C, Bjornsti M-A. 2002 Active site mutations in DNA topoisomerase I distinguish the cytotoxic activities of camptothecin and the indolocarbazole, rebeccamycin. J Biol Chem 277:3813–3822.
18. Urasaki Y, Laco G, Takebayashi Y, Bailly C, Kohlhagen G, Pommier Y. 2001 Use of camptothecin-resistant mammalian cell lines to evaluate the role of topoisomerase I in the antiproliferative activity of the indolocarbazole, NB-506, and its topoisomerase I binding site. Cancer Res 61:504–508.
19. Lee MP, Brown SD, Chen A, Hsieh T-S. 1993 DNA topoisomerase I is essential in *Drosophila melanogaster*. Proc Natl Acad Sci USA 90:6656–6660.
20. Morham SG, Kluckman KD, Voulomanos N, Smithies O. 1996 Targeted disruption of the mouse topoisomerase I gene by camptothecin selection. Mol Cell Biol 16:6804–6809.
21. Goto T, Wang JC. 1985 Cloning of yeast TOP1, the gene encoding DNA topoisomerase I, and construction of mutants defective in both DNA topoisomerase I and DNA topoisomerase II. Proc Natl Acad Sci USA 82:7178–7182.
22. Castano IB, Heathpagliuso S, Sadoff BU, Fitzhugh DJ, Christman MF. 1996 A novel family of Trf (DNA topoisomerase I-related function) genes required for proper nuclear segregation. Nucleic Acids Res 24:2404–2410.
23. Eng W-K., Faucette L, Johnson RK, Sternglanz R. 1988 Evidence that DNA topoisomerase I is necessary for the cytotoxic effects of camptothecin. Mol Pharmacol 34:755–760.
24. Bjornsti M-A, Benedetti P, Viglianti GA, Wang JC. 1989 Expression of human DNA topoisomerase I in yeast cells lacking yeast DNA topoisomerase I: restoration of sensitivity of the cells to the antitumor drug camptothecin. Cancer Res 49:6318–6323.

25. Nitiss J, Wang JC. 1988 DNA topoisomerase-targeting antitumor drugs can be studied in yeast. Proc Natl Acad Sci USA 85:7501–7505.
26. Tissenbaum HA, Guarente L. 2002 Model organisms as a guide to mammalian aging. Dev Cell 2:9–19.
27. Wahl GM, Carr AM. 2001 The evolution of diverse biological responses to DNA damage: insights from yeast and p53. Nat Cell Biol 3:E277–E286.
28. Ma D. 2001 Applications of yeast in drug discovery. Prog Drug Res 57:117–162.
29. Cyert MS. 2001 Genetic analysis of calmodulin and its targets in *Saccharomyces cerevisiae*. Annu Rev Genet 35:647–672.
30. Shaw JD, Cummings KB, Huyer G, Michaelis S, Wendland B. 2001 Yeast as a model system for studying endocytosis. Exp Cell Res 271:1–9.
31. Kitagawa K, Hieter P. 2001 Evolutionary conservation between budding yeast and human kinetochores. Nat Rev Mol Cell Biol 2:678–687.
32. Forsburg SL. 2001 The art and design of genetic screens: yeast. Nat Rev Genet 2:659–668.
33. Sikorski RS, Hieter P. 1989 A system of shuttle vectors and yeast host strains designed for efficient manipulation of DNA in *Saccharomyces cerevisiae*. Genetics 122:19–27.
34. Schneider JC, Guarente L. 1991 Vectors for expression of cloned genes in yeast: regulation, overproduction, and underproduction. In: Methods in enzymology. Guthrie C, Fink GR, ed. Academic Press, Inc., California, 373–388.
35. Rothstein R. 1991 Targeting, disruption, replacement, and allele rescue: integrative DNA transformation in yeast. In: Methods in enzymology. Abelson JN, Simon MI, ed. Academic Press, Inc., California, 281–301.
36. Cherry J, Adler C, Ball C, et al. 1998 SGD: *Saccharomyces* genome database. Nucleic Acids Res 26:73–80.
37. Costanzo MC, Hogan JD, Cusick ME, et al. 2000 The yeast proteome database (YPD) and caenorhabditis elegans proteome database (WormPD): comprehensive resources for the organization and comparison of model organism protein information. Nucleic Acids Res 28:73–76.
38. Rose MD, Broach JD. 1991 Cloning genes by complementation in yeast. In: Methods in enzymology. Abelson JN, Simon MI, ed. Academic Press, Inc., California, 195–230
39. Kauh EA, Bjornsti M-A. 1995 *SCT1* mutants suppress the camptothecin sensitivity of yeast cells expressing wild-type DNA topoisomerase I. Proc Natl Acad Sci USA 92:6299–6303.
40. Reid RJD, Fiorani P, Sugawara M, Bjornsti M-A. 1999 *CDC45* and *DPB11* are required for processive DNA replication and resistance to DNA topoisomerase I-mediated DNA damage. Proc Natl Acad Sci USA 96:11440–11445.
41. Reid RJD, Benedetti P, Bjornsti M-A. 1998 Yeast as a model organism for studying the actions of DNA topoisomerase-targeted drugs. BBA 1400:289–300.
42. Knab AM, Fertala J, Bjornsti M-A. 1993 Mechanisms of camptothecin resistance in yeast DNA topoisomerase I mutants. J Biol Chem 268:22322–22330.
43. Bauer BE, Wolfger H, Kuchler K. 1999 Inventory and function of yeast ABC proteins: about sex, stress, pleiotropic drug and heavy metal resistance. BBA 1461:217–236.
44. Balzi E, Goffeau A. 1995 Yeast multidrug resistance: the PDR network. J Bioenerg Biomembr 27:71–76.

45. Reid RJD, Kauh EA, Bjornsti M-A. 1997 Camptothecin sensitivity is mediated by the pleiotropic drug resistance network in yeast. J Biol Chem 272:12091–12099.
46. Simon JA, Szankasi P, Nguyen DK, et al. 2000 Differential toxicities of anticancer agents among DNA repair and checkpoint mutants of *Saccharomyces cerevisiae*. Cancer Res 60:328–333.
47. Knab AM, Fertala J, Bjornsti M-A. 1995 A camptothecin-resistant DNA toposiomerase I mutant exhibits altered sensitivities to other DNA topoisomerase poisons. J Biol Chem 270:6141–6148.
48. Redinbo MR, Stewart L, Kuhn P, Champoux JJ, Hol WGJ. 1998 Crystal structures of human topoisomerase I in covalent and noncovalent complexes with DNA. Science 279:1504–1513.
49. Stewart L, Redinbo MR, Qiu X, Hol WGJ, Champoux JJ. 1998 A model for the mechanism of human topoisomerase I. Science 279:1534–1541.
50. Redinbo MR, Stewart L, Champoux JJ, Hol WGJ. 1999 Structural flexibility in human topoisomerase I revealed in multiple non-isomorphous crystal structures. J Mol Biol 292:685–696.
51. Carey JF, Schultz SJ, Sisson L, Fazzio TG, Champoux JJ. 2003 DNA relaxation by human topoisomerase I occurs in the closed clamp conformation of the protein. Proc Natl Acad Sci USA 100:5640–5645.
52. Woo MH, Lasasso C, Guo H, Pattarello L, Benedetti P, Bjornsti M-A. 2003 Locking the DNA topoisomerase I protein clamp inhibits DNA rotation and induces cell lethality. Proc Natl Acad Sci USA 100:13767–13772.
53. Roca J, Berger JM, Harrison SC, Wang JC. 1996 DNA transport by a type II topoisomerase: direct evidence for a two-gate mechanism. Proc Natl Acad Sci USA 93:4057–4062.
54. Classen S, Olland S, Berger JM. 2003 Structure of the topoisomerase II ATPase region and its mechanism of inhibition by the chemotherapeutic agent ICRF-187. Proc Natl Acad Sci USA 100:10629-10634.
55. Alsner J, Svestrup JQ, Kjeldsen E, Sorensen BS, Westergaard O. 1992 Identification of an N-terminal domain of eukaryotic DNA topoisomerase I dispensibel for catalytic activity but essential for in vivo function. J Biol Chem 267:12408–12411.
56. Bjornsti M-A, Wang JC. 1987 Expression of yeast DNA topoisomerase I can complement a conditional-lethal DNA topoisomerase I mutation in *Esherichia coli*. Proc Natl Acad Sci USA 84:8971–8975.
57. Andersen FF, Andersen KE, Kusk M, et al. 2003 Recombinogenic flap ligation mediated by human topoisomerase I. J Mol Biol 330:235–246.
58. Lisby M, Olesen JR, Skouboe C, et al. 2001 Residues within the N-terminal domain of human topoisomerase I play a direct role in relaxation. J Biol Chem 276:20220–20227.
59. Staker BL, Hjerrild K, Feese MD, Behnke CA, Burgin AB Jr, Stewart L. 2002 The mechanism of topoisomerase I poisoning by a camptothecin analog. Proc Natl Acad Sci USA 99:15387–15392.
60. Stewart L, Ireton GC, Champoux JJ. 1999 A functional linker in human topoisomerase I is required for maximum sensitivity to camptothecin in a DNA relaxation assay. J Biol Chem 274:32950–32960.
61. Fiorani P, Bruselles A, Falconi M, Chillemi G, Desideri A, Benedetti P. 2003 Single mutation in the linker domain confers protein flexibility and camptothecin resistance to human topoisomerase I. J Biol Chem 278:43268-43275.

62. Urasaki Y, Laco GS, Pourquier P, et al. 2001 Characterization of a novel topoisomerase I mutation from a camptothecin-resistant human prostate cancer cell line. Cancer Res 61:1964–1969.
63. Li XG, Haluska P, Hsiang YH, Bharti AK, Liu LF, Rubin EH. 1997 Involvement of amino acids 361 to 364 of human topoisomerase I in camptothecin resistance and enzyme catalysis. Biochem Pharm 53:1019–1027.
64. Jensen AD, Svestrup JQ. 1996 Purification and characterization of human topoisomerase I mutants. Eur J Biochem 236:389–394.
65. Rubin E, Pantazis P, Bharti A, Toppmeyer D, Giovanella B, Kufe D. 1994 Identification of a mutant human topoisomerase I with intact catalytic activity and resistance to 9-nitro-camptothecin. J Biol Chem 269:2433–2439.
66. Hann CL, Carlberg AL, Bjornsti M-A. 1998 Intragenic suppressors of mutant DNA topoisomerase I-induced lethality diminish enzyme binding of DNA. J Biol Chem 273:31519–31527.
67. Fiorani P, Amatruda JF, Silvestri A, Butler RH, Bjornsti M-A, Benedetti P. 1999 Domain interactions affecting human DNA topoisomerase I catalysis and camptothecin sensitivity. Mol Pharmacol 56:1105–1115.
68. Benedetti P, Fiorani P, Capuani L, Wang JC. 1993 Camptothecin resistance from a single mutation changing glycine 363 of human DNA topoisomerase I to cysteine. Cancer Res 53:4343–4348.
69. Fertala J, Vance JR, Pourquier P, Pommier Y, Bjornsti M-A. 2000 Substitutions of Asn-726 in the active site of yeast DNA topoisomerase I define novel mechanisms of stabilizing the covalent-enzyme DNA intermediate. J Biol Chem 275:15246–15253.
70. Fujimori A, Gupta M, Hoki Y, Pommier Y. 1996 Acquired camptothecin resistance of human breast cancer MCF-7/C4 cells with normal topoisomerase I and elevated DNA repair. Mol Pharmacol 50:1472–1478.
71. Fujimori A, Harker WG., Kohlhagen G, Hoki Y, Pommier Y. 1995 Mutation at the catalytic site of topoisomerase I in CEM/C2, a human leukemia cell line resistant to camptothecin. Cancer Res. 55:1339–1346.
72. Megonigal MD, Fertala J, Bjornsti M-A. 1997 Cell cycle arrest and lethality produced by alterations in the catalytic activity of yeast DNA topoisomerase I mutants. J Biol Chem 272:12801–12808.
72a. Lynn RM, Bjornsti M-A, Caron PR, Wang JC. 1989 Peptide sequencing and site-directed mutagenesis identify tyrosine-727 as the active site tyrosine of Saccharomyces cerevisiae DNA topoisomerase I. Proc Natl Acad Sci USA 86:3559–3563.
73. Hann C, Evans DL, Fertala J, Benedetti P, Bjornsti M-A, Hall DJ.. 1998 Increased camptothecin toxicity in mammalian cells expressing *Saccharomyces cerevisiae* DNA topoisomerase I. J Biol Chem 273:8425–8433.
74. Doyle LA, Yang W, Abruzzo LV, Krogmann T, Gao Y, Rishi AK, Ross DD. 1998 A multidrug resistance transporter from human MCF-7 breast cancer cells. Proc Natl Acad Sci USA 95:15665–15670.
75. Maliepaard M, van Gastelen MA, de Jong LA, et al. 1999 Overexpression of the BCRP/MXR/ABCP gene in a topotecan-selected ovarian tumor cell line. Cancer Res 59:4559–4563.
76. Bates SE, Robey R, Miyake K, Rao K, Ross DD, Litman T. 2001 The role of half-transporters in multidrug resistance. J Bioenerg Biomembr 33:503–511.
77. Zou L, Mitchell J, Stillman B. 1997 CDC45, a novel yeast gene that functions with the origin recognition complex and Mcm proteins in initiation of DNA replication. Mol Cell Biol 17:553–563.

78. Zou L, Stillman B. 2000 Assembly of a complex containing Cdc45p, replication protein A, and Mcm2p at replication origins controlled by S-phase cyclin-dependent kinases and Cdc7p-Dbf4p kinase. Mol Cell Biol 20:3086–3096.
79. Masumoto H, Sugino A, Araki H. 2000 Dpb11 controls the association between DNA polymerases alpha and epsilon and the autonomously replicating sequence region of budding yeast. Mol Cell Biol 20:2809–2817.
80. Nyberg KA, Michelson RJ, Putnam CW, Weinert TA. 2002 Toward maintaining the genome: DNA damage and replication checkpoints. Annu Rev Genet 36:617–656.
81. Fiorani P, Reid RJD, Schepis A, Jacquiau HR, Guo H, Thimmaiah P, et al. 2004 The deubiquitinating enzyme Doa4p protects cells from DNA topoisomerase I poisons. J Biol Chem 279:21271–21281.
82. Swaminathan S, Amerik AY, Hochstrasser M. 1999 The Doa4 deubiquitinating enzyme is required for ubiquitin homeostasis in yeast. Mol Biol Cell 10:2583–2594.
83. Papa FR, Amerik AY, Hochstrasser M. 1999 Interaction of the Doa4 deubiquitinating enzyme with the yeast 26S proteasome. Mol Biol Cell 10:741–756.
84. Ayscough KR, Eby JJ, Lila T, Dewar H, Kozminski KG, Drubin DG. 1999 Sla1p is a functionally modular component of the yeast cortical actin cytoskeleton required for correct localization of both Rho1p-GTPase and Sla2p, a protein with talin homology. Mol Biol Cell 10:1061–1075.

6 Preclinical Models for Evaluating Topoisomerase I-Targeted Drugs

Aarti S. Juvekar, PhD,
Joyce Thompson, MD,
Clinton F. Stewart, PharmD,
and Peter J. Houghton, PhD

CONTENTS

1. INTRODUCTION

Type I and II DNA topoisomerases are the targets for numerous clinically efficacious antitumor agents. Over the last decade, considerable effort has been expended in developing camptothecin (CPT) derivatives that selectively target DNA topoisomerase I (TOP-I) *(1)*. The prodrug irinotecan (CPT-11) is approved for treatment of colon carcinoma and has demonstrated significant activity against numerous other cancers in adults and

Camptothecins in Cancer Therapy
Edited by: V. R. Adams and T. G. Burke © Humana Press Inc., Totowa, NJ

children. Topotecan is approved for treatment of platinum- or taxane-resistant ovarian carcinoma and has demonstrated broad-spectrum activity *(2)*. Other analogs are in clinical development, such as D5198f and the homocamptothecins and liposomal formulations of CPT derivatives, and offer the potential for prolonged plasma exposures.

Agents targeting TOP-I in clinical trials have proceeded through the preclinical stages of identifying cytotoxic potency and confirmation of in vivo antitumor activity. Acceptable toxicity in rodents and other species, as mandated by regulatory agencies, had been studied before clinical evaluation. CPTs have demonstrated remarkable activity against animal models *(3)*. However, less dramatic clinical activity has been reported, resulting in the discontinuation of at least one agent, 9-aminocamptothecin (9-AC).

In this review, we examine this preclinical-clinical interface with respect to understanding the value and limitations of preclinical models. Hopefully, lessons learned regarding development of camptothecins can be applied to the future development of drugs that induce cytotoxicity through their interactions with TOP-I. This article will focus on preclinical models used to assess antitumor activity and toxicity for TOP-I–targeted drugs and how information derived from valid models may be used to direct the design of clinical trials.

2. EARLY STUDIES

CPT was studied extensively in the Cancer Chemotherapy National Service Center of the National Cancer Institute during the 1960s. It was formulated in carboxymethylcellulose and administered by intraperitoneal (ip) injection using the Walker 256 rat carcinosarcoma model as the test system. Relative to other drugs evaluated, camptothecin had relatively poor activity *(4)*. However, the sodium salt of CPT demonstrated significant activity in increasing survival time in several lymphocytic leukemias *(5)*. Based on a lack of cross-resistance to dichloromethotrexate, BCNU, cytosine arabinoside, 6-mercaptopurine, and other agents, it was proposed that CPT had a novel mechanism of action. In contrast to the significant activity observed in these preclinical models, CPT, evaluated as the sodium salt, was found to be ineffective in patients with advanced disseminated melanoma or gastrointestinal malignancies *(6,7)*. Severe toxicities included myelo-suppression, vomiting, diarrhea, and hemorrhagic cystitis and resulted in the discontinuation of the clinical trial of sodium CPT. Other studies in China, however, demonstrated activity of 10-hydroxycamptothecin in treatment of head-and neck-and bladder cancers (reviewed in ref. *8*).

Studies by the Liu laboratory defined TOP-I as the target for CPT and the observation that the CPTs caused trapping of TOP-I on DNA and induced single-strand breaks *(9,10)* served as an impetus to reexplore this class of agent. Although CPT is frequently referred to as an "inhibitor" of TOP-I, it actually functions to convert this cellular enzyme into a cellular toxin *(11)*. CPTs inhibit the religation step, effectively trapping covalently linked TOP-I on DNA after a single-strand nick has been made by the enzyme. In cells replicating DNA, this could result in a collision between an advancing replication fork and the covalently linked enzyme-DNA complex, leading to replication fork stalling or a double-strand DNA break. The mechanism leading to cell death remains to be characterized, although it is believed that double-strand DNA breaks can initiate a cascade leading to apoptosis. Thus increased levels of TOP-I would favor increased formation of DNA–TOP-I–drug complexes, which would increase the probability of a collision with the advancing replication fork and the generation of DNA damage. In the absence of DNA replication, the reversibly stabilized DNA–TOP-I covalent complexes are not toxic, unless suprapharmacological drug concentrations are used. Based on the mechanism of action, one would anticipate predominantly or exclusively S-phase cells would be sensitive to the CPTs *(12)*. Because many human cancers are characterized by having relatively low growth fractions, protracted infusions or repeated exposures to drug over a long period should optimize cell killing.

3. RODENT TUMOR MODELS

Syngenic transplanted rodent tumors have been used as the primary in vivo screen for the activity of the CPT analogs. For leukemic models, such as L1210 or P388, tumor cells are inoculated to the peritoneal cavity, and drugs are administered ip. End points for these experiments are the drug-induced increase in lifespan (ILS). Thus with increasing drug dose there is an increase in lifespan until ILS is reduced because of drug induced toxicity. These models are valuable in determining differences in efficacy between analogs. Although such tests have been described as "in vivo test tubes," an objective of such screens is to avoid elimination of active compounds (i.e., false negatives).

In developing a CPT derivative at SmithKlineBeecham, several in vivo criteria were established for selecting analogs for further development. These included (1) being as active as CPT in a panel of preclinical models and (2) minimizing the requirements for camptothecin as a starting material—therefore, the analog was required to demonstrate potency in vivo (i.e., a maximally tolerated dose, MTD) at similar or lower levels than CPT *(8)*. The analog 9-dimethylaminomethyl, 10-hydroxycampto-thecin (topotecan) demonstrated superior ILS in mice bearing L1210 leukemia compared with that achieved by camptothecin at their respective MTD (173 ± 16 versus 118 ± 6% ILS).

For reasons given previously, protracted therapy with TOP-I inhibitors theoretically should prove most efficacious. Thus, assuming reasonable oral bioavailability, oral administration may prove to be most practical in therapy of human cancer. Secondary evaluation of topotecan compared the efficacy of oral and intravenous (iv) administered drug in syngeneic mice bearing (1) advanced systemic (iv inoculated) L1210, (2) advanced systemic (iv inoculated) Lewis lung carcinoma,(3) subcutaneously implanted Lewis lung carcinoma, (4) systemic (iv) B16 melanoma, and (5) ip implanted M5076 reticulum cell sarcoma *(13)*. Drug was administered every 3 hours four times per day at 4- or 7-day intervals. Orally administered topotecan was comparable in efficacy to parenteral treatment in four of five tumor models tested. The M5076 sarcoma implanted ip responded to topotecan administered ip or subcutaneously, but not when given orally.

Irinotecan (CPT-11; 7-ethyl-10-(4-[1-piperidino]-1-piperidino)-carbonyloxy-(20S)camptothecin) is a prodrug activated in rodents by plasma carboxylesterases and has been extensively studied in syngenic tumors *(14–16)*. Irinotecan demonstrated significant activity by both parenteral and oral routes against disseminated models, including the intravenous inoculation of the highly metastatic B16-F10 melanoma and the spontaneous metastases from subcutaneous implants of murine colon 26. The most comprehensive study reported *(16)* evaluated irinotecan in 10 murine tumors and 1 human xenograft. All 11 tumors responded to irinotecan, with 8 of them being responsive at the Decision Network-2 level (in which treated/control volumes were <10%), the criteria used by the National Cancer Institute to justify further development. This work also showed no cross-resistance in vivo in P388/vincristine leukemic cells resistant to vincristine and in human breast carcinoma cells selected for resistance to docetaxel (Taxotere). Thus rodent models indicate that camptothecins have significant antitumor efficacy. However, rodents appear to be highly resistant to the toxic effects of CPTs. For example, pharmacokinetic data showed that plasma concentrations and exposures of SN-38 (7-ethyl,10-hydroxy-(20S)camptothecin), the active metabolite of irinotecan, were significantly higher in mice than can be achieved in patients. Although this problem is not unique to CPTs, it is particularly problematic to irinotecan, because metabolism in mice is very different from that in humans.

4. HUMAN XENOGRAFT MODELS

Since the early 1980s, human tumor xenografts grown in immune-incompetent mice have to a large extent replaced transplantable syngenic animal models. There remains debate over the predictive value of these tumor models, because there was poor correlation between drug activity against specific tumor types in mice and comparable tumor histologies in clinical trials *(17)*. In contrast, our experience using models of pediatric solid tumors have been highly predictive in identifying agents active against specific tumor types *(18,19)*. The minimum requirement for validation of these models is that they should parallel the chemosensitivity-chemoresistance profile of the clinical disease. Thus one would anticipate colon carcinomas would be less sensitive to chemotherapeutic agents than, for example, pediatric rhabdomyosarcoma.

The most frequent approach taken is to heterograft surgical specimens of tumor into mice that are congenitally immune deficient (athymic nude mice or severe combined immunodeficiency mice) or mice that have been immune-deprived to prevent graft rejection. Alternatively, cells initially propagated in vitro from human tumors may be injected into these mice subcutaneously, or iv, if disseminated disease is required. In certain circumstances (for example, evaluation of brain tumors), it may be important to assess the preclinical activity of a new drug under conditions that closely mimic the clinical situation, in which case the development of orthotopic models can be attempted by injecting cells into the analogous site within the host. However, conditions for tumor growth in the mouse may differ from patients and differences in drug disposition and metabolism in the mouse may significantly influence tumor responses. Thus orthotopic models still have intrinsic limitations characteristic of other preclinical in vivo models. Several lines representing a tumor type are generally required to accurately recapitulate the clinical situation and to conduct "preclinical phase II evaluation." We have used six tumor lines per tumor "model" (e.g., rhabdomyosarcoma, neuroblastoma). However, the exact number that accurately predicts clinical response rates has not been determined and may require at least 10 tumors per histiotype. In developing topotecan for the treatment of neuroblastoma, we found that a daily systemic exposure to 100 ng/hour/mL topotecan lactone gave objective regressions in four of six neuroblastoma xenograft models. Interestingly, targeting the same exposure using the same schedule of drug administration in children with stage IV neuroblastoma yielded a response rate of approximately 60%.

The initial study by Giovanella and colleagues *(3)* demonstrating the curative activity of 9-AC in chemorefractory colon cancer xenografts served to focus considerable attention on this class of anticancer agent *(3)*. Subcutaneous administration of drug was highly active, whereas subsequent studies with iv administration were relatively disappointing. Significant antitumor activity of camptothecin analogs has been confirmed using an extensive panel of human tumor xenografts possessing a broad pattern of biological properties and chemosensitivities *(20–34)* (Table 1). In contrast, standard agents used for clinical treatment of the appropriate tumor type, showed considerably less activity. 9-AC induced complete remissions in mice bearing xenografts of colon adenocarcinoma and malignant melanoma BRO xenografts. 9-Nitrocamptothecin (rubitecan), is converted to 9-AC and is currently under clinical investigation. 9-Nitrocamptothecin demonstrated superior therapeutic efficacy compared with 9-AC and CPT in a large number of human xenograft models *(21)*. Topotecan also demonstrated good antitumor activity when administered iv, ip, and orally against xenografts derived from various childhood solid tumors; of note topotecan induced a high percentage of complete regressions in rhabdomyosarcomas, neuroblastomas, and some brain tumors. Clinical studies support the predictive value of these models. Clinically, topotecan has elicited high response rates in rhabdomyosarcoma *(35)*, neuroblastoma (approximately 60%), and medulloblastoma (approximately 35%). In contrast, reduced activity was found against colon carcinoma xenografts *(22)*.

Irinotecan was a highly efficacious analog in preclinical studies and currently is the "gold standard" against which new analogs are compared. When administered by iv, ip, or oral routes, irinotecan showed substantial activity against a broad spectrum of human tumor xenografts, including human cancer xenograft lines unresponsive to many cytotoxic agents. High cure rates were obtained against MX-1 mammary tumor, rhabdomyosarcomas, neuroblastomas, colon cancers, and brain tumors. Activity was also retained against tumors selected for resistance to topotecan, vincristine, melphalan, busulphan, procarbazine, and cyclophosphamide. As mentioned previously, mice readily activate irinotecan to SN-38, and plasma systemic exposure to SN-38 in mice greatly exceeds that achieved in patients. Thus exposures to SN-38 associated with tumor regressions in mice may be far in excess of exposures achievable in patients (discussed in Section 5.).

Two water-soluble analogs of CPT, GI147211 and GI149893 (10,11-methylenedioxy, 7-substituted compounds), have been assessed in preclinical models of colon and mammary carcinoma. Antitumor effects were dose- and schedule-dependent, with a greater reduction in tumor volume achieved by protracted dosing. Concurrent experiments demonstrated that these agents were more effective than topotecan in suppressing tumor growth, although optimal schedules for topotecan were not compared in these studies *(27)*. As a liposomal formulation, GI147211 (designated NX211) has demonstrated good antitumor activity against more than 20 lines of tumor xenografts and yielded with minimal toxic effects.

Alternatively, it has been proposed that hydrophobic CPTs may have greater E-ring stability, and hence may exert longer plasma exposures of the lactone form. 7-[(2-trimethylsilyl)ethyl)]-20 (S)-camptothecin (Karenitecin) is under clinical development, as are other water-insoluble derivatives such as DB-67. Homocamptothecins with an expanded E-ring are also in clinical trials. Again, increased lactone stability was the rationale behind the synthesis of these E-ring-modified agents.

For many of the experiments reported in Table 1, systemic exposures in the mouse to lactone forms of the given CPT derivative far exceed exposures that can be achieved in patients at tolerated dose levels. The data presented demonstrate the relative sensitivity of a given tumor to a series of analogs administered to their MTD levels in the mouse. Such data may overestimate the potential for activity in patients. Without knowing the relative toxicity–systemic exposure relationship in humans, such data may have limited predictive value for selecting analogs for further development. Although determination of the therapeutic efficacy in murine models serve as a potential criterion to select among analogs (assuming that mouse toxicity accurately reflects dose limiting toxicity in patients), it may have relatively little value in predicting clinical antitumor activity. For example, irinotecan administered daily for 10 days (MTD approximately 40 mg/kg/day) causes objective regressions in approximately 50% of colon carcinoma models *(24)*. However, we now know that a dose of 1.25 mg/kg to mice generates plasma SN-38 exposures that are tolerated in patients when irinotecan is administered on the same schedule. Thus evaluating the effect of camptothecin at the MTD in mice significantly overpredicts clinical activity.

5. SCHEDULE-DEPENDENT ANTITUMOR ACTIVITY

Animal models have been useful for examining alternative schedules of drug administration. Obtaining information about the schedule dependency in relation to both the antitumor activity and host toxicity of an agent is one of the goals of preclinical studies. TOP-I inhibitors are S-phase-specific cytotoxins. It is assumed therefore that after a cytotoxic threshold is achieved, exposure time, rather than further dose escalation, is the important parameter for determining the tumor response. Consequently, protracted drug administration could increase antitumor activity. Recent clinical data support schedule-dependent activity *(36)*, and additional clinical data, even in phase I trials, show greater antitumor activity is associated with protracted schedules of administration *(19,37)*.

The importance of scheduling was first reported by Kawato *(20)*. Additional testing confirmed this observation *(21–23)*. These studies showed that, for similar total dosages, protracted schedules were more effective than were more intense treatments of shorter duration. Several groups have reported schedule-dependent activity of camptothecin analogs, although this finding does not appear to have been used in design of the initial clinical trials *(38)*. Schedule-dependency is illustrated in Fig. 1, where the responses of individual rhabdomyosarcoma Rh30 xenografts have been measured in mice receiving drug vehicle (control) or topotecan treatment. Both treatment groups received the same total dose of drug, the only difference being that topotecan was either given over 5 days or 10 days. Clearly, topotecan administered over 10 days was significantly more active than the same dose given over 5 days. Also, in xenograft models drugs such as topotecan and irinotecan appear to be "self-limiting." Above some dose level, further increases in dose per administration do not result in further antitumor activ-

Table 1
Responsiveness of Human Tumor Xenografts to Treatment With Camptothecin Analogs

Drug	*Xenograft tumor*	*Dose (mg/kg) and schedule*	*Comments*		*Reference*
9AC	Colon HT-29 Colon CASE Colon Sw48	10–12.5 mg/kg × 2 /week for 5–6 weeks SC	Highly effective	ADR, 5-FU, MTX nitrosoureas, ALK, less effective/ineffective	*3*
CPT11	Mammary MX-1 Gastric St-15 Gastric SC-6 Lung QG56 Colon Co-4	200 mg (TD) iv 400–00 mg (TD) q (4 days × 3) PO	Very significant antitumor activity against all tumors Curative against MX-1 CPT11 more effective as three injections than one single injection for same total dose.	ADR, 5FU, CDDP less effective	*20*
CAM 9AC 9NC	Melanoma BRO	4 mg × 2/week IM	Growth inhibition and tumor regression	BRO tumors unresponsive to ADR, 5-FU, VCR, VBL, MTX, nitrosourea, and ALK.	*21*
Topotecan	Six rhabdomyosarcoma lines Seven colon lines Three osteosarcoma lines	1.5–2.0 mg (days × 5)3 IV/PO 12.5 mg q (4 days × 4) IP	Complete regressions in rhabdomyosarcomas. Significant activity in osteosarcomas. Growth inhibition in several colon lines. Results suggest significant schedule dependency		*22*
9AC 9NC 9CL-CAM	Breast carcinoma		9AC effective. 9NC effective. 9CL-CAM not effective. Results were dose, schedule, and route of administration-dependent.	Short infusions (72 hours every 21 days) not effective. Long infusions (5 days every 7 days) very effective.	*23*

CPT11	Six rhabdoyosarcoma lines Seven colon lines	10–40 mg (days ×5)2 IV and [(days ×5)2]3 IV Complete responses in five	All tumors very sensitive Complete and partial regressions in five out of eight colon lines. resistant to VCR lines out of six rhabdomyosarocma	CPT 11 effective against two xenografts selected for resistance to topotecan and rhabdomyosarcoma lines and melphalan.	*24*
CPT11	TNB9 Neuroblastoma	15–59 mg q (4 days ×3) IP	Growth inhibition.	VCR, Aclarubicin, VP16, 5-FU, and THP-ADR, ineffective.	*25*
CPT11 Topotecan	Six rhabdomyosarcoma lines Eight colon lines Three brain tumor lines	CPT11: 2.5–10 mg[(days ×5)2]3 IV Topotecan: 0.5–1.5 mg (days ×5) 12 PO Concluded: Low-dose	CPT 11 highly active (complete regressions) against colon lines. Both drugs similar high activity against rhabdomyosarcomas and brain tumors. protracted scheduling of daily administration is equiefficacies than shorter, more intense, schedules	CPT 11 and topotecan active against tumors selected for resistance to VCR CPT11 active against tumor selected for resistance to melphalan	*26*
Topotecan G1147211 G1149893	Colon HT-79 Colon SW-48 Mammary MX-1 Prostate PC-	3 MTD divided into three doses infused q 4 hourly in 24 hours ×2/week for 5 weeks Topotecan:	G1147211: G1149893: Regressions >50% in HT79 and SW-48 Complete regressions in MX-1, growth inhibition in PC3. Growth inhibition only		*27*
CPT11	PNET SKNMC Neuroblastomas	27–40 mg (days ×5) IV and q (4 days ×3) IV	Very effective, high complete response rates.		*28*

(continued)

Table 1 (Continued)

Drug	*Xenograft tumor*	*Dose (mg/kg) and schedule*	*Comment*		*Reference*
	N835 NB8 NB3				
CPT11	Six neuroblastoma lines	10–40 mg (days ×5)2 IV 5–10 mg [(days ×5)2]3 IV 25–50 mg (days ×5)12PO	Highly efficacious Complete regression of all tumors on the protracted iv schedule and all tumors using oral schedule		*29,30*
CPT11	Nine Brain tumor lines Gliomas Ependymomas Medulloblastomas	40 mg (days ×5)2 IP	Tumor regression in every treated tumor line.	CPT11 active against tumors resistant to busulphan, procarbazine, cyclophos-phamide, and melphalan.	*31*
9AC	Prostate PC3	2 mg ×2/week for 3 weeks SC 0.35–1 mg (days ×5)3 PO	Inhibition and regression of tumor growth.	PC3 is a hormone refractory prostate line	*32*
Topotecan	Six neuroblastoma lines	0.36 2 mg [(days ×5)2]3 IV	Highly effective Complete regressions in all tumors.	Minimum daily systemic exposure related to objective response	*33*

CAM, camptothecin; 9AC, 9-aminocamptothecin; 9NC, 9-nitrocamptothecin; 9CL-CAM, 9-chlorocamptothecin; SC, subcutaneous; IM, intramuscular; IV, intravenous; PO, by mouth; IP, intraperitoneal.

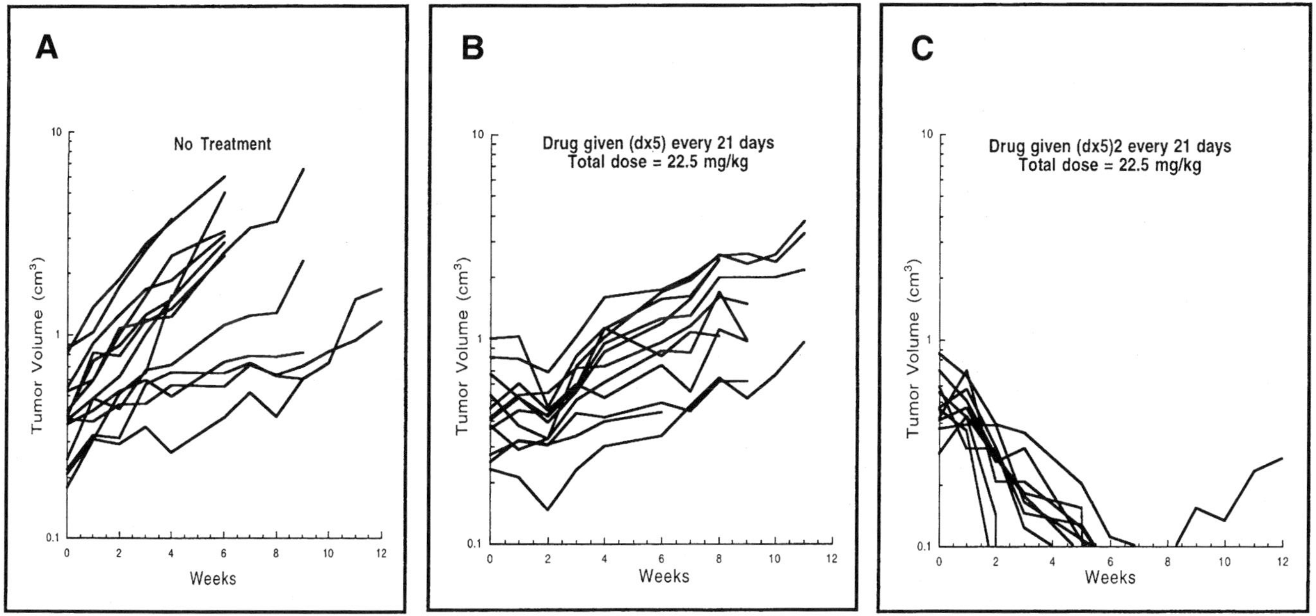

Fig. 1. Schedule-dependent antitumor activity of topotecan. Mice bearing Rh30 rhabdomyosarcoma xenografts were randomized into three groups of seven mice. Group A received no treatment (controls); group B received topotecan daily for 5 days at a dose of 1.5 mg/kg/day. Mice in group C received 0.75 mg/kg daily for 5 days on 2 consecutive weeks. Courses of treatment were repeated ever 21 days over 8 weeks for groups B and C. The total dose per 21-day course was 7.5 mg/kg for both treatment groups, and total drug per three cycles was 22.5 mg/kg. Each curve shows the growth of an individual tumor. In group B, topotecan caused disease stabilization, but most tumors progressed through treatment. In contrast, delivering the same dose of topotecan over 10 days induced complete responses with only a single tumor regrowth during the period of observation (12 weeks). (Houghton, unpublished data).

ity *(21)*. Similar results have been obtained with 9-AC and other CPT analoganalogs in various tumor models. Interestingly, administration of irinotecan using the (day × 5) 2 schedule every 21 days has demonstrated significant antitumor activity in a phase I clinical trial in children with tumors resistant to conventional therapy *(19,39)*.

6. MODELS OF RESISTANCE TO TOP-I INHIBITORS

Two CPT analogs, topotecan and irinotecan, are approved for treatment of refractory ovarian carcinoma and 5-fluorouracil refractory colon carcinoma, respectively. Thus new agents should demonstrate clear superiority over these established drugs to justify full development. Irinotecan is highly active against certain tumors that are intrinsically resistant to topotecan and against some xenografts selected *in situ* for acquired resistance to topotecan *(24)*. Several cell lines selected for resistance to camptothecin have been reported. In one line (CEM/C2), resistance is mediated by a mutation (Asn722Ser) in TOP-I *(39)*. In yeast, several mutations in TOP-I yield CPT resistance *(40)*. However, it is less certain in clinical tumors whether intrinsic or acquired resistance is the result of TOP-I mutations. Thus establishing xenograft models from cell lines in which resistance is caused by mutant enzyme may not necessarily recapitulate clinical resistance. At this time, mechanisms conferring CPT resistance in clinical cancers remain uncharacterized; however, the role of the breast cancer resistance–associated protein is associated in vitro with resistance to several camptothecin analogs *(41–44)*. Resistance to CPTs is undoubtedly complex, potentially analog-specific, and involves mechanisms proximal to DNA damage (i.e., accumulation/efflux), at the target level (mutation or activity of TOP-I) or distal to damage (repair processes). In several xenograft models, selection *in situ* for resistance to topotecan did not result in cross-resistance to irinotecan *(24)*. However, relatively few models of acquired resistance to CPT analogs have been reported. Relatively rapid development of an irinotecan-resistant neuroblastoma xenograft (NB-1691/CPT) has been reported *(45)*. Resistant tumors were derived after only four rounds of treatment/transplantation a stable irinotecan-resistant line was derived. This tumor is partially resistant to topotecan. Although the mechanism of resistance remains to be characterized, this tumor may represent a useful model for identifying novel TOP-I-targeted agents with characteristics significantly different from either irinotecan or topotecan.

7. TOXICITY

7.1. Hematopoietic Toxicity

The often dramatic preclinical activity of CPT analogs in xenograft models contrasts with the clinical activity observed in many phase II studies. As would be predicted from their S-phase activity, TOP-I inhibitors cause dose-limiting toxicity to rapidly renewing tissues such as hematopoietic tissues in humans and animals. Dose-limiting toxicity occurs at far lower systemic exposures in humans than in mice. Humans can tolerate only 11% as much topotecan per day as mice. This differential may be greater for irinotecan. Based on pharmacokinetic estimates of SN-38 systemic exposure at the MTD in patients receiving irinotecan every 7 days, it was estimated that the systemic exposure represented only 6% of the MTD in mice *(46)*. For myelosuppressive CPT analogs, failure to achieve drug exposures in patients that are curative in the murine models might be due to greater sensitivity of human myeloid progenitors. Using in vitro colony-forming assays, Erickson-Miller et al. *(47)* showed that hematopoietic progenitors of the myeloid lineage from humans, mice, and dogs exhibit differential sensitivity to the CPTs. The toxicity of CPT analogs to human and animal myeloid progenitors was quantified from the inhibition of marrow colony-forming unit–granulocyte macrophage (CFU-GM) colony. CPT lactone, topotecan, and 9-AC inhibited colony formation in a concentration-dependent manner. These results suggest that, because of greater sensitivity of the myelopoietic tissue, humans cannot tolerate exposures to CPTs that are curative in murine models. Relative to human myeloid progenitors, murine myeloid progenitors are relatively insensitive to all the compounds examined. The differences between mice and humans are large. For example, the concentration of topotecan causing a 50% reduction in CFUs was 46-fold lower for human cells when compared with murine progenitors. This differential was even greater (107-fold) for 9-AC *(47)*. The susceptibility of human CFU-GM to drug toxicity is more closely approximated by canine than by murine CFU-GM. This finding explains, in part, why even subcurative doses of CPTs may be severely myelotoxic in patients. The use of in vitro systems for predicting human tissue toxicity may have wider application to drug development *(48,49)*.

7.2. Gastrointestinal Toxicity

Irinotecan, administered on most of the schedules evaluated clinically, has been associated with an unanticipated and significant diarrhea. This is characterized by the early onset of symptoms and is probably a consequence of the acetylcholinergic activity of the bipiperidino side chain *(50)*. This toxicity is well controlled by atropine. However, delayed diarrhea is now recognized as a dose-limiting toxicity of this compound *(51)*. This toxicity was not anticipated from studies in rodents, in which diarrhea was not observed. Diarrhea may be caused by abnormalities of intestinal absorption or secretion, increased peristalsis, or drug-induced epithelial damage. The considerable interpatient variability in the severity of the diarrhea has made it difficult to explain the mechanism of irinotecan-associated diarrhea. This toxicity, however, is not unique to irinotecan. Delayed-onset diarrhea is the dose-limiting toxicity of topotecan administered orally to patients for 21 days. The etiology of this side effect of the CPTs is not yet clear, although several animal models have been established that attempt to simulate irinotecan-induced diarrhea.

7.2.1. Mouse Models

Ikuno et al. *(52)* observed characteristic changes in the intestinal mucosa of irinotecan-treated mice, including villous atrophy characterized by marked shortening of the villi, epithelial vacuolation of the ileum (associated with increased apoptosis), and goblet cell hyperplasia in the cecum. These structural and functional effects were postulated as the main causes of irinotecan-induced diarrhea and resulted in malabsorption and hypersecretion of mucin. Malabsorption in irinotecan-treated mice was thought to be caused by villous atrophy after crypt damage and apoptosis of absorptive cells in the small intestine. The goblet cell hyperplasia associated with excessive production of mucin in the cecum could be another contributing factor to the cause of diarrhea with irinotecan. A model of intestinal toxicity has been developed in the mouse; this has been used to identify potential modulators of irinotecan-induced diarrhea. Daily administration of very high dose levels (100 mg/kg) of irinotecan to mice resulted in loss of villi, epithelial vacuolation, decreased numbers of S-phase cells in the crypts, increased apoptotic cells, and reduced numbers of lymphocytes in the lamina propria. Oral administration of a synthetic bacterial lipopeptide, JBT 3002, encapsulated in phospholipid liposomes prevented irinotecan-induced damage to the intestinal epithelium and lamina propria *(53)*. Similarly, dietary supplementation with fish oil reduced gastrointestinal damage induced by irinotecan *(54)*.

7.2.2. Rat Models

Frequently, diarrhea is caused by the active secretion of electrolytes, especially chloride ions, suggesting this toxicity is independent of the action of irinotecan or the active metabolite, SN-38, on DNA–TOP-I. Relatively high concentrations of irinotecan caused eicosanoid-mediated chloride secretion in isolated rat colon *(55)*. Irinotecan-induced diarrhea was characterized in rats by assessing the relationship between intestinal toxicity and the activity of enzymes involved in the major metabolic pathways of this drug *(56)*. In rodents, irinotecan is converted to its active metabolite SN-38 by carboxylesterase; one possible mechanism for the diarrhea might include the structural and functional injuries to the intestinal tract resulting from the direct cytotoxic activity of the SN-38. Detoxification of SN-38 occurs by liver glucoronidation and conjugated SN-38 is secreted into the bile and in the feces. Conjugated metabolites may be further converted or processed to an active SN-38 by β-glucuronidase of the microflora resident in the large intestine. In this rat model, histological damage was most severe in the cecum, with a markedly decrease in the size and number of crypts and evidence of superficial mucosal erosion. The segmental differences in the degree of damage showed good correlation with the β-glucuronidase activity in the contents of the lumen, suggesting that this enzyme plays a key role in intestinal toxicity induced by irinotecan. Intestinal tissue carboxylesterase activity, which also converts irinotecan to its active form, showed poor correlation to the degree of tissue damage. Administration of antibiotics to sterilize the intestine exerted a protective effect against the diarrhea by completely inhibiting the β-glucuronidase activity of the intestinal flora and, accordingly, the formation of active SN-38. Rustum and colleagues *(57)* have also developed a rat model of irinotecan-induced gastrointestinal toxicity. In their study, very high dose levels of irinotecan (150–200 mg/kg daily × 3 iv) resulted in 86–100% lethality in treated animals and 93–100% incidence of severe diarrhea, which was associated with serious damage to the duodenal villi and colonic crypts. Interleukin-15 (100–400 μg/kg (3, 8, and 11 doses ip) completely protected against irinotecan-induced delayed diarrhea and lethality. The validity of these rodent models must, however, wait for confirmatory results in other models and, ultimately, clinical trials.

7.2.3. Hamster Models

The hamster has also been proposed as a model for irinotecan-induced intestinal toxicity *(58)*. Female Syrian hamsters were dosed ip with irinotecan (50 mg/kg/day) for 10 days and observed through day 20. By day 5, all treated animals had developed diarrhea and deaths occurred starting on day 7. Histological examination revealed a time-dependent loss of structural integrity in the jejunal and ileal mucosa; the typical columnar morphology of the epithelial cells was lost and the villi appeared corrugated. The epithelium was thinned and vacuolated in the colon within the first 5 days of treatment. Detection of proliferating cell nuclear antigen showed an increase in the number of labeled epithelial cells and labeling intensity in treated animals. The labeled cells were located further toward the tips of villi compared with control animals. Increased levels of proliferating cell nuclear antigen and loss of differentiation in cell morphology suggested that irinotecan induces a cell-cycle block in S-G2, with subsequent loss of physiologic function in hamster intestinal epithelium. Kobayashi et al. *(59)* have also studied the effect of pH on uptake of irinotecan, SN-38 lactone, and SN-38 carboxylate in isolated intestinal cells from Syrian hamsters. From these studies, it is proposed that uptake of lactone is by passive diffusion, whereas there may be an energy-dependent accumulation (transport) for carboxylate. Accumulation of irinotecan carboxylate showed saturation kinetics with apparent K_m approximately 50 μM in jejunal and ileal cells.

8. INTERSPECIES DIFFERENCES THAT COMPLICATE TRANSLATION OF PRECLINICAL RESULTS

8.1. Interspecies Differences in Drug Metabolism and Disposition

CPTs have demonstrated greater activity against model tumors in rodents than against tumors in patients. In part, this appears to be a consequence of the greater tolerance of the toxic effects of these agents in mice than in humans. Analysis of data from mice and rats showed that predicting clinical maximally tolerated doses for eight TOP-I inhibitors from rodent data would result in starting clinical trials very close to, or at dose levels exceeding, the human MTD *(60)*. In contrast, initial starting doses based on canine data would be safe. The plasma systemic exposures, expressed as an area under the concentration-time curve, for irinotecan and its active metabolite SN-38 in mice *(16,61)* and patients *(62–64)* are presented in Table 2. To facilitate comparison between schedules, systemic exposure has been expressed for each course of therapy, usually in a 21-day time frame at the highest nontoxic dose for mice and the MTD for humans. Not all investigators report both the lactone and total drug, hence it is difficult to directly compare the systemic exposure of irinotecan and SN-38 between studies. However, when given once weekly in humans, the systemic exposure to irinotecan and, particularly SN-38, is significantly greater in mice than in humans.

This raises the concern that studies with syngenic tumors or human xenograft models in mice may overpredict the potential clinical utility of this and other classes of anticancer drugs. For CPTs, the reasons for the interspecies differences are not well understood. Rather than use the mouse model to predict systemic drug exposures associated with toxicity, we have determined the systemic exposure associated with antitumor effect against the human tumor xenograft models. For a series of neuroblastoma xenografts, the daily systemic exposure to topotecan that caused objective regressions was determined when the drug was administered 5 days per week for 2 consecutive weeks *(33)*. Partial responses were achieved in each of six independently derived neuroblastoma lines at a daily topotecan lactone systemic exposure of 100 ng/mL/hour, whereas complete responses were achieved in four tumor lines. The results of these studies define the effective antitumor systemic exposure to the camptothecin analog. Current data from our studies in children indicate that exposure of 100 ng/mL/hour (achieved after a dose of 0.61 mg/kg in mice) results from a daily dose of approximately 3 mg/m^2 in children. For irinotecan, dose levels of approximately 1.25 mg/kg in mice yield SN-38 plasma systemic exposures achieved at doses of 20–30 mg/m^2 administered to children *(19)*. This difference is a consequence of very efficient activation of irinotecan by plasma carboxylesterase in mice. In contrast, activation of irinotecan in humans is poor.

Table 2
Comparison of Irinotecan and SN-38 Systemic Exposure (AUC) Between Mice and Humans

Reference		*Lactone Irinotecan (mg/mL/hour)*	*Lactone SN-38 (mg/mL/hour)*	*Total Irinotecan (mg/mL/hour)*	*Total SN-38 (mg/mL/hour*
Mice					
16	Irinotecan 52.5 mg/kg IV	NA	NA	62.5	34.5
61	Irinotecan 10 mg/kg IV [(days ×5)2]3	13.0	5.3	NA	NA
Humans					
62	Irinotecan 350 mg/m^2 IV once every 3 weeks	NA	NA	34.0	0.45
63	Irinotecan 100 mg/m^2 IV for 3 consecutive days every 3 weeks	NA	NA	27.9	0.96
64	Irinotecan 150 mg/m^2 week IV for 4 of 6 weeks	5.6	0.24	16.8	0.82
19	Irinotecan 20 mg/m^2 IV [(days ×5)2]3	4.0	1.4	NA	NA

Note: Total and lactone AUC have been calculated for the cumulative exposure for a 21-day cycle of therapy.
AUC, area under the curve; IV, intravenous; NA, not available.

Recently, a strain of mouse, designated *Es1*^{e}, deficient in plasma esterases, has been identified. Kinetic studies indicated that the activation of irinotecan to SN-38 by *Es1*^{e} mouse plasma in vitro is 600-fold less efficient, although extracts from organs indicated no difference in drug metabolism as compared with controls *(65)*. It is proposed that the *Es1*^{e} mouse may represent a more representative model of irinotecan drug activation *(66,67)*.

8.2. Protein Binding

Systemic exposure to CPT analogs represents total drug concentration, which consists of both drug bound to plasma protein and unbound drug. For drugs extensively bound to plasma proteins, such as SN-38, unbound drug concentrations correlate best with the indices of pharmacologic effect. Where there is significant interspecies variability in the plasma protein binding, comparison between unbound drug concentrations and toxicity in humans and animals may be more appropriate than the total drug concentration. Interspecies differences in drug protein binding are seen with the CPT analogs. CPT exists as a pentacyclic structure with a lactone moiety in the terminal E-ring. When used against purified TOP-I, the presence of a lactone ring is a structural requirement for activity. Factors influencing the lactone-carboxylate equilibrium may therefore be important determinants of drug activity. In addition to pH, presence of protein, particularly albumin, has been shown to be important to the stability of the lactone moiety *(68,69)*. Human serum albumin has a marked preference for the carboxylate form of CPT, greater than serum albumin from five other species. Thus binding of the carboxylate to albumin drives the equilibrium away from the active lactone form of the drug. Structural modifications to CPT, as seen with irinotecan, SN-38, and topotecan, diminish the interspecies differences in stabilization of the lactone. This is in contrast with 9-AC, in which the marked interspecies difference in stabilization of the carboxylate form was similar to that observed with CPT. Four hours after intragastric administration of camptothecin or 9-nitrocamptothecin, lactone forms compose 57–81% and 47–95% of the total drug, in mouse plasma, respectively. In contrast, the lactone composed only a minor component of total drug levels in plasma from humans treated orally with either drug *(70)*. This interspecies variability in protein stabilization of the carboxylate form is important for translation of data derived in rodents to clinical trials. These results also illustrate the importance of determining the systemic exposure to lactone forms of CPT analogs that induce objective regressions in xenograft models. This information may be valuable in understanding and designing phase II clinical trials *(71,72)*. Attempts to encapsulate and stabilize lactone forms of CPTs may also increase the therapeutic utility of drugs such as CPT or topotecan *(73,74)*.

9. FUTURE DIRECTIONS

Animal models, and human tumor xenografts in particular, have predicted dramatic clinical therapeutic activity of CPT drugs. Agents, such as topotecan and irinotecan, are clearly active in several adult and childhood cancers, as well as myelodysplastic syndromes. For analogs such as 9-AC, clinical results have been quite disappointing. Retrospective analysis of preclinical data for TOP-I inhibitors shows that such differences are caused by interspecies differences in drug disposition and host tolerance. For CPTs, mice tolerate significantly greater systemic exposure than can be achieved in patients at tolerated levels of toxicity. Further, the remarkable schedule dependency for antitumor activity seen in many preclinical models has not been adequately addressed in the design of clinical trials. When response rates for xenograft tumors are calculated for doses that yield clinically achievable systemic exposures, these models rather accurately predict the clinical results. Similarly, we would anticipate approximately 15–25% of colon carcinoma xenografts demonstrating objective responses (≥50% volume regression) using doses of irinotecan that in mice yield clinically achievable systemic exposures for SN-38. However, such information is not available when selecting between analogs at a relatively early stage in development. One way in which equi-efficacious analogs could be distinguished would be to introduce assays of differential species marrow toxicity at an early stage in development. This may allow identification of analogs with significant antitumor activity, but with little difference in species toxicity. Whether mouse transgenic models will obviate any of these issues remains to be determined. These models may have the advantage of development of spontaneous tumors, at more natural sites (e.g., medulloblastoma in the cerebellum). Thus transgenics may represent specialized models for drug evaluation. However, the problems of translating drug effects in rodent to human remain.

The TOP-I-targeted agents in clinical investigation are mainly based on a CPT structure. There are many more analogs in preclinical development. One focus in developing novel CPTs has been on stabilization of the E-ring lactone. This has been achieved by increasing the lipophilicity of CPTs by substitution on the 7-position with bulky alkyl, alkylamino, and alkylsilyl groups. A more novel approach has been synthesis of homocamptothecins, in which a seven-membered lactone E-ring has far greater stability. Interestingly, the homocamptothecin appears to change the sequence specificity of the drug-induced DNA cleavage by TOP-I *(75)*. However, differences in lipophilicity are more likely to result in alterations in the pharmaceutical properties of this class of agent, rendering longer plasma clearance times, and potentially allowing greater systemic exposure to active forms of these drugs. Because there are few clinical data to support the value of delivering

CPTs by prolonged continuous infusion, it is unclear if analogs with greater lactone stability will be more efficacious. Definitive activity in preclinical models with intrinsic or acquired resistance to current CPTs would be important in advancing such analogs to clinical testing. Perhaps of greater interest will be development of novel topoisomerase inhibitors based on the crystal structure of the DNA–TOP-I–DNA ternary complex.

New structures such as protoberberines *(76)*, indolocarbazoles (rebeccamycin analogs) *(77)*, and lipophilic epipodophyllotoxins have emerged as potential dual inhibitors of topoisomerases. Of particular interest is F11782, an ethylidene glucoside ester of epipodophyllotoxin that putatively inhibits the catalytic cycle of both type I and II enzymes, preventing their binding to DNA *(78)*. This agent has demonstrated significantly better activity against both syngenic and xenograft tumor models than etoposide *(79)*. However, direct comparison with irinotecan and topotecan has not been reported. Demonstration of activity of these newer inhibitors against CPT-resistant tumors would be an exciting development. Development and characterization of additional human tumor models resistant to CPTs would be valuable.

The full curative/therapeutic potential of these drugs will not be realized without compensating for the dose-limiting neutropenia and intestinal toxicity. Thus approaches to reducing myelosuppression, through use of hematopoietic growth factors, reconstitution with peripheral blood cell progenitors, or protecting marrow through transduction of CPT-resistant genes, appear rational. Attempts to modulate intestinal toxicity through administration of interleukin-15, or JBT 3002, or alkalinization of the intestinal lumen *(80)* may allow increased dose intensity, or (rationally) more protracted courses of treatment with these agents. Oral administration of topotecan and irinotecan is limited by poor bioavailability. In children and mice, approximately 24% of topotecan and approximately 9% of irinotecan is absorbed. Unabsorbed drug passing to the distal intestine may contribute to the greater gastrointestinal toxicity observed in patients treated with oral dosing. Recently, the use of agents that block the ABC-transporter, breast cancer resistance protein ABCG2, have been shown to increase oral bioavailability of CPTs *(81)*. Such modulators may allow effective oral therapy with these agents using protracted schedules of administration. Validation of animal models of intestinal toxicity is important. Design of clinical protocols that more accurately recapitulate optimal schedules and drug exposures determined in xenograft models also seems appropriate with these agents that are highly schedule-dependent in their antitumor activity. Clearly an understanding of the biochemical or molecular events that determine such dramatic schedule dependency will help in more effective clinical utilization of these agents, alone, or in combination with other cytotoxic agents.

ACKNOWLEDGMENTS

Work from these laboratories was supported by UPHS grants CA23099, CA 32613, CA21765 (Cancer Center Support CORE Grant), and by American Lebanese Syrian Associated Charities (ALSAC).

REFERENCES

1. Trask DK, Muller MT. Stabilization of type I topoisomerase-DNA covalent complexes by actinomycin D. Proc Natl Acad Sci USA 1988; 85:1417–1421.
2. Holland JF, Frei E III, Bast RC Jr, Kufe DW, Morton DL, Weichselbaum RR, eds. Cancer medicine, 4th ed. Williams & Wilkins, Pennsylvania, 1997.
3. Giovanella BC, Stehlin JS, Wall ME, et al. DNA topoisomerase 1-targeted chemotherapy of human colon cancer xenografts. Science 1989; 246:1046–1048.
4. DeWys WD, Humphreys SR, Goldin A. 1968 Studies on the therapeutic effectiveness of drugs with tumor weight and survival time indices of Walker 256 carcinosarcoma. Cancer Chemo Rept 52:229–242.
5. Gallo RC, Whang-Peng J, Adamson RH. 1971 Studies on the antitumor activity, mechanism of action, and cell cycle effects of camptothecin. J Natl Cancer Inst 46:789–795.
6. Gottlieb JA, Guarino AM, Call JB, Oliverio VT, Block JB. 1970 Preliminary pharmacologic and clinical evaluation of camptothecin sodium (NSC 100880). Cancer Chemother Rep 54: 461–470.
7. Moertel CG, Schutt AJ, Reitemeier RJ, Hahn RG. 1972 Phase II study of camptothecin (NSC-100880) in the treatment of advanced gastrointestinal cancer. Cancer Chemother Rep 56:95–101.
8. Kingsbury WD, Boehm JC, Jakas DR, et al. 1990 Synthesis of water soluble (aminoalkyl) camptothecin analogues: inhibition of topoisomerase I and antitumor activity. J Med Chem 4:98–107.
9. Hsiang YH, Hertzberg R, Hecht S, Liu LF. 1985 Camptothecin induces protein-linked DNA breaks via mammalian DNA topoisomerase I. J Biol Chem 260:14873–14878.
10. Chen AY, Liu LF. 1994 DNA topoisomerases: essential enzymes and lethal targets. Annu Rev Pharmacol Toxicol 34:191–218.
11. Nitiss J, Wang JC. 1988 DNA topoisomerase-targeted drugs can be studied in yeast. Proc Natl Acad Sci USA 85:7501–7505.
12. Liu LF. Topoisomerase-I targeted drugs. mechanism of inhibition and cytotoxicity. In Vth World Conference on Clinical Pharmacology and Therapeutics. Highlights of a satellite symposium: approaches to Cancer Treatment by Topoisomerase-I inhibitors. Taguchi T, Wang JC, eds. BIOMEDIS, Tokyo, 1992, 6–9.
13. McCabe FL, Johnson RK. 1994 Comparative activity of oral and parenteral topotecan in murine tumor models: efficacy of oral topotecan. Cancer Investig 12:308–313.
14. Kunimoto T, Nitta K, Tanaka T, et al. 1987 Antitumor activity of 7-ethyl-10-[4-(1-piperidino)-1-piperidino]-1-carbonyloxy-camptothecin, a novel water soluble derivative of camptothecin, against murine tumors. Cancer Res 47:5944–5947.
15. Matsuzaki T, Yokokura T, Mutai M, Tsuruo T. 1988 Inhibition of spontaneous and experimental metastasis by a new derivative of camptothecin, irinotecan, in mice. Cancer Chemother Pharmacol 21:308–312.

16. Bissery MC, Vrignaud P, Lavelle F, Chabot GG. 1996 Experimental antitumor activity and pharmacokinetics of the camptothecin analog irinotecan (CPT-11). Anti-Cancer Drugs 7:437–460.
17. Johnson JI, Decker S, Zaharevitz D, et al. 2001 Relationships between drug activity in NCI preclinical in vitro and in vivo models and early clinical trials. Br J Cancer 84:1424–1431.
18. Horowitz ME, Etcubanas E, Christensen ML, et al. 1988 Phase II testing of melphalan in children with newly diagnosed rhabdomyosarcoma: a model for anticancer drug development. J Clin Oncol 6:308–314.
19. Furman WL, Stewart CF, Poquette CA, et al. 1999 Direct translation of a protracted irinotecan schedule from xnograft model to phase I trial in children. J Clin Oncol 17:1815–1824.
20. Kawato Y, Furuta T, Aonuma M, Yasuoka M, Yokokura T, Matsumoto K. 1991 Antitumor activity of a camptothecin derivative against human tumor xenografts in nude mice. Cancer Chemother Pharmacol 28:192–198.
21. Pantazis P, Hinz HR, Mendoza JT, et al. 1992 Complete inhibition of growth followed by death of human malignant melanoma cells in vitro and regression of human melanoma xenografts in immunodeficient mice induced by camptothecins. Cancer Res 52:3980–3987.
22. Houghton PJ, Cheshire PJ, Myers L, Stewart CF, Synold TW, Houghton JA. 1992 Evaluation of 9-dimethylaminomethyl-l0-hydroxycamptothecin against xenografts derived from adult and childhood solid tumors. Cancer Chemother Pharmacol 31:229–239.
23. Pentazis P, Kozielski AJ, Vardeman DM, Petry ER, Giovanella BC. 1993 Efficacy of camptothecin congeners in the treatment of human breast carcinoma xenografts. Oncol Res 5:273–281.
24. Houghton PJ, Cheshire PJ, Hallman JC, Bissery MC, Mathieu-Boue A, Houghton JA. 1993 Therapeutic efficacy of the topoisomerase I inhibitor 7-ethyl-10-(4-[1-piperidino]-1-piperidino)-carbonyloxy-camptothecin against human tumor xenografts: lack of cross resistance in vivo in tumors with acquired resistance to the topoisomerase inhibitor 9-dimethylaminomethyl-10-hydoxycamptothecin. Cancer Res 53:2823–2829.
25. Komuro H, Li P, Tsuchida Y, et al. 1994 Effects of CPT11 (a unique DNA topoisomerase 1 inhibitor) on a highly malignant xeno-transplanted neuroblastoma. Med Pediatr Oncol 23:487–492.
26. Houghton PJ, Cheshire PJ, Hallman JD, et al. 1995 Efficacy of topoisomerase I inhibitors, topotecan and irinotecan, administered at low dose levels in protracted schedules to mice bearing xenografts of human tumors. Cancer Chemother Pharmacol 36:393–403.
27. Emerson DL, Besterman JM, Brown HR, et al. 1995 In vivo antitumor activity of two seven-substituted water soluble camptothecin analogues. Cancer Res 55:603–609.
28. Vassal G, Terrier-Lacombe MJ, Bissery MC, et al. 1996 Therapeutic activity of CPT-11, a DNA-topoisomerase I inhibitor, against peripheral primitive neuroectodermal tumour and neuroblastoma xenografts. Br J Cancer 74:537–545.
29. Thompson, J, Zamboni WC, Cheshire PJ, et al. 1997 Efficacy of systemic administration of irinotecan against neuroblastoma xenografts. Clin Cancer Res 3:423–431.
30. Thompson J, Zamboni WC, Cheshire PJ, et al. 1997 Efficacy of oral administration of irinotecan against neuroblastoma xenografts. Anti-Cancer Drugs 8: 313–322.
31. Hare CB, Elion GB, Houghton PJ, et al. 1997 Therapeutic efficacy of the topoisomerase I inhibitor 7-ethyl-10-(4-[1-piperidino]-1-piperidino)-carbonyl-

oxy-camptothecin against pediatric and adult central nervous system tumor xenografts. Cancer Chemother Pharmacol 393:187–191.
32. deSouza PL, Cooper MR, Imondi AR, Myers CE. 1997 9-aminocamptothecin: a topoisomerase I inhibitor with preclinical activity in prostate cancer. Clin Cancer Res 3:287–294.
33. Zamboni WC, Stewart CF, Thompson J, et al. 1998 The relationship between topotecan systemic exposure and tumor response in human neuroblastoma xenografts. J Natl Cancer Inst 90:505–511.
34. Thompson J, Stewart CF, Houghton PJ. 1998 Animal models for studying the action of topoisomerase I targeted drug. Biochimica Biophysica Acta 1400:301–319.
35. Pappo AS, Lyden E, Breneman J, et al. 2001 Up-front window trial of topotecan in previously untreated children and adolescents with metastatic rhabdomyosarcoma: an intergroup rhabdomyosarcoma study. J Clin Oncol 19:213–219.
36. Furman WL, Stewart CF, Kirstein M, et al. 2002 Protracted intermittent schedule of topotecan in children with refractory acute leukemia: a pediatric oncology group study. J Clin Oncol 20:1617–1624.
37. Cosetti M, Wexler LH, Calleja E, et al. 2002 Irinotecan for pediatric solid tumors: The Memorial Sloan-Kettering experience. J Ped Hematol Oncol 24:101–105.
38. Mugishima H, Matsunaga T, et al. 2002 Phase I study of irinotecan in pediatric patients with malignant solid tumors. J Ped Hematol Oncol 24:94–100.
39. Fujimori A, Harker WG, Kohlhagen G, Hoki Y, Pommier Y. 1995 Mutation at the catalytic site of topoisomerase I in CEM/C2, a human leukemia cell line resistant to camptothecin. Cancer Res 55:1339–1346.
40. Knab AM, Fertala J, Bjornsti MA. 1995 A camptothecin-resistant DNA topoisomerase I mutant exhibits altered sensitivities to other DNA topoisomerase poisons. J Biol Chem 270:6141–6148.
41. Bates SE, Robey R, Miyake K, Rao K, Ross DD, Litman T . 2001 The role of half-transporters in multidrug resistance. J Bioenerg Biomembr 33:503–511.
42. Maliepaard M, van Gastelen MA, Tohgo A, et al. 2001 Circumvention of breast cancer resistance protein (BCRP)-mediated resistance to camptothecins in vitro using non-substrate drugs or the BCRP inhibitor GF120918. Clin Cancer Res 7:935–941.
43. Scheffer GL, Maliepaard M, Pijnenborg AC, et al. 2000 Breast cancer resistance protein is localized at the plasma membrane in mitoxantrone- and topotecan-resistant cell lines. Cancer Res 60:2589–2593.
44. Kawabata S, Oka M, Shiozawa K, et al. 2001 Breast cancer resistance protein directly confers SN-38 resistance of lung cancer cells. Biochem Biophys Res Commun 280:1216–1223.
45. Thompson J, Stewart CF, Houghton PJ. Models for studying the action of topoisomerase-I targeted drugs. In: Cancer drug discovery and development. Tumor models in cancer research. Teicher BA, ed. Humana Press, New Jersey, 2002, 541–564.
46. Houghton PJ, Stewart CF, Zamboni WC, et al. 1996 Schedule- dependent efficacy of camptothecins in models of human cancer. Ann NY Acad Sci 803:188-201.
47. Erickson-Miller CL, May RD, Tomaszewski J, et al. 1997 Differential toxicity of camptothecin, topotecan and 9-aminocamptothecin to huma, canine, and murine myeloid progenitors (CFU-GM) in vitro. Cancer Chemo Pharmacol 39:467–472.
48. Parchment RE, Gordon M, Grieshaber CK, Sessa C, Volpe D, Ghielmini M. 1998 Predicting hematological toxicity (myelosuppression) of cytotoxic drug therapy from in vitro tests. Ann Oncol 9:357–364.

49. MacGregor JT, Collins JM, Sugiyama Y, et al. 2001 In vitro human tissue models in risk assessment: report of a consensus-building workshop. Toxicol Sci 59:17–36.
50. Morton CL, Wadkins RM, Danks MK, Potter PM. 1999 The anticancer prodrug CPT-11 is a potent inhibitor of acetylcholinesterase but is rapidly catalyzed to SN-38 by butyrylcholinesterase. Cancer Res 59:1458–1463.
51. Wiseman LR, Markham A. 1996 Irinotecan. Drugs. 52:606–623.
52. Ikuno N, Soda H, Watanabe M, Oka M. 1995 Irinotecan (CPT-11) and characteristic mucosal changes in the mouse ileum and cecum. J Natl Cancer Inst 87:1876–883.
53. Shinohara H, Killion JJ, Kuniyasu H, Kumar R, Fidler IJ. 1998 Prevention of intestinal toxic effects and intensification of irinotecan's therapeutic efficacy against murine colon cancer liver metastases by oral administration of the lipopeptide JBT 3002. Clin Cancer Res 4:2053–2063.
54. Hardman WE, Moyer MP, Cameron IL. 1999 Fish oil supplementation enhanced CPT-11 (irinotecan) efficacy against MCF7 breast carcinoma xenografts and ameliorated intestinal side-effects. Br J Cancer 81:440–448.
55. Sakai H, Diener M, Gartmann V, Takeguchi N. 1995 Eicosanoid-mediated Cl^- secretion induced by the antitumor drug, irinotecan (CPT-11), in the rat. Naunyn-Schmiedeberg's Arch Pharmacol 351:309–314.
56. Takasuna K, Hagiwara T, Hirohashi M, et al. 1996 Involvement of beta-glucuronidase in intestinal microflora in the intestinal toxicity of the antitumor camptothecin derivative irinotecan hydrochloride (CPT-11). Cancer Res 56: 3752–3757.
57. Cao S, Black JD, Troutt AB, Rustum YM. 1998 Interleukin 15 offers selective protection from irinotecan-induced intestinal toxicity in a preclinical animal model. Cancer Res 58:3270–3274.
58. Bacon JA, Petrella DK, Cramer CT, et al. 1996 Intestinal toxicity and changes in proliferating cell nuclear antigen (PCNA) levels in hamsters induced by a camptothecin analogue [abstract]. The Toxicologist
59. Kobayashi K, Bouscarel B, Matsuzaki Y, Ceryak S, Kudoh S, Fromm H. 1999 pH-dependent uptake of irinotecan and its active metabolite, SN-38, by intestinal cells. Int J Cancer 83:491–496.
60. Roy SK, Clark DL, Zheng H, McGuinn WD, Smith DD, Andrews PA. 1999 Predictive value of rodent and non-rodent toxicology studies in support of phase I trials of topoisomerase inhibitors. Proc American Assoc Cancer Res 40:737A.
61. Stewart CF, Zamboni WC, Crom WR, Houghton PJ. 1997 Disposition of irinotecan and SN-38 following oral and intravenous irinotecan dosing in mice. Cancer Chemother Pharmacol 40:259–265.
62. Abigerges D, Chabot GG, Armand J, Herait P, Gouyette A, Gandia D. 1995 Phase I and pharmacologic studies of the camptothecin analog irinotecan administered every three weeks in cancer patients. J Clin Oncol 13:210–221.
63. Catimel G, Chabot GG, Guastalla JP, et al. 1995 Phase I and pharmacokinetic study of irinotecan (CPT-11) administered daily for three consecutive days every three weeks in patients with advanced solid tumors. Ann Oncol 6:133–140.
64. Rothenberg ML, Kuhn JG, Burris HA, et al. 1993 Phase I and pharmacokinetic trial of weekly CPT-11. J Clin Oncol 11:2194–2204.
65. Morton CL, Wierdl M, Oliver L, et al. 2000 CPT-11 is primarily metabolized by ES-1-encoded plasma esterase in mice. Proc Am Assoc Cancer Res 41:819,5199a.
66. Morton CL, Wierdl M, Oliver L, et al. 2000Activation of CPT-11 in mice: identification and analysis of a highly effective plasma esterase. Cancer Res 60:4206–4210.

67. Morton CL, Taylor KR, Iacono L, et al. 2002 Metabolism of CPT-11 in esterase deficient mice. Proc Am Assoc Cancer Res 43:1231A.
68. Burke TG, Mi Z. 1994 The structural basis of camptothecin interactions with human serum albumin: impact on drug stability. J Med Chem 37:40–6.
69. Burke TG, Munshi CB, Mi Z, Jiang Y. 1995 The important role of albumin in determining the relative human blood stabilities of the camptothecin anticancer drugs [letter] [published erratum appears J Pharm Sci 84(12):1492]. J Pharm Sci. 84:518–519.
70. Liehr JG, Ahmed AE, Giovanella BC. 1996 Pharmacokinetics of camptothecins administered orally. Ann NY Acad Sci 803:157–163.
71. Kirstein MN, Houghton PJ, Cheshire PJ, et al. 2001 Relation between 9-aminocamptothecin systemic exposure and tumor response in human solid tumor xenografts. Clin Cancer Res 7:358–366.
72. Takimoto CH. 2001 Why drugs fail: of mice and men revisited. Clin Cancer Res 7:229–230.
73. Daud SS, Fetouh MI, Giovanella BC. 1995 Antitumor effect of liposome-incorporated camptothecin in human malignant xenografts. Anti-Cancer Drugs 6:83–93.
74. Burke TG, Gao X. 1994 Stabilization of topotecan in low pH liposomes composed of distearoylphosphatidylcholine. J Pharm Sci 83:967–969.
75. Bailly C, Lansiaux A, Dassonneville L, et al. 1999 Homocamptothecin, an E-ring-modified camptothecin analogue, generates new topoisomerase I-mediated DNA breaks. Biochemistry 38:15556–15563.
76. Sanders MM, Liu AA, Li TK, et al. 1998 Selective cytotoxicity of topoisomerase-directed protoberberines against glioblastoma cells. Biochem Pharmacol 56:1157–1166.
77. Bailly C, Qu X, Chaires JB, et al. 1999 Substitution at the F-ring N-imide of the indolocarbazole antitumor drug NB-506 increases the cytotoxicity, DNA binding, and topoisomerase I inhibition activities. J Med Chem 42:2927–2935.
78. Hill BT, Barrett JM, Perrin D, Gras S, Limouzy A, Chazottes E, van Hill B. 1999 Mechanism of action of F 11782, a novel catalytic dual inhibitor of topoisomerase I and II. Proc. Am Assoc Cancer Res 40:755A.
79. Kruczynski A, Astruc J, Chazottes E, et al. 1999 Preclinical antitumor activity of F 11782, a novel catalytic dual inhibitor of topoisomerase I and II. Proc Am Assoc Cancer Res 40:757A.
80. Kobayashi K, Takeda Y, Akiyama Y, et al. 1999 Reduced irinotecan-induced side-effects by the oral alkalinization. Proc Am Assoc Clin Oncol 18:1900a.
81. Schuetz JD, Leggas M, Sampath J, et al. 2002 Potent BCRP inhibition by the ErbB1 inhibitor ZD1839 (Iressa) dramatically enhances oral bioavailability of topotecan and irinotecan in mice. Proc Am Assoc Cancer Res 43:1351A.

7 Mechanisms of Resistance to Camptothecins

Zeshaan A. Rasheed, MD, PhD,
and Eric H. Rubin, MD

Contents

1. INTRODUCTION

Camptothecins (CPTs) are a group of antineoplastic agents that specifically target DNA topoisomerase I (TOP-I) and are known as "TOP-I poisons." The parent compound is a naturally occurring alkaloid found in the Chinese plant *Camptotheca accuminata.* This compound was first identified in the 1960s in a screen of plant extracts for antineoplastic drugs *(1).* Subsequently, many derivatives of the parent compound have been synthesized, including topotecan, irinotecan, 9-aminocamptothecin, 9-nitrocamptothecin, exatecan mesylate (DX-8951f), ST1481, and Karenitecin (BNP1350). Topotecan and irinotecan have been approved by the Food and Drug Administration for clinical use. Topotecan, a 10-hydroxyl modification of CPT, is approved for treatment of metastatic ovarian and small-cell

Camptothecins in Cancer Therapy
Edited by: V. R. Adams and T. G. Burke © Humana Press Inc., Totowa, NJ

lung cancer and for myeloid malignancies. Irinotecan (CPT-11) is a prodrug that is converted to the active compound SN-38 by plasma and cellular carboxylesterases, and is approved for use in the treatment of metastatic colorectal and rectal carcinomas. Food and Drug Administration approval for clinical use of both of these drugs was based on approximately 30% response rates with transient clinical responses *(2,3)*. However, based on studies in mouse xenograft models, these response rates are disappointing *(4–6)*. The mechanisms underlying *de novo* and acquired clinical resistance to CPTs are unclear. Similar to other drugs, clinical resistance to CPTs might be the result of inadequate metabolism and accumulation of drug in the tumor, alterations in the target (TOP-I), or alterations in the cellular response to the TOP-I–CPT interaction.

2. CELLULAR METABOLISM, ACCUMULATION, AND TRANSPORT OF CPTS

Cell culture data indicate that only brief exposures to submicromolar concentrations of CPT are required to target TOP-I and to kill proliferating cancer cells *(7)*. Additionally, the lactone form of CPT is the active form of the drug *(8)*. Achieving high enough intracellular concentrations of the active form of CPT is dependent on cellular uptake, metabolism, and efflux mechanisms (Table 1).

Few studies have addressed mechanisms of cellular CPT uptake. Both active and passive transport mechanisms are implicated in intestinal cell uptake of CPT *(9)*. Furthermore, active efflux by P-glycoprotein (P-gp) and multidrug resistance–associated protein (MRP) in mammalian intestinal cells may also limit the oral absorption of CPT-11 *(10)*. Another study found that ovarian cancer cells contain active transporters that are required for the influx of topotecan and SN-38 *(11)*.

In addition to uptake, cellular metabolism may be particularly important for the prodrug CPT-11, which is converted to its active form, SN-38, by cellular carboxylesterases *(12–15)*. Increased levels of cellular carboxylesterases correlate with increased cellular sensitivity to CPT-11 *(12,16)*. However, a recent study found that carboxylesterase-mediated sensitization of human tumor cells to CPT-11 cannot override BCRP-mediated drug resistance (which is further discussed in the following sections) *(17)*.

SN-38 is also conjugated and detoxified by UDP-glucuronosyltransferase (UGT) to yield an SN-38-glucuronide *(18)*. SN-38 glucuronidation is specifically catalyzed by human liver UGT1A1, UGT1A3, UGT1A6, and UGT1A9 isoforms *(19)* and is associated with increased efflux of the drug from colon cancer cells *(20)*. Furthermore, glucuronidation of CPTs has been associated with altered chemosensitivity of breast cancer cells and lung cancer cells *(21,22)*.

Table 1
Proteins Implicated in Cellular Resistance to CPTs

Process Protein	*Reference*
Cellular uptake	*9,11*
Metabolism Carboxylesterase	*12–15*
UDP-glucuronyltransferase	*18–20*
Cellular efflux P-glycoprotein	*24*
MRP2	*25*
BCRP	*26–30*

Several ATP-binding cassette (ABC) proteins have been implicated in efflux and cellular resistance to CPTs in yeast and mammalian cells. A screen for mutations that suppress the cytotoxic effects of CPT in yeast cells resulted in the identification of an ABC protein, Snq2, which confers resistance to CPT *(23)*. Furthermore, in mammalian cells, P-gp overexpression confers resistance to CPT derivatives, albeit to a lesser degree than to other substrates of P-gp, such as the anthracyclines *(24)*. Also, antisense oligonucleotides directed against the MRP2 gene can increase cellular sensitivity to CPT-11 and SN-38 *(25)*.

Recently, the BCRP gene (also known as MTX or ABCP), an ABC half-transporter *(26,27)*, was found to be overexpressed in cells selected for resistance to doxorubicin, mitoxantrone, or topotecan. Interestingly, these cells are cross-resistant to SN-38 and 9-aminocamptothecin, but not to CPT *(21,28–30)*. Additionally, in some human cells treated with anthracyclines a mutant form of BCRP (R482G/T) was preferentially selected, which exhibits greater resistance to anthracyclines and relative lower resistance to topotecan compared to the wild-type protein *(31,32)*. Furthermore, cells that overexpress both the native and mutant R482T form of BCRP are more resistant to and accumulate less 9-aminocamptothecin compared with a close analog, 9-nitrocamptothecin *(33)*. Similarly, another study showed that a lipophilic 7–modified CPT analogue (ST1481) is not a substrate for BCRP *(34)*. These results suggest that certain CPT analogs may be less susceptible to BCRP-mediated efflux. Furthermore, recent studies found that estrogen antagonists and agonists and novobiocin can enhance accumulation of CPT analogs in cells overexpressing BCRP, thereby overcoming BCRP-mediated drug resistance *(35,36)*.

To date, there are relatively few published studies of BCRP gene expression in clinical samples. BCRP seems to be expressed at low levels in breast cancer and leukemic cells *(37,38)*. Furthermore, the expression of BCRP in breast carcinoma cells does not seem to correlate with response to doxorubicin-based chemotherapy *(37)*, nor is it upregulated in patients with breast cancer that were previously treated with anthracyclines versus those patients that were not treated with these drugs *(39)*. Another recent study found that BCRP protein expression was increased in leukemia cells from three of four patients after an infusion of topotecan and arabinoside-C *(40)*. However, more clinical studies are needed to determine the role of BCRP overexpression and mutations in resistance to CPTs.

3. ALTERATIONS IN TOP-I THAT CONFER RESISTANCE TO CPTS

CPT causes DNA damage by stabilizing a normally transient covalent complex between TOP-I and DNA *(41)*. Furthermore, genetic studies in yeast identified TOP-I as a unique cellular target for the CPTs *(42–44)*. Therefore, it is not surprising that TOP-I mutations conferring resistance to CPT have been identified in various mammalian and yeast cells, and, more recently, in tumor tissue from a patient treated with irinotecan *(45)*. Most of the point mutations can be found clustered in three regions of the protein, including one near the catalytic tyrosine at position 723 *(46–55)* (Fig. 1). Furthermore, crystal structures of the TOP-I–DNA and TOP-I-DNA-topotecan covalent complexes and models of the TOP-I-DNA-drug ternary complex have enabled structural mapping of these mutations *(56–60)*. Structural models of the ternary complex implicate CPT in an intercalated position at the –1 and +1 base pairs of the cleavage site, with hydrogen bonding between the drug and both TOP-I and DNA, stabilizing the ternary complex. Mutations in the regions between amino acids 361–364, 533, and 722 explain resistance to CPT, because these regions of TOP-I are associated with the DNA and are in close proximity to the intercalated drug *(57)*.

Some TOP-I point mutations, including Y723F, Y727F, R364H, G503S, N722S, and F361S, which confer CPT resistance, are also implicated in resistance to the indolocarbazoles, a group of TOP-I–targeting compounds structurally unrelated to CPT *(61,62)*. These studies indicate that CPT and the indolocarbazoles may share binding sites in the TOP-I–DNA complex. In contrast, some TOP-I mutants, including N726S/A, that confer resistance to CPT retain sensitivity to the indolocarbazole rebeccamycin *(61)*. In addition to point mutations, a mutant TOP-I containing an internal duplication of residues 20–609 has been described in a murine cell line that is enzymatically resistant to the indolocarbazole, NB-506, and CPT *(63)*.

Recent studies also indicate that interactions between TOP-I and other proteins may affect cellular sensitivity to CPTs. The TOP-I–binding protein, nucleolin, may recruit TOP-I to the nucleolus as a result of the high rate of transcription in this region *(64)*. Studies of a nucleolin orthologue in yeast, Nsr1p, indicate that the absence of this protein is associated with relocalization of TOP-I from a predominantly nucleolar localization to a

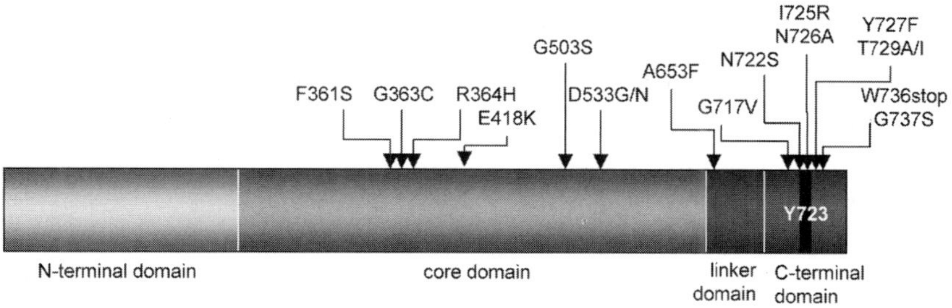

Fig. 1. Schematic of resistance-conferring mutations of TOP-I. The catalytic Y723 is indicated, as are the three main clusters of mutations.

diffuse nuclear localization in resistance to CPT *(65)*. Recently, nucleolin was found to redistribute from a predominantly nucleolar pattern to a speckled nuclear and perinuclear pattern in U937 cells exposed to CPT *(66)*. TOP-I is also known to move rapidly from the nucleolus to the nucleus after cellular exposure to CPT *(67,68)*. This relocalization has been associated with SUMO (small ubiquitin-like modifier) modification of TOP-I *(69)*. This event may decrease TOP-I–DNA interactions and thus minimize TOP-I–mediated DNA damage induced by CPT (*see* further discussion in the following sections). Notably, altered localization of topoisomerase IIα (top2α) (as a result of loss of nuclear localization sequences) was identified in mammalian cell lines resistant to the top2-targeting drugs etoposide and mitoxantrone, which presumably results in resistance by decreasing interactions between the enzyme and DNA *(70–73)*.

4. ALTERATIONS IN THE CELLULAR RESPONSE TO TERNARY COMPLEX FORMATION

CPT specifically targets TOP-I and induces the formation of CPT–TOP-I–DNA ternary complexes *(74)*. CPT cytotoxicity is S-phase selective and can be ameliorated in cell culture by treatment with the DNA polymerase inhibitor, aphidicolin *(75)*. Furthermore, collision of replication and transcriptional machinery with the ternary complex leads to double-stranded DNA breaks and is necessary for induction of cell death *(74,76)*. However, relatively little is known about the pathways downstream to CPT-TOP-I-DNA ternary complex formation that ultimately lead to repair of DNA damage or cell death.

Studies in yeast and cell culture models have implicated several DNA replication, DNA damage checkpoint, and DNA repair proteins in the response to cleavable complex formation (Table 2). Cellular exposure to CPT results in the activation of S-phase checkpoint proteins, such as Chk1

Table 2
Genes Implicated in the Cellular Response to CPT Induced DNA Damage

Process mutated gene	*Reference*
Checkpoint ATM, MEC1, MEC2	*79,81,115*
ATR	*78*
CHK1	*77*
RAD9, RAD17	*81,82*
DNA repair CAS, CSB	*116*
RAD6	*81*
TDP	*90*
TRF4	*117*
MSM2, MSM3, MSH2	*87,88,118*
XRCC	*91*
PNK1	*89*
DNA replication CDC45, DPB11	*83*
WRN	*84*
Ubiquitylation/sumoylation UBP1	*102*
DOA4	*103*
26S proteasome, ubiquitin	*101*
C9, SUMO	*104,119*

(77), ATR *(78)*, ATM *(79)*, and the DNA-dependent protein kinase (DNA-PK) multimer *(79,80)*. Furthermore, loss of function of Chk1 or ATR is associated with increased cellular sensitivity to CPT *(77,78)*. Several studies showed that loss of RAD9, a checkpoint protein that is activated by DNA damage and induces G_2 arrest, enhances TOP-I-induced cell death *(81,82)*. In addition to checkpoint proteins, proteins involved in DNA replication are also involved in CPT cytotoxicity. A yeast screen for conditional mutants with enhanced sensitivity to TOP-I-mediated DNA damage led to the identification of the yeast replication proteins, Dpb11p and Cdc45p, as important determinants of CPT sensitivity *(83)*. Dpb11p and Cdc45p are implicated in DNA polymerase switching from priming to processive replication *(83)*. Also, studies in murine cells implicate the loss of the Werner syndrome protein in CPT hypersensitivity *(84)*. The Werner protein is a helicase that interacts with TOP-I, and CO purifies with the DNA replication complex *(85,86)*.

With regard to repair of CPT-induced DNA damage, both mismatch repair and base excision repair systems are implicated (Table 2). Cells lacking the mismatch repair protein, MSH2, are hypersensitive to CPT *(87,88)*. Recently, Meijer et al. showed that a eukaryotic polynucleotide kinase, Pnk1, also plays a role in CPT-induced DNA damage repair, and cells lacking this gene are hypersensitive to CPT *(89)*. Additionally, Nash and colleagues identified a tyrosine-DNA phosphodiesterase that specifically cleaves TOP-I that is covalently linked to DNA *(90)*. Studies in yeast indicate that loss of tyrosine-DNA phosphodiesterase in the presence of mutant RAD9 confers hypersensitivity to CPT *(90)*. Importantly, although most of these studies indicate that loss of function of a DNA repair protein enhances cellular sensitivity, to date only a single study has demonstrated that overexpression of a DNA repair protein confers CPT hypersensitivity. Park et al. have shown that overexpression of a protein involved in base excision repair, X-ray repair cross-complementing gene I protein (XRCC), leads to CPT resistance in cells *(91)*.

Cellular processes, such as apoptotic pathways, downstream from DNA damage may also be important in the resistance to CPT *(92)*. Studies have shown that proapoptotic proteins, such as p53 and Bax, are upregulated after CPT treatment, whereas bcl-2 expression is decreased *(93)*. Additionally, CPT resistance has been associated with downregulation of apoptotic pathways involving Bcl-2, caspases, Akt, necrosis factor-κB (NF-κB), and transforming growth factor (TGF)-β *(94)*. Overexpression of bcl-2 and $p21^{Waf1/Cip1}$ have been associated with relative resistance to CPT *(92,95)*. Furthermore, CPT treatment of cells leads to the activation of caspases and cleavage of TOP-I, a substrate for caspase-3 *(93,96)*. Suppression of NF-κB leads to reduced CPT cytotoxicity by a p21-depenedent mechanism *(97)* and proteasome inhibition-mediated stabilization of NF-κB is associated with enhanced CPT cytotoxicity *(98)*. Finally, a recent study found that HER2 and HER3 cause a phosphoinositide-3 kinase–dependent activation of AKT that leads to CPT and multidrug resistance *(99)*. Taken together, these data indicate that proapoptotic and antiapoptotic proteins may regulate the cellular response to CPT.

Recently, posttranslational modifications of TOP-I were reported after CPT treatment of cells and may be involved in resistance. TOP-I is ubiquitylated and degraded after cells are treated with CPT, which appears to occur in the context of the ternary complex rather than free TOP-I *(100)*. Recently, tumor cells deficient in CPT-induced TOP-I downregulation were found to be more sensitive to CPT, implicating ubiquitylation of TOP-I as an important determinant of cellular sensitivity *(101)*. Additionally, CPT-induced TOP-I–DNA covalent complex formation results in transcriptional arrest and 26S proteasome-mediated degradation of TOP-I and the large subunit of RNA polymerase II. Degradation of the transcriptional machinery then initiates transcription-coupled repair. Furthermore, recovery from transcriptional arrest depends on degradation of TOP-I and functional transcription-coupled repair, affecting cellular sensitivity to CPT *(76)*. In yeast, two proteins related to the ubiquitylation pathway were discovered using genetic screens for mutants that alter CPT sensitivity. Overexpression of a ubiquitin specific protease, Ubp11, confers resistance to TOP-I–mediated DNA damage *(102)* and loss of DOA4, a 26S pro-teasome-associated C-terminal ubiquitin hydrolase, sensitizes cells to TOP-I–mediated DNA damage *(103)*.

TOP-I is also modified by SUMO after CPT treatment *(104)*. Sumoylation of TOP-I is associated with relocalization of the protein from the nucleolus to a more diffuse nuclear pattern after CPT treatment *(69)*, whereas, TOP-I mutants that cannot be sumoylated remain more concentrated in nucleoli of cells even after CPT treatment *(105)*. Together these studies strongly suggest that sumoylation regulates TOP-I localization in the nucleus and that sumoylation of TOP-I may function to decrease TOP-I–DNA interactions and thus minimize TOP-I–mediated DNA damage induced by CPT.

Although the mechanisms related to CPT-induced TOP-I ubiquitylation and sumoylation are unknown, recent studies of a TOP-I–binding protein, named topors, suggest that this protein may be involved *(106)*. Topors is a RING protein that functions in vitro as an E3 ubiquitin ligase *(107)* and as an E3-type SUMO ligase *(108)*. Moreover, topors sumoylates TOP-I in vitro *(108)*. In cells, topors is associated with promyelocytic leukemia (PML) nuclear bodies and rapidly disperses to a diffuse nuclear pattern on cellular treatment with CPT, similar to TOP-I *(109)*. It is possible that topors plays a role in the cellular response to CPT, and regulates the function of TOP-I after CPT-induced DNA damage (Fig. 2).

5. RESISTANCE TO CPT IN THE CLINICAL SETTING

More studies of clinical specimens are needed to determine whether the resistance mechanisms detected in yeast and cell culture models are clinically relevant. In addition, cellular metabolism, via carboxylesterases and UGTs, plays an important role in the cytotoxicity of CPT-11 in cell culture models. Little is known regarding the clinical relevance of this finding, although varied carboxylesterase activity has been reported in clinical specimens *(13,14)*. BCRP seems to be expressed at low levels in breast cancer cells and leukemic cells *(37,38)*. Recently, BCRP protein expression was found to increase in leukemia cells obtained from patients following infusion of topotecan and arabinoside-C in patients *(40)*. To date, altered expression of BCRP in clinical samples has not been proven to correlate with altered CPT sensitivity.

There is a limited number of clinical studies that have analyzed clinical specimens (tumor tissue or surrogates) for mutations in TOP-I and most have yielded negative results *(51,110)*. Recently, Tsurutani et al. reported a TOP-I mutation in a tumor specimen from a patient with large-cell carcinoma of the lung *(45)*. The mutation results in two changes, a stop codon at position 736 and a glycine to serine missense mutation at codon 737. Inter-

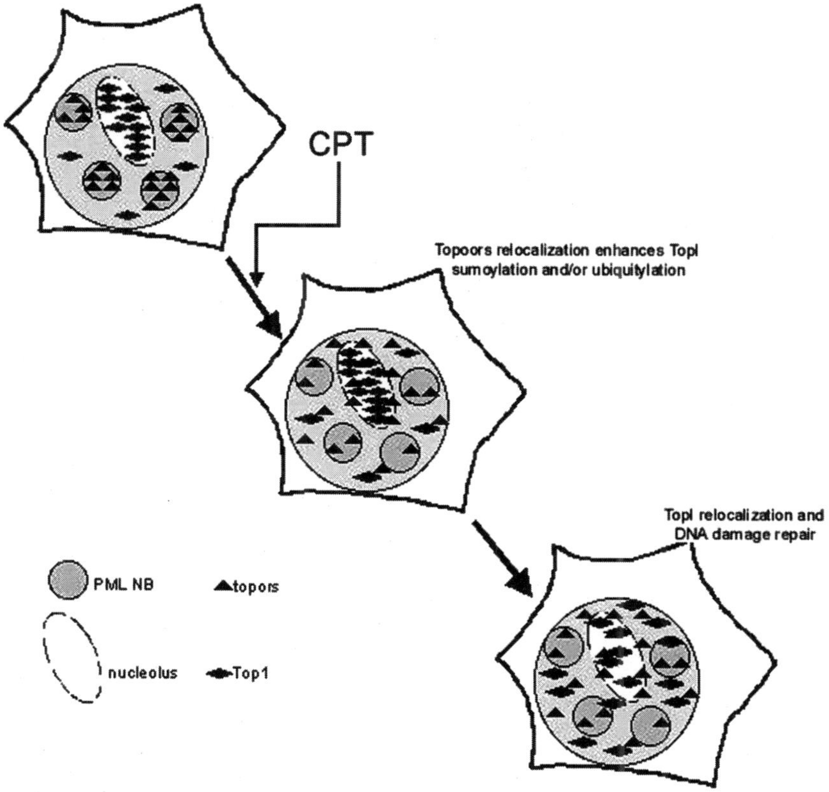

Fig. 2. Model of the regulation of TOP-I localization and its role in resistance to camptothecin (CPT). CPT treatment induces relocalization of TOP-I and topors to a diffuse nuclear pattern. The TOP-I topors complex may induce ubiquitylation or sumoylation of TOP-I in response to TOP-I–mediated DNA damage.

estingly, the patient with this mutation did not respond to a chemotherapy regimen consisting of cisplatin and irinotecan *(45)*. However, it remains to be determined if these mutations result in enzymatic resistance to CPT.

Other studies using clinical specimens found alterations in TOP-I and TOP-2α levels after treatment with CPT. Analyses in clinical study of 11 patients with nonhematological malignancies treated with oral CPT for 14 days showed decreases in TOP-I protein levels in nonmalignant peripheral blood mononuclear cells (PBMCs) that were not the result of cleavable complex formation, suggesting that TOP-I is degraded after CPT exposure in nonmalignant cells *(111)*. Analyses in a similar clinical study of nonmalignant PBMCs in patients treated with a 72-hour infusion of 9-aminocamptothecin (9-AC) also indicated decreases in TOP-I protein levels at 48 or 72 hours in two of three patients *(112)*. In contrast, two of four patients with leukemia who were treated with a 72-hour infusion of 9-AC showed no change in TOP-I protein levels in their malignant blast cells at 48 or 72 hours *(113)*, suggesting that if TOP-I degradation occurs in these cells, the timing is distinct from that of nonmalignant PBMCs. It is possible that the apparent difference in 9-AC–induced TOP-I degradation may relate to alterations in ubiquitin-proteasome pathways in malignant versus nonmalignant cells. These findings are consistent with the observation that malignant and nonmalignant cultured cells differ in their capacity to degrade TOP-I *(101)*. Interestingly, topors protein and mRNA expression are decreased in tumor tissues versus matched normal tissues, suggesting that topors may be involved in the apparent differences in CPT-induced TOP-I degradation in these tissues *(114)*.

Other mechanisms of CPT resistance that have been identified in yeast and cell culture models need to be evaluated clinically, including the role of TOP-I localization and specific repair processes. Pharmacogenetic and biochemical understanding of clinical CPT resistance will improve the use of CPTs in the treatment of malignancy.

ACKNOWLEDGMENTS

The authors would like to thank Drs. Leroy F. Liu and Ahamed Saleem for helpful discussions in writing this review.

REFERENCES

1. Wall ME, Wani MC. 1995 Camptothecin and taxol: discovery to clinic—thirteenth Bruce F. Cain Memorial Award Lecture. Cancer Res 55:753–760.
2. ten Bokkel Huinink W, Gore M, Carmichael J, et al. 1997 Topotecan versus paclitaxel for the treatment of recurrent epithelial ovarian cancer. J Clin Oncol 15:2183–2193.
3. Rothenberg ML, Eckardt JR, Kuhn JG, et al. 1996 Phase II trial of irinotecan in patients with progressive or rapidly recurrent colorectal cancer. J Clin Oncol 14:1128–1135.
4. Zamboni WC, Stewart CF, Cheshire PJ, et al. 1998 Studies of the efficacy and pharmacology of irinotecan against human colon tumor xenograft models. Clin Cancer Res 4:743–753.
5. Houghton PJ, Cheshire PJ, Hallman JD 2nd, et al. 1995 Efficacy of topoisomerase I inhibitors, topotecan and irinotecan, administered at low dose levels in protracted schedules to mice bearing xenografts of human tumors. Cancer Chemother Pharmacol 36:393–403.
6. Giovanella BC, Stehlin JS, Wall ME, et al. 1989 DNA topoisomerase I—targeted chemotherapy of human colon cancer in xenografts. Science 246:1046–1048.

7. Goldwasser F, Bae I, Valenti M, Torres K, Pommier Y. 1995 Topoisomerase I-related parameters and camptothecin activity in the colon carcinoma cell lines from the National Cancer Institute anticancer screen. Cancer Res 55:2116–2121.
8. Hertzberg RP, Caranfa MJ, Holden KG, et al. 1989 Modification of the hydroxy lactone ring of camptothecin: inhibition of mammalian topoisomerase I and biological activity. J Med Chem 32:715–720.
9. Gupta E, Luo F, Lallo A, et al. 2000 The intestinal absorption of camptothecin, a highly lipophilic drug, across Caco-2 cells is mediated by active transporter(s). Anticancer Res 20:1013–1016.
10. Luo FR, Paranjpe PV, Guo A, Rubin E, Sinko P. 2002 Intestinal transport of irinotecan in Caco-2 cells and MDCK II cells overexpressing efflux transporters Pgp, cMOAT, and MRP1. Drug Metab Dispos 30:763–770.
11. Ma J, Maliepaard M, Nooter K, et al. 1998 Reduced cellular accumulation of topotecan: a novel mechanism of resistance in a human ovarian cancer cell line. Br J Cancer 77:1645–1652.
12. Danks MK, Morton CL, Pawlik CA, Potter PM. 1998 Overexpression of a rabbit liver carboxylesterase sensitizes human tumor cells to CPT-11. Cancer Res 58: 20–22.
13. Ahmed F, Vyas V, Cornfield A, et al. 1999 In vitro activation of irinotecan to SN-38 by human liver and intestine. Anticancer Res 19:2067–2071.
14. Khanna R, et al. 2000 Proficient metabolism of irinotecan by a human intestinal carboxylesterase. Cancer Res 60:4725–4478.
15. Humerickhouse R, Lohrbach K, Li L, Bosron WF, Dolan ME. 2000 Characterization of CPT-11 hydrolysis by human liver carboxylesterase isoforms hCE-1 and hCE-2. Cancer Res 60:1189–1192.
16. Wierdl M, Wierdl M, Oliver L, et al. 2001 Sensitization of human tumor cells to CPT-11 via adenoviral-mediated delivery of a rabbit liver carboxylesterase. Cancer Res 61:5078–5082.
17. Wierdl, M, Wall A, Morton CL, et al. 2003 Carboxylesterase-mediated sensitization of human tumor cells to CPT-11 cannot override ABCG2-mediated drug resistance. Mol Pharmacol 64:279–288.
18. Ciotti M, Basu N, Brangi M, Owens IS. 1999 Glucuronidation of 7-ethyl-10-hydroxycamptothecin (SN-38) by the human UDP-glucuronosyltransferases encoded at the UGT1 locus. Biochem Biophys Res Commun 260:199–202.
19. Hanioka N, Ozawa S, Jinno H, Ando M, Saito Y, Sawada J. 2001 Human liver UDP-glucuronosyltransferase isoforms involved in the glucuronidation of 7-ethyl-10-hydroxycamptothecin. Xenobiotica 31:687–699.
20. Cummings J, Boyd G, Ethell BT, et al. 2002 Enhanced clearance of topoisomerase I inhibitors from human colon cancer cells by glucuronidation. Biochem Pharmacol 63:607–613.
21. Brangi M, Litman T, Ciotti M, et al. 1999 Camptothecin resistance: role of the ATP-binding cassette (ABC), mitoxantrone-resistance half-transporter (MXR), and potential for glucuronidation in MXR-expressing cells. Cancer Res 59:5938–5946.
22. Takahashi T, Fujiwara Y, Yamakido M, et al. 1997 The role of glucuronidation in 7-ethyl-10-hydroxycamptothecin resistance in vitro. Jpn J Cancer Res 88: 1211–1127.
23. Reid RJ, Kauh EA, Bjornsti MA. 1997 Camptothecin sensitivity is mediated by the pleiotropic drug resistance network in yeast. J Biol Chem 272:12091–12099.

24. Chen AY, Yu C, Potmesil M, Wall ME, Wani MC, Liu LF. 1991 Camptothecin overcomes MDR1-mediated resistance in human KB carcinoma cells. Cancer Res 51:6039–6044.
25. Koike K, Kawabe T, Tanaka T, et al. 1997 A canalicular multispecific organic anion transporter (cMOAT) antisense cDNA enhances drug sensitivity in human hepatic cancer cells. Cancer Res 57:5475–5479.
26. Kawabata S, Oka M, Shiozawa K, et al. 2001 Breast cancer resistance protein directly confers SN-38 resistance of lung cancer cells. Biochem Biophys Res Commun 280:1216–1223.
27. Honjo Y, Hrycyna CA, Yan QW, et al. 2001 Acquired mutations in the MXR/BCRP/ABCP gene alter substrate specificity in MXR/BCRP/ABCP-overexpressing cells. Cancer Res 61:6635–6639.
28. Maliepaard M, van Gastelen MA, de Jong LA, et al. 1999 Overexpression of the BCRP/MXR/ABCP gene in a topotecan-selected ovarian tumor cell line. Cancer Res 59:4559–4563.
29. Allen JD, Brinkhuis RF, Wijnholds J, Schinkel AH. 1999 The mouse Bcrp1/Mxr/Abcp gene: amplification and overexpression in cell lines selected for resistance to topotecan, mitoxantrone, or doxorubicin. Cancer Res 59:4237–4241.
30. Yang CH, et al. 2000 BCRP/MXR/ABCP expression in topotecan-resistant human breast carcinoma cells. Biochem Pharmacol 60:831–837.
31. Allen JD, Jackson SC, Schinkel AH. 2002 A mutation hot spot in the bcrp1 (abcg2) multidrug transporter in mouse cell lines selected for Doxorubicin resistance. Cancer Res 62:2294–2299.
32. Komatani H, Kotani H, Hara Y, et al. 2001 Identification of breast cancer resistant protein/mitoxantrone resistance/placenta-specific, ATP-binding cassette transporter as a transporter of NB-506 and J-107088, topoisomerase I inhibitors with an indolocarbazole structure. Cancer Res 61:2827–2832.
33. Rajendra R, Gounder MK, Saleem A, et al. 2003 Differential effects of the breast cancer resistance protein on the cellular accumulation and cytotoxicity of 9-aminocamptothecin and 9-nitrocamptothecin. Cancer Res 63:3228–3233.
34. Perego P, De Cesare M, De Isabella P, et al. 2001 A novel 7-modified camptothecin analog overcomes breast cancer resistance protein-associated resistance in a mitoxantrone-selected colon carcinoma cell line. Cancer Res 61:6034–6037.
35. Sugimoto Y, Tsukahara S, Imai Y, Sugimoto Y, Ueda K, Tsuruo T. 2003. Reversal of breast cancer resistance protein-mediated drug resistance by estrogen antagonists and agonists. Mol Cancer Ther 2:105–112.
36. Yang CH, Chen YC, Kuo ML. 2003 Novobiocin sensitizes BCRP/MXR/ABCP overexpressing topotecan-resistant human breast carcinoma cells to topotecan and mitoxantrone. Anticancer Res 23:2519–2523.
37. Kanzaki A, Toi M, Nakayama K, et al. 2001 Expression of multidrug resistance-related transporters in human breast carcinoma. Jpn J Cancer Res 92:452–458.
38. Ross DD, Karp JE, Chen TT, Doyle LA. 2000 Expression of breast cancer resistance protein in blast cells from patients with acute leukemia. Blood 96:365–368.
39. Faneyte IF, Kristel PM, Maliepaard M, et al. 2002 Expression of the breast cancer resistance protein in breast cancer. Clin Cancer Res 8:1068–1074.
40. Gounder M, et al. 2003 Sequential topoisomerase targeting in patients with leukemia: pharmacodynamic (PD) studies of phase I trial of topotecan/cytosine arabinoside (T/ara C) followed by etoposide. Proc Am Assoc Cancer Res

41. Hsiang YH, Hertzberg R, Hecht S, Liu LF. 1985 Camptothecin induces protein-linked DNA breaks via mammalian DNA topoisomerase I. J Biol Chem 260:14873–14878.
42. Bjornsti MA, Benedetti P, Viglianti GA, Wang JC. 1989 Expression of human DNA topoisomerase I in yeast cells lacking yeast DNA topoisomerase I: restoration of sensitivity of the cells to the antitumor drug camptothecin. Cancer Res 49:6318–6323.
43. Eng WK, Faucette L, Johnson RK. 1988 Evidence that DNA topoisomerase I is necessary for the cytotoxic effects of camptothecin. Mol Pharmacol 34:755–760.
44. Nitiss J, Wang JC. 1988 DNA topoisomerase-targeting antitumor drugs can be studied in yeast. Proc Natl Acad Sci USA 85:7501–7505.
45. Tsurutani J, Nitta T, Hirashima T, et al. 2002 Point mutations in the topoisomerase I gene in patients with non-small cell lung cancer treated with irinotecan. Lung Cancer 35:299–304.
46. Benedetti P, Fiorani P, Capuani L, Wang JC. 1993 Camptothecin resistance from a single mutation changing glycine 363 of human DNA topoisomerase I to cysteine. Cancer Res 53:4343–4348.
47. Chang JY, Liu JF, Juang SH, Liu TW, Chen LT. 2002 Novel mutation of topoisomerase I in rendering cells resistant to camptothecin. Cancer Res 62:3716–3721.
48. Fujimori A, Harker WG, Kohlhagen G, Hoki Y, Pommier Y. 1995 Mutation at the catalytic site of topoisomerase I in CEM/C2, a human leukemia cell line resistant to camptothecin. Cancer Res 55:1339–1346.
49. Kubota N, Kanzawa F, Nishio K, et al. 199. Detection of topoisomerase I gene point mutation in CPT-11 resistant lung cancer cell line. Biochem Biophys Res Commun 188:571–577.
50. Rubin E, Pantazis P, Bharti A, Toppmeyer D, Giovanella B, Kufe D. 1994 Identification of a mutant human topoisomerase I with intact catalytic activity and resistance to 9-nitro-camptothecin. J Biol Chem 269:2433–2439.
51. Takatani H, Oka M, Fukuda M, et al. 1997 Gene mutation analysis and quantitation of DNA topoisomerase I in previously untreated non-small cell lung carcinomas. Jpn J Cancer Res 88:160–165.
52. Tamura H, Kohchi C, Yamada R, et al. 1991 Molecular cloning of a cDNA of a camptothecin-resistant human DNA topoisomerase I and identification of mutation sites. Nucleic Acids Res 19:69–75.
53. Tanizawa A, Beitrand R, Kohlhagen G, Tabuchi A, Jenkins J, Pommier Y. 1993 Cloning of Chinese hamster DNA topoisomerase I cDNA and identification of a single point mutation responsible for camptothecin resistance. J Biol Chem 268:25463–25468.
54. Urasaki Y, Laco GS, Pourquier P, et al. 2001 Characterization of a novel topoisomerase I mutation from a camptothecin-resistant human prostate cancer cell line. Cancer Res 61:1964–1969.
55. Fiorani P, Bruselles A, Falconi M, Chillemi G, Desideri A, Benedetti P. 2003 Single mutation in the linker domain confers protein flexibility and camptothecin resistance to human topoisomerase I. J Biol Chem 278:43268–43275.
56. Redinbo MR, Stewart L, Kuhn P, Champoux JJ, Hol WG. 1998 Crystal structures of human topoisomerase I in covalent and noncovalent complexes with DNA. Science 279:1504–1513.

57. Staker BL, Hjerrild K, Feese MD, Behnke CA, Burgin AB Jr, Stewart L. 2002 The mechanism of topoisomerase I poisoning by a camptothecin analog. Proc Natl Acad Sci USA 99:15387–15392.
58. Stewart L, et al. 2001 Topotecan bound to human topoisomerase I at 2.0 A resolution. Proc Am Assoc Cancer Res 42(Suppl.):80–81.
59. Kerrigan JE, Pilch DS. 2001 A structural model for the ternary cleavable complex formed between human topoisomerase I, DNA, and camptothecin. Biochemistry 40:9792–9798.
60. Fan Y, Weinstein JN, Kohn KW, Shi LM, Pommier Y. 1998 Molecular modeling studies of the DNA-topoisomerase I ternary cleavable complex with camptothecin. J Med Chem 41:2216–2226.
61. Woo MH, Vance JR, Marcos AR, Bailly C, Bjornsti MA. 2002 Active site mutations in DNA topoisomerase I distinguish the cytotoxic activities of camptothecin and the indolocarbazole, rebeccamycin. J Biol Chem 277:3813–3822.
62. Urasaki Y, Laco GS, Pourquier P, et al. 2001 Use of camptothecin-resistant mammalian cell lines to evaluate the role of topoisomerase I in the antiproliferative activity of the indolocarbazole, NB-506, and its topoisomerase I binding site. Cancer Res 61:504–508.
63. Komatani H, Morita M, Sakaizumi N, et al. 1999 A new mechanism of acquisition of drug resistance by partial duplication of topoisomerase I. Cancer Res 59: 2701–2708.
64. Bharti AK, Olson MO, Kufe DW, Rubin EH. 1996 Identification of a nucleolin binding site in human topoisomerase I. J Biol Chem 271:1993–1997.
65. Edwards TK, Saleem A, Shaman JA, et al. 2000 Role for nucleolin/Nsr1 in the cellular localization of topoisomerase I. J Biol Chem 275:36181–36188.
66. Mi Y, Thomas SD, Xu X, Casson LK, Miller DM, Bates PJ. 2003 Apoptosis in leukemia cells is accompanied by alterations in the levels and localization of nucleolin. J Biol Chem 278:8572–8579.
67. Danks MK, Garrett KE, Marion RC, Whipple DO. 1996 Subcellular redistribution of DNA topoisomerase I in anaplastic astrocytoma cells treated with topotecan. Cancer Res 56:1664–1673.
68. Buckwalter CA, Lin AH, Tanizawa A, Pommier YG, Cheng YC, Kaufmann SH. 1996 RNA synthesis inhibitors alter the subnuclear distribution of DNA topoisomerase I. Cancer Res 56:1674–1681.
69. Mo YY, Yu Y, Shen Z, Beck WT. 2002. Nucleolar delocalization of human topoisomerase I in response to topotecan correlates with sumoylation of the protein. J Biol Chem 14:14.
70. Harker WG, Slade DL, Parr RL, Feldhoff PW, Sullivan DM, Holguin MH. 1995 Alterations in the topoisomerase II alpha gene, messenger RNA, and subcellular protein distribution as well as reduced expression of the DNA topoisomerase II beta enzyme in a mitoxantrone-resistant HL-60 human leukemia cell line. Cancer Res 55:1707–1716.
71. Mirski SE, Cole SP. 1995 Cytoplasmic localization of a mutant M(r) 160,000 topoisomerase II alpha is associated with the loss of putative bipartite nuclear localization signals in a drug-resistant human lung cancer cell line. Cancer Res 55:2129–2134.
72. Valkov NI, Gump JL, Engel R, Sullivan DM. 2000 Cell density-dependent VP-16 sensitivity of leukaemic cells is accompanied by the translocation of topoisomerase IIalpha from the nucleus to the cytoplasm. Br J Haematol 108:331–345.

73. Wessel I, Jensen PB, Falck J, Mirski SE, Cole SP, Sehested M. 1997 Loss of amino acids 1490Lys-Ser-Lys1492 in the COOH-terminal region of topoisomerase IIalpha in human small cell lung cancer cells selected for resistance to etoposide results in an extranuclear enzyme localization. Cancer Res 57:4451–4454.
74. Hsiang YH, Lihou MG, Liu LF. 1989 Arrest of replication forks by drug-stabilized topoisomerase I-DNA cleavable complexes as a mechanism of cell killing by camptothecin. Cancer Res 49:5077–5082.
75. D'Arpa P, Beardmore C, Liu LF. 1990 Involvement of nucleic acid synthesis in cell killing mechanisms of topoisomerase poisons. Cancer Res 50:6919–6924.
76. Desai SD, Zhang H, Rodriguez-Bauman A, et al. 2003 Transcription-dependent degradation of topoisomerase I-DNA covalent complexes. Mol Cell Biol 23: 2341–2350.
77. Wan S, Capasso H, Walworth NC. 1999 The topoisomerase I poison camptothecin generates a Chk1-dependent DNA damage checkpoint signal in fission yeast. Yeast 15:821–828.
78. Cliby WA, Lewis KA, Lilly KK, Kaufmann SH. 2002 S phase and G2 arrests induced by topoisomerase I poisons are dependent on ATR kinase function. J Biol Chem 277:1599–1606.
79. Wang H, Wang X, Zhou XY, et al. 2002 Ku affects the ataxia and rad 3-related/ CHK1-dependent S phase checkpoint response after camptothecin treatment. Cancer Res 62:2483–2487.
80. Shao RG, Cao CX, Zhang H, Kohn KW, Wold MS, Pommier Y. 1999. Replication-mediated DNA damage by camptothecin induces phosphorylation of RPA by DNA-dependent protein kinase and dissociates RPA:DNA-PK complexes. Embo J 18:1397–1406.
81. Simon JA, Szankasi P, Nguyen DK, et al. 2000. Differential toxicities of anticancer agents among DNA repair and checkpoint mutants of Saccharomyces cerevisiae. Cancer Res 60:328–333.
82. Megonigal MD, Fertala J, Bjornsti MA. 1997 Alterations in the catalytic activity of yeast DNA topoisomerase I result in cell cycle arrest and cell death. J Biol Chem 272:12801–12808.
83. Reid RJ, Fiorani P, Sugawara M, Bjornsti MA. 1999 CDC45 and DPB11 are required for processive DNA replication and resistance to DNA topoisomerase I-mediated DNA damage. Proc Natl Acad Sci USA 96:11440–11445.
84. Lebel M, Leder P. 1998 A deletion within the murine Werner syndrome helicase induces sensitivity to inhibitors of topoisomerase and loss of cellular proliferative capacity. Proc Natl Acad Sci USA 95:13097–13102.
85. Lebel M. 2001. Werner syndrome: genetic and molecular basis of a premature aging disorder. Cell Mol Life Sci 58:857–867.
86. Lebel M, Spillare EA, Harris CC, Leder P. 1999 The Werner syndrome gene product co-purifies with the DNA replication complex and interacts with PCNA and topoisomerase I. J Biol Chem 274:37795–37799.
87. Jacob S, Aguado M, Fallik D, Praz F. 2001 The role of the DNA mismatch repair system in the cytotoxicity of the topoisomerase inhibitors camptothecin and etoposide to human colorectal cancer cells. Cancer Res 61:6555–6562.
88. Pichierri P, Franchitto A, Piergentili R, Colussi C, Palitti F. 2001 Hypersensitivity to camptothecin in MSH2 deficient cells is correlated with a role for MSH2 protein in recombinational repair. Carcinogenesis 22:1781–1787.
89. Meijer M, Karimi-Busheri F, Huang TY, Weinfeld M, Young D. 2002 Pnk1, a DNA kinase/phosphatase required for normal response to DNA damage by gamma-

radiation or camptothecin in Schizosaccharomyces pombe. J Biol Chem. 277:4050–4055.
90. Pouliot JJ, Yao KC, Robertson CA, Nash HA. 1999 Yeast gene for a Tyr-DNA phosphodiesterase that repairs topoisomerase I complexes. Science. 286:552–555.
91. Park SY, Lam W, Cheng YC. 2002 X-ray repair cross-complementing gene I protein plays an important role in camptothecin resistance. Cancer Res. 62:459–465.
92 Nieves-Neira W, Pommier Y. 1999 Apoptotic response to camptothecin and 7-hydroxystaurosporine (UCN-01) in the 8 human breast cancer cell lines of the NCI Anticancer Drug Screen: multifactorial relationships with topoisomerase I, protein kinase C, Bcl-2, p53, MDM-2 and caspase pathways. Int J Cancer. 82:396–404.
93. Zhang XW, Xu B. 2000 Differential regulation of P53, c-Myc, Bcl-2, Bax and AFP protein expression, and caspase activity during 10-hydroxycamptothecin-induced apoptosis in Hep G2 cells. Anticancer Drugs. 11:747–756.
94. Reinhold WC, Kouros-Mehr H, Kohn KW, et al. 2003 Apoptotic susceptibility of cancer cells selected for camptothecin resistance: gene expression profiling, functional analysis, and molecular interaction mapping. Cancer Res. 63:1000–1011.
95. Walton MI, Whysong D, O'Connor PM, Hockenbery D, Korsmeyer SJ, Kohn KW. 1993 Constitutive expression of human Bcl-2 modulates nitrogen mustard and camptothecin induced apoptosis. Cancer Res. 53:1853–1861.
96. Samejima K, Svingen PA, Basi GS, et al. 1999 Caspase-mediated cleavage of DNA topoisomerase I at unconventional sites during apoptosis. J Biol Chem. 274:4335–4340.
97. Sakaida T, Iwadate Y, Yamaji S, et al. 2003 Acquisition of drug resistance by constitutive suppression of NF-kappaB in ras-transformed NIH3T3 mouse fibroblasts. Int J Oncol. 23:1071–1077.
98. Cusack JC Jr, Liu R, Houston M, et al. 2001 Enhanced chemosensitivity to CPT-11 with proteasome inhibitor PS-341: implications for systemic nuclear factor-kappaB inhibition. Cancer Res. 61:3535–3540.
99. Knuefermann C, Lu Y, Liu B, et al. 2003 HER2/PI-3K/Akt activation leads to a multidrug resistance in human breast adenocarcinoma cells. Oncogene. 22: 3205–3212.
100. Desai SD, Liu LF, Vazquez-Abad D, D'Arpa P. 1997 Ubiquitin-dependent destruction of topoisomerase I is stimulated by the antitumor drug camptothecin. J Biol Chem. 272:24159–24164.
101. Desai SD, Li TK, Rodriguez-Bauman A, Rubin EH, Liu LF. 2001 Ubiquitin/26S proteasome-mediated degradation of topoisomerase I as a resistance mechanism to camptothecin in tumor cells. Cancer Res. 61:5926–5932.
102. Byrne L, Bjornsti M. 2001 The ubiquitin C-terminal hydrolase, Ubp11p, suppresses camptothecin induced cell lethality. Proc Am Assoc Cancer Res. 42:415.
103. Fiorani P, Thimmaiah P, Bjornsti M. 2001 DOA4, a 26S proteosome-associated ubiquitin hydrolase, and the cortical actin cytoskeleton affect cell sensitivity to DNA topoisomerase I poisons. Proc Am Assoc Cancer Res. 42:717.
104. Mao Y, Sun M, Desai SD, Liu LF. 2000 SUMO-1 conjugation to topoisomerase I: A possible repair response to topoisomerase-mediated DNA damage. Proc Natl Acad Sci USA. 97:4046–4051.
105. Rallabhandi P, Hashimoto K, Mo YY, Beck WT, Moitra PK, D'Arpa P. 2002 Sumoylation of topoisomerase I is involved in its partitioning between nucleoli and nucleoplasm and its clearing from nucleoli in response to camptothecin. J Biol Chem. 277:40020–40026.

106. Haluska P Jr, Saleem A, Rasheed Z, et al. 1999 Interaction between human topoisomerase I and a novel RING finger/arginine-serine protein. Nucleic Acids Res. 27:2538–2544.
107. Rasheed ZA, et al. 2000 The topoisomerase I-binding protein, topors, may be a ubiquitin ligase. Proc Am Assoc Cancer Res. 41:210.
108. Rasheed ZA, et al. 2002 The RING protein, topors, functions as an E-type SUMO ligase for human topoisomerase. Proc Am Assoc Cancer Res. 43:1156.
109. Rasheed ZA, Saleem A, Ravee Y, Pandolfi PP, Rubin EH. 2002 The topoisomerase I-binding RING protein, topors, is associated with promyelocytic leukemia nuclear bodies. Exp Cell Res. 277:152–160.
110. Ohashi N, Fujiwara Y, Yamaoka N, Katoh O, Satow Y, Yamakido M. 1996 No alteration in DNA topoisomerase I gene related to CPT-11 resistance in human lung cancer. Jpn J Cancer Res. 87:1280–1287.
111. Gupta E, et al. 1998 Clinical evaluation of sequential topoisomerase targeting in the treatment of advanced malignancy. Cancer Therapeutics. 1:292–301.
112. Rubin E, Wood V, Bharti A, et al. 1995 A phase I and pharmacokinetic study of a new camptothecin derivative, 9-aminocamptothecin. Clin Cancer Res. 1:269–276.
113. Saleem, A., et al. 2000 Mechanisms of resistance to camptothecins. Ann N Y Acad Sci. 922:46–55.
114. Saleem A, et al. 2002 Topors functions as an E3-type SUMO ligase and is a candidate tumor suppressor gene on chromosome 9p13. Proc Am Assoc Cancer Res. 43(Suppl.):74.
115. Smith PJ, Makinson TA, Watson JV. 1989 Enhanced sensitivity to camptothecin in ataxia-telangiectasia cells and its relationship with the expression of DNA topoisomerase I. Int J Radiat Biol. 55:217–231.
116. Squires S, Ryan AJ, Strutt HL, Johnson RT. 1993 Hypersensitivity of Cockayne's syndrome cells to camptothecin is associated with the generation of abnormally high levels of double strand breaks in nascent DNA. Cancer Res. 53:2012–209.
117. Walowsky C, Fitzhugh DJ, Castano IB, Ju JY, Levin NA, Christman MF. 1999 The topoisomerase-related function gene TRF4 affects cellular sensitivity to the antitumor agent camptothecin. J Biol Chem. 274:7302–7308.
118. Pandit B, Roy M, Dutta J, Padhi BK, Bhoumik G, Bhattacharyya NP. 2001 Co-amplification of dhfr and a homologue of hmsh3 in a Chinese hamster methotrexate-resistant cell line correlates with resistance to a range of chemotherapeutic drugs. Cancer Chemother Pharmacol. 48:312–318.
119. Van Wardenburg R, Gibson A, Bjornsti M. 2002 Human homologues of yeast TAH genes that modulate cell sensitivity to camptothecin. Proc Am Assoc Cancer Res. 43:793.

8 Recent Advances in Camptothecin Drug Design and Delivery Strategies

Thomas G. Burke, PhD,*
Tian-Xiang Xiang, PhD,
Bradley D. Anderson, PhD,
and Lori J. Latus, MD

CONTENTS

1. INTRODUCTION

Camptothecin (CPT) (Fig. 1) and its related analogs are an expanding class of anticancer agents that have the potential to effect a broad and significant clinical impact *(1–15)*. Clinical interest in the CPTs is in large part based on their unique mode of action: these agents turn topoisomerase I (TOP-I), an enzyme that alleviates the torsional stress of supercoiled DNA, into an intracellular poison. The CPTs stabilize the covalent binding of TOP-I to its DNA substrate and the formation of these complexes leads to reversible, single-strand nicks. Initially, the nicks do not negatively affect the cellular viability; however, according to the fork collision model, the nicks are ultimately converted to irreversible and lethal double-strand breaks

*Deceased

Camptothecins in Cancer Therapy
Edited by: V. R. Adams and T. G. Burke © Humana Press Inc., Totowa, NJ

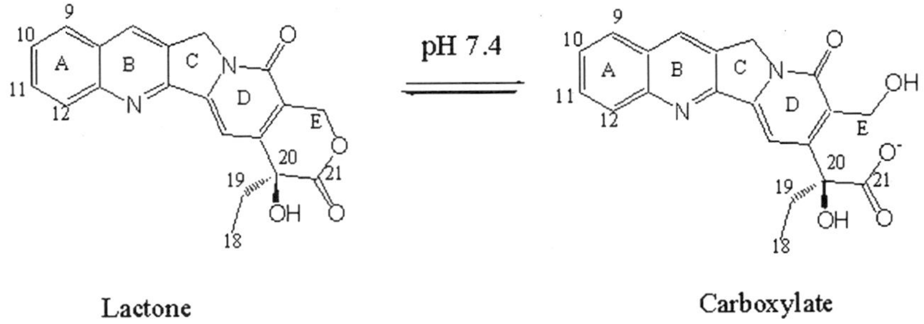

Fig. 1. Camptothecin hydrolysis at physiological pH.

during DNA synthesis. As a result of this mechanism of action, the CPTs are regarded as being S-phase specific agents and are therefore toxic to cells that are actively replicating DNA *(11,16,17)*. Because of their proliferating nature, cancerous cells spend more time in the S-phase relative to normal cells. Also, it has been shown that TOP-I is overexpressed in a variety of tumor lines *(8,15)*. Logically, the accelerated rate of cell replication and the overexpression of TOP-I provide a limited basis for selectivity through which the CPTs can generate greater cytotoxicity against cancerous cells than against normal cells.

The preclinical development and clinical utility of the CPTs have been obscured by their unique nature; they exhibit unusual reactivity and dynamics in vivo. With respect to reactivity, each of the clinically relevant CPT analogs shown in Fig. 2 possesses an α-hydroxy-δ-lactone pharmacophore. This moiety, at pH 7.0 and above, is extremely reactive and easily hydrolyzes to the carboxylate, or "ring opened," form (*see* Fig. 1). Although the lactone form of the CPTs has been shown to be the biologically active form, the carboxylate form is regarded as inactive *(18–20)*. As a consequence of the unstable α-hydroxy-δ-lactone pharmacophore, on dissolution in water the CPTs yield an equilibrium consisting of the two separate drug species: the biologically active lactone form and the biologically inactive carboxylate form generated on the hydrolysis of the parent drug *(14,18)*.

With respect to the unusual dynamics of these drugs in vivo, the extent of drug hydrolysis for several CPTs is intensified in human blood, because the equilibrium of active lactone form versus inactive carboxylate form is greatly affected by the presence of human serum albumin (HSA). Affected congeners include CPT, 9-aminocamptothecin, and 9-nitrocamptothecin. Taking advantage of the intensely fluorescent CPT lactone and carboxylate forms, time-resolved fluorescence spectroscopy has been implemented to directly measure the differential manner in which these two distinct drug forms interact with HSA *(21)*. Although the lactone form of CPT binds to HSA with moderate affinity, the carboxylate form of CPT tightly binds

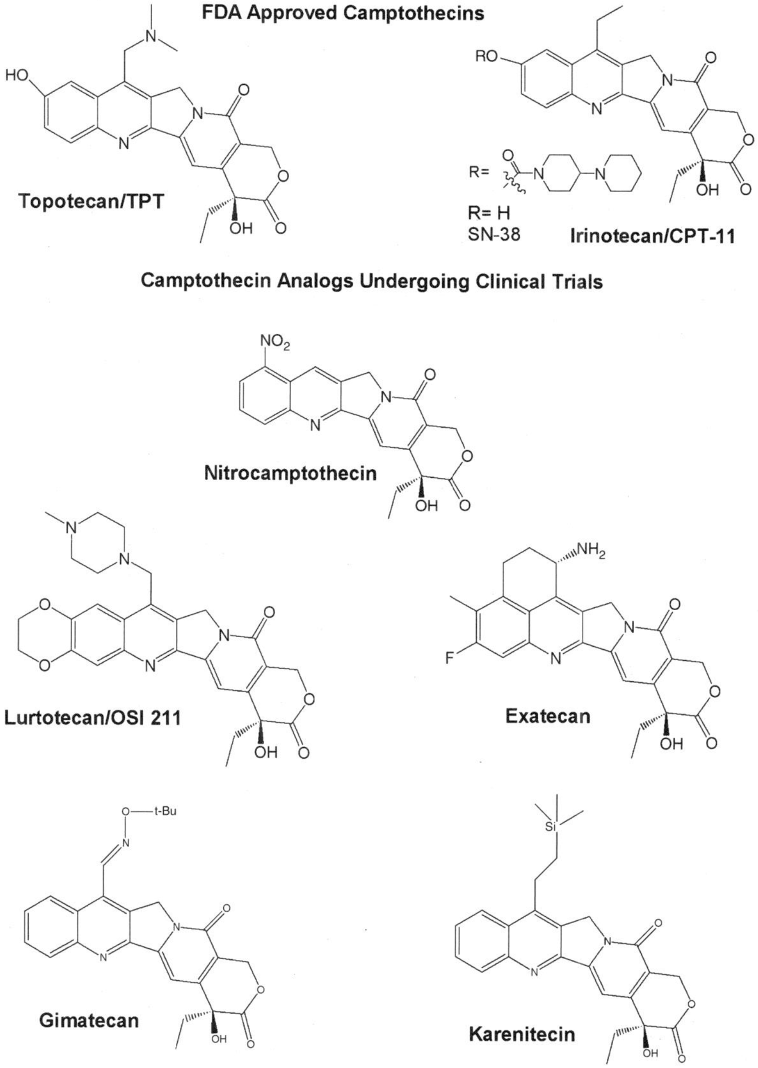

Fig. 2. Clinical candidates and Food and Drug Administration–approved analogs in the camptothecin family of antitumor agents.

HSA, resulting in a 150-fold increase in its affinity for this serum protein. After adding the lactone form of CPT to an aqueous solution containing HSA, the avid binding of the carboxylate form to HSA propels the chemical equilibrium to the right and ultimately leads to rapid and complete lactone ring hydrolysis. This extreme shift in the equilibrium is not observed when CPT lactone is added to an aqueous solution lacking HSA.

The labile nature of the CPT lactone pharmacophore, combined with high-affinity HSA interactions for specific CPT analogs, has confounded the clinical duplication of the impressive activity observed in preclinical studies, particularly those performed in murine models. For instance, that 9-aminocamptothecin was highly effective against human tumor xenografts in nude mice yet performed poorly in clinical studies may in part be due to the remarkable interspecies variations in albumin binding *(22,23)*. Indeed, physiologically relevant concentrations of HSA can attenuate, by 500- to 1000-fold, the anticancer activities (as measured by IC_{50} values) of CPT, 9-aminocamptothecin, and 9-nitrocamptothecin *(24,25)*. Thus, in humans, protein-binding interactions present a significant hurdle to realizing therapeutically effective lactone levels of these agents. Because prolonged exposures are requisite for therapeutic efficacy (owing to the S-phase-specificity of these drugs), rational analog design aimed at surmounting the distinctive in vivo reactivity and dynamics of the CPTs is a logical goal to pursue. In this chapter, we review several drug design and drug delivery approaches aimed at conserving the active lactone forms of the CPTs.

2. RATIONAL DRUG DESIGN

2.1. A,B-Ring Design Strategies for Elevating Active Lactone Levels in Blood and Tissue

In its initial clinical debut in 1972, CPT was first administered to patients as the "ring-opened" carboxylate (sodium salt form). This trial was initiated without any mechanistic understanding of drug action (i.e., without knowledge of the ultimate biological target of the compound and without the understanding that intact lactone functionality was required for anti-TOP-I activity) *(5,6,18)*. The necessity of a closed lactone ring for anti-TOP I activity was recognized in the 1980s and has since resulted in CPT development efforts focused on water-soluble, "closed-ring" congeners. Examples of such agents include topotecan and CPT-11 (*see* Fig. 2), which contain substituted A and B rings with water-solubilizing moieties (at the end of the molecule distal to the lactone moiety). With the expansion of these research and development efforts, it became apparent that the A and B rings of CPT could be modified by a variety of changes without negatively affecting the anti-TOP-I activity.

Although the anti-TOP-I activities of CPTs are frequently conserved with A,B-ring modification, changes in this portion of the drug strongly modulate human plasma and blood stabilities. Although >99.5 % of CPT and 9-aminocamptothecin convert to their carboxylate forms in human plasma *(26)*, agents such as topotecan, CPT-11, and SN-38 all display vastly improved stabilities (with equilibrium lactone of 12%, 21%, and 21%, respectively) *(24,27)*. Research has shown that the improved stabilities of

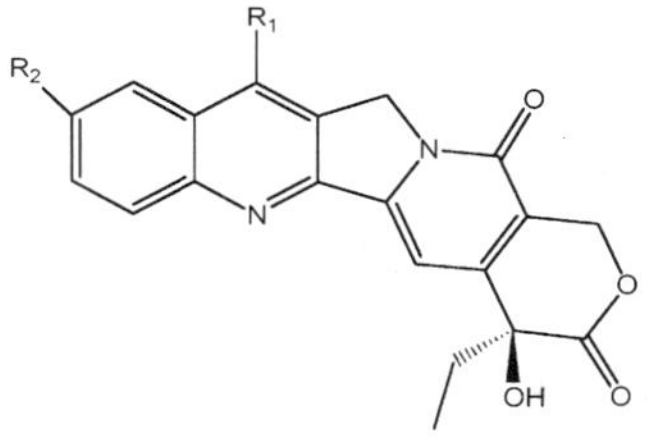

Compound	R_1	R_2
camptothecin	H	H
7-methylcamptothecin	$-CH_3$	H
7-ethylcamptothecin	$-C_2H_5$	H
7-propylcamptothecin	$-C_3H_7$	H
7-butylcamptothecin	$-C_4H_9$	H
DB-202	$-Si(CH_3)_2C(CH_3)_3$	H
DB-67	$-Si(CH_3)_2C(CH_3)_3$	OH
SN-38	$-C_2H_5$	OH

Fig. 3. Structures of several 7-modified and 7,10-modified camptothecins.

topotecan, CPT-11, and SN-38 relative to CPT and its 9-amino analog correlate well with their favorable interactions with HSA. Topotecan, SN-38, and CPT-11 contain structural functionalities in the A,B-rings that effectively prevent high-affinity binding of the carboxylate drug forms to HSA.

Recently the rational design of a dual 7,10-modified CPT has been described, an agent that displays markedly improved human blood stability and potent anti–TOP-I anticancer activity *(28)*. The new agent shown (Fig. 3) is 7-*t*-butyldimethylsilyl-10-hydroxy-camptothecin (DB-67). Prepared using the radical cascade approach *(29,30)*, the design of DB-67 was based on the following two considerations: (1) dual 7,10-substitution eliminates the highly specific binding of carboxylate form over lactone form by HSA *(21,26,27,31,32)* and (2) lactone ring stability is further enhanced by increased lipid bilayer partitioning *(21,33,34)*. Dual 7,10-substitution of CPT (in which the 10-substituent is a hydroxy group) vastly improves human plasma and blood stabilities *(27,35)*. SN-38 contains this dual 7-alkyl-10-hydroxy substitution pattern and it has been demonstrated that this modification prevents SN-38 from binding the high-affinity CPT carboxylate binding pocket on HSA *(27)*.

Table 1
Overall Association Constants for Camptothecin Analogues Interacting With Unilamellar Vesicles of Electroneutral DMPC, Negatively Charged DMPG in PBS Buffer at pH 7.4 and 37°C

Compound	$K_{DMPC}(M^{-1})$	$K_{DMPG}(M^{-1})$
20(S)-camptothecin	100	100
7-methyl-20(S)-camptothecin	150	180
7-ethyl-20(S)-camptothecin	250	300
7-propyl-20(S)-camptothecin	540	600
7-butyl-20(S)-camptothecin	940	—
DB-202	15500	1600
DB-67	2500	2800
SN-38	250	320

Binding isotherms were contructed using the method of fluorescence anisotropy titration, and K values were determined from the slopes of double-reciprocal plots. The K values are subject ot 10% uncertainty.

DMPC, dimyristoylphosphatidylcholine; DMPG, dimyristoyl-phospatidylglycerol; PBS, phosphate-buffered saline.

In addition to altered human albumin binding, lipophilicity also promotes CPT stability by favoring lactone partitioning into the membranes of red blood cells, thereby protecting the active lactone form from hydrolysis. Rational drug design efforts have focused on adding lipophilicity to CPT through 7-alkyl substitution. Figure 3 summarizes the structures of several 7-alkyl substituted CPTs, whereas Table 1 summarizes the overall association constants of the compounds interacting with small unilamellar vesicles of electroneutral dimyristoylphosphatidylcholine and negatively charged dimyristoyl-phosphatidylglycerol in phosphate-buffered saline at pH 7.4 and 37°C. The data contained in Table 1 indicate that increasing alkyl chain length at the 7-position (from methyl to butyl) increased membrane binding approximately 10-fold, whereas inclusion of a 7-*t*-butyldimethylsilyl functionality (DB-202) increased membrane binding an additional 10-fold over the butyl substitution.

After screening highly lipophilic 7-silylcamptothecins, otherwise known as silatecans, we observed that the key α-hydroxy-δ-lactone pharmacophore in DB-67 displays superior stability in human blood when compared with Food and Drug Administration–approved topotecan, CPT-11, and several other CPTs under clinical investigation *(28)*. A $t_{1/2}$ value of 130 minutes and a percent lactone at equilibrium value of 30 in human blood was observed for DB-67; the *t*-butyldimethylsilyl group enhances lipophilicity and thereby promotes drug associations with blood cells. DB-67 was found to be 25 times more lipophilic than CPT, 10 times more lipophilic than SN-38, and readily incorporates as its active lactone form into cellular and liposomal bilayers. In addition, the dual 7-alkylsilyl and 10-hydroxy substitution pattern in DB-67 blocks the associations of the carboxylate form of DB-67 with the high-affinity carboxylate binding pocket on HSA. Collectively, the enhanced lipophilicity and altered HSA interactions provide DB-67 with outstanding human blood stability when compared with other CPTs containing the conventional α-hydroxy-δ-lactone pharmacophore. DB-67 has also been shown to display potent anti-TOP-I activity and potent anticancer activity in vitro and in vivo *(28,36)*.

2.2. E-Ring Design Strategies Resulting in Intrinsically Potent Agents With Altered Hydrolysis Profiles

Lavergne, Bigg, and collaborators *(37,38)* developed an alternative medicinal chemistry approach to enhancing lactone ring stability. In 1997 they reported that an E-ring-expanded congener of CPT (otherwise known as homocamptothecin [Fig. 4]), prepared by homologation of the α-hydroxy lactone to a β-hydroxy lactone, displayed significantly enhanced human plasma stability. Interestingly, the homologation procedure allowed for the conservation of high anti-TOP-I activity *(37,38)*. Since the initial findings, other studies have shown that homocamptothecin and its related A,B-ring analogs display biological activities against a range of different cancers *(38–51)*.

Whereas the α-hydroxy lactone of CPT activates the lactone toward a nucleophilic attack, the presence of a β-hydroxy lactone prevents this type of facile activation of the lactone. The resulting β-hydroxy lactone is stable over a period of several hours. Because more than a decade of previous research suggested that any change to the E-ring portion of CPT significantly attenuated anticancer activity *(14,18,19,52)*, the finding that activity can be conserved through homologation of the α-hydroxy lactone to a β-hydroxy lactone E-ring received considerable attention.

The rational design and total synthesis of A,B,E-ring–modified 7-silylcamptothecins (homosilatecans) have also been described *(53)* and are shown in Fig. 4. Prepared by total synthesis using the cascade radical annulation approach *(29)*, the homosilatecan agents combine E-ring expansion (or homologation of the α-hydroxy lactone to a β-hydroxy lactone as described by Lavergne, Bigg, and coworkers) with A,B-ring modifications. Homosilatecans contain a silyl group at position 7 and, in some cases, modifications at the 10 position. Using high-performance liquid chromatography, homosilatecans were observed to be very blood stable (over several hours) *(53)*, significantly improving on the plasma and blood stability observed for homocamptothecin. Homo-silatecans displayed greater than 80% lactone levels after 3 hours of incubation, with homosilatecan lactone levels being substantially in excess of the blood lactone levels observed for clinically relevant CPTs at similar time points. Whereas marked interspecies

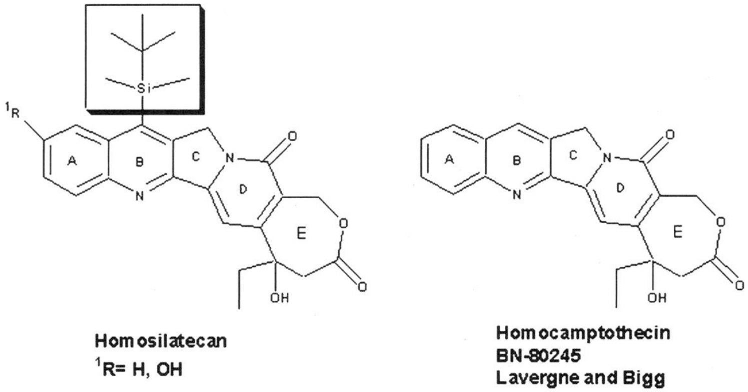

Fig. 4. Structural comparison of the homosilatecans and homocamptothecin.

variations in blood stabilities have been previously noted for agents such as CPT and 9-aminocamptothecin, no such variations occur for homosilatecans *(53)*. Thus it seems likely that successful treatment strategies achieved in animal models with homo-silatecans may be more readily translated to a clinical setting.

As described previously, rational design efforts can lead to the development of new analogs that display altered stabilities and high intrinsic potencies. Creation of homocamptothecin analogs through the insertion of a methylene group in the E-ring has been shown to be a convenient means of altering human blood stabilities and maintaining high intrinsic potencies. Moreover, the interesting biological properties of the E-ring-expanded analogs have prompted investigations of other changes to the E-ring. The synthesis of a novel E-ring-modified keto ether analog of CPT and homocamptothecin has been recently reported *(54)*. The new analog is an isomer of homocamptothecin that includes the α-hydroxy carbonyl functionality that CPT possesses and that is absent in the homocamptothecin structure. The new keto ether analog, which contains an E-ring that does not open in contrast to CPT and homocamptothecin analogs, was found to be inactive in cell culture assays. This initial finding suggests some degree of E-ring lability may be important for activity against the topoisomerase I target.

2.3. E-Ring Design Strategies Resulting in Prodrugs That Undergo Nonenzymatic Intramolecular Activation

There are two CPT analogs that are Food and Drug Administration approved, topotecan and irinotecan (CPT-11). CPT-11 is a prodrug that requires enzymatic activation via carboxylesterases to generate the active metabolite, SN-38. Between topotecan and SN-38, SN-38 possesses the greatest intrinsic human blood stability relative to the level of active lactone species of the drug. In whole blood, SN-38 displays 21% lactone at equilibrium whereas topotecan displays 12% lactone levels *(27)*. Despite the enhanced blood lactone levels of its active agent, the clinical utility of CPT-11 is negatively affected by its propensity to cause severe diarrhea, which is considered to be its major toxicity *(55)*.

The pharmacology of CPT-11 is complex and it is not entirely clear how this affects its tendency to cause severe diarrhea. First, as with all α-hydroxy-δ-lactone CPT congeners, the active metabolite SN-38 displays the typical reactivity that yields the inactive carboxylate versus active lactone equilibrium. Second, SN-38 is detoxified to SN-38 glucuronide (SN-38G) by the enzyme UGT1A1 *(56)*. Preliminary reports indicate that interpatient variation in glucuronidation of SN-38 correlates with the occurrence of dose limiting diarrhea: the higher the biliary index (the ratio of SN-38 to SN-38G), the greater the severity of the diarrhea *(57)*. Third, the reverse reaction, SN-38G>>SN-38, is catalyzed by bacterial glucuronidases in the intestine; the impact of the intestinal flora on this retroconversion can be modulated by antibiotics in some patients *(58)*. Last, a mere fraction of the administered CPT-11 drug is converted to SN-38 and, accordingly, the residual prodrug is either metabolized (CYP3A4, CYP3A5) or excreted (hepatic and renal modes of elimination) *(59)*. Carboxylesterases are ubiquitous enzymes. Prodrug conversion may therefore occur both in normal tissues, typically the liver, and at the tumor site, albeit with reduced efficiency relative to the liver. Moreover, because each patient exhibits a highly individual pharmacokinetic profile after CPT-11 administration, the extent of the toxicity cannot be predicted *a priori*. In view of multifarious processes that affect the ultimate activity of CPT-11, a reasonable hypothesis would be that simplification of the active SN-38 agent's pharmacology may result in improved efficacy and a more predictable toxicity profile. Recent reviews of CPT-11 *(55,60)* have underscored the need for approaches that reduce toxicities and improve efficacies for this agent.

A prodrug approach has been pursued in our laboratory that is based on nonenzymatic prodrug conversion and liposomal targeting of the prodrug to the tumor site. In patients, CPTs exhibit broad biodistribution to both tumor lesions and healthy tissue, with the latter resulting in myelosuppression and, as mentioned previously, dose-limiting diarrhea *(61)*. Previous research has indicated that such toxicities can be mitigated and tumor targeting enhanced by using liposomal core-loaded drug formulations *(62)*. Recently, we described a versatile prodrug strategy for loading the liposomal lumen with water-insoluble CPTs *(63)*. Before our work, research on core-loaded liposomal CPT formulations had been limited to the water-soluble CPTs topotecan, CPT-11, GG-211 (lurtotecan), and CDK-602. Each of these agents contains a basic amino group and loads into the core of premade small unilamellar vesicles using well-established ion gradient methods *(64,65)*.

Water-insoluble CPTs such as 7-ethyl-10-hydroxy-camptothecin (SN-38) and 7-*t*-butyl-dimethylsilyl-10-hydroxycamptothecin (DB-67) lack amino groups and do not load into liposomes using gradient driven processes. To prepare prodrugs of these agents that readily load into the core of liposomes and, unlike CPT-11, do not require enzymatic activation, we developed a procedure *(63)* that involves conversion of an active CPT analog to a 20-OR ω-aminoalkanoic acid ester prodrug in which $R = CO[CH_2]_nNH_2$ and $n = 1–3$. The basic amino group of the prodrug serves three roles. First, at pH ranges of 3.0 to 5.0, the amine enhances aqueous solubility. Second, it enhances responsiveness to a transmembrane ammonium sulfate gradient across the liposomal bilayer, thereby facilitating active loading of the agent into the liposomal aqueous core. Finally, at a physiological pH of 7.0 or above (the pH to be encountered after drug release), the nucleophilicity of the amine manifests itself and cyclization to the C-21 carbonyl carbon occurs. As shown in Fig. 5, the result of the reaction for the glycine ester is the formation of an unusual six-membered morpholine 2,5-dione ring 2 (or lactam intermediate). The lactam intermediate arose by intramolecular nucleophilic attack of the amino group on the lactone E-ring carbonyl carbon of CPT. This cyclization triggers a rapid and convenient nonenzymatic decomposition process that releases active CPT.

Accordingly, this novel liposomal approach (Fig. 6) offers a potential system for tumor-targeting prodrugs of many water-insoluble CPTs, including the highly lipophilic and clinically attractive analogs SN-38 and DB-67. The rate of formation of the active agent at the tumor site occurs by chemical activation and can be controlled through the selection of *n* (the length of the alkyl spacer group). Whereas other CPT prodrugs such as CPT-11 and camptothecin-20(S)-alkylesters *(66,67)* require enzymatic activation, the 20-OR ω-aminoalkanoic acid ester prodrugs described in our work feature pH-mediated self-activation. Such nonenzymatic activation suggests these prodrugs will be well-suited for liposomal targeting to tumor tissue. Because of the inefficiency of CPT-11 metabolism to the active agent SN-38 in the human body, chemically activated 20-OR ω-aminoalkanoic acid ester prodrugs of SN-38 may also be of potential utility prepared as an intravenous injectable without liposomal formulation.

3. DRUG DELIVERY STRATEGIES

3.1. Cyclodextrin Formulations of CPTs

Although increased lipophilicity and reduced interaction with HSA for CPT analogs such as DB-67 can markedly improve their human blood sta-

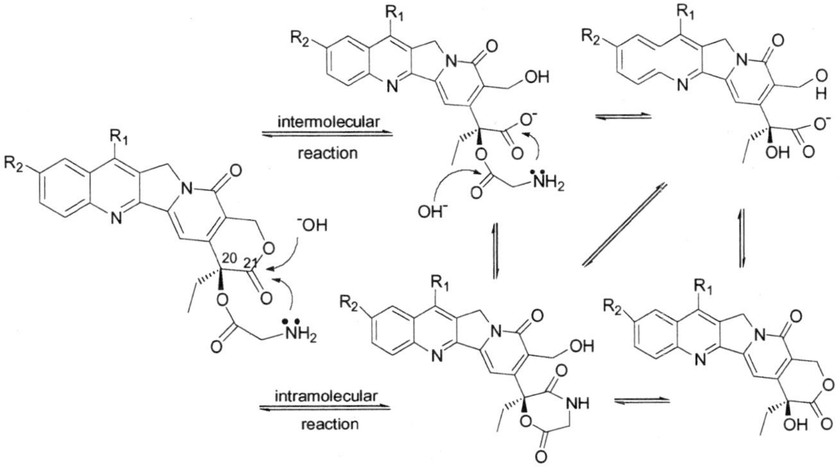

Fig. 5. 20-OR ω-aminoalkanoic acid ester prodrugs featuring pH-mediated self-activation with the formation of a novel lactam intermediate.

bility and anti-TOP-I activity, these CPT analogs in their lactone form usually possess much poorer water solubility, making their parenteral formulation a real challenge. In the past, poor solubility has prevented the extensive use of highly lipophilic CPT analogs in the clinical treatment of cancer. In recent years, several approaches have been explored including liposomes *(33,34)*, microspheres *(68–70)*, and complexation with cyclo-dextrin derivatives *(71–75)*. Cyclodextrins have been widely used to improve solubility, stability, and bioavailability of a variety of poorly soluble and labile drugs *(76–82)*. Kang and coworkers have recently investigated the solubility and stability of the lactone-ring intact CPT as a function of concentrations of various α-, β-, and γ-cyclodextrins *(74)*. The phase-solubility measurements show a linear increase in the solubility of CPT with increasing concentration of CDs with the 1:1 stability constants ($K_{1:1}$) being in the range of 41 to 910 M^{-1}. The stability of CPT in a pH 7.4 buffer also increases linearly with an increase in the concentration of dimethyl-β-CD (DM-CD). The observed pseudo–first-order hydrolysis rate constants (k_{obs}) for the free and complexed CPT are $19.7 \times 10^{-5}/s^{-1}$ and $1.97 \times 10^{-5}/s^{-1}$, respectively, corresponding to an increase in half-life of CPT from 0.98 to 9.8 hours. Cytotoxicity studies against the human-derived myeloid THP-1 leukemia cell line have shown DM-CD/CPT and hydroxypropyl-CD/CPT complexes to be about twofold more active than free CPT, presumably because of an increase in the stability of the complexed CPT against hydrolysis *(74)*. Cyclodextrins can form even more stable complexes with the lactone-ring–

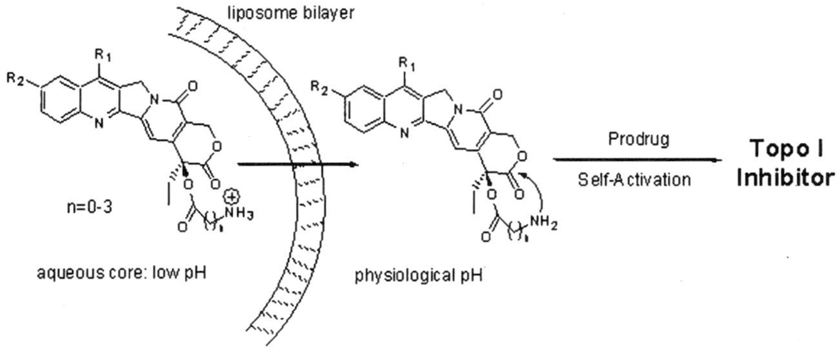

Fig. 6. Liposomes provide a means of targeting amine-containing prodrugs. The low pH within the liposomal core slows prodrug decomposition until it is released from the particle and encounters physiological pH, which initiates the decomposition reaction.

closed DB-67 with 1:1 stability constants ($K_{1:1}$) of $8.5 \times 10^3/M^{-1}$ and $5.8 \times 10^3/M^{-1}$ for sulfobutyl ether (SBE-CD) and 2-hydroxypropyl β-cyclodextrins (HP-CD), respectively, and a 1:2 stability constant ($K_{1:2}$) of $3.8 \times 10^4/M^{-1}$ for the neutral HP-CD *(75)*. The 1:1 stability constants for the lactone-ring-opened DB-67 with SBE-CD and HP-CD are 34- and 3.4-fold lower, respectively. The presence of 20% (w/v) SBE-CD or HP-CD reduces the rate of lactone-ring–opening hydrolysis at pH 7.4 by 1.6-fold and 1.8-fold, respectively, presumably because of the inclusion of the lactone ring in the 1:2 complex with HP-CD and the negatively charged ether groups in SBE-CD that may repel attacking OH^- ions near the lactone ring. Comparative studies on CPT and DB-67 indicated that the hydrophobic substituent in DB-67, silatecan 7-*t*-butyldimethylsilyl, is included within the CD cavity and another binding site at the lactone-ring is most plausible, because steric hindrance may prevent the binding of two cyclodextrins near the A and B rings. In spite of the remarkable solubilization of DB-67 by cyclodextrins, it is still not sufficient to achieve a desired concentration of 2 mg/mL for parenteral administration. Xiang and Anderson recently reported a method for preparing stable supersaturated aqueous solutions for DB-67 and, potentially, for other lipophilic CPT analogs *(75)*. In this approach, a concentrated alkaline aqueous solution of DB-67 carboxylate is mixed with an acidified cyclodextrin solution. The slow conversion from DB-67 carboxylate to the lactone form after the mixing prevents rapid precipitation of DB-67 for several days such that the mixture could be lyophilized for long-term storage and reconstituted to yield a clear, stable solution for parenteral administration. In separate studies, water-soluble cyclodextrin polymers are used as carriers that release CPT analogs and other drugs at their site of action under controlled conditions *(72)*.

3.2. Liposomal Formulations

Because of the presence of both aqueous and lipid bilayer compartments, liposomes possess both utility and versatility in stabilizing the lactone form of the CPTs *(27,38,51,56)*. Essentially, all CPTs are capable of associating with membranes *(38,51,56)*, and some proportion of core-loaded CPT drugs will integrate within the lipid bilayer (a higher fraction for lipophilic drugs such as DB-67 and a lower fraction for water-soluble agents such as topotecan). CPT agents that reside within the bilayer typically do so in the lactone form, thus bilayer associations can promote and stabilize the active form of CPTs. In addition, many CPT agents with reduced lipophilicity can be loaded into the liposome core and stabilized via pH reduction of the aqueous core milieu *(56)*.

Liposomes are a clear example of how the reactive nature of the CPTs can be modulated and the therapeutic efficacy of these agents can be potentially augmented. Drug-laden liposomal particles offer several distinct advantages. First, prolonged plasma exposures can be achieved, particularly via the use of stealth liposomes *(58)*. The Doxil (liposome-encapsulated doxorubicin) formulation (Alza), which implements Stealth liposome technology (Alza), incorporates 5% polyethyleneglycol (PEG)-linked distearoyl-phosphatidyl-ethanolamine in the liposome. In circulation, the lipid-conjugated PEG dually functions to prevent opsonization and extend the lifetime of the liposome *(83–85)*. Second, tumor lesions can be passively or actively targeted, thus elevating the levels of active drug at the tumor site. With respect to passive tumor targeting, studies have shown that Doxil and DaunoXome (liposome-encapsulated daunorubicin, Gilead) target tumors by exploiting the leaky tumor vasculature (also known as enhanced permeability and retention) *(86)*, which facilitates particle accumulation. An excellent example of passive tumor targeting and therapeutic response using liposomes is the treatment of Kaposi's sarcoma, which exhibits enhanced permeability and retention *(86)*. Finally, the liposomes can be engineered to act as drug storage depots such that protracted exposure to drug at the tumor locale can be optimized. Overall, the interest in using liposomes to stabilize CPTs and target their delivery to specific tissues has grown. To underscore this point, select investigations of liposomal CPT products are described in the following sections.

The most developed example of a liposomal CPT product is 7-[(4-methylpiperazino)methyl]-10,11-(ethylenedioxy)-(20S)-camptothecin trifluoroacetate [GI-147211C], which has been prepared in a lipid matrix similar to that of Doxil. In addition, GI-147211C (Gilead) has been encapsulated in a lipid matrix similar to that of DaunoXome. Both matrices consist of unilamellar liposomes made of phosphatidylcholines with saturated fatty acid chains and cholesterol. Such resilient bilayers serve two functions: drug leakage reduction and opsonization deterrence. Independent studies, which are described in the following section, have indicated that the liposomal encapsulation of GI-147211C (in either matrix) enhances the therapeutic index several-fold *(87)*. These results concur with studies of liposomal formulations of topotecan in which encapsulated topotecan was more efficacious than free drug *(88)*.

Preclinical studies in murine models have clearly documented the protective effects of the liposomal carrier on the stabilization of active GI-147211C and the prolongation of plasma exposure time. Because GI-147211C is an amphipathic agent, maintenance of the lactone species occurs on two fronts: stabilization of active drug via drug lactone intercalation of the lipid bilayer of the liposome and drug lactone conservation via pH adjustment of the core environment. Ultimately, GI-147211C within the bilayer can exit, or "leak" out of, the liposome; such leakage from liposomal GI-147211C formulations has been observed both in phosphate buffer and in plasma *(87)*.

Nevertheless, liposomal formulations of GI-147211C can modify drug biodistribution and concomitantly reduce drug accretion in normal tissues. Free GI-147211C causes potent general toxicity, which ultimately restricts the amount of GI-147211C that can be safely administered *(89–93)*. Thus, to delineate the therapeutic and pharmacokinetic differences between liposomal GI-147211C (in a lipid matrix similar to the Doxil) and free GI-147211C, in vivo murine studies were performed *(87)*. With respect to the plasma pharmacokinetics, notably enhanced blood circulation time for the liposomal formulation relative to free GI-147211C were noted; on dose correction, the area under the curve and C_{max} for the liposomal formulation (10 mg/kg) were 1250-fold and 35-fold higher, respectively, than the corresponding values for the free GI-147211C (8.72 mg/kg). With respect to evaluating therapeutic efficacy, a nude mouse xenograft model (H29 human colon carcinoma) was employed. The liposomal GI-147211C formulation (1 mg/kg liposomal GI-147211C) exhibited a 20-fold enhancement in antitumor activity relative to the nonliposomal GI-147211C (20 mg/kg GI-147211C). Treatment with free GI-147211C did not induce complete responses where as the liposomal GI-147211C caused complete remissions at doses that were fivefold lower than the maximally tolerated dose of nonliposomal GI-147211C *(96)*. Between the free and liposomal GI-147211C, the toxicities were comparable. However, the liposomal formulation revealed a fourfold increase in toxicity; this is likely related to the plasma pharmacokinetics described previously. Despite this increased toxicity, the therapeutic index of the liposomal GI-147211C was enhanced fivefold over that of the free GI-147211C *(87)*. This net gain in therapeutic index is outstanding and presents the possibility that in humans liposomal GI-147211C, or perhaps other liposomal CPT formulations, may display a similarly impressive enhancement of therapeutic index.

In addition to liposomal formulations of CPTs intended for intravenous administration, liposomal aerosols of 9-nitrocamptothecin have proven to be remarkably effective in the treatment of subcutaneous xenografts of human cancers in nude mice *(94)*. The anticancer properties of a liposomal aerosol of 9-nitrocamptothecin (formulated in dilauroylphosphatidylcholine and nebulized to provide a particle size of 1.6 microns mean diameter) were evaluated in nude mice bearing either human breast, colon, or lung cancer xenografts. The 9-nitrocamptothecin liposome aerosol was very effective in the treatment of each cancer type; most noteworthy is that these the results were obtained using doses significantly less than those used in mice receiving CPT agents via other routes of administration *(94)*. Also, in the case of locally advanced lung cancer, aerosol delivery could potentially provide a facile means of realizing focused treatment because it would direct high therapeutic doses to the target organ and potentially reduce undesirable systemic toxicity. However, it is also interesting to note that pharmacokinetic studies performed in the Knight laboratory have shown that aerosolized liposomal CPT, when inhaled by mice, promptly reached high concentrations in the lungs, followed by immediate distribution to the liver and other viscera, indicating that aerosol delivery of liposomal CPTs may useful in treating cancer systemically.

In closing, preclinical and clinical research clearly indicate that the combination of medicinal chemical and drug delivery approaches has been highly important in improving the therapeutic index of CPT-based therapies. Future research and development efforts will likely continue, if not intensify, in this regard. Specifically, we anticipate that a greater number of lactone-stable analogs will emerge, targeted delivery and long-circulating liposomal CPT formulations will be pursued clinically, and delivery systems with optimal drug retention and release profiles will be refined.

REFERENCES

1. Takimoto CH, Wright J, Arbuck SG. 1998 Clinical applications of the camptothecins. Biochim Biophys Acta 1400:107–119.
2. Takimoto CH, Arbuck SG. The camptothecins. In: Cancer chemotherapy and biotherapy. Chabner BA, Longo DA, eds. Lippincott-Raven Publishers, Pennsylvania, 1996, 463–484.
3. Garcia-Carbonero R, Supko JG. 2002 Current perspectives on the clinical experience, pharmacology, and continued development of the camptothecins. Clin Cancer Res 8:641–661.
4. Wall ME, Wani MC, Cook CE, Palmer KH. 1966 Plant antitumor agents. I. The isolation and structure of camptothecin, a novel alkaloidal leukemia and tumor inhibitor from *Camptotheca Acuminata*. J Am Chem Soc 88:3888–3889.
5. Wani MC, Nicholas AW, Manikumar G, Wall ME. 1987 Plant antitumor agents. 25. Total synthesis and antileukemic activity of ring A substituted camptothecin analogs. Structure-activity correlations. J Med Chem 30:1774–1779.

6. Wani MC, Nicholas AW, Wall ME. 1987 Plant antitumor agents. 28. Resolution of a key tricyclic synthon, 5′(RS)-1,5-dioxo-5′-ethyl-5′-hydroxy-2′H,5′H,6′H-6′-oxopyrano[3′ ,4′- f]delta 6,8-tetrahydro-indolizine: total synthesis and antitumor activity of 20(S)- and 20(R)-camptothecin. J Med Chem 30:2317–2319.
7. Kaneda N, Nagata H, Furuta T, Yokokura T. 1990 Metabolism and pharmacokinetics of the camptothecin analogue CPT-11 in the mouse. Cancer Res 50:1715–1720.
8. Giovanella BC, Stehlin JS, Wall ME, et al. 1989 DNA topoisomerase I–targeted chemotherapy of human colon cancer in xenografts. Science 246:1046–1048.
9. Kingsbury WD, Boehm JC, Jakas DR, et al. 1991 Synthesis of water-soluble (aminoalkyl)camptothecin analogs: inhibition of topoisomerase I and antitumor activity. J Med Chem 34:98–107.
10. Rowinsky EK, Grochow LB, Hendricks CB, et al. 1992 Phase I and pharmacologic study of topotecan: a novel topoisomerase I inhibitor. J Clin Oncol 10:647–656.
11. Houghton PJ, Cheshire PJ, Myers L, Stewart CF, Synold TW, Houghton JA. 1992 Evaluation of 9-dimethylaminomethyl-10-hydroxycamptothecin against xenografts derived from adult and childhood solid tumors. Cancer Chemother Pharmacol 31:229–239.
12. Blaney SM, Balis FM, Cole DE, et al. 1993 Pediatric phase I trial and pharmacokinetic study of topotecan administered as a 24-hour continuous infusion. Cancer Res 53:1032–1036.
13. Slichenmyer WJ, Nelson WG, Slebos RJ, Kastan MB. 1993 Loss of a p53-associated G1 checkpoint does not decrease cell survival following DNA damage. Cancer Res 53:4164–4168.
14. Hsiang YH, Hertzberg R, Hecht S, Liu LF. 1985 Camptothecin induces protein-linked DNA breaks via mammalian DNA topoisomerase I. J Biol Chem 260:14873–14878.
15. Potmesil M, Hsiang YH, Liu LF, et al. 1988 Resistance of human leukemic and normal lymphocytes to drug-induced DNA cleavage and low levels of DNA topoisomerase II. Cancer Res 48:3537–3543.
16. Kessel D, Bosmann HB, Lohr K. 1972 Camptothecin effects on DNA synthesis in murine leukemia cells. Biochim Biophys Acta 269:210–216.
17. Li LH, Fraser TJ, Olin EJ, Bhuyan BK. 1972 Action of camptothecin on mammalian cells in culture. Cancer Res 32:2643–2650.
18. Jaxel C, Kohn KW, Wani MC, Wall ME, Pommier Y. 1989 Structure-activity study of the actions of camptothecin derivatives on mammalian topoisomerase I: evidence for a specific receptor site and a relation to antitumor activity. Cancer Res 49:1465–1469.
19. Hertzberg RP, Caranfa MJ, Holden KG, et al 1989. Modification of the hydroxy lactone ring of camptothecin: inhibition of mammalian topoisomerase I and biological activity. J Med Chem 32:715–720.
20. Hsiang YH, Liu LF. 1988 Identification of mammalian DNA topoisomerase I as an intracellular target of the anticancer drug camptothecin. Cancer Res 48:1722–1726.
21. Mi Z, Burke TG. 1994 Differential interactions of camptothecin lactone and carboxylate forms with human blood components. Biochemistry 33:10325–10336.
22. Hochberg F, Grossman SA, Mikkelson T, Calabresi P, Fisher J, Piantadosi S. For the NABTT CNS Consortium, Baltimore, MD. 1998 Efficacy of 9-aminocamptothecin (9-AC) in adults with newly diagnosed glioblastoma multiforme (GBM) and recurrent high grade astrocytomas (HGA). Proc Am Soc Clin Oncol 17:388.
23. Takimoto CH, Dahut W, Harold N, et al. 1996 Clinical pharmacology of 9-aminocamptothecin. Ann NY Acad Sci 803:324–326.

24. Mi Z, Malak H, Burke TG. 1995 Reduced albumin binding promotes the stability and activity of topotecan in human blood. Biochemistry 34:13722–13728.
25. Zimmer SG, Burke TG. 2000 Human serum albumin markedly diminishes the blood stabilities and anticancer activities of several clinically relevant camptothecins. Proc Am Soc Clin Oncol 19:200A.
26. Burke TG, Mi Z. 1993 Preferential binding of the carboxylate form of camptothecin by human serum albumin. Anal Biochem 212:285–287.
27. Burke TG, Mi Z. 1994 The structural basis of camptothecin interactions with human serum albumin: impact on drug stability. J Med Chem 37:40–46.
28. Bom D, Curran DP, Kruszewski S, et al. 2000 The novel silatecan 7-*tert*-butyldimethylsilyl-10-hydroxycamptothecin displays high lipophilicity, improved human blood stability, and potent anticancer activity. J Med Chem 43:3970–3980.
29. Josien H, Ko S-B, Bom D, Curran DP.. 1998 A general synthetic approach to the (20*S*)-camptothecin family of antitumor agents by a regiocontrolled cascade radical cyclization of aryl isonitriles. Chem Eur J 4:67–83.
30. Josien H, Bom D, Curran DP, Zheng YH, Chou TC. 1997 7-Silylcamptothecins (silatecans): a new family of camptothecin antitumor agents. Bioorg Med Chem Lett 7:3189–3194.
31. Burke TG, Munshi CB, Mi Z, Jiang Y. 1995 The important role of albumin in determining the relative human blood stabilities of the camptothecin anticancer drugs [letter] [published erratum appears in J Pharm Sci 1995 Dec;84(12):1492]. J Pharm Sci 84:518–519.
32. Mi Z, Burke TG. 1994 Marked interspecies variations concerning the interactions of camptothecin with serum albumins: a frequency-domain fluorescence spectroscopic study. Biochemistry 33:12540–12545.
33. Burke TG, Staubus AE, Mishra AK. 1992 Liposomal stabilization of camptothecin's lactone ring. J Am Chem Soc 114:8318–8319.
34. Burke TG, Mishra AK, Wani MC, Wall ME. 1993 Lipid bilayer partitioning and stability of camptothecin drugs. Biochemistry 32:5352–5364.
35. Burke TG, Mi Z. 1993 Ethyl substitution at the 7 position extends the half-life of 10-hydroxycamptothecin in the presence of human serum albumin. J Med Chem 36:2580–2582.
36. Pollack IF, Erff M, Bom D, Burke TG, Strode JT, Curran DP. 1999 Potent topoisomerase I inhibition by novel silatecans eliminates glioma proliferation in vitro and in vivo. Cancer Res 59:4898–4905.
37. Lavergne O, Lesueur-Ginot L, Pla Rodas F, Bigg DCH. 1997 BN80245: an E-ring modified camptothecin with potent antiproliferative and topoisomerase I inhibitory activities. Bioorg Med Chem Lett 7:2235–2238.
38. Lavergne O, Lesueur-Ginot L, Pla Rodas F, et al.. 1998 Homocamptothecins: synthesis and antitumor activity of novel E-ring-modified camptothecin analogs. J Med Chem 41:5410–5419.
39. Chauvier D, Morjani H, Manfait M. 2002 Ceramide involvement in homocamptothecin- and camptothecin-induced cytotoxicity and apoptosis in colon HT29 cells. Int J Oncol 20:855–863.
40. Bailly C, Laine W, Baldeyrou B, et al. 2001 A novel B-ring modified homocamptothecin, 12-Cl-hCPT, showing antiproliferative and topoisomerase I inhibitory activities superior to SN-38. Anticancer Drug Des 16:27–36.
41. Lansiaux A, Facompre M, Wattez N, et al. 2001 Apoptosis induced by the homocamptothecin anticancer drug BN80915 in HL-60 cells. Mol Pharmacol 60:450–461.

42. Demarquay D. 2001 The homocamptothecin BN 80915 is an higly potent orally active topoisomerase I poison. Anticancer Drugs 12:9–19.
43. Chauvier D, Chourpa I, Bigg DC, Manfait M. 2000 Kinetics of in vitro hydrolysis of homocamptothecins as measured by fluorescence. Ann N Y Acad Sci 922: 314–316.
44. Demarquay D, Coulomb H, Huchet M, et al. 2000 The homocamptothecin, BN 80927, is a potent topoisomerasse I poison and topoisomerase II catalytic inhibitor. Ann N Y Acad Sci 922:301–302.
45. Lavergne O. 2000 Homocamptothecins: E-ring modified CPT analogs. Ann N Y Acad Sci 922:100–111.
46. Urasaki Y. 2000 Activity of a novel camptothecin analogue, homocamptothecin, in camptothecin-resistant cell lines with topoisomerase I alterations. Cancer Res 60:6577–6580.
47. Lavergne O, Demarquay D, Bailly C, et al. 2000 Topoisomerase I-mediated antiproliferative activity of enantiomerically pure fluorinated homocamptothecins. J Med Chem 43:2285–2289.
48. Philippart P. 2000 Homocamptothecin, an E-ring-modified camptothecin, exerts more potent antiproliferative activity than other topoisomerase I inhibitors in human colon cancers obtained from surgery and maintained in vitro under histotypical culture conditions. Clin Cancer Res 6:1557–1562.
49. Bailly C, Lansiaux A, Dassonneville L, et al. 1999 Homocamptothecin, an E-ring-modified camptothecin analogue, generates new topoisomerase I-mediated DNA breaks. Biochemistry 38:15556–15563.
50. Lavergne O, Harnett J, Rolland A, et al. 1999 BN 80927: a novel homocamptothecin with inhibitory activities on both topoisomerase I and topoisomerase II. Bioorg Med Chem Lett 9:2599–2602.
51. Lesueur-Ginot L, Demarquay D, Kiss R, et al. 1999 Homocamptothecin, an E-ring modified camptothecin with enhanced lactone stability, retains topoisomerase I-targeted activity and antitumor properties. Cancer Res 59:2939–2943.
52. Hsiang YH, Liu LF, Wall ME, et al.. 1989 DNA topoisomerase I-mediated DNA cleavage and cytotoxicity of camptothecin analogs [published erratum appears in Cancer Res 1989 Dec 1;49(23):6868]. Cancer Res 49:4385–4389.
53. Bom D, Curran DP, Chavan AJ, et al. 1999 Novel A,B,E-ring-modified camptothecins displaying high lipophilicity and markedly improved human blood stabilities. J Med Chem 42:3018–3022.
54. Du W, Curran DP, Bevins RL, Zimmer SG, Zhang J, Burke TG. 2002 Synthesis and evaluation of a novel E-ring modified alpha-hydroxy keto ether analogue of camptothecin. Bioorg Med Chem 10:103–110.
55. Ratain MJ. 2002 Irinotecan dosing: does the CPT in CPT-11 stand for "can't predict toxicity"? J Clin Oncol 20:7–8.
56. Iver L, King CD, Whitington PF. 1998 Genetic predisposition to the metabolism of irinotecan (CPT-11): Role of uridine diphosphated glucuronosyltransferase isoform 1A1 in the glucuronidation of its active metabolite (SN-38) in human liver microsomes. J Clin Invest 101:847–854.
57. Gupta E, Lestingi TM, Mick R, Ramirez J, Vokes EE, Ratain MJ. 1994 Metabolic fate of irinotecan in humans: correlation of glucuronidation with diarrhea. Cancer Res 54:3723–3725.
58. Kehrer DF, Sparreboom A, Verweij J, et al. 2001 Modulation of irinotecan-induced diarrhea by cotreatment with neomycin in cancer patients. Clin Cancer Res 7:1136–1141.

59. Humerickhouse R, Lohrbach K, Li L, Bosron WF, Dolan ME. 2000 Characterization of CPT-11 hydrolysis by human liver carboxylesterase isoforms hCE-1 and hCE-2. Cancer Res 60:1189–1192.
60. Bleiberg H, Cvitkovic E. 1996 Characterisation and clinical management of CPT-11 (irinotecan)-induced adverse events: the European perspective. Eur J Cancer 32A(Suppl. 3):S18–S23.
61. Arun B, Frenkel EP. 2001 Topoisomerase I inhibition with topotecan: pharmacologic and clinical issues. Expert Opin Pharmacother 2:491–505.
62. Barenholz Y. 2001 Liposome application: problems and prospects. Curr Opin Coll Inter Sci 6:66–77.
63. Liu X, Lynn BC, Zhang J, et al. 2002 A versatile prodrug approach for liposomal core-loading of water-insoluble camptothecin anticancer drugs. J Am Chem Soc 124:7650–7651.
64. Tardi P, Choice E, Masin D, Redelmeier T, Bally M, Madden TD. 2000 Liposomal encapsulation of topotecan enhances anticancer efficacy in murine and human xenograft models. Cancer Res 60:3389–3393.
65. Sadzuka Y, Hirotsu S, Hirota S. 1999 Effective irinotecan (CPT-11)-containing liposomes: intraliposomal conversion to the active metabolite SN-38. Jpn J Cancer Res 90:226–232.
66. Cao Z, Harris N, Kozielski A, Vardeman D, Stehlin JS, Giovanella B. 1998 Alkyl esters of camptothecin and 9-nitrocamptothecin: synthesis, in vitro pharmacokinetics, toxicity, and antitumor activity. J Med Chem 41:31–37.
67. Cao Z, Pantazis P, Mendoza J, et al. 2000 Structure-activity relationship of alkyl camptothecin esters. Ann N Y Acad Sci 922:122–135.
68. Ertl B, Platzer P, Wirth M, Gabor F. 1999 Poly(D,L-lactic-co-glycolic acid) microspheres for sustained delivery and stabilization of camptothecin. J Control Rel 61:305–317.
69. Shenderova A, Burke TG, Schwendeman SP. 1999 The acidic microclimate in poly(lactide-co-glycolide) microspheres stabilizes camptothecins. Pharm Re 16:241–248.
70. Shenderova A, Burke TG, Schwendeman SP. 1997 Stabilization of 10-hydroxycamptothecin in poly(lactide-co-glycolide) microsphere delivery vehicles. Pharm Res 14:1406–1414.
71. Underberg WJ, Goossen RM, Smith BR, Beijnen JH. 1990 Equilibrium kinetics of the new experimental anti-tumour compound SK&F 104864-A in aqueous solution. J Pharm Biomed Anal 8:681–683.
72. Kosak KM. 2001 Cyclodextrin polymer compositions as drug carriers. US patent 6,048,736.
73. Rubinfeld J, Wrenn SM. 2001 Preparation of camptothecin complexes with cyclodextrins for pharmaceuticals. PCT Int. Appl. WO 20010744401.
74. Kang J, Kumar V, Yang D, Chowdhury PR, Hohl RJ 2002. Cyclodextrin complexation: influence on the solubility, stability, and cytotoxicity of camptothecin, an antineoplastic agent. Euro J Pharm Sci 15:169–170.
75. Xiang TX, Anderson BD. 2002 Stable supersaturated aqueous solutions of silatecan 7-t-butyldimethylsilyl-10-hydroxycamptothecin via chemical conversion in the presence of a chemical modified b-cyclodextrin. Pharm Res 19:1215–1222.
76. Darrington RT, Xiang TX, Anderson BD. 1990 Inclusion complexes of purine nucleoside with cyclodextrins. I. Complexation and stabilization of a dideoxypurine nucleoside with 2-hydroxypropyl-beta-cyclodextrin. Int J Pharm 59:35–44.

77. Tinwalla AY, Hoesterey BL, Xiang TX, Lim K, Anderson BD. 1993 Solubilization of thiazolobenzimidazole using a combination of pH adjustment and complexation with 2-hydroxypropyl-beta-cyclodextrin. Pharm Res 10:1136–1143.
78. Thompson DO. 1997 Cyclodextrins-enabling expcipients: their present and future status. Crit Rev Ther Drug Carrier Sys 14:1–104.
79. Szente L, Szetjili J. 1999Highly soluble cyclodextrin derivatives: chemistry, properties, and trends in development. Adv Drug Deliv Rev 36:17–28.
80. Li P, Zhao L, Yalkowsky SH. 1999 Combined effect of cosolvent and cyclodextrin on solubilization of nonpolar drugs. J Pharm Sci 88:1107–1111.
81. Zhao L, Li P, Yalkowsky SH. 1999Solubilization of fluasterone. J Pharm Sci 88:967–969.
82. Loftsson T, Gudmundsdottir H, Sigurjonsdottir JF, et al. 2001 Cyclodextrin solubilization of benzodiazepines: formulation of midazolam nasal spray. Int J Pharm 212:29–40.
83. Papahadjopoulos D, Allen TM, Gabizon A, et al. 1991 Sterically stabilized liposomes: improvements in pharmacokinetics and antitumor therapeutic efficacy. Proc Natl Acad Sci USA 88:11460–11464.
84. Gabizon A, Papahadjopoulos D. 1988 Liposome formulations with prolonged circulation time in blood and enhanced uptake by tumors. Proc Natl Acad Sci USA 85:6949–6953.
85. Woodle MC, Newman MS, Working PK. 1995 Biological properties of sterically stabilized liposomes. CRC Press, Florida.
86. Forssen EA, MaleBrune R, AdlerMoore JP, et al. 1996 Fluorescence imaging studies for the disposition of daunorubicin liposomes (daunoxome) within tumor tissue. Cancer Res 56:2066–2075.
87. Colbern GT, Dykes DJ, Engbers C, et al. 1998 Encapsulation of the topoisomerase I inhibitor GL147211C in pegylated (STEALTH) liposomes: pharmacokinetics and antitumor activity in HT29 colon tumor xenografts. Clin Cancer Res 4:3077–3082.
88. Madden TD, Demir AS, Zimmer S, Redelmeier TE, Bally MB, Burke T. 1998 Encapsulation of camptothecin class topoisomerase I inhibitors in lipid-based delivery systems. Physical formulation, evaluation of drug stability and plasma elimination in a murine model, and comparison of antitumor efficacy against murine L1210 and B16 tumors. Pharmaceut Res 15:S-140.
89. Dancey J, Eisenhauer EA. 1996 Current perspectives on camptothecins in cancer treatment [editorial]. Br J Cancer 74:327–338.
90. Gerrits CJ, Creemers GJ, Schellens JH, et al. 1996 Phase I and pharmacological study of the new topoisomerase I inhibitor GI147211, using a daily x 5 intravenous administration. Br J Cancer 73:744–750.
91. Eckhardt SG, Baker SD, Eckardt JR, et al. 1998 Phase I and pharmacokinetic study of GI147211, a water-soluble camptothecin analogue, administered for five consecutive days every three weeks. Clin Cancer Res 4:595–604.
92. Eckhardt SG, Baker SD, Eckhardt JR, et al. 1995 Phase I and pharmacokinetic study of the topoisomerase I inhibitor GG211. Proc. Am Soc Clin Oncol 14:476.
93. O'Dwyer P, Cassidy J, Kunka R, et al. 1995 Phase I trial of GG211, a new topoisomerase inhibitor, using a 72 hour continuos infusion. Proc Am Soc Clin Oncol 14:471.
94. Knight V, Koshkina NV, Waldrep JC, Giovanella BC, Gilbert BE. 1999 Anticancer effect of 9-nitrocamptothecin liposome aerosol on human cancer xenografts in nude mice. Cancer Chemother Pharmacol 44:177–186.

II Clinical Perspectives

9 Clinical Experience With 9-Aminocamptothecin

Lessons for New Drug Development

Chris H. Takimoto, MD, PhD

CONTENTS

1. INTRODUCTION

In preclinical studies first published in 1989 by Giovanella and colleagues, 9-aminocamptothecin (9-AC) demonstrated highly promising antitumor activity against human colorectal cancer xenografts *(1)*. This led to an extensive drug development program for 9-AC initially under the guidance of the National Cancer Institute, and later in cooperation with pharmaceutical industry sponsors. However, despite this impressive preclinical activity, 9-AC has not demonstrated clinically useful antitumor activity to date. Thus, in contrast to its more successful brethren, irinotecan and topotecan, 9-AC is no longer under active clinical development. Nonetheless, testing of other novel and new camptothecin derivatives remains an active area of pharmacological research. Thus a careful review of the early clinical and pharmacological trials of 9-AC may help us to understand why 9-AC has not shown more meaningful antitumor activity and may also provide important lessons for the future drug development of novel camptothecins and other topoisomerase I (TOP-I) targeting agents.

Camptothecins in Cancer Therapy
Edited by: V. R. Adams and T. G. Burke © Humana Press Inc., Totowa, NJ

2. HISTORICAL BACKGROUND

In 1986, Drs. Wani and Wall first synthesized the water-insoluble camptothecin derivative, 9-AC *(2)*. Subsequent laboratory studies revealed that 9-AC was a potent inhibitor of TOP-I *(3,4)*, and its ability to interfere with this enzyme correlated with its in vivo cytotoxic activity against murine L1210 leukemia cells *(3,5)*. In 1989, Giovanella and colleagues published their impressive results in the journal *Science* documenting the activity of 9-AC in human colon cancer xenografts models in nude mice *(1)*. 9-AC was highly active with minimal systemic toxicity and generated better antitumor responses than a number of different anticancer agents including 5-fluorouracil, doxorubicin, melphalan, methotrexate, vincristine, vinblastine, and others *(1)*. Interest in clinically developing this compound was further heightened by the demonstration of a broad range of activity against a diverse group of human tumor xenografts including malignant melanoma *(6)*, acute leukemia *(7)*, central nervous system tumors *(8)*, and ovarian *(9)*, prostate *(10)*, breast *(11)*, and bladder cancers *(12)*.

In animal studies, the principal dose-limiting toxicities of 9-AC were neutropenia and gastrointestinal toxicity. Preclinical pharmacological studies also revealed that brief intravenous infusions generating high peak concentrations for short periods were toxic and relatively inactive against human tumor xenografts. Instead, subcutaneous administration of 9-AC as a suspension in Tween-80 resulted in sustained plasma concentrations of 9-AC lactone in the nanomolar range and generated antitumor responses *(13)*.

3. CLINICAL DEVELOPMENT

In 1989, the US National Cancer Institute selected 9-AC as a high-priority compound for further clinical development. However, clinical trials with this agent were delayed because of difficulties in formulating this compound resulting from poor aqueous solubility. In 1993, 9-AC was successfully formulated in dimethylacetamide, polyethylene glycol, and phosphoric acid for use in phase I clinical trials. Later, in 1995, Pharmacia & Upjohn developed a newer colloidal dispersion formulation of 9-AC that was superior in stability and in compatibility with standard intravenous infusions. This newer colloidal dispersion formulation has been used in the more recent clinical studies of this agent.

3.1. Phase I Trials

Because preclinical studies highlighted the importance of prolonged exposures to 9-AC lactone, the first phase I trials of 9-AC dimethylacetamide used a continuous 72-hour intravenous infusion administered every 2 *(14)* or every 3 *(15,16)* weeks (Table 1). Both schedules yielded similar toxicity

Table 1
9-Aminocamptothecin (9-AC) Phase I Clinical Trials

Recommended phase II regimen	*9-AC formulation*	*Principal toxicities*	*Reference*
0.84 mg/m^2/day CIV × 3 days every 2 weeks, or	DMA	Neutropenia	*14*
1.13 mg/m^2/day CIV × 3 days every 2 weeks with G-CSF		Neutropenia and some thrombocytopenia	
1.08 mg/m^2/day CIV × 3 days every 3 weeks	DMA	Neutropenia and some thrombocytopenia	*15*
1.3 mg/m^2/day CIV × 3 day every 3 weeks	CD	Neutropenia	*16*
0.48 mg/m^2/day CIV × 5 days weekly for 3 of 4 weeks	DMA	Neutropenia Diarrhea	*17*
0.6 mg/m^2/day CIV × 5 days weekly for 2 of 3 weeks	CD	Neutropenia	
0.4 mg/m^2/day CIV × 7 days every 4 weeks	DMA	Neutropenia and some thrombocytopenia	*51*
0.51-0.6 mg/m^2/day CIV × 7 days every 4 weeks	CD		
1.65 mg/m^2 CIV over 24 hours weekly for 4 of 5 weeks	CD	Neutropenia	*18*
1.1 mg/m^2/day IV over 30 minutes daily × 5 days every 3 weeks	CD	Neutropenia	*19*
Oral Preparations			
No recommended oral dose daily × 5 every 2 weeks	CD (oral)	No dose-limiting toxicity determined	*20*
0.84 mg/m^2 orally daily × 14 days every 3 weeks	PEG-1000	Myelosuppression and diarrhea	*21*
Specialized phase I studies			
Pediatric patients			
1.25 mg/m^2/day CIV × 3 days every 3 weeks	DMA	Neutropenia Thrombocytopenia	*26*
Acute leukemia1.4 mg/m^2/day CIV over 7 days	CD	Mucositis	*27*

IV, intravenous; CIV, continuous intravenous infusion; G-CSF, granulocyte-colony-stimulating factor; DMA, dimethylacetamide; CD, colloidal dispersion.

profiles with dose escalation limited by neutropenia and, less commonly, thrombocytopenia. Other toxicities included mild to moderate fatigue, anemia, nausea and vomiting, diarrhea, alopecia, and mucositis. In contrast to irinotecan, severe diarrhea was not observed on the 72-hour infusion schedules. Additional schedules of 9-AC administration tested in a phase I clinical trials include prolonged 120-hour infusions given weekly for 2 or 3 consecutive weeks followed by a week rest period *(17)* and a weekly 24-hour infusion given for 4 of every 5 weeks *(18)* (Table 1). For most of these regimens, the major dose-limiting toxicity was still myelosuppression; however, diarrhea became more pronounced when prolonged administration schedules were tested *(17)*.

More recently, a short 15-minute infusion given daily for 5 days every 3 weeks was developed for clinical testing *(19)*. On this schedule, neutropenia and thrombocytopenia were dose limiting and the recommended phase II dose was 1.1 mg/m^2/day infused over 15 minutes daily for 5 days every 3 weeks. The colloidal dispersion formulation of 9-AC has also been administered to patients orally over a dose range of 0.2 to 0.68 mg/m^2/day daily *(20)*. However, in this study, no recommended phase II oral dose was determined because of large interpatient variability in the area-under-the-concentration versus time curve. Another oral study used 9-AC formulated as a polyethylene glycol 1000 capsule with much greater success *(21)*. Administration of 9-AC capsules over a dose range of 0.25 to 1.5 mg/m^2/day for 14 days every 3 weeks resulted in a recommended phase II dose of 1.1 mg/m^2/day. Neutropenia and thrombocytopenia were dose limiting, and the oral bioavailability of 9-AC in capsular form was a relatively consistent 48 ± 17.8%.

3.2. Clinical Pharmacology

All camptothecin derivatives, including 9-AC, contain a terminal lactone ring that rapidly hydrolyzes in aqueous solutions to form the more hydrophilic open-ring carboxylic acid species. Under nonacidic conditions, the equilibrium for this reaction very much favors a less active carboxylate form. The pharmacokinetics of the lactone and carboxylate species of 9-AC have been extensively examined (Table 2). Overall, the amount of active lactone 9-AC circulating in plasma is quite low relative to the total (lactone + carboxylate) 9-AC, with most studies reporting a lactone-to-total 9-AC plasma ratio of less than 0.16. This value is lower than the active lactone forms of topotecan (0.16–0.2) *(22)* or irinotecan (0.51) *(23,24)* that circulate in plasma. In addition, the plasma half-life for 9-AC lactone species is relatively short, ranging from 4.5 to 10 hours *(18,19,25–27)*. Urinary excretion of unchanged drug ranges from 8.6 to 32.1% of the administered dose *(19,25)*.

Table 2
9-Aminocamptothecin Clinical Pharmacology

Dose and schedule	*Formulation*	*Compound*	*Terminal half-life (hours)*	*Volume of distribution at steady-state* *(L/m^2)*	*CL* *($L/hour/m^2$)*	*Urinary excretion (%)*	*Percent lactone in plasma (%)*	*Reference*
0.12–1.8 mg/m^2/day IV over 72 hours	DMA	Lactone	4.47 ± 0.53	195 ± 114	24.5 ± 7.3	NR	8.7 ± 4.7	*25*
		Total	8.38 ± 2.1	23.6 ± 10.6	NR	32.1 ± 8.3 (over 24 hours)		
1.08 mg/m^2/day IV over 72 hours	DMA	Lactone	42.2 ± 34.4	12.6 ± 3.6	55.2 ± 18.0	NR	NR	*15*
0.86–1.49 mg/m^2/day IV over 72 hours*	DMA	Lactone	7.1 ± 3.5	135.3 ± 52.5	NR	NR	10.8 ± 3.6	*26*
		Total	8.1 ± 3.8	21.2 ± 13.3	NR	NR		
0.7–1.9 mg/m^2/day IV over 24 hours	CD	Lactone	10.7 ± 6.7	111.0 ± 72.3	18.0 ± 9.0	NR	7.99	*18*
0.9–1.55 mg/m^2/day IV over 72 hours	CD	Lactone	22.5 ± 8.5	325 ± 145	30.3 ± 4.5	NR	NR	*16*
0.45–1.4 mg/m^2/day CIV over 7 days	CD	Lactone	4.3 ± 2.7	58.4 ± 23.3	11.3 ± 4.9	NR	NR	*27*
0.48 mg/m^2/day CIV over 5 days	DMA	Lactone	NR	NR	12.3 ± 7.1	NR	13.8	*17*
		Total	NR	NR	1.65 ± 0.87	NR		
0.7–1.9 mg/m^2/day IV over 24 hours	CD	Lactone	10.7 ± 6.7	111.0 ± 72.3	18.0 ± 9.0	NR	7.99	*18*
		Total	7.7± 4.6	17.7 ± 6.0	2.36 ± 1.24	8.6 ± 4.0	NR	

IV, intravenous,; CIV, continuous intravenous infusion; DMA, dimethylacetamide formulation; CD, colloidal dispersion formulation; NR, not reported.

*Pediatric patients.

In a pharmacological study of 9-AC in brain cancer patients, subjects receiving anticonvulsant medications tolerated much higher doses of 9-AC consistent with an increased clearance of drug *(28)*. One possible explanation is that 9-AC hepatic clearance may be increased by enzyme induction caused by antiepileptic drugs such as phenytoin, carbamazepine, phenobarbital, primidone, felbamate, and valproic acid. However, hepatic metabolites of 9-AC have not been characterized *(29)*. An alternative explanation is that these same enzyme inducing antiepileptic agents may also result in the increase expression of transport proteins leading to increased 9-AC clearance and biliary excretion *(30)*.

Large interpatient variation in the plasma kinetics of 9-AC has been consistently observed in most studies, which is similar to clinical pharmacological studies of other camptothecin derivatives such as topotecan *(31)* and irinotecan *(23,24)*. In pharmacodynamic studies, moderate to strong correlations between dose-limiting myelosuppression and 9-AC steady state plasma concentrations *(25,30)* or overall area under the concentration-time curve (AUC) *(18,19,32)* have been observed.

3.3. Antitumor Activity

The antitumor activity of 9-AC administered as a 72-hour infusion has been examined in a variety of different tumors (Table 3). In phase II studies in advanced colorectal cancer, administration of 9-AC at 1.2 to 1.4 mg/m^2/day over 72 hours every 2 weeks to 16 previously untreated patients resulted in no objective responses *(33)*. However, the myelosuppressive toxicity of this regimen was substantial, with grade 4 neutropenia seen in 56% of patients and febrile neutropenia documented in 31% *(33)*. No objective antitumor activity was also seen in another trial examining 9-AC administered at 0.84 mg/m^2/day over 72 hours every 2 weeks in 17 untreated colorectal cancer patients *(34)*. In contrast, in advanced platinum refractory ovarian cancer patients, 72-hour infusions of 9-AC were active generating response rates of 21% *(35)* and 19% *(36)*. Activity in relapsed or refractory lymphoma patients was also observed *(37)*. Administration of 9-AC at 0.96 mg/m^2 over 72 hours every 3 weeks with granulocyte colony-stimulating factor to 40 patients with advanced lymphoma resulted in a partial response rate of 25% (95% confidence interval [CI] 13–41%) and a median survival of 12.5 months. In advanced cutaneous T-cell lymphoma, 9-AC at 1.1 mg/m^2/day every 2 weeks with granulocyte colony-stimulating factor resulted in partial responses in 2 of 12 patients for an overall rate of 17%, but myelosuppressive toxicity was high and 3 patients died from neutropenia and sepsis *(38)*. Minimal activity has also been reported in non-small-cell lung, central nervous system, and breast cancers (Table 3).

More prolonged infusion schedules administering 9-AC over 120 hours weekly for 3 of 4 weeks have also been tested in a limited number of studies. In 17 previously untreated advanced colorectal cancer patients, administration of 0.48 mg/m^2/day for 120 hours weekly for 3 of 4 weeks again resulted in no objective responses *(39)*. In lung cancer, administration of 120-hour infusions of 9-AC to stage IIIB and IV non-small-cell lung cancer patients generated only a single response in 12 previously untreated patients and produced a 1-year survival rate of 28% (95% CI = 5–58%) and a median survival of 10.2 months *(40)*.

The rights to this agent were transferred in 1997 from the Pharmacia & Upjohn Company to the IDEC Pharmaceutical Corporation. In this same year, phase II testing of 9-AC was initiated using a 1.1 mg/m^2 intravenous infusion daily for a 5-day schedule *(19)*. The results of phase II testing of 9-AC on this schedule have not been formally reported; however, in 1999 IDEC notified the US government that it was stopping the development of 9-AC based on preliminary phase II results *(41)*. Thus, despite showing impressive activity in preclinical models of colorectal cancer, 9-AC did not produce clinically meaningful antitumor activity of 9-AC in patients with this disease. Modest activity has been observed in refractory lymphoma patients and in women with platinum-refractory ovarian cancer, but the overall phase II activity of 9-AC on any schedule has been largely disappointing.

4. LESSONS FOR NEW DRUG DEVELOPMENT

This lack of clinically useful antitumor activity raises several key questions. First, why were the preclinical animal xenograft studies of 9-AC so promising initially given the later clinical findings? Second, what pharmacological characteristics make camptothecin derivatives such as topotecan and irinotecan so much more clinically successful than 9-AC?

The first question was explored in detail in an interesting study by Kirstein et al. *(42)*. Careful analysis of the pharmacological characteristics of 9-AC in nude mouse experiments were compared with the clinical pharmacological findings seen in early human studies of 9-AC. They adopted a novel approach first suggested by Minderman and colleagues *(43)*. This involved rigorously defining the minimally effective dose of 9-AC that caused objective tumor regressions in animals (MEDOR). However, Kirstein and colleagues expanded the MEDOR concept to include a minimally effective threshold exposure to 9-AC in plasma defined in terms of the AUC, thereby generating a new parameter that could more easily be applied across species to preclinical and clinical studies. The administration of 9-AC daily for 5 days for 2 consecutive weeks generated a MEDOR AUC of 690–1580 ng/mL/hour in the nude mouse experiments *(42)*. The mouse MEDOR AUC was then compared with the AUC profiles generated in humans in Phase I clinical trials. Unfortunately, dose-limiting myelosuppressive toxicity in humans limited the 9-AC AUC to a substantially lower range of 126–493 ng/mL/hour. The greater sensitivity of human bone marrow to 9-AC limited

Table 3
9-Aminocamptothecin Phase II Clinical Trials

Tumor type	*9-AC regimen*	*Evaluated patients*	*Previous therapy for advanced disease*	*Response rate (%)*	*Response type*	*Median duration of response (months)*	*Median duration of survival (months)*	*Reference*
Colorectal	1.42 mg/m^2/day IV for 72 hours every 2 weeks + GCSF	14	Yes	0 (95% CI 0–20)	0 PR	NR	9.5 (95% CI 7.3–12.9)	*33*
Colorectal	0.84 mg/m^2/day IV for 72 hours every 2 weeks	17	No	0	0 PR	NR	NR	*34*
Colorectal	0.48 mg/m^2/day IV for 120 hours weekly for 3 of 4 weeks	17	No	0	0 PR	NR	8 (0.75–14.5)	*39*
Nonsmall-cell lung	1.42 mg/m^2/day IV for 72 hours every 2 weeks + GCSF	54	No	9 (95% CI 3–19)	5 PR	2.25–7.0	5.4	*52*
Nonsmall-cell lung	0.6 mg/m^2/day IV for 120 hours weekly for 2 of 3 weeks	12	No	8 (95% CI 0–21)	1 PR	NR	10.2	*40*
Refractory Hodgkin's and non-Hodgkin's lymphoma	0.96 mg/m^2/day IV for 72 hours every 3 weeks ± G-CSF	40	Yes	25 (95% CI 13–41)	10 PR	5 (r 1–10)	12.5	*37*
Central nervous system	0.85–1.78 mg/m^2/day IV for 72 hours + 2 weeks	39	NR	3	1 PR	NR	NR	*53*
Head and neck	0.85–1.0 mg/m^2/day IV for 72 hours + 2 weeks	14	No	0	0 PR	NR	6 (1–9+)	*54*

Ovarian	0.84–1.13 mg/m^2/day IV for 72 hours + 2 weeks with GCSF	28	Yes	21	6 PR	NR	NR	*35*
Ovarian	0.84 mg/m^2/day IV for 72 hours + 2 weeks	27	Yes	19 (95% CI 6–38)	5 PR	NR	NR	*36*
Breast	1.1 mg/m^2/day IV for 72 hours every 2 weeks + GCSF	15	Yes	13	2 PR	3.5-5	NR	*55*
Cutaneous T-cell lymphoma	1.1 mg/m^2/day IV for 72 hours every 2 weeks +GCSF	12	Yes	17	2 PR	NR	5	*38*

IV, intravenous; G-CSF, granulocyte-co;ony stimulating factor; PR, partial response; NR, not reported; CI, confidence interval.

the plasma AUC in humans to levels below the minimally effective exposures range required for optimal anticancer activity. Even modest decreases in achievable systemic exposure can mean the difference between success and failure for drugs, such as the camptothecins, that have steep dose response curves and narrow therapeutic indices. This analysis is also quite consistent with previous findings showing that mouse bone marrow progenitor cells are 6 to 11 times more resistant to 9-AC than their human counterparts *(44)*. These studies predict, *a priori,* that maximal achievable concentrations of 9-AC in plasma would be lower in humans compared with mice because of marked differences in host tolerance to toxic drug effects. Kirstein and colleagues recommended that careful pharmacokinetic and pharmacodynamic studies be performed both in preclinical experiments and in early clinical trials. Better communication between preclinical scientists and physicians designing and conducting phase I clinical trials may further help to streamline the drug development process.

The second question of which pharmacological characteristics of topotecan and irinotecan make them more clinically useful than 9-AC is difficult to answer with certainty. Differences in the clinical pharmacology of these camptothecin derivatives are quite prominent. For example, both irinotecan and topotecan are much more water-soluble than 9-AC and are easier to formulate in pharmaceutical preparations. Furthermore, the lactone forms of both of these camptothecins are more stable than 9-AC in plasma with higher percentage of the active lactone species circulating in plasma after intravenous administration *(25)*. For topotecan it is 16–20% *(22)*, irinotecan (SN-38) 51–64% *(23,24)*, and for 9-AC approximately 9% *(25)*. The tight protein binding of the open ring 9-AC carboxylate to plasma albumin, which tends to destabilize the lactone species *(45)*, may explain this difference. In contrast, the protein binding of topotecan is much less, and for SN-38, plasma protein binding interactions actually tend to favor the stability of the active lactone species *(46)*. Another kinetic difference is found in the half-lives of these agents. The half-life of SN-38 is relatively long, 11 ± 3 hours, whereas for topotecan it is 3.01 ± 0.54 hours and for 9-AC it is 4.5 ± 0.5 hours. For this reason, irinotecan can be given as a relatively short infusion over 90 minutes every 3 weeks *(23,24)*, whereas topotecan and 9-AC are administered on consecutive days or as prolonged infusions over many days.

Additional differences at the molecular level of action may also be important in distinguishing between the different camptothecin analogues. For example, SN-38 is highly potent as an inhibitor of TOP-I and generates cleavable complexes in colon cancer cells that are more stabile than those generated by 9-AC or topotecan *(47)*. Molecular resistance mechanisms may also differ. P-glycoprotein-associated multidrug resistance may have some impact on the activity of some of these agents. Multidrug resistant

(MDR)-expressing cell lines are ninefold more resistant to topotecan and twofold more resistant to 9-AC *(48)* compared with parental wild-type cells. In contrast, irinotecan and SN-38 are not effective substrates for the MDR drug efflux pump *(49)* and cross-resistance between irinotecan and vincristine or doxorubicin is not observed in P388 leukemia cells expressing the MDR phenotype *(50)*.

In summary, 9-AC is more similar to topotecan than irinotecan. For example, both 9-AC and topotecan are not a prodrugs, they are a weak MDR substrates and both have relatively short half-lives in plasma after intravenous administration. Topotecan and 9-AC both exhibit dose-limiting toxicities consisting of myelosuppression rather than diarrhea and both have shown activity in ovarian cancer. Consequently, 9-AC was simply not unique enough to justify its further clinical development as a novel TOP-I-targeting agent.

5. CONCLUSIONS

The great promise of 9-AC seen in preclinical studies has not resulted in clinically useful antitumor activity. The reasons for this failure have been reviewed and provide some insights into further drug development in this area. However, there are no easy answers. Fundamentally, we still need to have a much better understanding of the pharmacology of these agents. Important and as-yet poorly understood issues include how these different camptothecins function at the molecular level, what are their key determinants of antitumor response, and what are their clinically relevant mechanisms of drug resistance? Despite these challenges, there is no doubt that TOP-I is a validated molecular target for anticancer therapy and the future drug development efforts are sure to result in new generations of useful and better agents that target this enzyme.

REFERENCES

1. Giovanella BC, Stehlin JS, Wall ME, et al. 1989 DNA topoisomerase I—targeted chemotherapy of human colon cancer in xenografts. Science 246:1046–1048.
2. Wani MC, Nicholas AW, Wall ME. 1986 Plant antitumor agents. 23. Synthesis and antileukemic activity of camptothecin analogues. J Med Chem 29:2358–2363.
3. Jaxel C, Kohn KW, Wani MC, Wall ME, Pommier Y. 1989 Structure-activity study of the actions of camptothecin derivatives on mammalian topoisomerase I: evidence for a specific receptor site and a relation to antitumor activity. Cancer Res 49:1465–1469.
4. Kingsbury WD, Boehm JC, Jakas DR, et al. 1991 Synthesis of water-soluble (aminoalkyl)camptothecin analogues: inhibition of topoisomerase I and antitumor activity. J Med Chem 34:98–107.
5. Hsiang YH, Liu LF, Wall ME, et al. 1989 DNA topoisomerase I-mediated DNA cleavage and cytotoxicity of camptothecin analogues. Cancer Res 49:4385–4389.

6. Pantazis P, Hinz HR, Mendoza JT, et al. 1992 Complete inhibition of growth followed by death of human malignant melanoma cells in vitro and regression of human melanoma xenografts in immunodeficient mice induced by camptothecins. Cancer Res 52:3980–3987.
7. Jeha S, Kantarjian H, O'Brien S, Vitek L, Beran M. 1998 Activity of oral and intravenous 9-aminocamptothecin in SCID mice engrafted with human leukemia. Leuk Lymph 32:159–164.
8. Potmesil M, Vardeman D, Kozielski AJ, Mendoza J, Stehlin JS, Giovanella BC. 1995 Growth inhibition of human cancer metastases by camptothecins in newly developed xenograft models. Cancer Res 55:5637–5641.
9. Pantazis P, Kozielski AJ, Mendoza JT, Early JA, Hinz HR, Giovanella BC. 1993 Camptothecin derivatives induce regression of human ovarian carcinomas grown in nude mice and distinguish between non-tumorigenic and tumorigenic cells in vitro. Int J Cancer 53:863–871.
10. de Souza PL, Cooper MR, Imondi AR, Myers CE. 19979-Aminocamptothecin: a topoisomerase I inhibitor with preclinical activity in prostate cancer. Clin Cancer Res 3:287–294.
11. Pantazis P, Kozielski AJ, Vardeman DM, Petry ER, Giovanella BC. 1993 Efficacy of camptothecin congeners in the treatment of human breast carcinoma xenografts. Oncol Res 5:273–281.
12. Keane TE, El-Galley RE, Sun C, et al. 1998 Camptothecin analogues/cisplatin: an effective treatment of advanced bladder cancer in a preclinical in vivo model system. J Urol 160:252–256.
13. Potmesil M, Arbuck SG, Takimoto CH, Liebes L, Hochster H. 1996 9-Aminocamptothecin and beyond. Preclinical and clinical studies. Ann N Y Acad Sci 803:231–246.
14. Dahut W, Harold N, Takimoto C, et al. 1996 Phase I and pharmacologic study of 9-aminocamptothecin given by 72-hour infusion in adult cancer patients. J Clin Oncol 14:1236–1244.
15. Rubin E, Wood V, Bharti A, et al. 1995 A phase I and pharmacokinetic study of a new camptothecin derivative, 9- aminocamptothecin. Clin Cancer Res 1:269–276.
16. Eder JP, Jr., Supko JG, Lynch T, et al. 1998 Phase I trial of the colloidal dispersion formulation of 9-amino-20(S)- camptothecin administered as a 72-hour continuous intravenous infusion. Clin Cancer Res 4:317–324.
17. Thomas RR, Dahut W, Harold N, et al. 2001 A phase I and pharmacologic study of 9-aminocamptothecin administered as a 120-h infusion weekly to adult cancer patients. Cancer Chemother Pharmacol 48:215–222.
18. Siu LL, Oza AM, Eisenhauer EA, et al. 1998 Phase I and pharmacologic study of 9-aminocamptothecin colloidal dispersion formulation given as a 24-hour continuous infusion weekly times four every 5 weeks. J Clin Oncol 16:1122–1130.
19. Herben VM, van Gijn R, Schellens JH, et al. 1999 Phase I and pharmacokinetic study of a daily times 5 short intravenous infusion schedule of 9-aminocamptothecin in a colloidal dispersion formulation in patients with advanced solid tumors. J Clin Oncol 17:1906–1914.
20. Mani S, Iyer L, Janisch L, et al. 1998 Phase I clinical and pharmacokinetic study of oral 9-aminocamptothecin (NSC-603071). Cancer Chemother Pharmacol 42:84–87.
21. de Jonge MJ, Punt CJ, Gelderblom AH, et al. 1999 Phase I and pharmacologic study of oral (PEG-1000) 9-aminocamptothecin in adult patients with solid tumors. J Clin Oncol 17:2219–2226.

22. Rowinsky EK, Grochow LB, Hendricks CB, et al. 1992 Phase I and pharmacologic study of topotecan: a novel topoisomerase I inhibitor. J Clin Oncol 10:647–656.
23. Rowinsky EK, Grochow LB, Ettinger DS, et al. 1994 Phase I and pharmacological study of the novel topoisomerase I inhibitor 7-ethyl-10-[4-(1-piperidino)-1-piperidino]carbonyloxycamptothecin (CPT-11) administered as a ninety- minute infusion every 3 weeks. Cancer Res 54:427–436.
24. Rothenberg ML, Kuhn JG, Burris HA, et al. 1993 Phase I and pharmacokinetic trial of weekly CPT-11. J Clin Oncol 11:2194–2204.
25. Takimoto CH, Dahut W, Marino MT, et al. 1997 Pharmacodynamics and pharmacokinetics of a 72-hour infusion of 9- aminocamptothecin in adult cancer patients. J Clin Oncol 15:1492–1501.
26. Langevin AM, Casto DT, Thomas PJ, et al. 1998 Phase I trial of 9-aminocamptothecin in children with refractory solid tumors: a pediatric oncology group study. J Clin Oncol 16:2494–2499.
27. Vey N, Kantarjian H, Tran H, et al. 1999 Phase I and pharmacologic study of 9-aminocamptothecin colloidal dispersion formulation in patients with refractory or relapsed acute leukemia. Ann Oncol 10:577–583.
28. Grossman SA, Hochberg F, Fisher J, et al. 1998 Increased 9-aminocamptothecin dose requirements in patients on anticonvulsants. NABTT CNS Consortium. The new approaches to brain tumor therapy. Cancer Chemother Pharmacol 42:118–126.
29. Takimoto CH, Dahut W, Harold N, et al. 1996 Clinical pharmacology of 9-aminocamptothecin. Ann N Y Acad Sci 803:324–326.
30. Minami H, Lad TE, Nicholas MK, Vokes EE, Ratain MJ. 1999 Pharmacokinetics and pharmacodynamics of 9-aminocamptothecin infused over 72 hours in phase II studies. Clin Cancer Res 5:1325–1330.
31. Grochow LB, Rowinsky EK, Johnson R, et al. 1992 Pharmacokinetics and pharmacodynamics of topotecan in patients with advanced cancer. Drug Metab Dispos 20:706–713.
32. de Jonge MJ, Verweij J, Loos WJ, Dallaire BK, Sparreboom A. 1999 Clinical pharmacokinetics of encapsulated oral 9-aminocamptothecin in plasma and saliva. Clin Pharmacol Ther 65:491–499.
33. Saltz LB, Kemeny NE, Tong W, Harrison J, Berkery R, Kelsen DP. 1997 9-Aminocamptothecin by 72-hour continuous intravenous infusion is inactive in the treatment of patients with 5-fluorouracil-refractory colorectal carcinoma. Cancer 80:1727–1732.
34. Pazdur R, Diaz-Canton E, Ballard WP, et al. 1997 Phase II trial of 9-aminocamptothecin administered as a 72-hour continuous infusion in metastatic colorectal carcinoma. J Clin Oncol 15:2905–2909.
35. McCarthy N, Sarosy G, Minasian L, et al. 1999 Phase II and pharmacokinetic (PK) study of 9-aminocamptothecin (9AC) in recurrent epithelial ovarian cancer [abstract]. Proc Am Soc Clin Oncol 18:363a.
36. Speyer J, Hochster H, Mandeli J, Runowicz C, Krook J, Wadler S. 1999 Phase II study of 72 hr 9-amino-camptothecin (9AC) infusion in second-line therapy of ovarian cancer (a NYGOG and ECOG study) [abstract]. Proc Am Soc Clin Oncol 18:363a.
37. Wilson WH, Little R, Pearson D, et al. 1998 Phase II and dose-escalation with or without granulocyte colony- stimulating factor study of 9-aminocamptothecin in relapsed and refractory lymphomas [published erratum appears in J Clin Oncol 1998;16(8):2895]. J Clin Oncol 16:2345–2351.

38. Argiris A, Heald P, Kuzel T, et al. 2001 Phase II trial of 9-aminocamptothecin as a 72-h infusion in cutaneous T-cell lymphoma. Invest New Drugs 19:321–326.
39. Pazdur R, Medgyesy DC, Winn RJ, et al. 1998 Phase II trial of 9-aminocamptothecin (NSC 603071) administered as a 120-hr continuous infusion weekly for three weeks in metastatic colorectal carcinoma. Invest New Drugs 16:341–346.
40. Vokes EE, Gordon GS, Rudin CM, et al. 2001 A phase II trial of 9-aminocaptothecin (9-AC) as a 120-h infusion in patients with non-small cell lung cancer. Invest New Drugs 19:329–333.
41. IDEC Pharmaceuticals Corporation. Letter to Stockholders, July 22, 1999. San Diego, California.
42. Kirstein MN, Houghton PJ, Cheshire PJ, et al. 2001 Relation between 9-aminocamptothecin systemic exposure and tumor response in human solid tumor xenografts. Clin Cancer Res 7:358–366.
43. Minderman H, Cao S, Rustman YM. 1998 Rational design of irinotecan administration based on preclinical models. Oncology (Huntingt) 12:22–30.
44. Erickson-Miller CL, May RD, Tomaszewski J, et al. 1997 Differential toxicity of camptothecin, topotecan and 9- aminocamptothecin to human, canine, and murine myeloid progenitors (CFU- GM) in vitro. Cancer Chemother Pharmacol 39:467–472.
45. Mi Z, Malak H, Burke TG. 1995 Reduced albumin binding promotes the stability and activity of topotecan in human blood. Biochemistry 34:13722–13728.
46. Burke TG, Mi Z. 1994 The structural basis of camptothecin interactions with human serum albumin: impact on drug stability. J Med Chem 37:40–46.
47. Tanizawa A, Fujimori A, Fujimori Y, Pommier Y. 1994 Comparison of topoisomerase I inhibition, DNA damage, and cytotoxicity of camptothecin derivatives presently in clinical trials. J Natl Cancer Inst 86:836–842.
48. Chen AY, Yu C, Potmesil M, Wall ME, Wani MC, Liu LF. 1991 Camptothecin overcomes MDR1-mediated resistance in human KB carcinoma cells. Cancer Res 51:6039–6044.
49. Jansen WJ, Hulscher TM, van Ark-Otte J, Giaccone G, Pinedo HM, Boven E. 1998 CPT-11 sensitivity in relation to the expression of P170-glycoprotein and multidrug resistance-associated protein. Br J Cancer 77:359–365.
50. Tsuruo T, Matsuzaki T, Matsushita M, Saito H, Yokokura T. 1988 Antitumor effect of CPT-11, a new derivative of camptothecin, against pleiotropic drug-resistant tumors in vitro and in vivo. Cancer Chemother Pharmacol 21:71–74.
51. Hochster H, Liebes L, Speyer J, et al. 1997 Phase I and pharmacodynamic study of prolonged infusion 9-amino-camptothecin (9AC) in two formulations [abstract]. Proc Am Soc Clin Oncol 16:704.
52. Vokes EE, Ansari RH, Masters GA, et al. 1998 A phase II study of 9-aminocamptothecin in advanced non-small-cell lung cancer. Ann Oncol 9:1085–1090.
53. Hochberg F, Grossman SA, Mikkelsen T, Calabresi P, Fisher J, Piantadosi S. 1998 Efficacy of 9-aminocamptothecin (9-AC) in adults with newly diagnosed glioblastoma multiforme (GBM) and recurrent high grade astrocytomas [abstract]. Proc Am Soc Clin Oncol 17:388a.
54. Lad T, Rosen F, Arietta R, Kuebler JP, Vokes E. 1998 Phase II trial of 9-aminocamptothecin (9AC/DMA) in patients with advanced squamous cell head and neck cancer [abstract]. Proc Am Soc Clin Oncol 17:392a.
55. Kraut EH, Balcerzak SP, Young D, et al. 2000 A phase II study of 9-aminocamptothecin in patients with refractory breast cancer. Cancer Invest 18:28–31.

10 Clinical Studies of Rubitecan (9-Nitro 20(S) Camptothecin)

Hilary Hewes, MD,
Judith A. Smith, PharmD,
and Claire Verschraegen, MD

CONTENTS

1. INTRODUCTION

Camptothecin (CPT) compounds are one of the newer classes of anticancer agents introduced over the past decade. Early investigational trials with the parent compound, CPT, derived from the bark of the *Camptotheca accuminata* tree, was introduced into clinical trials in the late 1970s. Because of its poor water solubility, CPT was formulated in sodium bicarbonate, which opened the 20(S) lactone ring and caused significant toxicity and inconsistent clinical activity. Hence, clinical development of camptothecin as an anticancer agent was halted *(1)*.

Under physiological conditions in humans, CPT analogs undergo a reversible, nonenzymatic, pH-dependent hydrolysis from the active lactone, closed ring form of the drug to the inactive carboxylate, open-ring form. CPTs have limited lactone stability that has contributed to the vari-

Camptothecins in Cancer Therapy
Edited by: V. R. Adams and T. G. Burke © Humana Press Inc., Totowa, NJ

ability in pharmacokinetic and pharmacodynamic results. Plasma protein-binding has been implicated in the limited clinical activity of the CPT analogs. In presence of human albumin, CPT analogs primarily bind to the albumin in the inactive carboxylate form, pulling the drug equilibrium away from the active lactone form *(2)*. These limitations initiated efforts to discover improved CPT analogs. The common approach has been to improve the aqueous solubility of newer CPT analogs to provide for convenient intravenous administration at pH values predominantly favoring the active lactone form of the drug. These efforts were successful in the development and Food and Drug Administration approval of two semisynthetic compounds: topotecan for the treatment of patients with cisplatin-refractory ovarian carcinoma and irinotecan (CPT-11) in combination with fluorouracil and leucovorin for the treatment of advanced colon carcinoma *(3–9)* (Table 1). Several other water-soluble CPT analogs are currently in various stages of preclinical or clinical development *(10–12)*.

There are many trials of chemotherapy combinations including CPT analogs, and, in most cases, there is synergistic activity between the topoisomerase-I inhibitor and DNA-damaging agents, such as alkylators, platinum, and antimetabolites *(13)*. However, clinical results are less than expected from the preclinical data and the search for the CPT analog that would be metabolized adequately in humans is still ongoing *(14)*. To accomplish this goal, there is a need for a better understanding of the biochemistry, pharmacokinetics, and pharmacodynamics of the CPT analogs in humans. 9-Nitro 20 (S)-camptothecin (9NC, RFS 2000, Rubitecan, or Orathecin®) has shown very promising activity in animal models; therefore, was selected for clinical trials *(15)*. In this chapter, we discuss the clinical development of rubitecan.

2. RUBITECAN

Rubitecan is a water-insoluble analog of CPT that has improved lactone stability relative to its precursor, 9-aminocamptothecin (9-AC), and can be manufactured at a considerably lower cost. The structure of rubitecan is similar to 9-AC but with a nitro group on ring A, C9 position (Fig. 1). Rubitecan has anticancer activity *per se*, but a small amount (<10%) is spontaneously converted to 9-AC in human plasma *(16)*. Neither of these two analogs maintains large concentrations of intact lactone ring in plasma, but rubitecan administered orally on a continuous basis does have substantial antitumor activity *(15)*.

2.1. Animal Studies

In preclinical studies, rubitecan has demonstrated activity against human ovarian and malignant melanoma cells in the human xenograft-nude mouse model when administered intramuscularly or by continuous intravenous infusion in the range of 1 to 4 mg/kg/day *(15,17–19)*. Oral administration,

Table 1
FDA-Approved Camptothecin Analogs

	Topotecan	*Irinotecan*
Trade name	Hycamtin	Camptosar
Chemical name	S-10-[(dimethylamino)methyl]-4-ethyl-4,9-dihydroxy-1H-pyrano[3=,4=:6,7]indolizino 1,2-b-quinoline-3,14-(4H,12H)-dione monohydrochloride	4S-4-11-diethyl-4-hydroxy-9-[(4-piperidino) carbonyloxyl]1H-pyranol[3=,4=:6,7] indolizinol[1,2-b]quinolone-3,14-(4H,12H)-dione hydrochloride trihydrate
FDA indication	Second-line treatment of ovarian cancer and small-cell lung cancer	Second-line treatment of metastatic colon carcinoma in 5-FU refractory patients. First-line treatment in combination with 5-FU + leucvorin treatment of colorectal cancer.
FDA approved dose	1.5 mg/m^2/days × 5 days q 3 weeks	125mg/m^2 q week × 4 weeks followed by 2 weeks rest (6-week cycle)
Mean percent Lactone AUC to total drug AUC	36%	38%
Dose adjustments	Renal impairment decrease dose 50%	Not necessary.
Common toxicity	Nausea, vomiting, neutropenia, thrombocytopenia, anemia, alopecia, microscopic hematuria, and proteinuria	Diarrhea, neutropenia, anemia, thrombocytopeni, abdominal cramps, nausea and vomiting, elevated serum transaminases, and elevated bilirubin

5-FU, 5-fluorouracil; AUC, area under the curve.

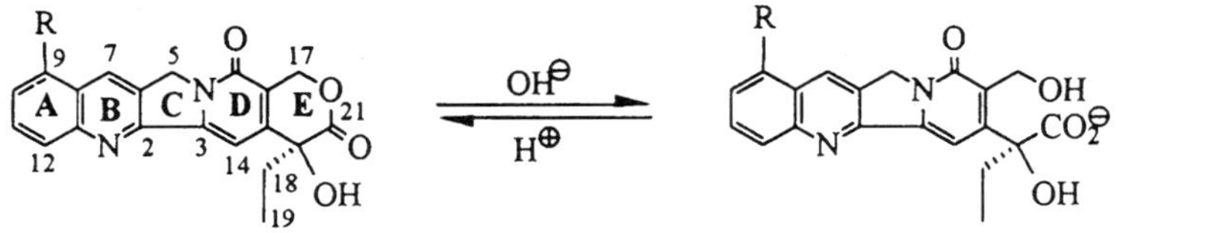

1: R = H, Camptothecin (Lactone)
2: R = NO_2, 9NC (Lactone)
3: R = H, Camptothecin (Carboxylate)
4: R = NO_2, 9NC (Carboxylate)

Fig. 1. Structure of 9-nitrocamptothecin.

through direct injection of cotton seed oil suspensions of rubitecan through the abdominal wall into the stomach in a dosage of 1.0 mg/kg/day, 5 days weekly for several weeks, is as effective against several human tumor xenografts *(18)*. For clinical trials, an oral formulation of rubitecan in a hard gelatin capsule was developed to circumvent the problems of infusing a non–water-soluble compound *(16)*.

In different preclinical studies, the maximum tolerated dose (MTD) of rubitecan was determined in mice and dogs. Nude mice received increasing doses of rubitecan by intrastomach injection until the MTD was established for the schedule of 5 days on, 2 days off. MTD for dogs was then extrapolated from these data, tested, and levels of the drug in plasma were determined by high-pressure liquid chromatography. MTD in mice for the previously mentioned schedule was 1 mg/kg/day, and in dogs 1 mg/kg/day at a schedule of 4 days on, 3 days off. Treatment of the human cancer xenografts in nude mice at these MTDs resulted in 100% growth inhibition of 30 of 30 tumors tested and total disappearance in 24 of 30. The trial focused on several of the most common human cancers, including breast, colorectal, pancreatic, ovarian, prostate, lung, and melanoma *(20)*.

One study analyzed the pharmacokinetic and tissue distribution of inhaled CPT formulated in Dilauroylphosphatic-dylcholine (DLPC) liposomes. C57BL/6 mice with subcutaneous Lewis lung carcinoma, Swiss nu/nu mice with human lung carcinoma xenografts, and BALB/c mice without tumors were used. After 30 minutes of inhalation of CPT liposome aerosol, drug was deposited in the lungs (310 ng/g) and was followed promptly by the appearance of high concentrations in the liver (192 ng/g), with lesser amounts appearing in other organs. Drug concentration in the brain was 61 ng/g. These results demonstrate a prompt pulmonary and later systemic distribution of CPT after liposome aerosol administration, and therefore support future trials involving aerosolized rubitecan in the treatment of lung, liver, kidney, and brain cancer in humans *(21)*.

2.2. Rubitecan and Radiation

Preclinical studies of combination of rubitecan with radiation are ongoing. One study examined the effect of combined radiation and rubitecan in the treatment of locally advanced pancreatic cancer in 3-month old nude homozygous Swiss mice. Pancreatic cancer cells were obtained from the American Type Culture Collection, and each mouse was injected with 10 million cells subcutaneously in the right hind leg. All mice received intragastric injections of rubitecan 5 days per week for 6 weeks. Radiation in the form of electron beam radiation was given, with the first treatment initiated in the same week in which the rubitecan was started, in three fashions: 500 rads once per week only during the first 2 weeks of treatment, 200 rads weekly for 3 weeks, or 100 rads weekly for 5 weeks. Mice were randomized into groups receiving treatments of rubitecan alone, rubitecan plus radiation, radiation alone, and control. Tumors were measured weekly and the mice were followed for 15–18 weeks after tumor injection. Results showed that the combined effect of the two treatments was less than the additive effect of the two treatments alone in the groups given 500 and 200 rads, and that those given 100 rads had a combination effect equivalent to the additive effect of the two treatments alone. The data suggest that spreading out the periods of radiation treatments and administering the radiation at lower doses is more effective *(22)*.

A second study examined the combination of RFS-2000 and ionizing radiation in vitro and in vivo to determine the possible radiation enhancing potential of rubitecan in human cancer cells. The in vitro study included H460 human lung carcinoma cells plated and treated with RFS-2000 for various lengths of time. Sublethal damage recovery was analyzed by using two split doses of radiation. For the in vivo study, H460 cell xenografts were used in nude mice, with tumors grown subcutaneously on the flank. The mice were then treated with rubitecan (1 mg/kg) or radiation (2 Gy) for 5 consecutive days, and tumor growth was measured for each treatment group. The in vitro results included radiation enhancement for incubation times between 4 and 24 hours with 10 n*M* 9-NC, and incubation with 10 n*M* rubitecan inhibited sublethal damage recovery by a factor of 2. In the in vivo experiments, rubitecan was shown to enhance the effects of fractionated radiotherapy (enhancement factor 1.64). These results suggest that the use of rubitecan can enhance the effects of radiation therapy in human lung cancer cases, and that the mechanism of the effect may involve inhibition of sublethal damage recovery *(23)*.

3. CLINICAL TRIALS

3.1. Phase I Studies

To determine the MTD, the first phase I study was performed in patients with advanced cancer refractory to conventional chemotherapy. Rubitecan was administered orally with escalating doses to cohorts of five patients beginning at 1 mg/m^2/day for 5 consecutive days every week for 4 weeks. Increments were 0.5 mg/m^2/day for each cohort. Toxicity was evaluated in

28 patients diagnosed with various malignancies. Each patient could be dose-escalated, if they tolerated the first 4 weeks of therapy without side effects. Seven patients received 1 mg/m^2/day for 28 weeks,; 10 patients, 1.5 mg/m^2/day for 68 weeks; and 26 patients, 2 mg/m^2/day for 159 weeks. At 1.5 mg/m^2/day or higher, the dose-limiting toxicity was hematologic, with grade 4 anemia in eight patients (29%); neutropenia in seven patients (25%) and thrombocytopenia in five patients(18%). Grade 2 or higher toxic effects occurred at each dose level—nausea and vomiting in 15 patients (54%), diarrhea in nine patients (32%), chemical cystitis in seven patients (25%), neutropenic sepsis in six patients (21%), and weight loss in five patients (18%) ($n = 28$). Responses were observed after 24 weeks of therapy in five patients with pancreatic, breast, ovarian, and hematologic tumors. Fourteen patients had disease stabilization and one patient received treatment up to 18 months. The MTD of rubitecan given orally has been estimated at 1.5 mg/m^2/day for 5 consecutive days weekly. Rubitecan may be tolerated for sustained periods, but has the potential for significant hematological, gastrointestinal, and urinary bladder toxicity. Significant antitumor activity was observed, warranting further clinical investigations *(24)*.

As trials of rubitecan have progressed forward into phase III for treatment of pancreatic cancer (*see* Subheading 3.4.), further phase I trials were conducted to assess the relationship between daily dosing, food intake, number of days of treatment, and toxicity.

In one study, rubitecan was administered according to one of two schedules: patients on schedule A received a starting dose of 2.0 mg/m^2/day for 5 days weekly twice repeated every 4 weeks. Second and third dose cohorts were 2.7 mg/m^2/day and 2.4 mg/m^2/day, respectively. At 2.0 mg/m^2/day, one of six patients had a dose-limiting toxicity (DLT) (febrile neutropenia). At 2.7 mg/m^2/day, two of five patients had DLT (febrile neutropenia and grade 4 thrombocytopenia). At the MTD of 2.4 mg/m^2/day, one of six patients had DLT (febrile neutropenia causing death). The starting dose of schedule B (1.7 mg/m^2/day) was 30% lower than the MTD on schedule A and was given daily for 14 days every 4 weeks. On schedule B, zero of six patients had DLT at 1.7 mg/m^2/day. In addition, even at the same dose/cycle (2.4 mg/m^2/cycle), there was less toxicity on schedule B compared with A, despite a 40% increase in the number of days of treatment. These results suggest that daily dose may be of greater influence on toxicity than dose/cycle or number of days of treatment *(25)*.

One other phase I trial explored the use of intraperitoneal infusion of 9-AC in patients with cancer in the peritoneal cavity. Patients were enrolled if they had known nodules in the peritoneal cavity that did not exceed 1 cm in diameter. 9-AC was given in six fractions over 12 days, with doses ranging from 1.25 to 13.5 mg/m^2 in cycles repeated every 28 days. Twelve patients received 31 cycles of 9-AC. The repeated intraperitoneal treatment was generally well tolerated, with DLT of neutropenia encountered at the highest dose level in two patients; a lower dose of 9 mg/m^2 was well tolerated. Seven patients were able to be evaluated: two patients had objective evidence of clinical benefit and only one had progressive disease. These results suggest that evaluation of intraperitoneal administration of rubitecan in patients with tumors involving primarily the peritoneal cavity may be warranted *(26)*.

An innovative phase I study testing the aerosol delivery of rubitecan has been completed. In this study, rubitecan is liposomated primarily to achieve the correct particle size required for deposition in the alveoli during nebulization, but also in the hope that the liposomal formulation will protect the molecule from being converted rapidly to carboxylate. The aerosol delivery allows an arterial distribution of rubitecan through the pulmonary artery system. Systemic levels are achieved. The bioavailability of this route of administration appears to be higher than after oral administration. DLTs were chemical pharyngitis and fatigue. No hematologic toxicity was seen. Responses were seen in two patients with endometrial cancer *(27)*.

3.2. Phase I Combination Studies

Phase I combination studies are now being performed, with cisplatin *(28)*, gemcitabine *(29)*, and with capecitabine *(30)*.

The first study evaluated a new escalation scheme for the combination of rubitecan and cisplatin, again in patients with advanced malignancies. Patients were given 28-day courses of therapy, beginning with intravenous cisplatin on day 1, followed by oral rubitecan daily for 5 days per week for 3 weeks. The study had a two-arm crossing (not crossover) design. Arm 1 consisted of a fixed dose of cisplatin (50 mg/m^2) and increasing doses of rubitecan (starting at 0.5 mg/day); arm 2 used a fixed dose of rubitecan (1.5 mg/day) and increasing doses of cisplatin (starting dose 20 mg/m^2). Crossing level was cisplatin 50 mg/m^2 and rubitecan 1.5 mg/day. At DLT, the dose was decreased by one level for the escalated drug, and the fixed drug was then escalated. Arm 1 enrolled 22 patients; 3 patients were treated at the crossing level and 29 patients underwent therapy under arm 2. Toxicities included grade >1 nausea/vomiting (16 patients) that was dose-limiting at the crossing dose level. Hematological toxicities included the DLT of prolonged thrombocytopenia in arm 1, and grade 4 neutropenia in arm 2. Results included prolonged stabilization of disease (>6 months) and tumor marker improvement in patients with pancreatic, cholangioma, cervical, renal, and ovarian carcinomas. Recommended phase II doses range from cisplatin 70 mg/m^2 and rubitecan 1.25 mg to 40 mg/m^2 and 2 mg of each drug, respectively, allowing for flexibility in dosing while maintaining a fairly well tolerated combination of therapy *(31)*.

In one study of rubitecan and gemcitabine combination, 1000 mg/m^2 of gemcitabine was administered on days 1 and 8 of a 21-day cycle either over

30 minutes, or at a rate of 10 mg/m²/minute, with increasing dose of rubitecan, from 0.75 to 1.25 mg/m² on days 1–5 and 8–12. In the continuous infusion arm, hematologic DLTs were observed at very low doses, and this arm was closed. Twenty-one patients with refractory or recurrent malignancies were treated in the standard gemcitabine arm. The MTD was defined as rubitecan 1 mg/m² and gemcitabine 1000 mg/m² administered intravenously over 30 minutes on days 1 and 8, given every 21 days. DLT was myelosuppression including neutropenia and thrombocytopenia. Other side effects included diarrhea, nausea, vomiting, and fatigue. Five patients had stable disease among 18 assessable patients with lung and breast cancers *(29)*.

A second similar study supported these results. In this phase I trial, patients were given escalating doses of rubitecan (doses ranging 1.0 mg/m²/day to 1.5 mg/m²/day) days 1–5 with a fixed dose of gemcitabine (1000 mg/m² intravenously over 30 minutes) for 3 consecutive weeks every 28 days. Of the nine patients enrolled to date, 35 courses of the combination treatment have been completed. No DLTs have been reported to date, and the most significant toxicities include grade 3 nausea/vomiting and grade 3 neutropenia. The authors recommend a phase II dose of rubitecan at 1.5 mg/m²/day in combination with the previously discussed dose of gemcitabine *(32)*.

A third study exploring the combination of rubitecan and gemcitabine involved patients with unresectable pancreatic cancer. Patients were eligible if they had prior gemcitabine therapy, provided there were no dose reductions. Rubitecan was administered as a single oral dose for 5 consecutive days each week, and gemcitabine was give intravenously over 30 minutes on days 5, 12, and 19 of each 28-day cycle. Nine patients were enrolled, each receiving a dose of rubitecan between 1.0 and 1.5 mg/m² and gemcitabine between 600 and 1000 mg/m². Toxicities included grade 3 anorexia, nausea, vomiting, fatigue, and abnormal liver tests, and grade 4 myelosuppression. A partial response was seen in a patient treated at the 1.5/800 level. The patient gained 27 pounds and had an 87% decrease in the size of liver metastases, with a fall in CA19-9 from 588 to 38 IU. Another patient treated at the 1/600 level had stable disease for 8 months *(33)*.

A recent publication reported the combination of rubitecan with capecitabine in patients with refractory, metastatic solid tumors. Capecitabine was administered two times per day for a total daily dose of 1300 mg/m² × 14 days followed by a 1-week break. Rubitecan was given daily 5 days per week for 2 weeks at a starting dose of 0.5 mg/m². Twenty-one patients were assessable for toxicity and response. DLTs included nausea and emesis, described as grade 2–3 in 3 of 14 patients; the MTD of rubitecan was determined at 0.75 mg/m². The incidence of hand-foot syndrome, stomatitis, diarrhea, and myelosuppression did not exceed that expected with capecitabine alone. Although stable disease was observed in 43% of patients for a median duration of 11 weeks, no objective responses were seen *(30)*.

Combination Phase I studies of rubitecan with radiation are ongoing.

3.3. Phase II Studies

A wide range of phase II studies have been started (Table 2), and several have now yielded peer reviews.

3.3.1. Ovarian Cancer

A phase II study of oral rubitecan was completed in patients with advanced Mullerian (ovarian, fallopian, or primary peritoneal) cancer refractory to platinum-based therapy. All patients were heavily pretreated and had refractory cancers. The median number of previous chemotherapy regimens was greater than three. The objective of the study was to determine the activity of a daily oral dose of rubitecan. Rubitecan dose was 1.5 mg/m^2/day for 4 consecutive days every week. Increments of 0.25 mg/day were authorized in patients who did not experience significant side effects. Of 29 patients evaluated, a 7% remission rate was observed. Thirty-four percent of patients had stable disease. The median survival was 8 months. Toxicity was evaluated in 31 patients. Grade 3 or 4 hematological toxicity consisted of anemia in 10 patients (32%), neutropenia in 8 patients(26%), and thrombocytopenia in 3 patients(10%). Grade >2 nonhematological toxic effects were nausea and vomiting in 26 patients(84%), diarrhea in 12 patients (39%), weight loss in 7 patients (22%), chemical cystitis in 6 patients(19%), and neutropenic sepsis in 6 patients (19%). Rubitecan was tolerated for sustained periods in some patients (up to 47 weeks). The observed 8-month survival in such a refractory patient population is noteworthy *(34)*.

3.3.2. Pancreatic Cancer

In the first phase II study evaluating the efficacy of rubitecan in treating patients with advanced pancreatic cancer, patients received rubitecan at 1.5 mg/m^2/day orally for 5 days per week for at least 8 weeks (two courses). Patients were analyzed for changes in tumor size by computed tomography scan, changes in serum CA 19-9 tumor marker levels, quality of life, and survival. Of 107 patients with advanced adenocarcinoma of the pancreas enrolled in the study, only 60 patients were able to be assessed; 47 patients did not receive the minimum two courses of treatment necessary to observe a response, usually because of poor performance status with early progression of disease. Response rate was 31.7% for patients evaluated, and the intent to treat response rate was 18%. Primary dose-limiting toxicities were myelosuppression with grade ≥3 anemia in 21% of patients, neutropenia in 14%, and thrombocytopenia in 7%. Nonhematological side effects (any grade) included nausea and vomiting (44% of patients), diarrhea (31%), and interstitial cystitis (22%). No deaths were attributed to rubitecan. Median survival for different subsets of patients is shown in Table 3 *(35)*.

A similar study was undertaken in Europe to evaluate the potential benefit of rubitecan administration in patients with advanced pancreatic cancer. Nineteen patients with locally advanced or metastatic adenocarcinoma were

Table 2
Completed or Ongoing Phase II Studies of Rubitecan

Organ site
Metastatic melanoma
Nonsmall-cell lung cancer
Progressive or rapidly advanced colorectal cancer
Hormone refractory prostate cancer
Recurrent, platinum resistant, and refractory ovarian cancer
Sarcomas
Unresectable hepatocellular carcinoma
Refractory metastatic breast cancer
Cancer of biliary tract
Advanced metastatic urothelial tract tumors
Glioblastoma multiforme
Advanced small-cell lung cancer
Cervical cancer
Head and neck cancer
Acute myeloid leukemia (AML)
Lymphoma
Myeloma

enrolled, and patients were given rubitecan orally five times per week, once per day. The endpoints of this study were toxicity, objective response rate, subjective response rate (i.e., pain control, performance status, and body weight), and survival. Of 14 patients assessable for response, 28.6% had an objective response, whereas a symptomatic improvement was observed in 92.9%. Overall median survival was 21 weeks (31 weeks in the group of 14 patients evaluated for response), and the 1-year survival was 16.7% (23.1% in the 14 assessable patients). Seven patients (36.8%) experienced toxicity severe enough to necessitate an interruption of rubitecan, all related to a prior dose increase, whereas milder toxicity was observed in eight patients (42.1%) *(36)*.

Because of the excellent response seen in some patients with pancreatic cancer, further studies of rubitecan for this disease have been started. So far, few data are available. One abstract has been published of a confirmatory study of the 1.5 mg/m^2/day of rubitecan for 5 days every 7 days given to 52 very refractory patients with a response rate of 9%, and a serologic remission rate, described as a 50% reduction in CA19-9, of 18%. Patients were encouraged to drink three liters of fluid per day to help reduce the incidence of previously reported cystitis. Only one patient (2%) was noted to have cystitis, suggesting that oral hydration is markedly effective in preventing

Table 3
Survival of Patients With Pancreatic Cancer Treated With Rubitecan

Subset of patients	*Number of patients*	*Survival (months)*
All	107	6.5
Evaluable	60	8.7
Responders	19	18.6
Stable disease	19	9.7
Progressive disease	22	6.8
Untreated	57	7.3
Previously treated	50	4.7
Previously treated with gemcitabine	33	4.7

this toxicity. Other side effects were similar to what was reported in the Phase I studies *(37)*.

3.3.3. Myelodysplasia

Rubitecan has been studied in patients with chronic myeloid leukemia, chronic myelomonocytic leukemia, and refractory anemia with excess blasts. The dose of rubitecan was 2 mg/m^2/day, Monday through Friday, every week. One of the eight Philadelphia-positive chronic myeloid leukemia patients had a complete cytogenetic remission. Of nine Philadelphia-negative chronic myeloid leukemia, two complete responses and four partial responses were observed. Among seven chronic myelomonocytic leukemia patients, there were two partial responses, and one patient with refractory anemia with excess blasts had a complete response. Diarrhea and nausea were the main side effects. Treatment dose could be increased in 7 patients, but 12 patients needed some treatment interruption to alleviate side effects *(38)*.

3.3.4. Breast Cancer

Of 18 patients with refractory breast cancer treated with rubitecan, 16 were evaluated for antitumor activity. There were no complete or partial responses. The investigators observed two patients with a minor response and three with disease stabilization. Side effects were similar to what has been described in former studies. Pharmacokinetic and pharmacodynamic studies were performed, but results have not yet been published *(39)*.

3.3.5. Colorectal Cancer

A randomized, open-label phase II study was performed in patients with advanced colorectal cancer. A crossover design was used to determine the intrapatient variation of the bioavailability and pharmacokinetics of the anticancer agent depending on the timing of food intake in relation to the oral drug administration (*see* Section 4.). Patients with previously untreated metastatic disease received rubitecan given orally at a dose of 1.5 mg/m^2/day, to be increased up to 2.0 mg/m^2/day for 5 consecutive days per week until disease progression. Nineteen patients entered the trial. A total number of 35 treatment cycles (median 2, range 1–4) were administered. All patients were evaluated for safety. The toxicity profile of rubitecan was generally mild to moderate, with sporadic cases of grade 4 toxicities, and diarrhea, leukopenia, and neutropenia reported. None of the 15 evaluated patients achieved an objective response, and the majority had early disease progression, suggesting that despite a good tolerance, rubitecan is clinically inactive in colorectal cancer at the currently recommended dose and schedule *(40)*.

3.3.6. Glioblastoma multiforme

The antitumor activity and safety of RFS2000 given once daily at 1.5 mg/m^2/day was investigated as first-line chemotherapy treatment for patients with advanced glioblastoma multiform. Seventeen patients were entered onto the trial, and 15 patients were considered eligible. A total of 49 cycles (range 1–8) were administered. Grade 3-4 toxicity was observed in five patients, with neutropenia and thrombocytopenia being common toxicities. The response rate was poor, with 5 patients experiencing tumor stabilization and 10 progressing. These results do not support the further evaluation of RFS2000 as a single agent in patients with recurrent glioblastoma multiforme *(41)*.

3.3.7. Melanoma

A phase II trial was conducted to assess the efficacy of rubitecan therapy in patients with metastatic cutaneous and uveal melanoma. Twenty-eight patients were enrolled in the trial, with 14 patients diagnosed with each of the two types of melanoma. Rubitecan was administered orally at a starting dose of 1.5 mg/m^2/day for 5 consecutive days of each week. No complete or partial responses were observed, although stabilization of disease was achieved in four individuals (15%) for durations of 3, 4, 6, and 8 months, respectively. Hematologic toxicity was moderate, and gastrointestinal side effects were common: 43% of the patients experienced grade 3 or 4 diarrhea and 18% reported grade 3 or 4 vomiting. No patients developed chemical cystitis with gross hematuria. Rubitecan at the dose and schedule studied in this trial was toxic without significant activity against metastatic melanoma of cutaneous or uveal origin *(42)*.

3.3.8. Soft-Tissue Sarcomas

In patients with gastrointestinal leiomyosarcomas and other soft-tissue sarcomas (STS), rubitecan was administered orally at 1.5 mg/m^2 per day ×

5 days every week to a total of 56 patients. Response evaluation was performed at 8 weeks, and those with stable or responding disease continued treatment until maximal response was achieved. Seventeen patients were enrolled on the gastrointestinal leiomyosarcoma arm; only one minor response, lasting less than 8 weeks was noted in a patient with liver metastases, and this arm was terminated. Thirty-nine patients were entered on the other soft-tissue sarcoma arm. Of these patients, three patients (8%) achieved a partial response for durations of 4, 6, and 13 months, respectively. Fourteen patients had stable disease for a median of 4 months (range 2–8 months). Two patients died of disease during the first 2 months. In terms of toxicity, four patients required hospitalization for nausea, vomiting, and dehydration. Grade 3 toxicities included diarrhea (8%), fatigue (19%), anorexia (2%), nausea (4%), vomiting (6%), neutropenia (8%), and thrombocytopenia (8%). Rubitecan is well tolerated but inactive in gastrointestinal leiomyosarcomas and has minimal activity in previously treated patients with soft-tissue sarcomas *(43)*.

3.3.9. Chordoma

An evaluation of the potential sensitivity of chordoma to rubitecan was recently initiated Nine patients with radiographically evident, unresectable, or metastatic chordoma were enrolled. A dosage of 1.25 mg/m^2/day orally for 5 days per week was used, and all patients were evaluated for response. One near-complete response of 251 days' duration was observed; however, the patient elected to discontinue therapy. Three patients have shown stability of disease (median response 174 days), and disease-free progression at 3 and 6 months was 66% and 33%, respectively. Only minor toxicities were reported. This early study suggests that rubitecan may have activity against advanced chordoma and will hopefully be followed by further studies *(44)*.

3.3.10. Gastric Cancer

The effect of rubitecan on gastric or gastroesophageal junction adenocarcinoma was studied in patients with measurable, unresectable, local, or metastatic disease. Patients had received no more than one prior chemotherapy regimen. Thirty-five patients have been enrolled, and received 1.5 mg/m^2/day of rubitecan for 5 days, followed by 2 days of rest, for 8 weeks. Patients were continued on treatment until progression or limiting toxicity was noted. Eight patients did not complete the full 8 weeks of therapy and were not evaluated. Of the 27 patients currently assessable, 3 achieved a partial response, 2 had a minor response, 6 patients had stable disease, and 16 showed progressive disease. Toxicities included grade 3 or 4 neutropenia, anemia, fatigue, myalgia, nausea, vomiting, and diarrhea; however, these toxicities were low in frequency and, in general, therapy was well tolerated. These preliminary results suggest that further studies of rubitecan with gastric carcinoma are warranted *(45)*.

3.3.11. Urothelial Tract Cancers

Rubitecan was tested in 21 patients with advanced metastatic urothelial tract tumors who had failed first-line treatment. Dosage was similar to other studies with 1.5 mg/m^2/day for 5 days followed by 2 days of rest with one cycle arbitrarily defined as a 3-week period. Among the 19 patients available for evaluation, 1 confirmed partial remission was noted and 6 patients had stable disease. Sixteen patients stopped treatment for progressive disease, and three for hematological toxicity. Grade 3 or 4 hematologic toxicities included eight patients with neutropenia, four with thrombocytopenia, and four patients with anemia. Other nonhematologic side effects were similar to those observed in other described studies *(46)*.

3.3.12. Non-small-Cell Lung Cancer

There has been one study of rubitecan in patients with refractory or relapsed non-small-cell lung cancer. Dosages of the drug were similar to the above studies. A total of 29 patients were enrolled; however, 3 patients never received the medication and 14 of 26 patients received less than 6 weeks of therapy because of a combination of toxicity or tumor progression. No major responses were observed. One patient had a 32% tumor reduction and another showed stability for 8 months. Major toxicities were similar to the previous studies and included febrile neutropenia, fatigue, diarrhea, and anemia. Significant hematuria was seen in four patients *(47)*.

3.3.13. Small-Cell Lung Cancer

A study enrolled patients with progressive or recurrent small-cell lung cancer who were then stratified into patients with response to previous chemotherapy and those refractory to prior therapy. Rubitecan was given at the dose of 1.5 mg/m^2/day on a 5 days on, 2 days off schedule, and one cycle was defined as a 3-week period. Fifteen sensitive and 22 refractory patients were enrolled. Common toxicities included febrile neutropenia, grade 4 thrombocytopenia, and grade 3–4 anemia, diarrhea, vomiting, and nausea. Five sensitive and six refractory patients had stable disease (median 16 weeks), and no objective responses have been observed. These results do not support further evaluation of rubitecan as a single agent of small-cell lung cancer for second-line therapy *(48)*.

3.4. Phase III Studies

There are only three ongoing phase III studies in pancreatic cancer. The first trial is in chemotherapy-naive patients and the other trials are in patients in whom chemotherapy failed. Rubitecan is compared with gemcitabine. The second trial is comparing rubitecan with 5-fluorouracil in patients in whom gemcitabine chemotherapy failed. A third study is comparing rubitecan with best appropriate therapy in multiply treated patients. These trials are ongoing and results have not been reported. Based on the results of the third trial, rubitecan has been placed on fast track by the Food and Drug Administration.

4. PHARMACOKINETICS PARAMETERS

In the first Phase I study of rubitecan, the main pharmacology objective was to demonstrate that rubitecan was absorbed in the intestine, and second, to determine what plasma level of drug could be obtained. Fourteen patients had plasma levels of total drug and lactone form measured by high-performance liquid chromatography analysis on the first day of rubitecan administration. Limited pharmacokinetic sampling of drug plasma concentrations was completed for the preliminary evaluation of the pharmacokinetic profile. The pharmacokinetic sampling time points included before infusion, 30 minutes, and 1, 2, 4, and 6 hours after drug administration. Four patients had additional pharmacokinetic sampling at 8, 18, 34, and 45 days of continuous administration of rubitecan. Another four patients had pharmacokinetic sampling for the first time while on treatment at days 8, 21, 28, or 56. On the first day of treatment, the rubitecan lactone maximum plasma concentration was 15.5 ng/mL (range 2.8–70 ng/mL) seen at a median of 1 hour (range 0.5–6 hours). The median maximum plasma concentration of the total drug occurred at a median of 4 hours (range 2–6 hours) and was 111 ng/mL (range 6.4–517 ng/mL). The mean percentage of the area under the curve (AUC) of the lactone form versus the AUC of the total drug was 14.7% (SD ± 14.3%). Plasma levels of rubitecan measured in patients on treatment (days 8–56) were similar to those observed in naive patients, with a median peak level of lactone of 10 ng/mL (range 1.8–74 ng/mL). There is a second peak around 6 to 8 hours after drug administration that may be related to an enterohepatic cycle *(24)*.

As early phase I studies revealed optimal dosing schedules, other studies helped to develop an optimal pharmacokinetic sampling schedule for rubitecan for use in phase II–III trials when administered daily for 5 days per week (Table 4). Concentration-time data of rubitecan and 9-AC were obtained from 14 patients who had received 1.5 mg/m^2/day rubitecan orally. Optimal sampling points were selected on the basis of the assessed population pharmacokinetic parameters using a D-optimality algorithm. The absorption rate constant, apparent volume of distribution, and apparent clearance of rubitecan were 0.81 $hour^{-1}$, 50 L, and 1.7 L/hour, respectively. For 9-AC, the corresponding values of the apparent volume of distribution and the elimination rate constant were 51 L and 0.102 $hour^{-1}$. Variability of the parameters within individuals ranged from 38% to 49%. For the first dose, optimal sampling points were 1, 3, 5, 8, and 24 hours after dosing, allowing an optimal sampling schedule to be derived for the assessment of the pharmacokinetic parameters of the rubitecan and its metabolite 9-AC *(49)*.

Table 4
Pharmacokinetics of Rubitecan

Reference	*Dose ($mg/m^2/day$)*	C_{maxlac} *(ng/mL)*	C_{maxtd} *(ng/mL)*	T_{maxlac} *(hour)*	T_{maxtd} *(hour)*	AUC_{lac} *(ng/mL/hour)*	$AUC_{td(0–24)}$ *(ng/mL/hour)*	*Ratio* $AUC_{lac/td}$ *(%)*	$T_{1/2lac}$ *(hour)*	$T_{1/2td}$ *(hour)*	*Comments*
40	1.5		57.3		3.1		774.7				Fasting
40	1.5		28.9		6.3		473.2				After a meal
52	2.0					183		25			
50	1.5	9.7	117	4.8	5.0			8	19.2	14.1	
24	1.0–2.0	15.5	111	1	4.0			14.7			
34	1.5	4.6	104.6	3.3	5.3		1505.6	6.2		14.1	On day 1

During the phase II study enrolling patients with Mullerian cancers, a more detailed pharmacology study was performed to look at the accumulation of drug during 1, 2, and 3 days of treatment with rubitecan 1.5 mg/m^2/day (three cohorts of three patients). Blood samples were obtained at predose and at 0.5, 1, 2, 4, 6, 8, 12, 16, 20, and 24 hours on day 1 for the first cohort; on days 1 and 2 for the second cohort; on days 1–3 for the third cohort; and every 4 hours thereafter, up to 72 hours after the last dose of rubitecan. After the first dose, the total drug maximum plasma concentration values ranged from 61 to 167 ng/mL. The total drug AUC values ranged from 624 to 2838 ng/mL/hour. The intestinal absorption of rubitecan appeared to be delayed with time to maximum plasma concentration for total drug ranged from 4 to 8 hours after the first dose. The mean terminal elimination half-life ($t_{1/2}$) was 10.6 hours after a single dose. The ranges of total drug maximum plasma concentration, and AUC values observed in patients receiving multiple doses of rubitecan were similar to the first cohort. The interpatient variability observed was fairly consistent between cohorts. The drug accumulation recorded on day 2 was similar to the drug accumulation seen on day 3 (mean accumulation index on day 2 was 1.53 (range 0.9–2.14); and on day 3 was 1.48 (range 1.14–1.99). The lactone concentrations were substantially lower than the total drug concentrations in the plasma and constituted about 0–20% of the total drug concentrations. The concentrations of lactone and the total concentration of the drug plus its metabolites in ascites were obtained from a patient who received a single dose of rubitecan. Although the lactone concentrations were undetectable, total concentrations in the fluid ranged from 1.4 to 4.4 ng/mL. Because of the slow elimination rate from the ascites, the ratio of ascites to plasma concentration of the total form increased as a function of time from 3.5% at 10 hours after dosing to 126% at 70 hours after dosing.

With rubitecan, the level of exposure to the lactone form is less than 10% of the total drug exposure. The pharmacokinetics of rubitecan appears to be nonlinear as demonstrated by rubitecan accumulation overtime, as suggested by the disproportional increase in AUCs with prolonged administration. No pharmacodynamic relationship could be determined between the rubitecan pharmacokinetic parameters and toxicity or response to rubitecan. These findings are similar to those observed in different trials of other CPT derivatives. The implications of the plasma lactone:total drug ratio in the therapeutic efficacy of rubitecan treatment cannot be conclusively defined. Rubitecan is highly protein-bound in the plasma. In addition, because of the lipophilic nature of rubitecan, the compound is retained intracellularly, especially in red blood cells. This intracellular pool of rubitecan may constitute a reserve of drug that is slowly released into the plasma. This phenomenon may also contribute to the toxicity of rubitecan. Therefore, the biological activity of rubitecan may depend on factors other than drug plasma concentration.

In a corroborating study that was performed at the Cancer Therapy and Research Center in San Antonio, similar interpatient variability was observed. Maximum plasma concentration (C_{max}) on day 1 was 117 ng/mL for the total drug and 9.7 ng/mL for the lactone. Time to maximum plasma concentration occurred at 5 and 4.8 hours, respectively. These results were not substantially different after one cycle of treatment (day 26). After administration of rubitecan, most of the drug remains in the nitro form and undergoes primarily nonrenal elimination. About 10% of rubitecan was irreversibly converted to 9-AC. Hence, an accumulation of 9-AC overtime was observed with the ratio of 9-AC/rubitecan increased on day 26 *(50)*.

The effect of food intake on the gastrointestinal absorption of rubitecan was tested in patients with colorectal cancers. Two single oral doses of rubitecan 1.5 mg/m^2 were given in a randomized fashion either after an overnight fasting period or immediately after a high-calorie breakfast, and crossed over to the alternative schedule after a 1-week washout period to patients with untreated advanced colon cancer. Pharmacokinetics were studied. Fourteen patients were evaluated for pharmacokinetic analysis. The bioavailability of rubitecan was found to be strongly dependent on the timing of food intake with a fasted-to-fed ratio for C_{max} of 1.98 (two-tailed $p < 0.001$; analysis of variance), $T_{(max)}$ 0.49 ($p < 0.001$), AUC (0–8 hours) 2.52 ($p < 0.001$), and AUC (0–24 hours) 1.64 ($p = 0.003$). These results demonstrate that the bioavailability is strongly dependent on the timing of food intake in relation to the oral administration of the drug. In future prospective trials in other tumor types, feeding conditions should be predetermined to reduce the variability of pharmacokinetic parameters *(40)*.

As mentioned previously, the possibility of an aerosol version of rubitecan delivery offers an exciting alternative mode of delivery. Of the six patients in the first cohort (6.7 μg/kg/day, which is equivalent to 0.26 mg/m^2/day), five volunteered for pharmacokinetic studies *(27)*. 9NC measured as total 9NC was detected in plasma at the first timepoint, midway through the 1-hour aerosol exposure. Total 9NC plasma concentrations continued to increase for 2 to 3 hours from the start of treatment reaching a mean peak concentration of 37.7 ng/mL (SD ± 20.2) at 2 hours (range 13.6–58.0 ng/mL). Mean clearance of 9NC was biphasic with a $T_{1/2\alpha}$ of 1.9 hours (SD ± 1.4) and a $T_{1/2\beta}$ of 16.4 hours (±10.5). The AUC of the lactone form measured in the last two patients comprised only 3.2% and 3.5% of the total 9NC *(51)*.

5. CONCLUSIONS AND PERSPECTIVES

The topoisomerase I inhibitors are a new class of anticancer agents that have shown activity against a wide range of hematological and solid tumors. The lactone form of the molecule is essential for the antitumor activity. Serum pH value and human serum albumin concentration are important factors in the stability of the open, active lactone form of CPT analogs. In xenograft nude mouse models of human tumors, water-soluble CPTs (TPT and CPT-11) have somewhat less activity than do water-insoluble agents (9-AC and rubitecan) (Dr. B. Giovanella, personal communication). This difference has not been demonstrated in clinical trials.

Phase I and II clinical trials have demonstrated antitumor activity of rubitecan in a wide range of solid tumors, including chemotherapy-resistant tumors. The current recommended schedule of rubitecan administration is 1.5 mg/m^2/day for 5 consecutive days every week. Tumor types that may be sensitive to rubitecan are pancreatic, gastric, ovarian, and chordoma. Although symptomatic improvement and long-term stability of disease is commonly observed, overall response rates are modest in most tumor types. Development of chemotherapy combination regimens and radiotherapy combinations with rubitecan are expected. Whether rubitecan will be a candidate for a new drug approval awaits the results of the phase III studies in patients with pancreatic cancer.

ACKNOWLEDGMENTS

Supported in part by Grant MO1 RR02558.

REFERENCES

1. Muggia FM, Creaven PJ, Hansen HH, Cohen MH, Selawry OS. 1972 Phase I clinical trial of weekly and daily treatment with camptothecin (NSC-100880): correlation with preclinical studies. Cancer Chemother Rep 56:515–521.
2. Verschraegen CF, Kudelka AP, Kavanagh JJ. 1998 Topoisomerase-I inhibitors in gynaecologic tumours. [Review]. Ann Acad Med (Sing) 27:683–687.
3. Rothenberg ML. 199CPT-11: an original spectrum of clinical activity. Semin Oncol 23:21–26.
4. Saltz LB, Cox JV, Blanke C, et al. 200Irinotecan plus fluorouracil and leucovorin for metastatic colorectal cancer. Irinotecan Study Group [see comments]. New Engl J Med 343:905–914.
5. Kudelka AP, Tresukosol D, Edwards CL, et al. 1996 Phase II study of intravenous topotecan as a 5-day infusion for refractory epithelial ovarian carcinoma. J Clin Oncol 14:1552–1557.
6. Ardizzoni A, Hansen H, Dombernowsky P, et al. 1997 Topotecan, a new active drug in the second-line treatment of small-cell lung cancer: a phase II study in patients with refractory and sensitive disease. The European Organization for Research and Treatment of Cancer Early Clinical Studies Group and New Drug Development Office, and the Lung Cancer Cooperative Group. J Clin Oncol 15: 2090–2096.
7. Bleiberg H, Cvitkovic E. 1996 Characterisation and clinical management of CPT-11 (irinotecan)-induced adverse events: the European perspective [review]. Eur J Cancer 32A(Suppl. 3):S18–23.
8. Rowinsky EK, Grochow LB, Hendricks CB, et al. 1992 Phase I and pharmacologic study of topotecan: a novel topoisomerase I inhibitor. J Clin Oncol 10:647–656.

9. von Pawel J, Schiller JH, Shepherd FA, et al. 1999 Topotecan versus cyclophosphamide, doxorubicin, and vincristine for the treatment of recurrent small-cell lung cancer. J Clin Oncol 17:658–667.
10. Wiseman LR, Markham A. 1996 Irinotecan. A review of its pharmacological properties and clinical efficacy in the management of advanced colorectal cancer. Drugs 52:606–623.
11. Dancey J, Eisenhauer EA. 1996 Current perspectives on camptothecins in cancer treatment [editorial]. Br J Cancer 74:327–338.
12. Garcia-Carbonero R, Supko JG. 2002 Current perspectives on the clinical experience, pharmacology, and continued development of the camptothecins. Clin Cancer Res 8:641–661.
13. Arbuck SG, Takimoto CH. 1998 An overview of topoisomerase I-targeting agents [review]. Semin Hematol 35:3–12.
14. Kohn KW, Pommier Y. 2000 Molecular and biological determinants of the cytotoxic actions of camptothecins. Perspective for the development of new topoisomerase I inhibitors. Ann NY Acad Sci 922:11–26.
15. Giovanella BC, Hinz HR, Kozielski AJ, Stehlin JS Jr, Silber R, Potmesil M. 1991 Complete growth inhibition of human cancer xenografts in nude mice by treatment with 20-(S)-camptothecin. Cancer Res 51:3052–3055.
16. Hinz HR, Harris NJ, Natelson EA, Giovanella BC. 1994 Pharmacokinetics of the in vivo and in vitro conversion of 9-nitro-20(S)-camptothecin to 9-amino-20(S)-camptothecin in humans, dogs, and mice. Cancer Res 54:3096–3100.
17. Pantazis P, Kozielski AJ, Mendoza JT, Early JA, Hinz HR, Giovanella BC. 1993 Camptothecin derivatives induce regression of human ovarian carcinomas grown in nude mice and distinguish between non-tumorigenic and tumorigenic cells in vitro. Int J Cancer 53:863–871.
18. Pantazis P, Kozielski A, Rodriguez R, et al. 1994 Therapeutic efficacy of camptothecin derivatives against human malignant melanoma xenografts. Melanoma Res 4:5–10.
19. Pantazis P, Early JA, Kozielski AJ, Mendoza JT, Hinz HR, Giovanella BC. 1993 Regression of human breast carcinoma tumors in immunodeficient mice treated with 9-nitrocamptothecin: differential response of nontumorigenic and tumorigenic human breast cells in vitro. Cancer Res 53:1577–1582.
20. Giovanella BC, Stehlin JS, Hinz HR, Kozielski AJ, Harris NJ, Vardeman DM. 2002 Preclinical evaluation of the anticancer activity and toxicity of 9-nitro-20(S)-camptothecin (Rubitecan). Int J Oncol 20:81–88.
21. Koshkina NV, Gilbert BE, Waldrep JC, Seryshev A, Knight V. 1999 Distribution of camptothecin after delivery as a liposome aerosol or following intramuscular injection in mice. Cancer Chemother Pharmacol 44:187–192.
22. Kemp KR, Liehr JG, Giovanella B. 2000 Combined radiation and 9-nitrocamptothecin (rubitecan) in the treatment of locally advanced pancreatic cancer. Ann NY Acad Sci 922: 320–323.
23. Amorino GP, Hercules SK, Mohr PJ, Pyo H, Choy H. 2000 Preclinical evaluation of the orally active camptothecin analog, RFS-2000 (9-nitro-20(S)-camptothecin) as a radiation enhancer. Int J Radiat Oncol Biol Phys 47:503–509.
24. Verschraegen CF, Natelson EA, Giovanella BC, et al. 1998 A phase I clinical and pharmacological study of oral 9-nitrocamptothecin, a novel water-insoluble topoisomerase I inhibitor. Anti-Cancer Drugs 9:36–44.

25. Zamboni W, Jung L, Jin R, et al. 2001 Phase I & pharmacokinetic (PK) study of intermittently administered 9-nitrocampothecin (9NC, Rubitecan) in patients with advanced malignancies. Proc Am Soc Clin Oncol 20:A411.
26. Alberts DS, Markman M, Armstrong D, Rothenberg ML, Muggia F, Howell SB. 2002 Intraperitoneal therapy for stage III ovarian cancer: a therapy whose time has come! J Clin Oncol 20:3944–3946.
27. Verschraegen CF, Gilbert BE, Loyer E, Huaringa AJ, Walsh G, Newman RA, et al. 2004. Clinical evaluation of the delivery and safety of aerosolized liposomal 9-nitro-20(s)-camptothecin in patients with advanced pulmonary malignancies. Clin Cancer Res 10:2319–2326.
28. Verschraegen CF, Vincent M, Abbruzzese J, et al. 2000 Phase I study of 9-nitro-20(S)-camptothecin (Rfs 2000) in combination with cisplatin for patients with advanced malignancies. Ann NY Acad Sci 922:345–348.
29. Fracasso PM, Rader JS, Govindan R, et al. 2002 Phase I study of rubitecan and gemcitabine in patients with advanced malignancies. Ann Oncol 13:1819–1825.
30. Michaelson MD, Ryan DP, Fuchs CS, et al. 2003 A phase I study of 9-nitrocamptothecin given concurrently with capecitabine in patients with refractory, metastatic solid tumors. Cancer 97:148–154.
31. Lenzi R, Verschraegen C, Kudelka A, et al. 2002 New escalation scheme for phase I study of drug combination: 9-nitro-20(S)-camptothecin (RFS 2000) with cisplatin for patients (pts) with advanced malignancies. Proc Am Soc Clin Oncol 21:A392.
32. Goetz AD, Rowinksy EK, Tolcher A, et al. 2003 Phase I and pharmacokinetic (PK) study of escalating doses of rubitecan in combination with weekly gemcitabine in patients with advanced solid malignancies. Proc Am Soc Clin Oncol 22:A626.
33. Szarka CE, Babb JS, Cheng JD, et al. 2001 Phase I study of rubitecan and gemcitabine in patients with unresectable pancreas cancer. Proc Am Soc Clin Oncol 20:A2289.
34. Verschraegen CF, Gupta F, Loyer E, et al. 1999 A phase II clinical and pharmacological study of oral 9-nitrocamptothecin in patients with refractory epithelial ovarian, tubal or peritoneal cancer. Anti-Cancer Drugs 10:375–383.
35. Stehlin JS, Giovanella BC, Natelson EA, et al. 1999 A study of 9-nitrocamptothecin (RFS-2000) in patients with advanced pancreatic cancer. Int J Oncol 14:821–831.
36. Konstadoulakis MM, Antonakis PT, Tsibloulis BG, et al. 2001 A phase II study of 9-nitrocamptothecin in patients with advanced pancreatic adenocarcinoma. Cancer Chemother Pharmacol 48:417–420.
37. Rivkin S, Burris III H, Gerstein H, et al. 2000 A phase II study of rubitecan (RFS 2000, 9 NC, 9-nitro-20(S)-camptothecin) in patients with refractory pancreatic cancer. ASCO Proc 19:262a.
38. Cortes J, O'Brien S, Giles F, et al. 2000 9-nitro-20-(S)-camptothecin (9-NC, RFS2000) in chronic myeloid leukemia (CML), chronic myelomonocytic leukemia (CMML) and myelodysplastic syndromes (MDS). Proc Am Soc Clin Oncol 19:7a.
39. Miller KD, Soule SE, Haney LG, et al. 2004 A phase II pharmacokinetic and pharmacodynamic trial of 9-nitrocamptothecin (9-NC) in patients (pts.) with metastatic breast cancer. Invest New Drugs 22:69–73.
40. Schoffski P, Herr A, Vermorken JB, et al. 2002 Clinical phase II study and pharmacological evaluation of rubitecan in non-pretreated patients with metastatic colorectal cancer-significant effect of food intake on the bioavailability of the oral camptothecin analogue. Eur J Cancer 38:807–813.

41. Raymond E, Campone M, Stupp R, et al.; EORTC Early Clinical Studies Group (ECSG); Brain Tumor Studies Group (BTSG); New Drug Development Program (NDDP). 2002 Multicentre phase II and pharmacokinetic study of RFS2000 (9-nitro-camptothecin) administered orally 5 days a week in patients with glioblastoma multiforme. Eur J Cancer 38:1348–1350.
42. Ellerhorst JA, Bedikian AY, Smith TM, Papadopoulos NE, Plager C, Eton O. 2002 Phase II trial of 9-nitrocamptothecin (RFS 2000) for patients with metastatic cutaneous or uveal melanoma. Anti-Cancer Drugs 13:169–172.
43. Patel SR, Beach J, Papadopoulos N, et al. 2003 Results of a 2-arm phase II study of 9-nitrocamptothecin in patients with advanced soft-tissue sarcomas. Cancer 97:2848–2852.
44. Mace JR, Chandler W, Paulino A, Zalupski M, Dunn R, Baker LH. 2002 Response of chordoma to a protracted schedule of 9-nitrocamptothecin: an update. Proc Am Soc Clin Oncol 21:A1626.
45. Ebrahimi B, Phan A, Yao JC, et al. 2002 Phase II clinical trial of Rubitecan against advanced gastric adenocarcinoma. Proc Am Soc Clin Oncol 21:150a.
46. Jonge, MD, Droz JP, Paz-Ares L, et al. 2002 Open label phase II study on RFS 2000 in advanced/metastatic urothelial tract tumors. Eur J Cancer 38:A142.
47. Fidias P, Supko J, Boral A, et al. 2001 A phase II and pharmacokinetic study of RFS-2000 (9-nitrocamptothecin) in patients with refractory or relapsed non-small cell lung cancer. Proc Am Soc Clin Oncol 20:A2839.
48. Bennouna J, Jonge MD, Favaretto A, et al. 2003 Phase II multicentre study of RFS 2000 (9-nitro-camptothecin) administered orally as a 5-day on-2-day off schedule in patients with advanced small cell lung cancer. Proc Am Soc Clin Oncol 22:A2754.
49. Schoemaker NE, Mathot RA, Schoffski P, Rosing H, Schellens JH, Beijnen JH. 2002 Development of an optimal pharmacokinetic sampling schedule for rubitecan administered orally in a daily times five schedule. Cancer Chemother Pharmacol 50:514–517.
50. Denis LJ, Tolcher A, Rizzo J, et al. 2000 Pharmacokinetic profile of 9-nitorcamptothecin following oral administration daily for 5 consecutive days every week. Proc Am Assoc Cancer Res 41:538.
51. Gilbert B, Newman R, Zamboni W, Knight V, Verschraegen C. 2001 Pharmacokinetics of multiple 9-nitro-camptothecin (9-NC) liposome aerosols during a phase I study: levels of total and lactone-forms, and its conversion to 9-amino-camptothecin (9-AC). Proc Am Soc Clin Oncol 20:A2111.
52. Zamboni WC, Jung LL, Egorin MJ, et al. 2002 Phase I studies of intermittently administered 9-nitrocamptothecin (9NC): relationship between daily dose and toxicity. Proc Am Soc Clin Oncol A390.

11 Irinotecan

Current Clinical Status and Pharmacological Aspects

Laurent P. Rivory, PhD

Contents

1. INTRODUCTION

Irinotecan (Fig. 1), also known as CPT-11, is a semisynthetic derivative of 20(S)camptothecin *(1)*, a pentacyclic alkaloid first identified in extracts of the Chinese shrub *Camptotheca acuminata*. The mechanism of action of camptothecin has been covered in other chapters of this book and need not be revisited here. However, it is pertinent to point out that CPT-11 itself is only a very weak stabilizer of the cleavable complex formed between DNA and topoisomerase I (TOP-I) and requires conversion to an active metabolite, SN-38 *(2)*. The latter is one of the most potent TOP-I poisons known, which may be a result of the prolonged half-life of interaction with the cleavable complex *(3)*. In vivo, the activation of CPT-11 to SN-38 is carried out by carboxylesterases *(4–8)*. In turn, SN-38 can be conjugated to SN-38 β-glucuronide *(9,10)*. CPT-11 is also metabolized to an aminopentanocarboxylic (APC), metabolite (*see* Fig. 1), and other minor, mostly inactive, products by cytochrome P450 3A4/5 *(11–14)*.

Camptothecins in Cancer Therapy
Edited by: V. R. Adams and T. G. Burke © Humana Press Inc., Totowa, NJ

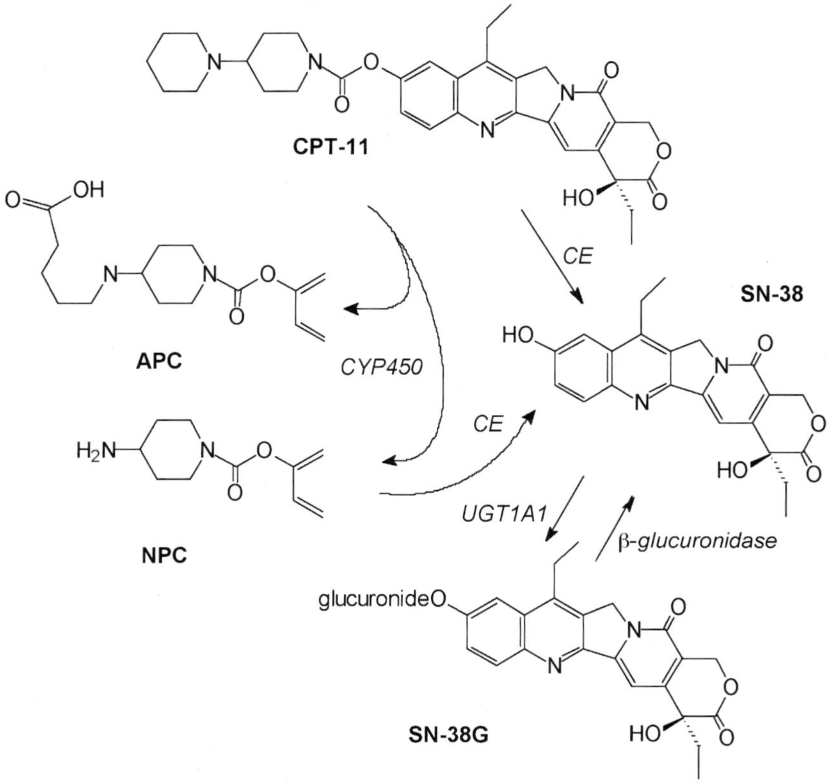

Fig. 1. The major pathways for the metabolism of CPT-11. CE, carboxylesterase; UGT1A1, UDP-glucuronosyl transferase 1A1; CYP450, cytochrome P450 3A.

CPT-11, as a single agent, has been investigated extensively against a variety of tumor types. It is the only camptothecin derivative to have clinically significant activity against colorectal adenocarcinoma and has been registered in many countries (Camptosar, Pharmacia & Upjohn, Kalamazoo, MI; Campto, Rhone-Poulenc Rorer, Antony, France) for the treatment of advanced forms of this disease not responsive to 5-fluorouracil (5-FU)-based therapy *(15–19)*. Recently, CPT-11 was approved by the Food and Drug Administration for first-line use with 5-FU and leucovorin based on Phase III studies of this combination versus 5-FU/leucovorin alone *(20,21)*.

Schedules that have been in clinical trials include treatment once every 2 *(22–24)* or 3 weeks *(25–27)*, once per week for 4 of 6 weeks *(28)* or 3 of 4 weeks *(29)*, daily for 3 consecutive days every 3 weeks *(30,31)*, 6 days of continuous infusion every 3–4 weeks *(32)*, and a variety of other protocols *(33)*. The daily doses have ranged from 40 mg/m^2 (continuous infusion) to 750 mg/m^2 (every 3 weeks).

The encouraging activity of CPT-11 was initially somewhat dampened by the presence of a spectrum of side effects consisting of myelosuppression, acute cholinergic syndrome, and delayed diarrhea. The most troublesome of these, the delayed diarrhea, has since become more manageable through aggressive supportive therapy with loperamide at the first signs of change in bowel habit *(16,27,34–36)*.

Recent and current clinical studies with CPT-11 include its evaluation in the adjuvant treatment of colorectal cancer, new indications such as central nervous system (CNS) and pediatric malignancy, other gastrointestinal tumors (pancreas, stomach, rectum), and attempts to improve its safety. Arguably, however, the new frontier of CPT-11 is in the treatment of lung cancer. Studies of the combination of CPT-11 with cisplatin and etoposide have demonstrated exciting activity in nonsmall-cell lung cancer (NSCLC) and small-cell lung cancer (SCLC), respectively.

2. CURRENT CLINICAL STATUS

Irinotecan was originally discovered by Japanese investigators of the Yakult Institute as part of a large scale screening of esters of SN-38 *(1)*. The product was developed by Daichi Pharmaceutical Company and licensed to Rhone-Poulenc Rorer (now Aventis) in France and Upjohn (now Pharmacia) in the United States. Many schedules were investigated on behalf of both companies; the weekly regimen was selected for Phase II development in the United States and the every-3-week protocol for development in Europe.

The currently registered product is supplied as a slightly acidic solution of CPT-11 in a sorbitol/lactic acid excipient for intravenous administration after dilution in normal or dextrose saline. The feasibility of oral administration was initially demonstrated using the intravenous formulation *(37)*. Recently, powder-filled capsules have been evaluated in a Phase I study of the oral route. The recommended Phase II dose for this formulation is 50 mg/m^2/day for 5 days every 3 weeks *(38)*.

2.1. Colorectal Adenocarcinoma

During the initial Phase I studies, some activity against advanced colorectal adenocarcinoma was observed. Phase II studies demonstrated modest but clinically significant activity with these schedules in patients with advanced colorectal carcinoma who progressed shortly after or during treatment with 5-FU *(15,18,39)*. Objective responses were observed in these studies (13.3, 10.8, and 13.7%, respectively) as were improvements or stabilization of weight, performance status, and pain. An interesting universal observation was the high percentage of patients who had disease stabilization as their best response (40.4 and 44.2%, respectively). This has sparked discussions as to whether minor responses, which are not usually considered significant in typical phase II studies, may actually predicate a likely survival advantage for drugs such as CPT-11 even in the absence of high rates of major responses *(40)*. Also, although patients responded early on in treatment *(16)*, some responses occurred as late as 24 weeks *(17)*.

The use of CPT-11 as a single agent in previously untreated metastatic colorectal adenocarcinoma revealed response rates that were comparable or slightly greater than for patients with prior exposure to 5-FU, indicating little if any cross-resistance between 5-FU and CPT-11 *(17,34)*. The benefit of CPT-11 in advanced colorectal cancer after 5-FU failure was subsequently confirmed in phase III randomized studies. Cunningham et al. demonstrated significant differences in 1-year survival and reduced patient deterioration (assessed from quality of life, weight loss, and pain-free survival) when patients were administered CPT-11 (350 mg/m^2 every 3 weeks) as compared with best supportive care *(19,41)*. The same regimen was shown to be superior to continuous 5-FU infusion in the same setting with modest but clinically significant increases in 1-year survival (45 versus 32%) and median survival (10.8 versus 8.5 months) *(42)*. Furthermore, although CPT-11 drug acquisition costs are greater than for 5-FU, there is an overall slight saving because of reductions in drug administration and medical care costs as well as years of survival gained *(43–45)*.

Because of its activity against colorectal cancer as a single agent, CPT-11 was an obvious candidate to study for the combination chemotherapy of this disease. The combination of CPT-11 (125 mg/m^2, 90-minute infusion), 5-FU (500 mg/m^2, intravenous [iv] bolus) with low-dose leucovorin (20 mg/m^2, iv bolus) every week is now regarded as standard first-line therapy in the United States for patients with advanced or recurrent disease *(21)* and has greater activity than either 5-FU/leucovorin or CPT-11 alone given in comparable regimens. The objective response rates in this study were 50% for the combination arm versus 29% for the 5-FU/leucovorin and CPT-11–only arms. Median overall survival was significantly prolonged ($p = 0.03$) with a hazard ratio of 0.78 (95% confidence interval: 0.63–0.97), although the absolute difference was only approximately 2 months *(21)*. The superiority of the combination has also been shown with different regimens of administration of the combination *(20)*.

There remains some potential for the further fine-tuning of CPT-11/fluoropyrimidine regimens for colorectal cancer. Other schedules of CPT-11, 5-FU, and leucovorin have been investigated, including a biweekly regimen *(46)*. Also, the question as to whether to use these agents in a concomitant or sequential fashion in the clinic is the subject of current study *(47)*. The other possibility is to substitute 5-FU with new-generation fluoropyrimidines such as capecitabine and tegafur. This may enable completely oral therapy when the oral formulation of CPT-11 becomes available.

In relation to single-agent efficacy, there has been some debate as to whether the every-3-week schedule (350 mg/m^2 every 3 weeks) has favorable activity in comparison to the weekly one (125 mg/m^2 every week for 4 of 6 weeks). Preliminary results of a randomized study examining this question indicate that the safety aspects are very similar in the second-line setting *(48)*, although further follow-up is required for analyses of response rate and survival. The 350 mg/m^2 every 3 weeks appears to result in reduced incidence of grade 3 or 4 delayed diarrhea, although this may be partly because of the significant percentage of patients on this arm treated at a reduced starting dose (300 mg/m^2). In many countries, CPT-11 is registered and can be used with either regimen at the discretion of the treating physician.

One of the other issues being elucidated is which patients are most likely to benefit from treatment with CPT-11. In common with many other cytotoxic agents, those with good performance status and normal hemoglobin have had the highest response rates and the longest progression-free survival in trials *(49)*. Interestingly, although those with poor performance status are more prone to delayed diarrhea, toxicity was a favorable prognostic indicator of response in both the US and the French phase II studies *(15,49)*. Indeed, Ychou et al. have suggested that escalations in dose might be considered in good-performance patients who have little in the way of antiproliferative toxicity early on in their treatment *(50)*.

The combination of CPT-11 with other agents with activity in colorectal cancer (i.e., capecitabine, raltitrexed, oxaliplatin, mitomycin C) is being pursued *(51–53)*. In particular, there is preliminary evidence from Phase I studies for significant activity with the combination of CPT-11 (200 mg/m^2, 2-hour infusion) with oxaliplatin (85 mg/m^2, 30-minute infusion) *(52)*. In 12 patients treated at the recommended phase II dose listed previously, grade 3/4 toxicities encountered were peripheral neuropathy (25%), delayed diarrhea (17%), and neutropenia (33%). A phase II study using a slightly different regimen of 85 mg/m^2 oxaliplatin days 1 and 15 plus 80 mg/m^2 CPT-11 days 1, 8, and 15 yielded a response rate of 46% in 36 pretreated (5-FU) patients able to be evaluated *(54)*.

2.2. Other Gastrointestinal Malignancies

The combination of CPT-11 with cisplatin was investigated early in the development of CPT-11 in Japanese phase I trials. Recent studies of this combination (CPT-11 65 mg/m^2, cisplatin 30 mg/m^2) given weekly for 4 of 6 weeks have shown strong clinical activity in chemotherapy-naive patients with advanced or metastatic esophageal cancer *(54)*. A different schedule (CPT-11 70 mg/m^2, days 1 and 15, cisplatin 80 mg/m^2, day 1 repeated every 4 weeks) has been tested for metastatic gastric cancer in both previously treated and chemotherapy-naive patients *(55,56)*. A higher response rate and slightly prolonged survival was noted for patients who had not received prior chemotherapy *(55)*.

There have been encouraging reports for the activity of a gemcitabine/CPT-11 combination against pancreatic adenocarcinoma and this in now the subject of a randomized phase III study *(57)*. CPT-11 has been evaluated for the treatment of other gastrointestinal malignancies (i.e., hepatocellular carcinoma, biliary adenocarcinoma) with mixed results *(58,59)*.

2.3. Lung Cancer

Lung cancer was also one of the early indications investigated with CPT-11 in Japan *(60,61)*. Some activity was noted in a variety of schedules and this led to the rapid development of combination chemotherapy for recurrent NSCLC and SCLC *(62)*. The combination of CPT-11 (60 mg/m^2) and cisplatin (30 mg/m^2) in a weekly regimen has shown some activity against lung cancer after progression on platinum therapy *(63)*. The response rate of 29% is comparable to other commonly used combinations.

2.3.1. Non-Small-Cell Lung Cancer

A recent phase I/II study of the combination of cisplatin, ifosfamide, and CPT-11 in previously untreated advanced NSCLC (IIIB and IV) showed an overall response rate of 62% *(64)*. The recommended phase II regimen was 70 mg/m^2 cisplatin (day 1), 1.5 g/m^2 ifosfamide (days 1–4), and 60 mg/m^2 CPT-11 (days 1, 8, and 15) every 4 weeks with granulocyte colony-stimulating factor support. The overall median survival was 393 days.

The camptothecins act as radiosensitizers *(65–67)*. A phase I/II study of the combination of radiotherapy (40 Gy to tumor and lymph nodes, followed by 20-Gy boost to the primary) with CPT-11 (weekly for 6 weeks) resulted in significant activity against locally advanced NSCLC. However, severe esophagitis and pneumonitis may limit the usefulness of this regimen even when CPT-11 is administered at 45 mg/m^2 *(68)*. Pneumonitis during concurrent radiochemotherapy with weekly CPT-11 may occur in as many as 70% of patients when the lower lung fields are included *(69)*.

2.3.2. Small-Cell Lung Cancer

A high response rate (71%) was observed by Masuda et al. *(70)* in the second-line treatment of SCLC (after platinum and etoposide/anthracycline), which is normally considered as a setting with little chemosensitivity. CPT-11 was administered days 1, 8, and 15 of a 4-week cycle (70 mg/m^2) with etoposide on days 1–3 (80 mg/m^2). The most commonly encountered toxicity (grade 3/4) was neutropenia in spite of the use of prophylactic granulocyte colony-stimulating factor (2 μg/kg/day, days 4–21).

Other combinations being pursued in the treatment of lung cancer include CPT-11/docetaxel *(71,72)* and CPT-11, carboplatin, and paclitaxel *(73)*. The latter regimen yielded an objective response rate of 61% in locally advanced and metastatic NSCLC but was also accompanied by significant toxicity with 30% of patients experiencing febrile or septic neutropenia.

2.4. Central Nervous System

CPT-11 has activity against CNS malignancy. In a study using the weekly regimen (125 mg/m^2), Freidman et al. observed a response rate of 15% and frequent disease stabilization in patients with advanced glioma *(74)*. There was a remarkable absence of severe toxicity in this population. This is likely to be due to an induction of metabolism of CPT-11 via the cytochrome P450 system (*see* Drug Interactions). This has led to the practice of intrapatient dose escalation. However, there are concerns that this may not translate into higher clinical activity because of possible nonlinearity of activation to SN-38 (*see* Section 4.1.). Therefore, a better strategy might be to use lower doses of CPT-11 in combination chemotherapy. One particularly promising combination is that of CPT-11 with alkylating agents such as BCNU and temozolomide *(75–77)*. These combinations are schedule-dependent but have yielded supra-additive tumor response rates in animal models. They are being explored in Phase I studies.

2.5. Carcinoma of the Cervix

Some activity was noted against squamous cell carcinoma of the cervix in Phase I trials; this has been pursued in phase II trials *(78,79)*. However, treatment must be undertaken with caution because many of these patients receive pelvic radiotherapy as part of their management, which leads to increased rates of gastrointestinal toxicity.

2.6. Other Malignancy

CPT-11 has displayed significant activity as a single agent against many other cancers *(30,33,80)*. Unfortunately, many of these trials have been small, and quantitative estimation of the benefit of CPT-11 in these often unreliable *(80)*. Phase I studies have been performed in the pediatric setting *(81–83)*, and phase II studies are ongoing.

3. CLINICAL/MOLECULAR CORRELATIONS

Because the camptothecins are TOP-I poisons, it could be anticipated that cancer cells overexpressing TOP-I would be more susceptible to CPT-11 *(84,85)*. However, it is becoming clear from studies with various experimental systems that downstream events after the stabilization of the cleavable complex are also critical *(86)*. Nevertheless, in view of the activity of CPT-11 in advanced colorectal cancer, it is pertinent to discuss the activity of TOP-I in this malignancy. The expression and activity of TOP-I in colorectal cancer have been studied using a variety of techniques. In terms of Western blotting, colorectal tissue contains more of the enzyme than its normal counterparts *(85)* or other malignancies *(87)* and may be correlated with stage *(85)*. Increased expression in some tumors could be related to increased gene copy numbers resulting from amplification of oncogene-containing elements that also include the TOP-I gene *(88)*.

Catalytic activity has also been measured in tumor samples *(89)* and shown to correlate with immunodetectable protein *(87)*. However, a recent study with a large series of specimens has demonstrated no clear differences between TOP-I activity in tumor and surrounding normal tissue *(90)*. There was also no association between activity and staging, although liver metastases tended to have lower activity than matched primary tumors *(90)*. One of the problems with these studies is determining which methodology best reflects the propensity of the cells to form TOP-I-mediated cleavable complexes. Indeed, although the formation of these complexes correlates moderately well with camptothecin cytotoxicity in cell lines, the expression of topoisomerase as assessed by either mRNA or Western blotting does not *(86)*. In a study of topotecan pharmacodynamics, neither tumor response nor toxicity correlated with the formation of cleavable complexes in peripheral blood mononuclear cells harvested during treatment *(91)*. Cleavable complexes occur in a transient fashion, even during continuous drug exposure, as a result of ubiquitination and redistribution of TOP-I to the cytoplasm *(92,93)*. Therefore, measuring the quantity of tumor-cleavable complexes formed during chemotherapy with CPT-11, even if it were feasible, might not lead to useful prognostic information.

The selection of CPT-11 in the treatment of individual patients could be reasonably based on molecular markers that predict for low likelihood of response with other agents. In the case of 5-FU, for example, there is some evidence that overexpression of the target, thymidylate synthase, correlates with reduced response rates and survival *(94,95)*. Because CPT-11 has no clinically apparent cross-resistance with 5-FU, a strategy that has been proposed is to treat first-line patients with 5-FU when thymidylate synthase expression is low. In the presence of elevated thymidylate synthase expression, CPT-11 could be chosen as an up-front regimen. However, given that first-line treatment with CPT-11, 5-FU, and leucovorin is now considered a standard regimen for colorectal cancer, at least in the United States, this strategy may not provide any clinical advantage.

The antitumor activity of CPT-11 is also likely to be influenced by activation, inactivation, and transport pathways active in tumors. In general, the relevance of these has not been well established with respect to anticancer activity. Some of the relevant data available are discussed further in the following section.

4. PHARMACOLOGY

The spontaneous but reversible opening of the hydroxy lactone ring complicates the pharmacology of all alpha hydroxy lactone camptothecins. Many of the studies of CPT-11, as with camptothecin, have not sought to differentiate the properties of the two species. Nevertheless, it is clear that the carboxylate and lactone forms are chemically very different and have different properties in terms of pharmacokinetics and pharmacodynamics (reviewed in *(96)*). For example, it is now well recognized that the closed lactone form is the species involved in stabilization of the cleavable complex and that part of the unfavorable profile of 20(*S*)camptothecin as used in the early clinical trials was its formulation as the carboxylate salt. Because the two forms are not often specifically investigated, the terminology used in the section below will only use the terms *lactone* and *carboxylate* when the specific species have been investigated. Otherwise, the concentrations will refer to total drug (lactone + carboxylate).

4.1. Activation

CPT-11 is a carbamate ester prodrug of SN-38 that requires activation in vivo *(2)*. This reaction has been shown to be mediated by carboxylesterases, which are present in many normal tissues and in tumor *(4–8)*. Mice and rats have a high capacity for activation of CPT-11 in plasma. In contrast, conversion in human plasma is extremely limited *(97)*. Instead, most of the activation is mediated by the liver and appears to involve two separate carboxylesterases *(7,98)*. The high-affinity carboxylesterase has a Km of approximately 2 μ*M* when the early non–steady-state reaction is examined. This enzyme, therefore, is likely to be responsible for most of the activation of CPT-11 at clinically relevant doses *(7)*. The saturation of this reaction has implications for the clinical pharmacokinetics of CPT-11 (*see* Section 5.).

The human esterases are particularly inefficient *(5,6,99)* and deacylation-limited *(5)*, but cleave the lactone form of CPT-11 preferentially *(8)*. The experimental and clinical implications of deacylation-limited activation of CPT-11 have been discussed *(99)*.

Ideally, a pro-drug should be preferentially activated in the target tissue, but relatively little is known on the conversion of CPT-11 in tumor tissue. Studies to date have shown that tumor activation rates are comparable, albeit slightly less, than matched normal samples *(90,100)*. One of the problems faced in the characterization of the formation of SN-38 in human tissues is that the steady-state rate is but a fraction of the initial velocity because the reaction is significantly deacylation-limited. This means that the enzyme kinetic parameters become highly dependent on the time course chosen. The presence of CPT-11–converting activity in the intestinal mucosa *(90,100,101)* may be of relevance to the development of an oral formulation.

The other product of CPT-11 activation is 4-piperidinopiperidine (*see* Fig. 1) and this compound may have activity against cancer cell lines *(102)*, albeit at concentrations several orders greater than those measured in patients *(103)*.

4.2. Oxidative Metabolism

CPT-11 undergoes significant oxidative metabolism in vivo to APC and aminopiperidino (NPC) metabolites. APC is a major plasma metabolite in patients *(13,103–105)*, whereas NPC, despite being a major product of hepatic microsomal oxidation *(106)*, is significantly less abundant *(105)*. Both are produced by the cytochrome P450 3A family *(11,12,14,107)*. Several monohydroxy metabolites have also been observed in plasma, urine, and bile and in microsomal incubations *(13,107–109)*. The putative pathways and the relevance of the products to the clinical activity of CPT-11 have been discussed *(99)*.

4.3. Conjugation of SN-38

SN-38 is conjugated by UDP-glucuronosyltransferase 1A1 (UGT 1A1) at the exposed C-10 hydroxyl position *(110)*. Most of the circulating plasma SN-38 is in this inactive form of SN-38 *(104,108,111–113)*. Because SN-38 and bilirubin are both substrates of UGT 1A1, administration of CPT-11 may cause transient increases in unconjugated bilirubin *(114)*. Pretreatment plasma concentrations of unconjugated bilirubin have been reported to correlate with the degree of subsequent myelosuppression *(114)*. Although SN-38G is inactive, it is hydrolyzed by bacterial β-glucuronidases in the gastrointestinal tract, releasing active drug and contributing to the enterohepatic recirculation of SN-38 *(115–117)*. This may play a role in initiating the delayed diarrhea (*see* Section 6.). Also, we have recently demonstrated that glucuronidases possibly represent a significant reactivation pathway for the production of SN-38 within the tumour *(118)*.

Increased glucurono conjugation of SN-38 has been demonstrated in a cell line selected in vitro for resistance to SN-38 *(119)*, but the clinical aspects of this mechanism remain to be investigated.

4.4. Transport

Rat studies and vesicular membrane experiments have shown that the canalicular multispecific organic anion transporter also known as MRP-2 is responsible, solely or in part, for the biliary excretion of CPT-11, SN-38, and SN-38G *(120–123)*. In particular, P-glycoprotein may be responsible for the high-affinity component of the transport of the carboxylate form of CPT-11 *(120)*. Thus the ATP binding cassette transporters, of which P-glycoprotein and MRP-2 are examples, are not only important in relation to the phenomenon of multidrug resistance but also to the disposition of CPT-11 and its metabolites. Recently, an additional ATP binding cassette transporter, BCRP (breast cancer resistance protein), has been described that imparts cross-resistance between mitoxantrone and several other cytotoxic agents, including SN-38 *(124,125)*. Its presence in the blood-brain barrier *(126)* may explain to some extent the lack of penetration of SN-38 into the CNS when CPT-11 is administered parenterally *(127)*.

5. CLINICAL PHARMACOLOGY

5.1. Clinical Pharmacokinetics

The pharmacokinetics of CPT-11 and some of its metabolites have been already extensively reviewed *(128,129)*. After iv administration, CPT-11 concentrations peak, as expected, at the end of the infusion, but at this time the carboxylate form accounts already for approximately 50% of the total drug *(130)*. The continuing hydrolysis and possibly increased disappearance of the lactone form mean that by approximately 2 hours after infusion, the ratio of CPT-11 lactone to total drug has reached an equilibrium value of approximately 25% *(130,131)*. The pharmacokinetic parameters for CPT-11 and its principal metabolites are shown in Table 1 and 2, respectively. The pharmacokinetics of CPT-11 and its metabolites are highly variable between patients, although intrapatient variability is modest *(113)*. This is, however, consistent with the number of metabolic routes involved. Available analyses do not indicate any evidence of induction or inhibition of any of the metabolic pathways.

CPT-11 has a large volume of distribution, particularly the lactone form, indicating rapid and extensive uptake into most tissues.

The concentrations of APC rise and peak soon after the end of infusion and then decline with a very similar terminal half-life to that of CPT-11. As mentioned previously, the concentrations of NPC are very low in plasma, and this metabolite does not appear to be quantitatively important in this matrix *(105)*.

Concentrations of SN-38 rise during the infusion and peak soon after although some patients show evidence of a flatter, more delayed, profile *(104,130)*. SN-38 in plasma is 50–70% in its active lactone form *(130–133)*, probably through the effects of differential activation *(8)* and protein-binding *(134)*. Concentrations of SN-38 are usually much lower than those of CPT-11, although this is dependent on the regimen used. During initial studies of CPT-11, the area under the curve (AUC) ratio of total SN-38 to CPT-11 was occasionally highest at the lower CPT-11 doses *(28,104)*, suggesting nonlinearity of activation. Short infusions (30–90 minutes) of CPT-11 yielded a molar ratio of the AUC of total SN-38 to CPT-11 of the order of 0.03 to 0.07 *(26,28,104,128,129)*, whereas prolonged infusions (4-, 5-, and 14-day continuous iv) yielded ratios as high as 0.24 *(135)*. Likewise, the

Table 1
Plasma Pharmacokinetic Parameters of Total CPT-11

Reference	*No. of patients*	*Infusion durations (hours)*	*Dose (mg/m^2)*	*$t_{1/2}$ (hours)*	*CL ($L/hours/m^2$)*	*Vd_{SS} (L/m^2)*
161	17	1.5	50–150	3.0	13.3	—
32	24	2.0	25–40	26.5	7.9	—
28	17	1.5	50–180	7.9	15.3	—
29	26	0.5, 1.5	50–145	9.3	15.0	142
169	31	1.5	100–345	5.2	21.0	148
25	60	0.5	100–750	14.2	15.0	157
31	21	0.5	100–345	—	15.2	—
131	12	1.5	100	6.8	18.8	—
113	47	0.5	350	—	15.2	—
160	19	0.5, 1.5	115–600	6.3	16.1	102
197	40	1.5	145	8.8	14.6	136
104	19	0.5, 1.5	115–600	6.3	16.1	102
105	10	1.5	200	13.5	14.0	138
159	45	1.5	80–300	12.1	17.6	262*
143	8	1.5	125	14.6	12.4	297

* Vd_{SS} expressed as L.

daily regimens used in children (daily × 5 for 2 weeks) produced an apparently increased activation *(136,137)* in comparison to the high dose every-3-weeks regimen *(138)*.

In general, although the plasma pharmacokinetics of SN-38 and SN-38G are highly variable between patients, their terminal half-lives are long (approximately 12 hours), and the concentrations of SN-38G usually exceed those of SN-38 *(104,111–113)*. The plasma pharmacokinetics of SN-38G parallel those of SN-38 in most patients (Fig. 2A), suggesting that glucuronidation of SN-38 is the rate limiting step in its elimination *(111)*. Indeed, the ratio of the concentrations of these two compounds is relatively constant until the very late time points at which the SN-38G concentrations decline comparatively faster *(139)*. This may reflect increased competition with bilirubin for glucurono-conjugation by UGT1A1.

4-PP, the other product of activation has concentrations that also peak soon after the infusion and decay very slowly *(103)*. The terminal half-life has been estimated to be approximately 30–40 hours, but the sampling was not sufficiently protracted to yield an accurate estimate. It is unclear what the mechanism is behind the very protracted pharmacokinetic profile for 4-PP, but it may represent prolonged activation of CPT-11. Indeed, CPT-11

Table 2
Plasma Pharmacokinetic Parameters for Total SN-38, SN-38G, and APC

Reference	No. of patients	Dose (mg/m^2)	SN38 $t_{1/2}$ (hours)	SN38 AUC (mM/hour)	SN-38G $t_{1/2}$ (hours)	SN-38G AUC (mM/hour)	AUC ratio SN-38G/SN-38	APC $t_{1/2}$ (hours)	APC AUC (mM/hour)
104	19	115	13	0.7	13	4.7	7.6	7.6	11.0
	300–350	17	1.2	12	5.0	5.6	6.7	26.0	
	500	11	1.4	13	11.0	8.0	8.2	36.0	
	600	7.1	2.4	5.6	11.0	4.2	4.9	108.0	
105	10	200	23.8	1.4	23.5	8.0	7.0	15.1	5.9
159	45	175	19.0	0.2	24.6	7.7	32.0	8.1	6.5
	200	23.8	1.1	23.5	8.0	7.0	15.1	5.9	
	230	19.9	1.8	20.8	8.0	4.5	9.6	6.8	
	260	20.9	0.7	21.5	8.0	11.0	8.7	7.4	
	300	29.1	1.2	27.9	12.5	10.9	13.0	9.5	
143	8	125	28.5	1.0	35.5	3.4	3.5	17.8	5.3

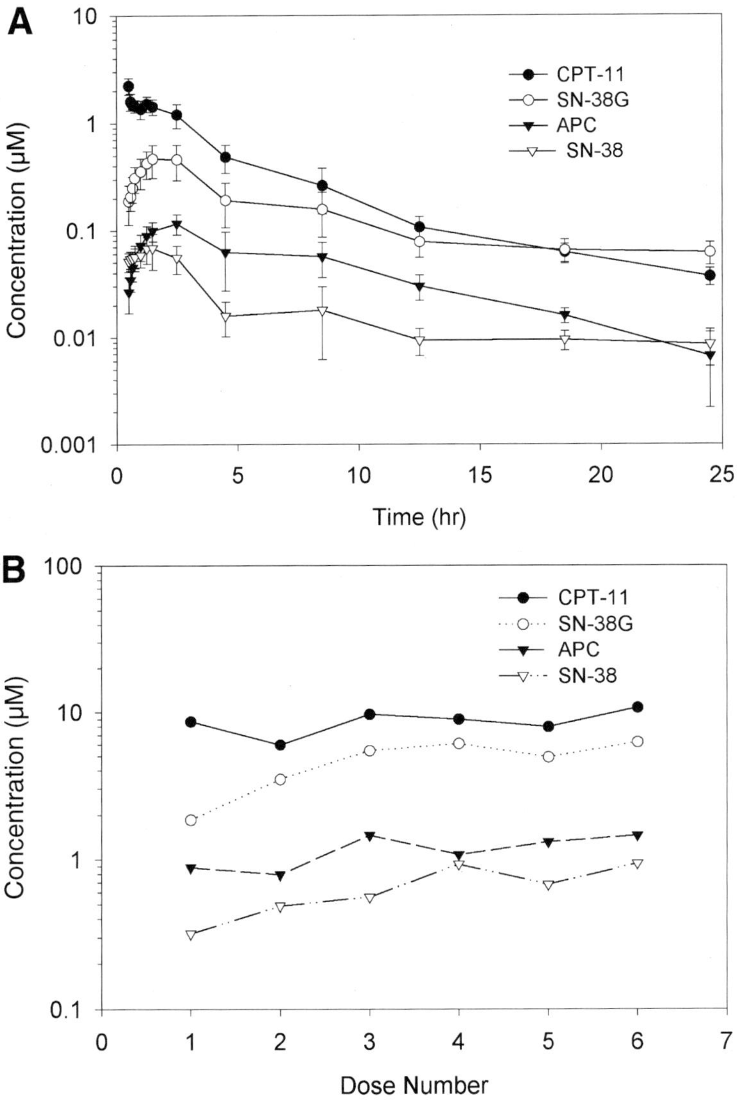

Fig. 2. **(A)** Mean plasma concentrations of CPT-11 and its principal metabolites in a patient receiving six consecutive doses of CPT-11 (115 mg/m^2) in a weekly regimen *(104)*. Note that SN-38 and its glucuronoconjugate (SN-38G) have prolonged and parallel terminal elimination phases. **(B)** The areas under the curve of these compounds after each administration and the kinetics of SN-38 and SN-38G are clearly interrelated in both situations.

is inefficiently converted to SN-38 but, paradoxically, this may be a positive factor in determining the clinical activity of this drug because of the "slow-release" effect that results from the large volume of distribution and long mean residence time of CPT-11 *(99)*. Low-dose protracted regimens, aside from considerations in terms of antitumor activity of schedule-dependent drugs, have an advantage in terms of the efficiency of the conversion to SN-38.

5.2. Pharmacokinetic/Pharmacodynamic Correlations

Several investigators have attempted to correlate the pharmacokinetics of CPT-11 and SN-38 with the toxicity experienced with CPT-11 treatment. Chabot et al. used the combined results of three French phase I studies to examine this question *(129)*. They analyzed the results corresponding to 97 first cycles of treatment with doses ranging from 33 to 750 mg/m^2. The percent drop in leucocytes and neutrophils was significantly correlated to CPT-11 AUC, CPT-11 CL, and SN-38 AUC. However, in most cases, the r^2 values were of the order of 0.2 to 0.3. Canal et al. also found significant correlations between the percentage fall in neutrophils and the AUC of both CPT-11 and SN-38 in 47 patients treated with 350 mg/m^2 CPT-11 *(113)*. Again, however, the r^2 values were 0.2–0.3. These results illustrate that toxicity increases with increased exposure to CPT-11 and its active metabolite. However, there remains a large degree of variability of the extent of side effects at any specific exposure.

As stated previously, one of the major toxicities is the late diarrhea and pharmacokinetic/pharmacodynamic (PK/PD) studies have provided conflicting answers. An early study, investigating the use of CPT-11 with the weekly regimen found that a putative marker of biliary excretion of SN-38, the so-called "biliary index," correlated with the severity of delayed diarrhea experienced by patients treated at 100–145 mg/m^2 with the weekly regimen *(112)*. This biliary index is calculated from:

$$BI = AUC_{CPT\text{-}11} * AUC_{SN\text{-}38}/AUC_{SN\text{-}38G}$$

One would expect that reduced conjugation ($\uparrow AUC_{SN-38}/AUC_{SN-38G}$) with increased dose of CPT-11 (↑CPT-11 AUC) to raise the biliary index and predict for the severity of side effects. Thus there is apparent theoretical support from these observations. However, there was no correlation between the biliary index and diarrhea with a 350 mg/m^2 three-weekly protocol *(113)*, although this may have been due to the low number of toxic episodes encountered after the implementation of high-dose loperamide *(113)*. Similarly negative results were reported for the weekly regimen in a larger trial with a starting dose of 125 mg/m^2 *(140)*. Nevertheless, there is now strong support for increased toxicity in individuals with genetically related deficiencies in the glucurono-conjugation of SN-38 (this is covered in more detail in the Section 5.4.).

In a preliminary study, we investigated the relationship between the "trough" concentrations of SN-38 and SN-38G in patients and the severity of side effects using a ultrasensitive assay *(141)*. Toxicity was most prominent in those in whom the plasma concentrations of either compound remained elevated relative to the population median *(142)*. This would suggest that patients who don't achieve significant "drug-free" periods are more at risk from treatment. However, the safety profile of the every-3-week regimen appears similar to the weekly protocol *(48)*, which would appear to be at odds with our observation.

5.3. Mass Balance and Excretion

Mass balance studies of CPT-11 reflect the multiplicity of pathways of metabolism and elimination of this drug. After the administration of 100 μCi of ^{14}C-CPT-11 (labeled on the C-7 ethyl group) along with a conventional 125 mg/m^2 dose, approximately 65% of the dose of the radioactivity was excreted in the feces *(143)*. Urinary excretion was essentially complete within 48 hours and accounted for the remaining dose. In comparison, fecal excretion continued for 7–8 days and consisted mostly of unchanged drug (32% of dose), SN-38, and APC (approximately 8% each). Presumably, much of this excretion is via the bile. In the radiolabel study, one patient had a biliary T-tube diversion and radioactivity in the bile collection accounted for 30% of the dose with an additional 15% recovered in the feces. Although some of the radioactivity recovered from the feces probably represents an inability to recover all the biliary drainage with T-tube diversions, there remains the possibility of direct intestinal secretion of drug. Indeed, 15% of the CPT-11 mass balance was found in the feces of bile-exteriorized rats despite the fact that drug was administered intravenously *(144)*. In T-tube–diverted patients, all known metabolites can be detected in the bile *(108,143)*. In the radiolabel study, SN-38G in the bile represented 2.7 % of the dose *(143)*, whereas this metabolite is not normally found in the feces to any appreciable extent *(105,143)*. The disparity between these findings is most likely the result of high β-glucuronidase activity in feces *(105)*.

The mass balance data also give an idea of the importance of the pathways of metabolism. In the study of Slatter et al., approximately 50% of the dose was excreted as unchanged CPT-11 *(143)*. The total of urine and fecal SN-38 plus SN-38G was only of the order of 12%. Therefore, as mentioned previously, activation to SN-38 species is a relatively inefficient process and CPT-11 is, therefore, only modestly activated in humans. The total formation of APC was 11% and NPC 1.5% indicating that oxidative metabolism is at least as important as activation to SN-38 from a mass balance point of view. A multitude of other minor products make up an additional small fraction of the mass balance *(143)*, but it is not clear whether these are contaminants, degradation products, or genuine metabolites *(108,109,143,145)*.

5.4. Special Populations

Gilbert's disease, which is a mild and often undiagnosed chronic hyperbilirubinemia, is linked to a genetic polymorphism of *UGT1A1*, the predominant isoform involved in the conjugation of bilirubin *(110)*. Affected individuals usually are homozygous for a variant allele that features an additional TA repeat in the promoter region (*UGT1A1**28). Genotype/phenotype correlations have been demonstrated with both bilirubin and SN-38 as substrates in vitro *(146)*. Case studies of patients with Gilbert's disease (on basis of history of unconjugated hyperbilirubinemia) have been reported, and these individuals have greatly reduced glucurono-conjugation of SN-38 as revealed by the AUC ratio of the conjugate to the free SN-38 *(147)*. Importantly, the toxicity of CPT-11 appears to be significantly increased in these patients, in keeping with this reduced ability to deactivate SN-38. The toxicity of CPT-11 has been shown to be increased in not only those with the *UGT1A1**28 allele, but also those with a polymorphism in the coding region (*UGT1A1**27), although the numbers were small in the latter category *(148)*. The pharmacokinetics of SN-38 have been shown to be modified according to the *UGT1A1* genotype in several pharmacokinetic studies *(149,150)*.

Aside from genetic abnormalities of SN-38 conjugation, other syndromes can also lead to impaired detoxification of SN-38. As mentioned previously, bilirubin is glucurono-conjugated by the same UGT isoform, and conditions that lead to increased heme turnover could interfere with CPT-11 metabolism. Wasserman found, in a preliminary study, that pretreatment unconjugated bilirubin correlated with neutropenia *(114)*. Elevations in serum bilirubin also often accompany hepatobiliary dysfunction. In this case, increased bilirubin probably reflects also a reduced excretion of CPT-11 and its metabolites by the biliary route rather than conjugation *per se (151)*. Guidelines recommend that patients with total bilirubin outside the normal range should be treated with great caution.

Nevertheless, patients with severe liver dysfunction retain significant ability to eliminate CPT-11, presumably through metabolism and renal elimination. In a recent study, patients with elevated alkaline phosphatase and bilirubin were found to have reduced clearance of CPT-11 *(152)*. The latter declined in a nonlinear fashion with increasing hepatic dysfunction reaching an asymptotic value of approximately 4 L/m^2/hour (as compared to approximately 15 L/m^2/hour in normal patients). This would suggest that renal excretion, which accounts for 20–25% of the elimination of unchanged CPT-11 *(143)*, represents a major route of elimination in patients with liver disease. Maintaining adequate renal function may be of great importance in this group *(153)*. This may explain the observation that raised serum creatinine is a risk factor for delayed diarrhea *(49)*.

5.5. Drug–Drug Interactions

In a study of CPT-11 in adult malignant glioma, the AUC of CPT-11 administered weekly at 125 mg/m^2 was only 40% of that achieved in patients with colorectal cancer *(74)*. The AUCs of SN-38 and SN-38G were even more dramatically decreased, consistent with a change from activation to deactivation metabolism. However, APC concentrations in the plasma may not necessarily increase dramatically *(154)*. Most patients in these trials were treated with phenytoin, phenobarbital, carbamazepine, or dexamethasone (or in combination), all of which are known inducers of CYP3A. Therefore, although CYP450-mediated metabolism accounts for a modest fraction (approximately 15 %) of the CPT-11 excretion mass balance, the effects of induction/inhibition of CYP450 appear to be considerable *(74,154)* and may affect the therapeutic index of this drug.

Other drug–drug interactions with CPT-11 in the oxidative pathway could theoretically arise with other inhibitors of CYP3A4, such as the macrolide antibiotics. A recent study has shown that ketoconazole, a known potent CYP3A4 inhibitor, does not significantly modify CPT-11 clearance when administered at a dose of 200 mg daily for 2–3 days. However, the pattern of metabolism is greatly modified and is diverted away from the oxidative formation of APC toward activation to SN-38 *(155)*.

The interactions with cyclosporin A *(156)* and valproic acid *(157)* have been investigated in preclinical models. Cyclosporin is an inhibitor of canalicular multispecific organic anion transporter and P-glycoprotein and a substrate of CYP3A4. The effect of cyclosporin pretreatment to rats injected with CPT-11 resulted in an average increase of 340, 360, and 200% in the AUCs of CPT-11, SN-38, and SN-38G, respectively. In the case of valproic acid, administration of 200 mg/kg of sodium valproate caused a 99% reduction in SN-38 conjugation *(157)*. Phenobarbital, on the other hand, led to increased conjugation, presumably through the upregulation of UGT1A1. The possibility of using some of these modulating agents is currently being investigated in the clinical setting.

Several Phase I studies of combinations containing CPT-11 have been carried out. When studied, the pharmacokinetics of CPT-11 or the other drugs have not been modified *(51,72,158–160)*. The only exception might be a study of CPT-11, carboplatin, and paclitaxel in which the unexpected severity of toxicity of the combination prompted the authors to speculate on a possible pharmacokinetic interaction *(73)*.

6. SIDE EFFECTS

As mentioned previously, CPT-11 presented a novel profile of side effects in early studies. Along with nausea and vomiting and myelosuppression (mostly neutropenia), the spectrum included an acute cholinergic syndrome and delayed diarrhea. The latter was sometimes severe in early studies and constituted a dose-limiting toxicity in many of these *(28)*. In early studies, it was implicated in several treatment-related deaths *(161)*.

6.1. Cholinergic Syndrome

The cholinergic syndrome occasionally observed with CPT-11 consists of vomiting and diarrhea accompanied by abdominal cramps, diaphoresis, and accommodation disturbances *(162)*. It is usually transient, is readily reversed by atropine *(28)*, and does not, therefore, constitute a dose-limiting toxicity.

It has been claimed to be mediated by ganglionic stimulation on the basis of a structural similarity between the bipiperidino side chain of CPT-11 and a known stimulant of nicotinic receptors of autonomic ganglia, dimethylphenylpiperazinium iodide *(162)*. However, we have recently confirmed that CPT-11 is a potent inhibitor of acetyl cholinesterase, particularly when in the lactone form *(163)*. The inhibition was shown in vitro to be instantaneously reversed on dilution and this, when combined with the short-lived nature of CPT-11 lactone in vivo, probably explains its transient nature. This side effect is more frequently encountered with the 350 mg/m^2 regimen when premedication with atropine is not used and typically involves 60–70% of patients, although few reactions are considered as severe *(48)*. Nevertheless, combinations of CPT-11 with other drugs capable of inhibiting acetyl cholinesterase may lead to increased severity of symptoms *(164)*.

6.2. Late-Onset Diarrhea

Late-onset or delayed diarrhea presents as loose stools some time after the administration of CPT-11. To differentiate this from the acute cholinergic syndrome, diarrhea is classified as delayed when it occurs at least 24 hours after the administration of CPT-11. In phase II trials using the three weekly protocol, the median time of onset was 5 days after infusion but ranged from 1 to 19 days after treatment *(36)*. Pivotal US Phase II studies using the weekly regimen found a more delayed toxicity with a median time of onset of 11 days *(16,18,165)* such that this toxicity was usually manifest 3–4 days after the second injection of a treatment course. The median duration of an episode of delayed diarrhea has been found to be approximately 3–5 days although the entire episode is often longer in those patients with grade 3 or grade 4 symptoms *(17,165)*.

Early trials reported delayed diarrhea to be noncumulative *(25)*, but several subjects developed severe chronic and apparently cumulative toxicity in a Phase I trial of the three weekly schedule *(26)*. Overall, delayed diarrhea is clearly dose-related, with increases in both severity and incidence with higher doses *(112)*. Although delayed diarrhea appears to be an idiosyncratic toxicity of CPT-11, it was also observed in early trials of camptothecin

(166) and has been encountered in the testing of other analogs. Recent clinical trials of orally administered camptothecin analogs have revealed that most, if not all, can induce gastrointestinal toxicity *(167)*. For example, delayed diarrhea was found to be the dose-limiting toxicity associated with protracted oral administration of both camptothecin *(167)* and topotecan *(168)*. In contrast, this toxicity is rare or nonexistent after intravenous administration *(169)*, even with protracted infusion regimens *(170,171)*. Therefore, it is likely that part of the difference between camptothecins is their disposition of active drug into the intestinal lumen, and that it is the concentrations of the cytotoxic species in this compartment that correlate with gastrointestinal injury *(172)*.

The morbidity of delayed diarrhea was particularly high in the early phase II studies of CPT-11. For example, in the European phase II study of CPT-11 for advanced colorectal adenocarcinoma, the every-3-week schedule (350 mg/m^2) resulted in delayed diarrhea in 87% of patients and 57% of cycles. Grade 3/4 diarrhea occurred in 39% and 12% of patients and cycles, respectively *(173)*. In the pivotal US phase II studies, 37% *(16)* and 56% *(34)* of the initially recruited patients developed grade 3 or grade 4 delayed diarrhea. The incidence of grade 4 delayed diarrhea was eventually reduced to 5% and 9% in the two studies, respectively, after implementing aggressive loperamide therapy and dose reductions in subsequent administrations to affected patients. Similar treatment strategies have also been used for the every-3-week protocol and a recent study has found that a starting dose of 500 mg/m^2 is feasible *(27)*. The incidence of grade 4 diarrhea in this latter study and using the 500 mg/m^2 starting dose was approximately 6%.

The delayed diarrhea as been described as secretory with a possible exudative component *(174)*. Both its frequency and severity are increased in the elderly (>65 years) and in patients previously treated with abdominal/pelvic irradiation *(17)*. On the other hand, previous chemotherapy does not seem to be a predisposing factor *(17)*. Pharmacokinetics of CPT-11, SN-38, and SN-38G are not significantly different in the aged *(140)* and thus do not explain the apparently heightened susceptibility of these patients.

Reduced gastrointestinal transit times are observed in a fraction of cases *(174)*, whereas intestinal absorption is apparently normal, as estimated from *d*-xylose absorption and fecal fat content *(174)*. Fecal clearance of α_1-antitrypsin appears to be consistently elevated indicating a possible mucosal injury or exudative phenomenon.

Early experiments using animal models demonstrated that SN-38 and SN-38 glucuronide participate in significant enterohepatic recirculation with the glucuronide being released by bacterial and mucosal glucuronidase activity *(101,117)*. Naturally occurring β-glucuronides used in traditional oriental medicine (*Kampo* medicine) are potent inhibitors of the glucuronidase-catalyzed release of SN-38 from SN-38G *(115)* and these play a protective role against delayed diarrhea in a rat model *(117)*. Conversely, the corresponding aglycones of these compounds are inhibitors of the glucuronidation of SN-38 *(116)*. Hence, *Kampo* glucuronides could contribute in two ways to the inhibition of the enterohepatic recycling of SN-38, namely by initially inhibiting the liberation of SN-38 and then, as aglycones, inhibit *de novo* glucuronidation of SN-38 *(115)*. However, these compounds also have antidiarrhea effects in other model systems *(175)* and their effects are also likely to be modulated by as-yet unknown mechanisms.

High-dose antibiotic regimens have been used to deplete the glucuronidase-secreting gastrointestinal flora in rats, resulting in a markedly improved cecal histopathology and a reduction in delayed diarrhea *(117,176)*. The plasma pharmacokinetics of CPT-11 and its metabolites are not affected by antibiotic sterilization of the large intestine, whereas concentrations of free SN-38 within the lumen are reduced *(177)*. However, the situation regarding the hydrolysis of SN-38G in man is not as clear, although it is evident that significant SN-38G hydrolytic activity is present in human feces, as mentioned previously *(105,178)*.

There is very little information available regarding the histopathology of the bowel in affected patients, although two patients with grade 4 bloody diarrhea were found to have acute colitis with edema and inflammatory infiltrate on colonoscopy/biopsy *(25)*. Others have found mild superficial erosion of the colon mucosa *(179,180)*. Occasionally, lesions have been suggestive of pseudomembranous colitis; these have been confirmed by culture of *Clostridium difficile (27)*. CPT-11 has been shown to cause an acute enhancement of chloride secretion in rat colon tissue through a thromboxane A–dependent mechanism *(181,182)*, possibly in response to eicosanoids generated by the subepithelial tissue. Thus a secretory component of delayed diarrhea could arise from the release of cyclo-oxygenase metabolites (thromboxanes and prostaglandins) generated by local inflammation and early mucosal injury. However, we could detect no such acute effect using human colon mucosa preparations (Brzuszczak et al., unpublished observations). Rather, the time course and the histopathology suggest the involvement of a delayed, local inflammatory response that may be aggravated by the release of local cytokines *(183)*. The demonstration that thalidomide *(184)* and budesonide *(179)* can prevent or ameliorate the delayed diarrhea to some extent is in support of such a mechanism. Anti-inflammatory cytokines *(185)* or their inducers, such as JBT-3002 *(186,187)*, could prove useful in the prevention of the delayed diarrhea. However, it remains to be established that these strategies do not affect the antitumor activity of CPT-11. Likewise, other possible strategies such as the protecting agent glutamine *(188)*, fish oil *(189)*, and activated charcoal *(190)* need to be further evaluated for their possible utility.

There is no known specific antidote to delayed diarrhea, and heavy reliance is made on supportive treatment. As mentioned previously, the aggressive use of loperamide is the standard for managing delayed diarrhea, although some patients do not appear to respond. Octreotide and budesonide have been used in some loperamide-refractory incidences of delayed diarrhea *(179,191)*. The current high-dose regimen advocated is a starting dose of 4 mg loperamide followed by 2 mg every 2 hours until 12 hours after the last stool has been passed. Substitution of 4 mg loperamide every 4 hours during the night is permitted.

The mechanism of action of loperamide against diarrhea in general is thought to be mediated through a reduction in gut motility because of its μ-opioid agonist effects *(192)*. However, loperamide is also effective against some forms of secretory diarrhea, possibly through actions of calmodulin inhibition and calcium blocking *(192)*.

6.3. Nausea/Vomiting

CPT-11 is emetogenic, and some prophylactic cover for nausea and vomiting is required. In most patients it is recommended that 10 mg dexamethasone be administered iv in combination with a 5-HT_3 blocker (tropisetron, ondansetron) at least 30 minutes before commencing the infusion.

6.4. Other Toxicity

Less frequent drug-related events include: thrombocytopenia *(135)*, toxic death *(78,161,193)*, major hepatic dysfunction *(147,193,194)*, bradycardia *(195)*, pneumonitis *(60,62)*, and tumor lysis syndrome *(196)*.

7. FUTURE DIRECTIONS

From a clinical perspective, it is likely that CPT-11 will eventually move into the adjuvant setting for colorectal adenocarcinoma. In this respect, it is vital that new strategies be evaluated for their ability to reduce side effects—delayed diarrhea in particular. Although loperamide has had a substantial impact on the extent and severity of this toxicity, there are still occasional patients who present with severe refractory oeadiarrhea. The most promising strategies revolve around reducing an apparent cytokine-mediated exacerbation of mucosal injury. It is important that these strategies be shown not interfere with the antitumor activity of CPT-11 or introduce idiosyncratic side effects of their own.

CPT-11 appears particularly promising as a component of combination chemotherapy for NSCLC. The development of doublets for this indication is a worthwhile area of research. However, the optimal combination make take some time to define because of the large number of other agents with good activity in this setting (e.g., cisplatin, docetaxel, gemcitabine, vinorelbine) as well as the endless permutations possible with different schedules.

The area of CNS malignancy is another area of promise, although the drug–drug interactions between CPT-11 and the anticonvulsants may be troublesome. The induction of liver CYP3A4 by dexamethasone, phenobarbital, and phenytoin, in particular, appear to shift the metabolism from activation to inactivation. Because the activation pathway appears to be saturable clinically, this problem cannot be expected to be rectified by increasing doses. A move away from aromatic anticonvulsants to sodium valproate may also not provide a solution to this problem because of possible drug interactions with the glucuronidation of SN-38. Gabapentin might be a worthwhile alternative and should perhaps be the first-line anticonvulsant therapy for those likely to proceed to chemotherapy. The intrahepatic competition for available CPT-11 by activation and deactivation pathways may to lead to other drug–drug interactions with substrates and inhibitors of CYP3A4.

REFERENCES

1. Sawada S, Okajima S, Aiyama R, et al. 1991Synthesis and antitumor activity of 20(S)-camptothecin derivatives: carbamate-linked, water-soluble derivatives of 7-ethyl-10-hydroxycamptothecin. Chem Pharm Bull. 39:1446–1450.
2. Kawato Y, Aonuma M, Hirota Y, Kuga H, Sato K. 1991 Intracellular roles of SN-38, a metabolite of the camptothecin derivative CPT-11, in the antitumor effect of CPT-11. Cancer Res. 51:4187–4191.
3. Tanizawa A, Fujimori A, Fujimori Y, Pommier Y. 1994 Comparison of topoisomerase I inhibition, DNA damage, and cytotoxicity of camptothecin derivatives presently in clinical trials. J Natl Cancer Inst. 86:836–842.
4. Tsuji T, Kaneda N, Kado K, Yokokura T, Yoshimoto T, Tsuru D. 1991 CPT-11 converting enzyme from rat serum: purification and some properties. J Pharmacobiodyn. 14:341–349.
5. Rivory LP, Bowles MR, Robert J, Pond SM. 1996 Conversion of irinotecan (CPT-11) to its active metabolite, 7-ethyl-10-hydroxycamptothecin (SN-38), by human liver carboxylesterase. Biochem Pharmacol. 52:1103–1111.
6. Satoh T, Hosokawa M, Atsumi R, Suzuki W, Hakusui H, Nagai E. 1994 Metabolic activation of CPT-11, 7-ethyl-10-[4-(1-piperidino)-1- piperidino]carbonyloxycamptothecin, a novel antitumor agent, by carboxylesterase. Biol Pharm Bull. 17:662–664.
7. Slatter JG, Su P, Sams JP, Schaaf LJ, Wienkers LC. 1997 Bioactivation of the anticancer agent CPT-11 to SN-38 by human hepatic microsomal carboxylesterases and the in vitro assessment of potential drug interactions. Drug Metab Dispos. 25:1157–1164.
8. Haaz MC, Rivory LP, Riche C, Robert J. 1997 The transformation of irinotecan (CPT-11) to its active metabolite SN-38 by human liver microsomes. Differential hydrolysis for the lactone and carboxylate forms. Naunyn Schmiedebergs Arch Pharmacol. 356:257–262.

9. Atsumi R, Suzuki W, Hakusui H. 1991 Identification of the metabolites of irinotecan, a new derivative of camptothecin, in rat bile and its biliary excretion. Xenobiotica. 21:1159–1169.
10. Haaz MC, Rivory L, Jantet S, Ratanasavanh D, Robert J. 1997 Glucuronidation of SN-38, the active metabolite of irinotecan, by human hepatic microsomes. Pharmacol Toxicol. 80:91–96.
11. Santos A, Zanetta S, Cresteil T, et al. 2000 Metabolism of irinotecan (CPT-11) by CYP3A4 and CYP3A5 in humans. Clin Cancer Res. 6:2012–2020.
12. Haaz MC, Rivory L, Riche C, Vernillet L, Robert J. 1998 Metabolism of irinotecan (CPT-11) by human hepatic microsomes: participation of cytochrome P-450 3A and drug interactions. Cancer Res. 58:468–472.
13. Rivory LP, Riou JF, Haaz MC, et al. 1996 Identification and properties of a major plasma metabolite of irinotecan (CPT-11) isolated from the plasma of patients. Cancer Res. 56:3689–3694.
14. Haaz MC, Riche C, Rivory LP, Robert J. 1998 Biosynthesis of an aminopiperidino metabolite of irinotecan [7-ethyl-10-[4-(1-piperidino)-1-piperidino]carbonyloxycamptothecine] by human hepatic microsomes. Drug Metab Dispos. 26:769–774.
15. Rothenberg ML, Cox JV, DeVore RF, et al. 1999 A multicenter, phase II trial of weekly irinotecan (CPT-11) in patients with previously treated colorectal carcinoma. Cancer. 85:786–795.
16. Rothenberg ML, Eckardt JR, Kuhn JG, et al. 1996 Phase II trial of irinotecan in patients with progressive or rapidly recurrent colorectal cancer. J Clin Oncol. 14:1128–1135.
17. Rougier P, Bugat R, Douillard JY, et al. 1997 Phase II study of irinotecan in the treatment of advanced colorectal cancer in chemotherapy-naive patients and patients pretreated with fluorouracil-based chemotherapy. J Clin Oncol. 15:251–260.
18. Pitot HC, Wender DB, O'Connell MJ, et al. 1997 Phase II trial of irinotecan in patients with metastatic colorectal carcinoma. J Clin Oncol. 15:2910–2919.
19. Cunningham D, Pyrhonen S, James RD, et al. 1998 Randomised trial of irinotecan plus supportive care versus supportive care alone after fluorouracil failure for patients with metastatic colorectal cancer. Lancet. 352:1413–1418.
20. Douillard JY, Cunningham D, Roth AD, et al. 2000 Irinotecan combined with fluorouracil compared with fluorouracil alone as first-line treatment for metastatic colorectal cancer: a multicentre randomised trial. Lancet. 355:1041–1047.
21. Saltz LB, Cox JV, Blanke C, et al. 2000 Irinotecan plus fluorouracil and leucovorin for metastatic colorectal cancer. Irinotecan Study Group. New Engl J Med. 343:905–914.
22. Shimada Y, Yoshino M, Wakui A, et al. 1993 Phase II study of CPT-11, a new camptothecin derivative, in metastatic colorectal cancer. CPT-11 Gastrointestinal Cancer Study Group. J Clin Oncol. 11:909–913.
23. Shimada Y, Rougier P, Pitot H. 1996 Efficacy of CPT-11 (irinotecan) as a single agent in metastatic colorectal cancer. Eur J Cancer. 32A(Suppl. 3):S13–S17.
24. Rothenberg ML, Kuhn JG, Schaaf LJ, et al. 1998 Alternative dosing schedules for irinotecan. Oncology. 12:68–71.
25. Abigerges D, Chabot GG, Armand JP, Herait P, Gouyette A, Gandia D. 1995 Phase I and pharmacologic studies of the camptothecin analog irinotecan administered every 3 weeks in cancer patients. J Clin Oncol. 13:210–221.
26. Rowinsky EK, Grochow LB, Ettinger DS, et al. 1994 Phase I and pharmacological study of the novel topoisomerase I inhibitor 7-ethyl-10-[4-(1-piperidino)-1-piperidino]carbonyloxycamptothecin (CPT-11) administered as a ninety-minute infusion every 3 weeks. Cancer Res. 54:427–436.

27. Merrouche Y, Extra JM, Abigerges D, et al. 1997 High dose-intensity of irinotecan administered every 3 weeks in advanced cancer patients: a feasibility study. J Clin Oncol. 15:1080–1086.
28. Rothenberg ML, Kuhn JG, Burris HA, et al. 1993 Phase I and pharmacokinetic trial of weekly CPT-11. J Clin Oncol. 11:2194–2204.
29. de Forni M, Bugat R, Chabot GG, et al. 1994 Phase I and pharmacokinetic study of the camptothecin derivative irinotecan, administered on a weekly schedule in cancer patients. Cancer Res. 54:4347–4354.
30. Tsuda H, Takatsuki K, Ohno R, et al. 1994 Treatment of adult T-cell leukaemia-lymphoma with irinotecan hydrochloride (CPT-11). CPT-11 Study Group on Hematological Malignancy. Br J Cancer. 70:771–774.
31. Catimel G, Chabot GG, Guastalla JP, et al. 1995 Phase I and pharmacokinetic study of irinotecan (CPT-11) administered daily for three consecutive days every three weeks in patients with advanced solid tumors. Ann Oncol. 6:133–140.
32. Ohe Y, Sasaki Y, Shinkai T, et al. 1992 Phase I study and pharmacokinetics of CPT-11 with 5-day continuous infusion. J Natl Cancer Inst. 84:972–974.
33. Ohno R, Okada K, Masaoka T, et al. 1990 An early phase II study of CPT-11: a new derivative of camptothecin, for the treatment of leukemia and lymphoma. J Clin Oncol. 8:1907–1912.
34. Conti JA, Kemeny NE, Saltz LB, et al. 1996 Irinotecan is an active agent in untreated patients with metastatic colorectal cancer. J Clin Oncol. 14:709–715.
35. Armand JP, Ducreux M, Mahjoubi M, et al. 1995 CPT-11 (irinotecan) in the treatment of colorectal cancer. Eur J Cancer. 31A:1283–1287.
36. Abigerges D, Armand JP, Chabot GG, et al. 1994 Irinotecan (CPT-11) high-dose escalation using intensive high-dose loperamide to control diarrhea. J Natl Cancer Inst. 86:446–449.
37. Drengler RL, Kuhn JG, Schaaf LJ, et al. 1999 Phase I and pharmacokinetic trial of oral irinotecan administered daily for 5 days every 3 weeks in patients with solid tumors. J Clin Oncol. 17:685–696.
38. Pitot H, Adjei AA, Reid JM, et al. 2001 A phase I and pharmacokinetic study of a powder-filled capsule (PFC) formulation of oral irinotecan (CPT-11) given daily for 5 days every 3 weeks in patients with advanced solid tumors [abstract]. Proc Am Soc Clin Oncol. 20:102a.
39. Van Cutsem E, Cunningham D, Ten Bokkel Huinink WW, et al. 1999 Clinical activity and benefit of irinotecan (CPT-11) in patients with colorectal cancer truly resistant to 5-fluorouracil (5-FU). Eur J Cancer. 35:54–59.
40. Allen M, Cunningham D, Schmitt C. 1998 The importance of stabilization as an endpoint in the treatment of metastatic colorectal carcinoma: recent quality of life studies. Anti-Cancer Drugs. 9:783–790.
41. Cunningham D, Glimelius B. 1999 A phase III study of irinotecan (CPT-11) versus best supportive care in patients with metastatic colorectal cancer who have failed 5-fluorouracil therapy. V301 Study Group. Semin Oncol. 26:6–12.
42. Rougier P, Van Cutsem E, Bajetta E, et al. 1998 Randomised trial of irinotecan versus fluorouracil by continuous infusion after fluorouracil failure in patients with metastatic colorectal cancer. Lancet. 352:1407–1412.
43. Iveson TJ, Hickish T, Schmitt C, Van Cutsem E. 1999 Irinotecan in second-line treatment of metastatic colorectal cancer: improved survival and cost-effect compared with infusional 5-FU. Eur J Cancer. 35:1796–1804.
44. Levy-Piedbois C, Durand-Zaleski I, Juhel H, Schmitt C, Bellanger A, Piedbois P. 2000 Cost-effectiveness of second-line treatment with irinotecan or infusional 5-fluorouracil in metastatic colorectal cancer. Ann Oncol. 11:157–161.

45. Schmitt C, Blijham G, Jolain B, Rougier P, Van Cutsem E. 1999 Medical care consumption in a phase III trial comparing irinotecan with infusional 5-fluorouracil (5-FU) in patients with metastatic colorectal cancer after 5-FU failure. Anti-Cancer Drugs. 10:617–623.
46. Ducreux M, Ychou M, Seitz JF, et al. 1999 Irinotecan combined with bolus fluorouracil, continuous infusion fluorouracil, and high-dose leucovorin every two weeks (LV5FU2 regimen): a clinical dose-finding and pharmacokinetic study in patients with pretreated metastatic colorectal cancer. J Clin Oncol. 17:2901–2908.
47. Goldberg RM, Erlichman C. 1998 Irinotecan plus 5-FU and leucovorin in advanced colorectal cancer: North American trials. Oncology. 12:59–63.
48. Fuchs C, Miller L, Moore M, et al. 2000 Phase III comparison of two CPT-11 dosing regimens (weekly x 4 every-6-weeks Vs every-3-weeks) in second-line colorectal cancer (CRC) therapy: interim safety report [abstract]. Proc Am Soc Clin Oncol. 19:255a.
49. Freyer G, Rougier P, Bugat R, et al. 2000 Prognostic factors for tumour response, progression-free survival and toxicity in metastatic colorectal cancer patients given irinotecan (CPT-11) as second-line chemotherapy after 5FU failure. CPT-11 F205, F220, F221 and V222 study groups. Br J Cancer. 83:431–437.
50. Ychou M, Kramar A, Raoul J, et al. 2000 Final results of a study using CPT-11 high dose (500 mg/m2) as first line chemotherapy in patients with metastatic colorectal cancer (MCRC) [abstract]. Proc Am Soc Clin Oncol. 19:249a.
51. Ford HE, Cunningham D, Ross PJ, et al. 2000 Phase I study of irinotecan and raltitrexed in patients with advanced gastrointestinal tract adenocarcinoma. Br J Cancer. 83:146–152.
52. Wasserman E, Cuvier C, Lokiec F, et al. 1999 Combination of oxaliplatin plus irinotecan in patients with gastrointestinal tumors: results of two independent phase I studies with pharmacokinetics. J Clin Oncol. 17:1751–1759.
53. Hejna M, Kostler WJ, Raderer M, et al. 2000 Phase II study of second-line oxaliplatin, irinotecan and mitomycin C in patients with advanced or metastatic colorectal cancer. Anti-Cancer Drugs. 11:629–634.
54. Scheithauer W, Kornek GV, Raderer M, et al. 1999 Combined irinotecan and oxaliplatin plus granulocyte colony-stimulating factor in patients with advanced fluoropyrimidine/ leucovorin-pretreated colorectal cancer. J Clin Oncol. 17:902–906.
55. Boku N, Ohtsu A, Shimada Y, et al. 1999 Phase II study of a combination of irinotecan and cisplatin against metastatic gastric cancer. J Clin Oncol. 17:319–323.
56. Shirao K, Shimada Y, Kondo H, et al. 1997 Phase I-II study of irinotecan hydrochloride combined with cisplatin in patients with advanced gastric cancer. J Clin Oncol. 15:921–927.
57. Rocha Lima CM, Sherman CA, Brescia FJ, Brunson CY, Green MR. 2001 Irinotecan/gemcitabine combination chemotherapy in pancreatic cancer. Oncology. 15:46–51.
58. Sanz-Altamira P, O'Reilly EM, Stuart K, et al. 2001 A phase II trial of irinotecan (CPT-11) for unresectable biliary tree carcinoma. Ann Oncol. 12:501–504.
59. O'Reilly EM, Stuart K, Sanz-Altamira P, et al. 2001 A phase II study of irinotecan in patients with advanced hepatocellular carcinoma. Cancer. 91:101–105.
60. Fukuoka M, Niitani H, Suzuki A, et al. 1992 A phase II study of CPT-11, a new derivative of camptothecin, for previously untreated non-small-cell lung cancer. J Clin Oncol. 10:16–20.
61. Masuda N, Fukuoka M, Kusunoki Y, et al. 1992 CPT-11: a new derivative of camptothecin for the treatment of refractory or relapsed small-cell lung cancer. J Clin Oncol. 10:1225–1229.

62. Masuda N, Fukuoka M, Takada M, et al. 1992 CPT-11 in combination with cisplatin for advanced non-small-cell lung cancer. J Clin Oncol. 10:1775–1780.
63. Nakanishi Y, Takayama K, Takano K, et al. 1999 Second-line chemotherapy with weekly cisplatin and irinotecan in patients with refractory lung cancer. Am J Clin Oncol. 22:399–402.
64. Fujita A, Takabatake H, Tagaki S, Sekine K. 2000 Phase I/II study of cisplatin, ifosfamide and irinotecan with rhG-CSF support in patients with stage IIIB and IV non-small-cell lung cancer. Cancer Chemother Pharmacol. 45:279–283.
65. Omura M, Torigoe S, Kubota N. 1997 SN-38, a metabolite of the camptothecin derivative CPT-11, potentiates the cytotoxic effect of radiation in human colon adenocarcinoma cells grown as spheroids. Radiother Oncol. 43:197–201.
66. Chen AY, Okunieff P, Pommier Y, Mitchell JB. 1997 Mammalian DNA topoisomerase I mediates the enhancement of radiation cytotoxicity by camptothecin derivatives. Cancer Res. 57:1529–1536.
67. Boothman DA, Wang M, Schea RA, Burrows HL, Strickfaden S, Owens JK. 1992 Posttreatment exposure to camptothecin enhances the lethal effects of x-rays on radioresistant human malignant melanoma cells. Int J Rad Oncol Biol Phys. 24:939–948.
68. Takeda K, Negoro S, Kudoh S, et al. 1999 Phase I/II study of weekly irinotecan and concurrent radiation therapy for locally advanced non-small cell lung cancer. Br J Cancer. 79:1462–1467.
69. Yamada M, Kudoh S, Hirata K, Nakajima T, Yoshikawa J. 1998 Risk factors of pneumonitis following chemoradiotherapy for lung cancer. Eur J Cancer. 34:71–75.
70. Masuda N, Matsui K, Negoro S, et al. 1998 Combination of irinotecan and etoposide for treatment of refractory or relapsed small-cell lung cancer. J Clin Oncol. 16:3329–3334.
71. Masuda N, Negoro S, Kudoh S, et al. 2000 Phase I and pharmacologic study of docetaxel and irinotecan in advanced non-small-cell lung cancer. J Clin Oncol. 18:2996–3003.
72. Adjei AA, Klein CE, Kastrissios H, et al. 2000 Phase I and pharmacokinetic study of irinotecan and docetaxel in patients with advanced solid tumors: preliminary evidence of clinical activity. J Clin Oncol. 18:1116–1123.
73. Natale RB, Socinski M, Sandler A, Israel VP, Miller L. 2000 Phase I/II trial of irinotecan, carboplatin, and paclitaxel in advanced or metastatic NSCLC. Oncology. 14:29–34.
74. Friedman HS, Petros WP, Friedman AH, et al. 1999 Irinotecan therapy in adults with recurrent or progressive malignant glioma. J Clin Oncol. 17:1516–1525.
75. Castellino RC, Elion GB, Keir ST, et al. 2000 Schedule-dependent activity of irinotecan plus BCNU against malignant glioma xenografts [published erratum appears in Cancer Chemother Pharmacol 2000;46(1):84]. Cancer Chemother Pharmacol. 45:345–349.
76. Coggins CA, Elion GB, Houghton PJ, et al. 1998 Enhancement of irinotecan (CPT-11) activity against central nervous system tumor xenografts by alkylating agents. Cancer Chemother Pharmacol. 41:485–490.
77. Patel V, Elion G, Houghton P, et al. 2000 Schedule-dependent activity of temozolomide plus CPT-11 against a human central nervous system tumor-derived xenograft. Clin Cancer Res. 6:4154–4157.
78. Lhomme C, Fumoleau P, Fargeot P, et al. 1999 Results of a European Organization for Research and Treatment of Cancer/Early Clinical Studies Group phase II trial of first-line irinotecan in patients with advanced or recurrent squamous cell carcinoma of the cervix. J Clin Oncol. 17:3136–3142.

79. Verschraegen CF, Levy T, Kudelka AP, et al. 1997 Phase II study of irinotecan in prior chemotherapy-treated squamous cell carcinoma of the cervix. J Clin Oncol. 15:625–631.
80. Rosen LS. 1998 Irinotecan in lymphoma, leukemia, and breast, pancreatic, ovarian, and small-cell lung cancers. Oncology. 12:103–109.
81. Blaney S, Berg SL, Pratt C, et al. 2001 A phase I study of irinotecan in pediatric patients: a pediatric oncology group study. Clin Cancer Res. 7:32–37.
82. Vassal G, Droz F, Frappaz D, et al. 1999 A phase I trial of irinotecan (CPT-11) in children [abstract]. Proc Am Soc Clin Oncol. 18:563a.
83. Vassal G, Pondarre C, Boland I, et al. 1998 Preclinical development of camptothecin derivatives and clinical trials in pediatric oncology. Biochimie. 80:271–280.
84. Niwa K, Misao R, Hanabayashi T, et al. 1994 Semi-quantitative analysis of DNA topoisomerase-I mRNA level using reverse transcription-polymerase chain reaction in cancer cell lines: its relation to cytotoxicity against camptothecin derivative. Jpn J Cancer Res. 85:869–874.
85. Giovanella BC, Stehlin JS, Wall ME, et al. 1989 DNA topoisomerase I–targeted chemotherapy of human colon cancer in xenografts. Science. 246:1046–1048.
86. Goldwasser F, Bae I, Valenti M, Torres K, Pommier Y. 1995 Topoisomerase I-related parameters and camptothecin activity in the colon carcinoma cell lines from the National Cancer Institute anticancer screen. Cancer Res. 55:2116–2121.
87. Husain I, Mohler JL, Seigler HF, Besterman JM. 1994 Elevation of topoisomerase I messenger RNA, protein, and catalytic activity in human tumors: demonstration of tumor-type specificity and implications for cancer chemotherapy. Cancer Res. 54:539–546.
88. McLeod HL, Keith WN. 1996 Variation in topoisomerase I gene copy number as a mechanism for intrinsic drug sensitivity. Br J Cancer. 74:508–512.
89. McLeod HL, Douglas F, Oates M, et al. 1994 Topoisomerase I and II activity in human breast, cervix, lung and colon cancer. Int J Cancer. 59:607–611.
90. Guichard S, Terret C, Hennebelle I, et al. 1999 CPT-11 converting carboxylesterase and topoisomerase activities in tumour and normal colon and liver tissues. Br J Cancer. 80:364–370.
91. Abbruzzese JL, Madden T, Sugarman SM, et al. 1996 Phase I clinical and plasma and cellular pharmacological study of topotecan without and with granulocyte colony-stimulating factor. Clin Cancer Res. 2:1489–1497.
92. Danks MK, Garrett KE, Marion RC, Whipple DO. 1996 Subcellular redistribution of DNA topoisomerase I in anaplastic astrocytoma cells treated with topotecan. Cancer Res. 56:1664–1673.
93. Desai SD, Liu LF, Vazquez-Abad D, D'Arpa P. 1997 Ubiquitin-dependent destruction of topoisomerase I is stimulated by the antitumor drug camptothecin. J Biol Chem. 272:24159–24164.
94. Salonga D, Danenberg KD, Johnson M, et al. 2000 Colorectal tumors responding to 5-fluorouracil have low gene expression levels of dihydropyrimidine dehydrogenase, thymidylate synthase, and thymidine phosphorylase. Clin Cancer Res. 6:1322–1327.
95. Johnston PG, Lenz HJ, Leichman CG, et al. 1995 Thymidylate synthase gene and protein expression correlate and are associated with response to 5-fluorouracil in human colorectal and gastric tumors. Cancer Res. 55:1407–1412.
96. Rivory LP, Robert J. 1995 Molecular, cellular, and clinical aspects of the pharmacology of 20(S)camptothecin and its derivatives. Pharmacol Ther. 68:269–296.

97. Guemei A, Cottrell J, Band R, et al. 2001 Human plasma carboxylesterase and butyrylcholinesterase enzyme activity: correlations with SN-38 pharmacokinetics during a prolonged infusion of irinotecan. Cancer Chemother Pharmacol. 47:283–290.
98. Humerickhouse R, Lohrbach K, Li L, Bosron WF, Dolan ME. 2000 Characterization of CPT-11 hydrolysis by human liver carboxylesterase isoforms hCE-1 and hCE-2. Cancer Res. 60:1189–1192.
99. Rivory LP. 2000 Metabolism of CPT-11. Impact on activity. Ann N Y Acad Sci. 922:205–215.
100. Ahmed F, Vyas V, Cornfield A, et al. 1999 In vitro activation of irinotecan to SN-38 by human liver and intestine. Anticancer Res. 19:2067–2071.
101. Kaneda N, Nagata H, Furuta T, Yokokura T. 1990 Metabolism and pharmacokinetics of the camptothecin analogue CPT-11 in the mouse. Cancer Res. 50:1715–1720.
102. Onishi Y, Oguro M, Kizaki H. 1997 A lymphoma cell line resistant to 4-piperidinopiperidine was less sensitive to CPT-11. Cancer Chemother Pharmacol. 39:473–478.
103. Dodds H, Clarke S, Findlay M, Bishop J, Robert J, Rivory L.2000 Clinical pharmacokinetics of the irinotecan metabolite 4-piperidinopiperidine and its possible clinical importance. Cancer Chemother Pharmacol. 45:9–14.
104. Rivory LP, Haaz MC, Canal P, Lokiec F, Armand JP, Robert J. 1997 Pharmacokinetic interrelationships of irinotecan (CPT-11) and its three major plasma metabolites in patients enrolled in phase I/II trials. Clin Cancer Res. 3:1261–1266.
105. Sparreboom A, de Jonge MJ, de Bruijn P, et al. 1998 Irinotecan (CPT-11) metabolism and disposition in cancer patients. Clin Cancer Res. 4:2747–2754.
106. Dodds HM, Haaz MC, Riou JF, Robert J, Rivory LP. 1998 Identification of a new metabolite of CPT-11 (irinotecan): pharmacological properties and activation to SN-38. J Pharmacol Exp Ther. 286:578–583.
107. Dodds H, Wunsch R, Gillam E, Rivory L. 1999 Further elucidation of the pathways involved in the catabolism of the camptothecin analogue irinotecan [abstract]. Proc Am Assoc Cancer Res. 40:110.
108. Lokiec F, du Sorbier BM, Sanderink GJ. 1996 Irinotecan (CPT-11) metabolites in human bile and urine. Clin Cancer Res. 2:1943–1949.
109. Dodds HM, Robert J, Rivory LP. 1998 The detection of photodegradation products of irinotecan (CPT-11, Campto, Camptosar), in clinical studies, using high-performance liquid chromatography/atmospheric pressure chemical ionisation/mass spectrometry. J Pharm Biomed Anal. 17:785–792.
110. Iyer L, King CD, Whitington PF, et al. 1998 Genetic predisposition to the metabolism of irinotecan (CPT-11). Role of uridine diphosphate glucuronosyltransferase isoform 1A1 in the glucuronidation of its active metabolite (SN-38) in human liver microsomes. J Clin Invest. 101:847–854.
111. Rivory LP, Robert J. 1995 Identification and kinetics of a beta-glucuronide metabolite of SN-38 in human plasma after administration of the camptothecin derivative irinotecan. Cancer Chemother Pharmacol. 36:176–179.
112. Gupta E, Lestingi TM, Mick R, Ramirez J, Vokes EE, Ratain MJ. 1994 Metabolic fate of irinotecan in humans: correlation of glucuronidation with diarrhea. Cancer Res. 54:3723–3725.
113. Canal P, Gay C, Dezeuze A, et al. 1996 Pharmacokinetics and pharmacodynamics of irinotecan during a phase II clinical trial in colorectal cancer. Pharmacology and Molecular Mechanisms Group of the European Organization for Research and Treatment of Cancer. J Clin Oncol. 14:2688–2695.

114. Wasserman E, Myara A, Lokiec F, et al. 1998 Bilirubin (Bil) and SN-38 metabolism: pharmacodynamics of CPT-11 [abstract]. Proc Am Soc Clin Oncol. 17:185a.
115. Narita M, Nagai E, Hagiwara H, Aburada M, Yokoi T, Kamataki T. 1993 Inhibition of beta-glucuronidase by natural glucuronides of kampo medicines using glucuronide of SN-38 (7-ethyl-10-hydroxycamptothecin) as a substrate. Xenobiotica. 23:5–10.
116. Yokoi T, Narita M, Nagai E, Hagiwara H, Aburada M, Kamataki T. 1995 Inhibition of UDP-glucuronosyltransferase by aglycons of natural glucuronides in kampo medicines using SN-38 as a substrate. Jpn J Cancer Res. 86:985–989.
117. Takasuna K, Kasai Y, Kitano Y, et al. 1995 Protective effects of kampo medicines and baicalin against intestinal toxicity of a new anticancer camptothecin derivative, irinotecan hydrochloride (CPT-11), in rats. Jpn J Cancer Res. 86:978–984.
118. Dodds H, Stewart CF, Cheshire PJ, Hanna SK, PJ H, Rivory LP. 2001 Primary versus secondary activation of CPT-11: a role for tumor glucuronidases? [abstract] Proc Am Assoc Cancer Res. 42:253.
119. Takahashi T, Fujiwara Y, Miyazaki M, et al. 1998 The role of glucuronidation in 7-ethyl-10-hydroxycamptothecin (SN-38) resistance [abstract]. Proc Am Soc Clin Oncol. 17:185a.
120. Chu XY, Kato Y, Sugiyama Y. 1997 Multiplicity of biliary excretion mechanisms for irinotecan, CPT-11, and its metabolites in rats. Cancer Res. 57:1934–1938.
121. Chu XY, Kato Y, Niinuma K, Sudo KI, Hakusui H, Sugiyama Y. 1997 Multispecific organic anion transporter is responsible for the biliary excretion of the camptothecin derivative irinotecan and its metabolites in rats. J Pharmacol Exp Ther. 281:304–314.
122. Chu XY, Kato Y, Ueda K, et al. 1998 Biliary excretion mechanism of CPT-11 and its metabolites in humans: involvement of primary active transporters. Cancer Res.; 58:5137–5143.
123. Sugiyama Y, Kato Y, Chu X. 1998 Multiplicity of biliary excretion mechanisms for the camptothecin derivative irinotecan (CPT-11), its metabolite SN-38, and its glucuronide: role of canalicular multispecific organic anion transporter and P-glycoprotein. Cancer Chemother Pharmacol. 42:S44–S49.
124. Brangi M, Litman T, Ciotti M, et al. 1999 Camptothecin resistance: role of the ATP-binding cassette (ABC), mitoxantrone-resistance half-transporter (MXR), and potential for glucuronidation in MXR-expressing cells. Cancer Res. 59:5938–5946.
125. Litman T, Brangi M, Hudson E, et al. 2000 The multidrug-resistant phenotype associated with overexpression of the new ABC half-transporter, MXR (ABCG2). J Cell Sci. 113:2011–2021.
126. Schellens JH, Maliepaard M, Scheper RJ, et al. 2000 Transport of topoisomerase I inhibitors by the breast cancer resistance protein. Potential clinical implications. Ann NY Acad Sci. 922:188–194.
127. Blaney SM, Takimoto C, Murry DJ, et al. 1998 Plasma and cerebrospinal fluid pharmacokinetics of 9-aminocamptothecin (9-AC), irinotecan (CPT-11), and SN-38 in nonhuman primates. Cancer Chemother Pharmacol. 41:464–468.
128. Chabot GG. 1997 Clinical pharmacokinetics of irinotecan. Clin Pharmacokinet. 33:245–259.
129. Chabot GG, Abigerges D, Catimel G, et al. 1995 Population pharmacokinetics and pharmacodynamics of irinotecan (CPT-11) and active metabolite SN-38 during phase I trials. Ann Oncol. 6:141–151.
130. Rivory LP, Chatelut E, Canal P, Mathieu Boue A, Robert J. 1994 Kinetics of the in vivo interconversion of the carboxylate and lactone forms of irinotecan (CPT-11) and of its metabolite SN-38 in patients. Cancer Res. 54:6330–6333.

131. Sasaki Y, Yoshida Y, Sudoh K, et al. 1995 Pharmacological correlation between total drug concentration and lactones of CPT-11 and SN-38 in patients treated with CPT-11. Jpn J Cancer Res. 86:111–116.
132. Herben V, Schellens J, Swart M, et al. 1999 Phase I and pharmacokinetic study of irinotecan administered as a low-dose, continuous intravenous infusion over 14 days in patients with malignant solid tumors. J Clin Oncol. 17:1897–1905.
133. Van Groeningen C, Van Der Vijgh W, Giaccone G, et al. 1997 Phase I clinical and pharmacokinetic study of 5 day CPT-11 hepatic arterial infusion (HAI) chemotherapy [abstract]. Proc Am Soc Clin Oncol. 16:219a.
134. Burke TG, Mi Z. 1994 The structural basis of camptothecin interactions with human serum albumin: impact on drug stability. J Med Chem. 37:40–46.
135. Takimoto C, Morrison G, Harold N, et al. 2000 Phase I and pharmacologic study of irinotecan administered as a 96-hour infusion weekly to adult cancer patients. J Clin Oncol. 18:659–667.
136. Furman W, Stewart C, Poquette C, et al. 1999 Direct translation of a protracted irinotecan schedule from a xenograft model to a phase I trial in children. J Clin Oncol. 17:1815–1824.
137. Ma MK, Zamboni WC, Radomski KM, et al. 2000 Pharmacokinetics of irinotecan and its metabolites SN-38 and APC in children with recurrent solid tumors after protracted low-dose irinotecan. Clin Cancer Res. 6:813–819.
138. Vassal G, Santos A, Pein F, Frappaz D, Mignard D, Doz F. 1997 Pharmacokinetics of irinotecan (CPT-11) and its metabolites in children [abstract]. Proc Am Assoc Cancer Res. 38:79.
139. Kehrer DF, Yamamoto W, Verweij J, de Jonge MJ, de Bruijn P, Sparreboom A. 2000 Factors involved in prolongation of the terminal disposition phase of SN-38: clinical and experimental studies. Clin Cancer Res. 6:3451–3458.
140. Schaaf L, Ichhpurani N, Elfring G, Wolf D, Rothenberg M, Von Hoff D. 1997 Influence of age on the pharmacokinetics of irinotecan (CPT-11) and its metabolites, SN-38 and SN-38 glucuronide (SN-38G), in patients with previously treated colorectal cancer [abstract]. Proc Am Soc Clin Oncol. 16:202a.
141. Rivory LP, Findlay M, Clarke S, Bishop J. 1998 Trace analysis of SN-38 in human plasma by high-performance liquid chromatography. J Chromatogr B Biomed Sci Appl. 714:355–359.
142. Rivory LP, Clarke S, Bishop J, O'Donnell A, Emmett L, Findlay M. 1996 Irinotecan (CPT-11): a preliminary investigation of the relationship between trough concentrations of the active metabolite, SN-38, and toxicity. 10th NCI-EORTC Meeting.
143. Slatter JG, Schaaf LJ, Sams JP, et al. 2000 Pharmacokinetics, metabolism, and excretion of irinotecan (CPT-11) following I.V. infusion of [(14)C]CPT-11 in cancer patients. Drug Metab Dispos. 28:423–433.
144. Kaneda N, Yokokura T. 1990 Nonlinear pharmacokinetics of CPT-11 in rats. Cancer Res. 50:1721–1725.
145. Dodds HM, Craik DJ, Rivory LP. 1997 Photodegradation of irinotecan (CPT-11) in aqueous solutions: identification of fluorescent products and influence of solution composition. J Pharm Sci. 86:1410–1416.
146. Iyer L, Hall D, Das S, et al. 1999 Phenotype-genotype correlation of in vitro SN-38 (active metabolite of irinotecan) and bilirubin glucuronidation in human liver tissue with UGT1A1 promoter polymorphism. Clin Pharmacol Ther. 65:576–582.
147. Wasserman E, Myara A, Lokiec F, et al. 1997 Severe CPT-11 toxicity in patients with Gilbert's syndrome: two case reports. Ann Oncol. 8:1049–1051.

148. Ando Y, Saka H, Ando M, et al. 2000 Polymorphisms of UDP-glucuronosyl-transferase gene and irinotecan toxicity: a pharmacogenetic analysis. Cancer Res. 60:6921–6926.
149. Ando Y, Saka H, Asai G, Sugiura S, Shimokata K, Kamataki T. 1998 UGT1A1 genotypes and glucuronidation of SN-38, the active metabolite of irinotecan. Ann Oncol. 9:845–847.
150. Iyer L, Janisch L, Das S, et al. 2000 UGT1A1 promoter genotype correlates with pharmacokinetics of irinotecan (CPT-11) [abstract]. Proc Am Soc Clin Oncol. 19:178a.
151. Raymond E, Vernillet L, Boige V, et al. 1999 Phase I and pharmacokinetic (PK) study of irinotecan (CPT-11) in cancer patients (pts) with hepatic dysfunction [abstract]. Proc Am Soc Clin Oncol. 18:165a.
152. Boige V, Vernillet L, Hua A, et al. 2000 Total plasma clearance of irinotecan (CPT-11) correlates with both alkaline phosphatase and bilirubin levels in patients with tumoral hepatic involvement [abstract]. Proc Am Assoc Cancer Res. 41:608.
153. Ong S, Clarke S, Bishop J, Dodds H, Rivory LP. 2001 Toxicity of irinotecan (CPT-11) and hepato-renal dysfunction. Anti-Cancer Drugs. 12:619–625.
154. Reid J, Buckner J, Schaaf L, et al. 1999 Pharmacokientics of irinotecan (CPT-11) in recurrent glioma patients: results of an NCCTG phase II trial [abstract]. Proc Am Soc Clin Oncol. 18:141a.
155. Kehrer DF, Verweij J, de Bruijn P, Sparreboom A. 2001 Modulation of irinotecan (CPT-11) metabolism in cancer patients by ketoconazole [abstract]. Proc Am Assoc Cancer Res. 42:538.
156. Gupta E, Safa AR, Wang X, Ratain MJ. 1996 Pharmacokinetic modulation of irinotecan and metabolites by cyclosporin A. Cancer Res. 56:1309–1314.
157. Gupta E, Wang X, Ramirez J, Ratain MJ. 1997 Modulation of glucuronidation of SN-38, the active metabolite of irinotecan, by valproic acid and phenobarbital. Cancer Chemother Pharmacol. 39:440–444.
158. de Jonge MJ, Verweij J, Planting AS, et al. 1999 Drug-administration sequence does not change pharmacodynamics and kinetics of irinotecan and cisplatin. Clin Cancer Res. 5:2012–2017.
159. de Jonge MJ, Sparreboom A, Planting AS, et al. 2000 Phase I study of 3-week schedule of irinotecan combined with cisplatin in patients with advanced solid tumors. J Clin Oncol. 18:187–194.
160. Saltz LB, Kanowitz J, Kemeny NE, et al. 1996 Phase I clinical and pharmacokinetic study of irinotecan, fluorouracil, and leucovorin in patients with advanced solid tumors. J Clin Oncol. 14:2959–2967.
161. Negoro S, Fukuoka M, Masuda N, et al. 1991 Phase I study of weekly intravenous infusions of CPT-11, a new derivative of camptothecin, in the treatment of advanced non-small-cell lung cancer. J Natl Cancer Inst. 83:1164–1168.
162. Gandia D, Abigerges D, Armand JP, et al. 1993 CPT-11-induced cholinergic effects in cancer patients. J Clin Oncol. 11:196–197.
163. Dodds H, Rivory L. 1999 The mechanism for the inhibition of acetylcholinesterases by irinotecan (CPT-11). Mol Pharmacol. 56:1346–1353.
164. Valencak J, Raderer M, Kornek GV, Henja MH, Scheithauer W. 1998 Irinotecan-related cholinergic syndrome induced by coadministration of oxaliplatin. J Natl Cancer Inst. 90:160.
165. Pitot HC. 1998 US pivotal studies of irinotecan in colorectal carcinoma. Oncology. 12:48–53.

166. Moertel CG, Schutt AJ, Reitemeier RJ, Hahn RG. 1972 Phase II study of camptothecin (NSC-100880) in the treatment of advanced gastrointestinal cancer. Cancer Chemother Rep. 56:95–101.
167. Natelson EA, Giovanella BC, Verschraegen CF, et al. 1996 Phase I clinical and pharmacological studies of 20-(S)-camptothecin and 20-(S)-9-nitrocamptothecin as anticancer agents. Ann NY Acad Sci. 803:224–230.
168. Creemers GJ, Gerrits CJ, Eckardt JR, et al. 1997 Phase I and pharmacologic study of oral topotecan administered twice daily for 21 days to adult patients with solid tumors. J Clin Oncol. 15:1087–1093.
169. Rowinsky EK, Grochow LB, Hendricks CB, et al. 1992 Phase I and pharmacologic study of topotecan: a novel topoisomerase I inhibitor. J Clin Oncol. 10:647–656.
170. Kantarjian HM, Beran M, Ellis A, et al. 1993 Phase I study of Topotecan, a new topoisomerase I inhibitor, in patients with refractory or relapsed acute leukemia. Blood. 81:1146–1151.
171. Kudelka AP, Tresukosol D, Edwards CL, et al. 1996 Phase II study of intravenous topotecan as a 5-day infusion for refractory epithelial ovarian carcinoma. J Clin Oncol. 14:1552–1557.
172. Araki E, Ishikawa M, Iigo M, Koide T, Itabashi M, Hoshi A. 1993 Relationship between development of diarrhea and the concentration of SN-38, an active metabolite of CPT-11, in the intestine and the blood plasma of athymic mice following intraperitoneal administration of CPT-11. Jpn J Cancer Res. 84:697–702.
173. Rougier P, Bugat R. 1996 CPT-11 in the treatment of colorectal cancer: clinical efficacy and safety profile. Semin Oncol. 23:34–41.
174. Saliba F, Hagipantelli R, Misset JL, et al. 1998 Pathophysiology and therapy of irinotecan-induced delayed-onset diarrhea in patients with advanced colorectal cancer: a prospective assessment. J Clin Oncol. 16:2745–2751.
175. Kase Y, Hayakawa T, Aburada M, Komatsu Y, Kamataki T. 1997 Preventive effects of Hange-shashin-to on irinotecan hydrochloride-caused diarrhea and its relevance to the colonic prostaglandin E2 and water absorption in the rat. Jpn J Pharmacol. 75:407–413.
176. Takasuna K, Hagiwara T, Hirohashi M, et al. 1996 Involvement of beta-glucuronidase in intestinal microflora in the intestinal toxicity of the antitumor camptothecin derivative irinotecan hydrochloride (CPT-11) in rats. Cancer Res. 56:3752–3757.
177. Takasuna K, Hagiwara T, Hirohashi M, et al. 1998 Inhibition of intestinal microflora beta-glucuronidase modifies the distribution of the active metabolite of the antitumor agent, irinotecan hydrochloride (CPT-11) in rats. Cancer Chemother Pharmacol. 42:280–286.
178. Schaaf L, Slatter J, Sams J, et al. 1999 Metabolism and excretion of irinotecan (CPT-11) following IV infusion of [14C]CPT-11 in patients with advanced solid tumor malignancy [abstract]. Proc Am Soc Clin Oncol. 18:164a.
179. Lenfers BH, Loeffler TM, Droege CM, Hausamen TU. 1999 Substantial activity of budesonide in patients with irinotecan (CPT-11) and 5-fluorouracil induced diarrhea and failure of loperamide treatment. Ann Oncol. 10:1251–1253.
180. Shinkai T, Arioka H, Kunikane H, et al. 1994 Phase I clinical trial of irinotecan (CPT-11), 7-ethyl-10-[4-(1-piperidino)-1-piperidino]carbonyloxy-camptothecin, and cisplatin in combination with fixed dose of vindesine in advanced non-small cell lung cancer. Cancer Res. 54:2636–2642.

181. Sakai H, Diener M, Gartmann V, Takeguchi N. 1995 Eicosanoid-mediated Cl- secretion induced by the antitumor drug, irinotecan (CPT-11), in the rat colon. Naunyn-Schmiedebergs Arch Pharmacol. 351:309–314.
182. Sakai H, Sato T, Hamada N, et al. 1997 Thromboxane A2, released by the antitumour drug irinotecan, is a novel stimulator of Cl- secretion in isolated rat colon. J Physiol. 505:133–144.
183. Goto S, Okutomi T, Suma Y, Kera J, Soma G, Takeuchi S. 1996 Induction of tumor necrosis factor by a camptothecin derivative, irinotecan, in mice and human mononuclear cells. Anticancer Res. 16:2507–2511.
184. Govindarajan R, Heaton KM, Broadwater R, Zeitlin A, Lang NP, Hauer-Jensen M. 2000 Effect of thalidomide on gastrointestinal toxic effects of irinotecan. Lancet. 356:566–567.
185. Cao S, Black JD, Troutt AB, Rustum YM. 1998 Interleukin 15 offers selective protection from irinotecan-induced intestinal toxicity in a preclinical animal model. Cancer Res. 58:3270–3274.
186. Shinohara H, Killion JJ, Kuniyasu H, Kumar R, Fidler IJ. 1998 Prevention of intestinal toxic effects and intensification of irinotecan's therapeutic efficacy against murine colon cancer liver metastases by oral administration of the lipopeptide JBT 3002. Clin Cancer Res. 4:2053–2063.
187. Shinohara H, Killion JJ, Bucana CD, Yano S, Fidler IJ. 1999 Oral administration of the immunomodulator JBT-3002 induces endogenous interleukin 15 in intestinal macrophages for protection against irinotecan-mediated destruction of intestinal epithelium. Clin Cancer Res. 5:2148–2156.
188. Savarese D, Al-Zoubi A, Boucher J. 2000 Glutamine for irinotecan diarrhea. J Clin Oncol. 18:450–451.
189. Hardman WE, Moyer MP, Cameron IL. 1999 Fish oil supplementation enhanced CPT-11 (irinotecan) efficacy against MCF7 breast carcinoma xenografts and ameliorated intestinal side-effects. Br J Cancer. 81:440–448.
190. Michael M, Brittain M, Nagai J, et al. 2001 A phase II study of activated charcoal to prevent irinotecan (CPT-11) induced diarrhea [abstract]. Proc Am Soc Clin Oncol. 20:405a.
191. Zidan J, Haim N, Beny A, Stein M, Gez E, Kuten A . 2001 Octreotide in the treatment of severe chemotherapy-induced diarrhea. Ann Oncol. 12:227–229.
192. Ooms LA, Degryse AD, Janssen PA. 1984 Mechanisms of action of loperamide. Scand J Gastroenterol Supp. 96:145–155.
193. Nikolic-Tomasevic Z, Jelic S, Popov I, Radosavljevic D. 2000 Colorectal cancer: dilemmas regarding patient selection and toxicity prediction. J Chemother. 12:244–251.
194. van Groeningen C, Van der Vijgh W, Baars J, Stieltjes H, Huibregtse K, Pinedo H. 2000 Altered pharmacokinetics and metabolism of CPT-11 in liver dysfunction: a need for guidelines. Clin Cancer Res. 6:1342–1346.
195. Miya T, Fujikawa R, Fukushima J, Nogami H, Koshiishi Y, Goya T. 1998 Bradycardia induced by irinotecan: a case report. Jpn J Clin Oncol. 28:709–711.
196. Boisseau M, Bugat R, Mahjoubi M. 1996 Rapid tumour lysis syndrome in a metastatic colorectal cancer increased by treatment (CPT-11). Eur J Cancer. 32A:737–738.
197. Gupta E, Mick R, Ramirez J, et al. 1997 Pharmacokinetic and pharmacodynamic evaluation of the topoisomerase inhibitor irinotecan in cancer patients. J Clin Oncol. 15:1502–1510.

12 Clinical Experience With Topotecan

Aimee K. Bence, PhD,
and Val R. Adams, PharmD

CONTENTS

1. OVERVIEW

Topotecan (Hycamtin, GlaxoSmithKline) is a water-soluble semisynthetic derivative of camptothecin (CPT), an alkaloid extracted from the stem wood of the Chinese tree *Camptotheca acuminata (1)*. As a result of its anticancer activity and favorable toxicity profile, in 1996, topotecan was approved for use in the United States as an antitumor agent in the treatment of recurrent ovarian cancer. In 1998, it was approved as a second-line treatment for patients with small-cell lung cancer (SCLC). Clinical trials have also assessed its activity in the treatment of myelodysplastic syndrome, pancreatic, head and neck, myeloma, prostate, renal cell, melanoma, gliomal, uterine, cervical, hepatocellular, gastric, and breast cancers. Numerous ongoing trials are evaluating the role of topotecan in combination chemotherapy. The current dosing regimen approved by the Food and Drug Administration (FDA) is a 30-minute intravenous (iv) infusion of 1.5 mg/m^2 daily for 5

Camptothecins in Cancer Therapy
Edited by: V. R. Adams and T. G. Burke © Humana Press Inc., Totowa, NJ

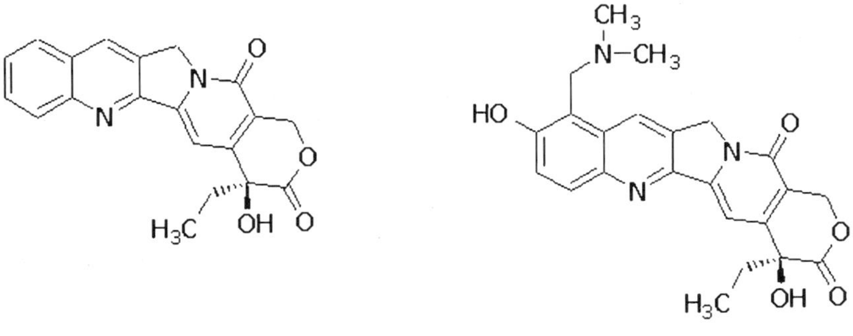

Camptothecin Topotecan

Fig. 1. Chemical structures of camptothecin and topotecan.

days, which is repeated every 3 weeks. Topotecan is available as a parenteral preparation and is supplied in vials containing 4 mg, which is reconstituted in 4 mL sterile water. The resulting 1 mg/mL solution is further diluted with a 5% dextrose or 0.9% saline solution before injection.

2. CHEMISTRY AND MECHANISM OF ACTION

As seen in Fig. 1, topotecan ((S)-9-[(dimethylamino)methyl]-10-hydroxy camptothecin) differs from CPT in that a basic side chain has been introduced at position 9 and a hydroxyl at position 10. These structural modifications increase the water solubility and biological activity of topotecan when compared with CPT. As with CPT, the lactone moiety in the E-ring of topotecan can undergo a nonenzymatic, reversible hydrolysis to the corresponding open-ring carboxylate. The hydrolysis of the lactone ring is pH-dependent; the lactone predominates in acidic conditions, whereas the carboxylic acid form predominates at neutral or basic pH. Because the lactone species is a much more potent anticancer agent than the carboxylic acid *(2,3)*, its in vivo concentration is an important determinant of the anticancer activity of topotecan.

The anticancer properties of topotecan result from its capacity to inhibit topoisomerase I (TOP-I) *(4)*. TOP-I is an essential nuclear enzyme that aids in DNA replication by relieving torsional strain. Topotecan disrupts the normal function of TOP-I by stabilizing the TOP-I–DNA complex and preventing the dissociation of TOP-I from DNA. Advancing DNA replication forks collide with the stable TOP-I-DNA-topotecan complex, resulting in double-strand breaks in DNA and cellular death *(5–7)*.

3. CLINICAL PHARMACOLOGY

3.1. Pharmacokinetics

As with all CPT analogs, the pharmacokinetics of topotecan are complicated by the rapid conversion of the lactone moiety to the open-ring carboxylic acid. At physiological pH, only 15–35% of the drug is in the lactone form and within 1 hour of administration, the predominant species is the carboxylic acid *(8–14)*. The pharmacokinetics of topotecan can be described by an open, two-compartment model, and a linear relationship exists between dose and mean peak phase concentrations and area under the concentration-time curve (AUC) *(9)*.

3.1.1. Absorption and Distribution

Only the iv administration of topotecan is approved for use by the FDA. However, recently, there has been an increased interest in the evaluation of other routes of administration. Most notably, oral formulations have been developed and assessed in clinical trials. Oral topotecan has a bioavailability of 32–44% with interpatient variability of 24–31% *(15–18)*. The peak plasma concentration occurs approximately 0.75 to 2 hours after oral administration *(15,19)*. No significant differences in the ratio of lactone to carboxylic acid were found when the oral route was compared with iv administration *(16,18)*. However, interpatient and intrapatient variability were found to be higher with oral topotecan than with the iv route *(19,20)*. Phase I studies also have evaluated intraperitoneal administration of topotecan. As indicated by a peritoneal to plasma AUC ratios of 31:1 and 54:1, intraperitoneal administration results in a significant pharmacological advantage compared to systemic exposure *(54,55)*.

Topotecan is distributed widely in the body, with a volume of distribution of approximately 50 L/m^2 (total drug) and 75 L/m^2 (lactone) *(8,13,21)*. Between studies however, there has been a significant variation in the reported volume of distribution *(9,12,22–26)*. Unlike other CPT derivatives, topotecan does not bind extensively to plasma proteins (7–31%) *(27,28)*. Topotecan has good central nervous system (CNS) penetration and crosses the blood–brain barrier more effectively than CPT *(29,30)*. In pediatric patients treated with a 24 (5.5–7.5 mg/m^2/day) or 72-hour (0.5–1.25 mg/m^2/day) continuous iv infusion of topotecan, the median penetration of drug into the cerebral spinal fluid was 29% for the 24-hour infusion and 42% for the 72-hour infusion *(31)*.

3.1.2. Metabolism and Elimination

As previously discussed, topotecan undergoes nonenzymatic hydrolysis of the lactone ring. This hydrolysis is the primary metabolic pathway for the clearance of topotecan. One minor metabolite, *N*-desmethyl topotecan, has been characterized, and small amounts (1–4%) of this metabolite have been detected in plasma, urine, and feces after iv administration of topotecan (1.0 mg/m^2 daily for 5 days every 3 weeks) *(32,33)*.

Topotecan (total drug) is rapidly cleared from the central compartment with a $t_{1/2}(\alpha)$ of 3–31 minutes and a terminal half-life of 1.8–4.5 hours after iv administration *(8,10,12–14,21,23)*. As a result of the short half-life of topotecan, the drug does not accumulate when it is administered by the approved regimen (1.5 mg/m^2 daily for 5 consecutive days once every 3 weeks) *(8)*. Mean total plasma clearance rates of topotecan have ranged from 7.5–34.8 L/m^2/hour and are not predictably influenced by age or dose *(21,23,34)*. Both topotecan and the carboxylic acid are renally eliminated, with 20–40% of the dose excreted in the first 24 hours after administration *(8,9,13,22)*.

Renal impairment reduces the plasma clearance of topotecan and is associated with lower maximum tolerated doses *(35)*. Many ovarian or SCLC patients with recurrent or relapsed disease are treated with cisplatin and may have decreased renal function. Consequently, renal status should be carefully considered when calculating the appropriate dose of topotecan. The standard 1.5 mg/m^2/day is appropriate for patients with normal renal function (24-hour creatinine clearance of greater than 60 mL/minute), regardless of prior therapy. Current guidelines recommend that patients with moderate renal impairment (24-hour creatinine clearance of 20–39 mL/minute) receive 50% of the recommended dose; the dose should be reduced from 1.5 mg/m^2/day to 0.75 mg/m^2/day *(35,36)*. The guidelines indicate that dose adjustment is not required for minimally treated patients with a serum creatinine of 40–59 mL/minute. However, in patients who have received extensive prior therapy and have renal dysfunction, the recommended doses are 1.0 mg/m^2/day (creatinine clearance 40–59 mL/minute) and 0.5 mg/m^2/day (creatinine clearance 20–39 mL/minute) *(36)*. Dosing guidelines for patients with a creatinine clearance of less than 20 mL/minute have not been established.

Topotecan also has been detected in the bile, suggesting that a biliary route of elimination may be involved in the clearance of topotecan *(13)*. However, no difference was observed in the clearance, terminal half-life, or volume of distribution in patients with impaired hepatic function (serum bilirubin 29–255 μmol/L) when compared with patients with normal bilirubin levels *(35)*. As a result, dose adjustments are not recommended for patients with hepatic dysfunction. Body weight and age do not appear to affect the pharmacokinetic parameters of topotecan, and dose adjustments for these covariates are not recommended *(24,34)*.

3.2. Administration

In the United States, the FDA has approved topotecan to be administered as 30-minute iv infusion of 1.5 mg/m^2 daily for 5 consecutive days every 3 weeks. Although this regimen has been widely used, clinical investigators have continued to study alternate regimens to optimize the dose and schedule of topotecan. Topotecan has been administered as a 30-minute infusion weekly (1.5–6.0 mg/m^2) *(37–39)*, a 24-hour infusion weekly (1.0–2.0 mg/m^2) *(14)*, a 24-hour infusion every 21 days (2.5–15 mg/m^2) *(9,25,40)*, a 3-day continuous infusion every 21 days (0.5–2.6 mg/m^2/d) *(41)*, a 5-day continuous infusion every 21 days (0.17–3.6 mg/m^2/d) *(42–44)*, and as a 21-day continuous infusion every 28 days (0.2–0.8 mg/m^2/d) *(45–47)*. Single iv doses given over 30 minutes of up to 22.5 mg/m^2 once every 3 weeks have been administered *(13)*. Although some of these schedules were well tolerated and resulted in objective responses, the FDA-approved, 5-day daily regimen is the standard of care. However, alternate dosing schedules warrant further consideration because they may have utility in a palliative setting or as a component of combination regimens.

Recently, there has been increased interest in evaluating oral administration of topotecan. The results of several clinical trials indicate that oral topotecan may be as effective as the iv form in treating recurrent SCLC and ovarian cancer. However, the toxicity profile of the oral route differs from that of iv topotecan. Notably, oral treatment may cause less myelotoxicity than iv administration *(48–50)*. A multicenter, randomized study evaluating oral versus iv topotecan found comparable response rates for iv (20%) and oral (13%) administration in relapsed epithelial ovarian cancer patients *(50)*. Similarly, response rates were comparable in patients with previously treated SCLC (23% oral vs 15% iv) *(48)*. As with iv administration of topotecan, several doses and schedules of oral topotecan have been evaluated, including daily oral treatment for 5 to 21 consecutive days and twice daily treatment for 10 or 21 days *(20,48,49,51–53)*. Current data from Phase II trials indicate that oral administration of 2.3 mg/m^2/day for 5 days once every 3 weeks is a well-tolerated and effective regimen *(48,50)*.

Several phase I studies have assessed the feasibility of administering intraperitoneal topotecan *(54,55)*. Unlike iv or oral administration, in which the dose-limiting toxicity is myelosuppression, the dose-limiting toxicities of intraperitoneal administration are hypotension, chills, and fever. Consequently, much higher doses can be safely administered, and intraperitoneal administration may allow for combination therapy with other cytotoxic drugs that are myelosuppressive.

Preclinical studies have evaluated the effectiveness of liposomal encapsulation of topotecan *(56–58)*. Topotecan formulated in sphingomyelin/cholesterol liposomes resulted in a sustained release of the lactone species over approximately 24 hours. The liposomal formulation protected the lactone from hydrolysis, which translated into increased survival rates in animal xenograft models when compared with free topotecan *(58)*. Intrathecal, intramuscular, transdermal, and subcutaneous administration of topotecan have also been investigated *(59,60)*.

3.3. Pharmacodynamics

Myelosuppression is the dose-limiting toxicity of both iv and oral topotecan, and the extent of myelosuppression correlates with total topotecan AUC. This correlation was seen with multiple administration regimens (a 30-minute infusion daily for 5 days once every 3 weeks, a 20-minute infusion once every 3 weeks, a 72-hour continuous infusion, and a 24-hour continuous infusion) *(8,9,13,14,22,61)*. Other pharmacokinetic parameters, including the time plasma concentration is higher than 10 nmol/L, predict toxicity. However, none appear to be more predictive than dose *(8,9,22)*. Consequently, routine monitoring of pharmacokinetic parameters does not appear to be warranted at this time.

3.4. Toxicity

3.4.1. Hematological

Myelosuppression is the dose-limiting toxicity of topotecan therapy for all iv doses and schedules. Reversible, noncumulative neutropenia and thrombocytopenia are the most frequent toxicities observed after topotecan administration; neutropenia usually occurs more often and is more severe than thrombocytopenia. The hematologic toxicities from four Phase II and III trials evaluating topotecan (1.5 mg/m^2/day) were compiled and analyzed *(36)*. Of the 454 advanced-stage ovarian cancer patients who were treated with topotecan, 81% experienced grade 4 neutropenia. In addition, 26% of the patients had grade 4 thrombocytopenia and 40% grade 4 anemia *(36)*. Similar results were seen when 107 SCLC patients were treated with 1.5 mg/m^2/day for 5 days once every 3 weeks. Grade 4 neutropenia and thrombocytopenia were reported in 70% and 29% of patients, respectively. The onset of neutropenia occurred 8–12 days after the start of topotecan therapy with the nadir occurring at approximately 12 days. Neutrophil counts recovered by 21 days after the initiation of therapy, allowing for retreatment at 3 weeks. The platelet nadir occurred at approximately day 15 and recovered by day 21 *(62)*.

Patients who have received prior chemotherapy or radiation or have impaired renal function have an increased risk of myelosuppression *(12,22,36,63)*. The topotecan dose should be reduced by 0.25 mg/m^2 per dose for patients who have grade 4 neutropenia or thrombocytopenia *(36)*. Granulocyte colony-stimulating factor (G-CSF) has been in used in combination with topotecan in an effort to increase the dose intensity. The data from these studies are conflicting. In one study, G-CSF support allowed the dose of topotecan to be increased 2.3-fold. Other researchers, however, found that dose escalation with G-CSF was not possible because thrombocytopenia and fatigue were dose-limiting *(12,25)*. Because the value of dose intensification in ovarian and SCLC is unclear *(64,65)*, it is uncertain whether there is clinical benefit in using G-CSF over dose reduction in SCLC and ovarian cancer patients *(66)*.

3.4.2. Other Toxicities

Nonhematological toxicities are generally mild to moderate in severity and are not dose-limiting. In large clinical trials in which topotecan was administered to ovarian and SCLC patients, alopecia was the most common nonhematological side effect reported, occurring in 56–82% of patients *(62,67,68)*. Nausea (40–78%), vomiting (24–64%), and fatigue (26–41%) were also frequently reported. Other less common toxicities seen after topotecan administration included skin rash, mild and transient elevations of liver function tests, abdominal pain, stomatitis, arthralgias, myalgias, microscopic hematuria, peripheral neuropathies, and diarrhea. Many of these toxicities could be effectively managed with supportive measures.

The schedule and route of administration affect the toxicity profile of topotecan. After treatment with intraperitoneal topotecan, the dose-limiting toxicities were hypotension, chills, and fever *(54)*. In contrast, mucositis and diarrhea were dose-limiting in leukemia patients receiving a 5-day continuous infusion of topotecan *(69)*. Diarrhea was also dose-limiting in patients treated with oral topotecan twice daily for 21 days *(53)*, but was not dose-limiting when topotecan was given by continuous infusion for 21 days or orally on a daily × 5 regimen *(49,70–72)*. Although the primary toxicity of the standard regimen is myelosuppression, these data indicate different toxicities may be dose-limiting for other routes and schedules of administration. Rare cases of life-threatening hypersensitivity reactions have been reported.

3.5. Drug Interactions

When topotecan and G-CSF were administered to patients on the same day, neutropenia and thrombocytopenia were more severe. Consequently, topotecan and G-CSF should not be administered concurrently *(22)*. Several drugs have been identified that can alter the pharmacokinetic properties of topotecan. Coadministration of phenytoin and topotecan increased the total drug and lactone clearance and increased the AUC of the topotecan metabolite, *N*-desmethyl topotecan *(73)*. Other drugs that induce hepatic cytochrome P450 enzymes, such as dexamethasone and phenobarbital, also increase the clearance of topotecan *(74)*. Additional studies characterizing of the effects of P450-inducing agents on topotecan pharmacokinetics are necessary. Preclinical studies demonstrated that when probenecid, which is known to inhibit renal tubular secretion, was administered to mice in combination with topotecan the systemic clearance of topotecan and total renal clearance were decreased *(75)*.

3.6. Mechanisms of Resistance

Little is known about the in vivo mechanisms of resistance to topotecan and other CPT analogs. Several resistance mechanisms, however, have been identified in vitro, including decreased cellular levels of TOP-I *(76,77)*, reduced TOP-I activity *(78,79)*, a decrease in the number of TOP-I-DNA–cleavable complexes *(78)*, migration of TOP-I out of the nucleolus *(80–82)*, and mutations of amino acids within the active site of TOP-I *(80–83)*. Topotecan is a substrate for the breast cancer resistance protein *(77,84,85)* and the P-glycoprotein multidrug transporter *(86,87)* resulting in decreased accumulation of topotecan in cells. The degree of P-glycoprotein–associated resistance for topotecan is, however, significantly less than that observed for other multidrug resistance substrates *(87–90)*. Enhanced topotecan efflux was observed in a tumor-resistant cell line that does not overexpress P-glycoprotein, suggesting that other efflux mechanisms, such as breast cancer resistance protein, may contribute to the development of topotecan resistance *(77,85)*. Although ongoing studies continue to accrue information about these pathways, the clinical relevance of these mechanisms of resistance in human tumors has yet to be elucidated.

4. SINGLE-AGENT ANTICANCER ACTIVITY OF TOPOTECAN

4.1. Ovarian Cancer

Topotecan is approved for use in patients with advanced ovarian cancer who are refractory to, or who relapsed after, receiving platinum-based therapy. Response rates of 14–23% have been observed in phase II noncomparator trials evaluating topotecan given daily for 5 days every 21 days to patients who have received a platinum-based chemotherapy regimen as first-line treatment (Table 1) *(68,72,91–94)*. The majority of the observed responses were partial responses, with complete responses seen in less than 5% of the patients. The median duration of response in these studies ranged from 18 to 45 weeks.

A phase III multicenter, randomized trial compared the standard topotecan regimen (1.5 mg/m^2/day for 5 days every 21 days) with paclitaxel (175 mg/m^2 infused over 3 hours every 21 days) in women with advanced epithelial ovarian cancer who had previously failed a platinum-based therapy. The results were originally published in 1997 *(67)* and have been subsequently updated *(95,96)*. At the conclusion of the study, 226 patients were able to be evaluated for response with 114 randomized to the paclitaxel arm and 112 randomized to the topotecan arm. No significant difference was found in the efficacy of these two agents; topotecan had a response rate of 20%, whereas the response rate of paclitaxel was 13%. Similarly, there was

Table 1
Summary of the Results From Phase II and III Trials With Topotecan Monotherapy in Ovarian Cancer

Previous treatments	*Dose*	*Number of evaluable patients*	*CR (%)*	*PR (%)*	*Median duration of response (weeks)*	*Median Duration of Survival (weeks)*	*Reference*
Phase II trials							
Cisplatin	1.5 mg/m^2	28		14	36	40	*92*
PAX+ platinum regimen	1.5 mg/m^2	130	1	13	18	47	*94*
Platinum regimen	1.5 mg/m^2	92	1	15	22	*68*	
Platinum regimen	1.5 mg/m^2	31		23		44	*91*
PAX+ platinum regimen	1.25 mg/m^2	28		14	18	24	*93*
Phase III trials							
Platinum regimen	1.5 mg/m^2	112	4	16	32	61	*95*
Platinum regimen	PAX (175 mg/m^2)	114	3	10	20	43	*95*
Platinum regimen	1.5 mg/m^2	235	5	12		57	*97*
Platinum regimen PLD	(50 mg/m^2)	239	4	16		60	*97*

CR, complete response; PR, partial response; PAX, paclitaxel; PLD, pegylated liposomal doxorubicin.
Note: Topotecan was administered as a 30 minute infusion daily for 5 days once every 3 weeks.

no significant difference in the overall median survival between topotecan and paclitaxel (61 and 43 weeks, respectively). Topotecan, however, did have a significantly longer median time to progression than paclitaxel (23 weeks and 14 weeks, respectively) and a significantly greater incidence of grade 4 neutropenia and thrombocytopenia.

Patients were eligible to cross over and receive the treatment in the alternate arm as third-line therapy. Overall, 110 patients crossed over; 61 patients crossed over from paclitaxel to topotecan and 49 patients crossed over from topotecan to paclitaxel. A partial response was observed in 13% of the patients that crossed over from paclitaxel to topotecan therapy. Of the patients that crossed over from the topotecan arm to the paclitaxel arm, 10% achieved a complete or partial response. The third-line therapies had comparable median time to progression (9 weeks for both arms) and median survival (40 and 48 weeks for topotecan and paclitaxel, respectively) indicating that topotecan and paclitaxel have a degree of non-cross-resistance.

The efficacy of topotecan was compared with pegylated liposomal doxorubicin (PLD) in a phase III trial of patients with recurrent ovarian cancer. Patients were randomized and either treated with topotecan (1.5 m/m^2/day for 5 days every 21 days) or PLD (50 mg/m^2 as a 1-hour infusion every 28 days). Of the 474 patients able to be evaluated, 17% had a response to topotecan (n = 235) and 20% responded to PLD therapy (n = 239). The survival times for topotecan and PLD were comparable (57 and 60 weeks, respectively). The frequency of grade 1, 2, and 3 toxicities were similar with both treatment regimens, but the incidence of grade 4 toxicity was significantly higher in the topotecan treatment arm (71%) than in the PLD arm (17%). This was due to the high frequency of grade 4 hematological toxicity in patients treated with topotecan *(97)*. Although PLD had comparable efficacy to topotecan as a salvage therapy for ovarian cancer, it had less toxicity and was dosed much less frequently, which may translate into improved patient convenience. These differences may increase the likelihood that PLD will be chosen over topotecan by prescribing physicians as second-line therapy.

Clinical trials of topotecan in patients with recurrent ovarian cancer demonstrate that response rates are higher in patients who initially responded to platinum-based therapy. In patients who were platinum-sensitive (relapsed more than 6 months after treatment) response rates were 10–29%, whereas in patients who had platinum-resistant disease (relapsed in less than 6 months) or platinum-refractory disease, response rates were 2–13% *(50,67,68,94,97)*. The Phase III trial comparing topotecan with PLD prospectively randomized patients who had platinum-sensitive and platinum-resistant tumors. Overall, 29% of the 111 platinum-sensitive patients had a response to topotecan compared with 6% for the 124 platinum-resistant patients *(97)*.

Other clinical trials have examined the efficacy of alternate dosing regimens of topotecan. In contrast to the standard daily × five regimen, a daily × three topotecan regimen (2 mg/m^2) was evaluated in women with recurrent ovarian cancer. In the 28 patients able to be evaluated, the overall response rate was 32% and stable disease was achieved in 18% of patients, which compares favorably with that observed in the daily × five regimen *(98)*. Response rates of 9–38% were observed in platinum-resistant ovarian cancer patients who received a 21-day continuous infusion of topotecan (0.3–0.5 mg/m^2/day) *(71,99)*. Weekly administration of topotecan (2–6 mg/m^2 weekly for 3 weeks followed by a rest week) resulted in partial responses in 25% of the 32 patients able to be evaluated *(39)*. A small randomized study comparing 24-hour continuous administration (1.75 mg/m^2 once weekly for 4 weeks) to the standard dosing regimen indicated that topotecan was significantly more effective when administered according to the approved regimen. In the 24-hour continuous infusion arm, 3% of the 32 patients had a partial response compared with 23% of the 31 patients in the standard dosing arm. However, overall survival was comparable in each arm (11 and 12 months for the daily × five and 24-hour infusion, respectively) *(91)*.

4.2. SCLC

In 1998, topotecan was approved for use as a second-line agent in the treatment of SCLC. Although numerous agents have been shown to have activity in the treatment of recurrent SCLC, topotecan is the only single-agent therapy currently approved in the United States. Because the response of SCLC to salvage therapy is usually influenced by the sensitivity of the patient to first-line therapy, most studies evaluating topotecan have stratified patients as refractory (patients whose disease was stable or progressed within 90 days of first-line therapy) or sensitive (patients who responded to first-line therapy, but relapsed more than 90 days after front-line therapy). In Phase II clinical trials, the overall response rates of topotecan (1.25–1.5 mg/m^2/day for 5 consecutive days once every 3 weeks) in refractory patients were 2–11%, with only 1 of 154 patients achieving a complete response. The median survival of patients in this subpopulation was 16–20 weeks (Table 2). In contrast, the overall response rates for sensitive patients were 14–37%, with a complete response observed in 2–13% of patients. The median survival for sensitive patients was 26–30 weeks *(70,100–102)*.

The drug combination cyclophosphamide, doxorubicin, and vincristine, used to treat recurrent SCLC, was chosen as the comparator therapy for the randomized, multicenter phase III trial with topotecan. Patients were eligible for this study if they had relapsed more than 60 days after receiving first-line therapy (the first-line therapy for most of the patients in the study was etoposide plus cisplatin). Overall, 211 patients able to be evaluated were enrolled in the study, with 107 patients randomized to receive topotecan

Table 2
Summary of the Results From Phase II and III Trials With Topotecan Monotherapy in Small-Cell Lung Cancer

Platinum sensitivity	*Dose*	*Number of evaluable patients*	*CR (%)*	*PR (%)*	*Median duration of survival (weeks)*	*Reference*
Phase II trials						
Resistant	1.5 mg/m^2	38		3	20	*101*
Sensitive	1.5 mg/m^2	36	8	11	27	*101*
Resistant	1.5 mg/m^2	47	2	4	20	*100*
Sensitive	1.5 mg/m^2	45	13	24	30	*100*
Resistant	1.5 mg/m^2	41		2	16	*70*
Sensitive	1.5 mg/m^2	57	2	12	26	*70*
Resistant	1.25 mg/m^2	28		11	20	*102*
Phase III Trials						
Sensitive	1.5 mg/m^2	107		24	25	*62*
Sensitive	CAV	104	1	17	25	*62*

CR, complete response; PR, partial response.
Notes: CAV, cyclophosphamide (1000 mg/m^2), doxorubicin (45 mg/m^2) and vincristine (2 mg on day 1) every 3 weeks. Topotecan was administered as a 30 minute infusion daily for 5 days once every 3 weeks.

(1.5 mg/m^2 as a 30-minute infusion daily for 5 days once every 3 weeks) and 104 patients randomized to the cyclophosphamide, doxorubicin, and vincristine (cyclophosphamide 1000 mg/m^2, doxorubicin 45 mg/m^2, and vincristine 2 mg on day 1 with the cycle repeated every 3 weeks) treatment arm. Patients in the topotecan arm had an overall response rate of 24% (no complete responders) compared with 18% in the cyclophosphamide, doxorubicin, and vincristine arm (one complete responder). The median duration of response, time to disease progression, and overall survival also were comparable. Patients treated with topotecan, however, had a significant increase in symptomatic improvement for four of the eight symptoms evaluated (dyspnea, anorexia, hoarseness, and fatigue) *(62)*.

The efficacy of topotecan has also been evaluated as a front-line therapy in chemotherapy-naive SCLC patients with extensive disease. Topotecan (2.0 mg/m^2/day for 5 days once every 3 weeks with G-CSF support) was administered to 48 patients. The partial response rate was 39%; none of the patients had a complete response. The median duration of response was 19 weeks and the overall median survival time was 40 weeks *(103)*. These results are comparable to other agents used as monotherapy for extensive stage SCLC, but are inferior to results seen with combination therapy *(104)*.

4.3. Other Malignancies

4.3.1. Hematological Malignancies

Several studies have demonstrated that topotecan may have utility in the treatment of a variety of hematological diseases including myelodysplastic syndrome (MDS), multiple myeloma, chronic myelomonocytic leukemia, acute myelocytic leukemia (AML), and acute undifferentiated leukemia. Forty-three multiple myeloma patients were treated with the conventional regimen of topotecan and a partial response rate of 16% was observed; there were no complete responders *(105)*. Complete remission rates of 27% and 37% were observed when patients with either chronic myelomonocytic leukemia ($n = 30$) or MDS ($n = 30$) were treated with a continuous infusion of topotecan (2.0 mg/m^2/day) for 5 days once every 21–28 days, respectively. The toxicity of the regimen, however, was high; in the first 4 weeks of therapy 20% of patients died as a result of complications arising from myelosuppression *(106)*. When 27 patients with refractory or relapsed acute leukemia were given a continuous infusion of topotecan (3.5–18 mg/m^2/day for 5 days once every 21–28 days), overall response rates of 18% were observed. Three patients (11%) had a complete response to this therapy *(43)*. A Phase I study evaluated a 5-day continuous infusion of topotecan (0.7–2.7 mg/m^2/day) in 17 patients with acute leukemia. One patient (6%) with chronic myelomonocytic leukemia in blast crisis achieved a complete response and one patient (6%) with AML had a partial response for an overall response rate of 12% *(42)*. In the subsequent phase II trial, 14 patients with either untreated or relapsed acute lymphocytic leukemia were treated with a 5-day continuous infusion of topotecan (2.1 mg/m^2/day). A complete response was found in only one patient for an overall response rate of 7% *(95)*. The response rates in these studies are noteworthy because many of these patients had failed prior therapies and were chemoresistant. phase I and II studies are evaluating several chemotherapy combinations that include topotecan. The data from these trials may lead to phase III studies in the future. Additional studies are clearly warranted to further elucidate the value of topotecan therapy in hematologic malignancies.

4.3.2. Pediatric Malignancies

Several phase II trials assessed topotecan in children with refractory non-CNS tumors. A 72-hour continuous infusion of topotecan (1.0–1.3 mg/m^2/day) was evaluated in 85 pediatric patients with refractory neuroblastoma and sarcomas of soft tissue and bone. The overall response rate was 2% *(107)*. Another phase II study evaluated topotecan therapy in 141 children with recurrent or progressive solid tumors. Patients were treated with 2 mg/m^2 of topotecan administered daily for 5 days once every 21 days. Complete and partial responses were observed in 2% and 1% of patients, respectively. Minor responses and stable disease were observed in 17% of patients, and the median duration of treatment for children in this study exceeded 8 months. This result is significant because phase II trials with other agents have not reported long-term duration of stable disease *(108)*. In a randomized phase II trial, 63 children with untreated neuroblastoma were either treated with two cycles of topotecan (2 mg/m^2/day for 5 days) or paclitaxel (350 mg/m^2 over 24 hours). Overall response rates of 37% were observed in the 32 patients receiving topotecan therapy compared with 16% for the 31 patients treated with paclitaxel *(109)*. These results favorably compare with other single-agent response rates. Combination chemotherapy, however, can result in up to a 90% complete response rate in patients with metastatic disease *(110)*. Ongoing studies are evaluating the role of topotecan in this setting.

Phase II trials also have been conducted in children with refractory CNS tumors. Pediatric patients with CNS tumors ($n = 45$) were treated with a 24-hour continuous infusion of topotecan (5.5–7.5 mg/m^2). Practically no activity was observed; only one patient (2%) had a partial response *(111)*. Similar results were seen in another study evaluating a 72-hour continuous infusion of topotecan (1.0–1.25 mg/m^2/day) in pediatric patients. In the 88 patients able to be evaluated, there were no complete or partial responses *(112)*. Although the response rates to topotecan were low, there were some patients in these studies who had an extended period of stable disease.

4.3.3. Non-Small-Cell Lung Cancer

Several phase II trials have evaluated the efficacy of topotecan using the standard dosing schedule of topotecan in patients with advanced nonsmall-cell lung cancer (NSCLC). Response rates between 0% and 15 % have been reported with a median survival of 8–9 months *(113–116)*. Notably, in the study with the highest response rates, subpopulation analysis indicated that patients with squamous cell carcinoma (5/14, 36%) were more likely to respond than were patients with non-squamous cell carcinoma (1/26, 4%) (114). To validate this result, additional patients with advanced squamous cell carcinoma were enrolled in the study; of 29 total patients able to be evaluated, 7 had partial responses (24%), with a median survival of 10 months *(117)*.

In addition to the daily × five regimen, clinical trials have also evaluated different dosing schedules and routes of administration in patients with NSCLC. Two studies examining a 21-day continuous infusion of topotecan found no advantage over the conventional 5-day dosing regimen *(115,118)*. Recently, the efficacy of 2.3 mg/m^2/day oral topotecan administered for 5 days once every 3 weeks was also evaluated. Although no complete or partial responses were observed, the overall median survival was 40 weeks and a palliative effect on disease-related symptoms was observed *(119)*. Consequently, the utility of topotecan warrants continued evaluation in NSCLC.

4.3.4. Gastrointestinal Malignancies

Topotecan has minimal activity in colorectal, pancreatic, esophageal, and gastric tumors. Unlike the CPT derivative irinotecan, which is active against colorectal tumors, clinical trials evaluating topotecan have failed to demonstrate a significant effect. When the standard dosing regimen of topotecan was used, response rates of 4–7% were observed *(120,121)*. Slightly higher doses of topotecan (3.5 mg/m^2/day for 5 days once every 3 weeks) with G-CSF support in fluoropyrimidine-refractory patients resulted in no responders and a median survival of only 16 weeks *(11)*. Poor response rates also have been observed in colorectal patients receiving a 21-day continuous infusion of topotecan (0.5–0.7 mg/m^2/day) *(46,68)*, and in patients with advanced gastric cancer treated with the standard dosing regimen *(122,123)*. Similarly, topotecan has limited efficacy in pancreatic cancer with response rates of 0–10% for the standard regimen and 8% in patients receiving a 0.5 mg/m^2/day 21-day continuous infusion *(124–126)*. No significant antineoplastic activity was observed when topotecan was given to esophageal carcinoma patients as either a 1.5 mg/m^2/day 24-hour continuous infusion or by the standard regimen *(127,128)*. Although these studies were performed in a small number of chemotherapy-resistant patients, enthusiasm for future research with topotecan in the treatment of gastrointestinal tumors is minimal.

4.3.5. CNS Malignancies

Because topotecan has good CNS penetration *(29,30)*, clinical trials have evaluated the activity of topotecan in CNS malignancies. Patients with newly diagnosed or recurrent malignant gliomas were treated with a continuous infusion of topotecan (2.6 mg/m^2) for 72 hours. Partial responses were seen in 9% of the 63 patients able to be evaluated. The response rates of patients with newly diagnosed disease and recurrent disease were 12% and 8%, respectively. Notably, none of the 28 patients with recurrent glioblastoma multiforme had a response to this therapy *(129)*. Other trials have evaluated the efficacy of topotecan when it is administered by the daily × five dosing schedule. Thirty-one patients with recurrent malignant glioma were treated (1.5 mg/m^2/day); 6% had either a complete or partial response *(130)*. Similarly, 33 patients with progressive glioma were treated (1.25–1.5 mg/m^2/day); 1 patient (3%) experienced a partial response to the therapy *(131)*. Although these response rates are dismal, they are consistent with the response rates observed for established therapies such as dacarbazine and temozolomide *(132,133)*.

4.3.6. Head and Neck Malignancies

The anticancer activity of topotecan also has been assessed in head and neck tumors. A phase II trial evaluated the efficacy of topotecan (1.5 mg/m^2 as a 24-hour continuous infusion on days 1, 8,15, and 22 of a 35-day cycle) in patients with metastatic or recurrent squamous cell carcinoma of the head and neck. Neither chemotherapy-naive (n = 16) nor previously treated patients (n = 16) responded to the therapy *(134)*. Similarly, no responses were observed when patients with recurrent metastatic squamous cell carcinoma of the head and neck were treated with the standard regiment of topotecan (n = 21) *(135)*. In another study evaluating the efficacy of the standard dosing regimen of topotecan, however, 14% of patients (n = 22) with advanced squamous cell cancer of the head and neck responded *(136)*.

4.3.7. Breast Cancer

Although many doses and schedules have been evaluated, topotecan has shown only modest efficacy in patients with advanced breast cancer. Response rates of 10% have been observed in two studies evaluating the effectiveness of the conventional regimen of topotecan in advanced breast cancer patients who had failed front-line therapy *(137,138)*. A 21-day continuous infusion of 0.6 mg/m^2/day every 4 weeks, a 30-minute infusion every 3 weeks (22.5 mg/m^2), and a 1.5 mg/m^2 24-hour continuous infusion every week resulted in response rates of 15%, 5%, and 0%, respectively

(118,139). Greater response rates (37%) were observed in a recent study evaluating the conventional dosing regimen in breast cancer patients with bidimensionally measurable brain metastases, suggesting that topotecan may be an effective treatment alternative for this patient population *(140)*.

4.3.8. Endometrial Cancer

An emerging use for topotecan may be in the treatment of metastatic or recurrent endometrial cancer. Historically, single-agent therapy has achieved an approximately 20% response rate *(141)*. Topotecan achieved a similar response rate (7.5% complete response, 12.5% partial response) in patients with advanced or recurrent endometrial cancer. The initial dose (1.5 mg/m^2 daily for 5 days every 3 weeks, 1.2 mg/m^2 for patients with prior radiation) was associated with unexpected toxicities, so the dose was reduced to 1.0 mg/m^2 daily for 5 days every 3 weeks (0.8 mg/m^2 for patients with prior radiation) *(142)*. Less impressive response rates were observed in another study in which patients were treated with a similar dose and schedule. Only 9% of patients had a partial or complete response, but 55% of patients achieved stable disease *(143)*. Several studies are ongoing that will clarify the potential use of topotecan in endometrial cancer.

4.3.9. Other Tumors

Topotecan has modest activity in the treatment of cervical cancer. Response rates from 12% to 19% have been observed in patients with recurrent disease *(144–146)*; chemotherapy-naive patients 19% had a complete or partial response *(147)*. Clinical trials assessing the anticancer activity of topotecan in prostate cancer *(148,149)*, malignant melanoma *(150)*, renal cell carcinoma *(150)*, and hepatocellular cancer *(151)* have also been conducted. Topotecan did not produce significant response rates in any of these trials.

5. TOPOTECAN IN COMBINATION THERAPY

5.1. Overview and Rationale

Combination therapy of active drugs from different classes has become a mainstay in the treatment of tumors. Ideally, drug combinations should contain agents that, when used alone, have the capacity to induce a complete response in some patients. If possible, drugs should be chosen that have different mechanisms of action, different toxicity profiles, different mechanisms of resistance, and have shown synergy in vitro. Each drug in the combination should be administered at its optimal dose and schedule. Using these criteria, topotecan is well suited for use in multiple-drug regimens because it has a unique mechanism of action and it is relatively non–cross-resistant with other anticancer agents. Preclinical studies have demonstrated that topotecan in combination with cisplatin, paclitaxel, radiation, and cyclophosphamide are synergistic, providing the rational support for the clinical evaluation of these combinations *(152–157)*. Clinical trials have evaluated the utility of topotecan in combination with platinum compounds, antimicrotubule agents, TOP-II inhibitors, alkylating agents, antimetabolites, anthracyclines, and radiation.

Sound clinical and mechanistic rationale formed the basis for the clinical trials evaluating the combination of platinum compounds and topotecan. Both cisplatin and topotecan are effective in treating ovarian and SCLC tumors. Indeed, cisplatin is a commonly used front-line therapy for these cancers. Despite their overlapping antitumor activity, the mechanism of action and principle dose-limiting toxicities of these agents do not overlap. Myelosuppression is the dose-limiting toxicity for topotecan, whereas nephrotoxicity and neurotoxicity are dose-limiting for cisplatin. As with cisplatin, paclitaxel is used as a front-line treatment of ovarian cancer and has been evaluated in combination with topotecan. However, the overlapping myelosuppression may limit the utility of this combination.

Topotecan has also been evaluated in combination with TOP-II inhibitors such as etoposide and doxorubicin. As with TOP-I, TOP-II is a nuclear enzyme that regulates DNA topology. Preclinical studies have shown that in athymic mice with a SW480 colon cancer xenograft, treatment with topotecan caused a transient and reversible increase in TOP-IIα levels. Sequential administration of a TOP-I inhibitor followed by a TOP-II inhibitor resulted in enhanced cytotoxicity *(158–160)*. These preclinical results formed the basis for the clinical trials of topotecan and TOP-II inhibitors and highlight the importance of sequencing issues in evaluating combination therapy regimens. Indeed, the sequence of administration is important in many of the topotecan drug combination regimens being evaluated. For instance, significantly higher rates of neutropenia and thrombocytopenia were observed when cisplatin (50 mg/m^2 on day 1) was given before topotecan (0.75 mg/m^2/day on days 1–5) compared with when it was given after topotecan (50 mg/m^2 on day 5). The increased toxicity may be caused, in part, by cisplatin-induced alterations in renal function that reduced the renal elimination of topotecan *(161)*. Although numerous clinical trials have evaluated topotecan with other cytotoxic agents to define the optimal dose and schedule of the drug combination, this discussion will focus primarily on how the results of Phase II and III clinical trials are defining the place of topotecan drug combinations in cancer therapy.

5.2. Topotecan Combination Therapy and Ovarian Cancer

Combination regimens with topotecan have been assessed as front-line therapies for the treatment of ovarian cancer. Topotecan was evaluated in a Phase II trial in combination with carboplatin and paclitaxel in 18 patients with advanced epithelial ovarian cancer. Topotecan (1.0 mg/m^2/day on days 1–3), carboplatin (AUC 5 on day 3), and paclitaxel (175 mg/m^2 on day 3) resulted in an overall response rate of 88%, with 28% of the patients achieving a complete response. Neutropenia was the major toxicity, with grade 3 or 4 toxicity occurring in 94% of the patients *(162)*. The response rate is better than those observed with carboplatin and paclitaxel in phase III studies (64–75%); however, the toxicity does not justify the benefit *(163,164)*. Rather than use all three drugs concurrently, two phase III trials are evaluating the sequential administration of six cycles of carboplatin and paclitaxel (carboplatin AUC 5 and paclitaxel 175 mg/m^2, 3-hour infusion) followed by observation or four cycles of topotecan (1.25 or 1.5 mg/m^2 per day × 5 days every 21 days). Both studies have completed enrollment, and preliminary results were recently presented. Based on the preliminary data, this sequential administration approach does not appear to prolong the progression-free survival; however, few events had occurred and further follow-up is planned *(165,166)*. The feasibility of administering sequential couplets of cisplatin and topotecan followed by paclitaxel and cisplatin as a front-line treatment was evaluated in 34 patients with advanced epithelial ovarian cancer. Four cycles of cisplatin (50 mg/m^2 on day 1) and topotecan (0.75 mg/m^2 on days 1–5 every 3 weeks) were followed by interval debulking of the tumor (if necessary). Subsequently, four cycles of paclitaxel (135 mg/m^2 on day 1) and cisplatin (75 mg/m^2 on day 2 every 3 weeks) were administered. The overall response rate was 78%. These results compare favorably with the response rate of 73% observed in the Gynecologic Oncology Group 111 trial that established paclitaxel and cisplatin as a front-line therapy in the treatment of advanced epithelial ovarian cancer *(167)*.

Some topotecan combinations have shown efficacy in patients with recurrent ovarian cancer. The combination of topotecan and gemcitabine has resulted in overall response rates of 12–64% *(168,169)*. However, these studies have had only limited number of patients; larger trials should be conducted to determine the efficacy of this combination. Topotecan also has been evaluated with paclitaxel. A 96-hour infusion of topotecan (2.8 mg/m^2) and paclitaxel (100 mg/m^2) was administered to 25 patients with recurrent ovarian cancer. After treatment, 28% of the patients had a partial response *(170)*. Similar response rates were observed when 36 patients received 1.25 mg/m^2 topotecan on days 1–3 and 600 mg/m^2 cyclophosphamide on day 1. A response was observed in 25% of patients and stable disease was achieved in another 44% *(171)*. These response rates are noteworthy considering the poor prognosis of this patient population. Currently, a large phase III trial (Gynecologic Oncology Group 0182-International Collaborative Ovarian Neoplasm 5) has been launched evaluating five different treatment regimens in chemotherapy-naive ovarian cancer patients: (Arm 1), standard regimen of carboplatin-paclitaxel (day 1); (Arm 2), standard carboplatin-paclitaxel (day 1) plus gemcitabine (days 1 and 8); (Arm 3), standard carboplatin-paclitaxel (day 1) plus PLD (every other cycle); (Arm 4), standard carboplatin-paclitaxel (day 1) plus topotecan (days 1–3) alternating with standard carboplatin-paclitaxel; and (Arm 5), carboplatin (day 8) plus gemcitabine (days 1 and 8) alternating with standard carboplatin-paclitaxel *(172,173)*. The results from this study may more clearly define the role of topotecan combination therapy as first-line chemotherapy in patients with ovarian cancer.

5.3. Topotecan Combination Therapy and Lung Cancer

5.3.1. SCLC

Because of topotecan's activity in recurrent SCLC, the role of topotecan in combination therapy as a first-line agent has been evaluated. The three drug combination (cisplatin, paclitaxel, and topotecan [with G-CSF support]) was assessed in chemotherapy-naive patients with extensive disease ($n = 37$). Patients were treated with cisplatin (40 mg/m^2), paclitaxel (85 mg/m^2), and topotecan (2.25 mg/m^2) on a weekly basis. G-CSF (5 μg/kg/day) was administered on days 3–5. The overall response rate was 81%, with 22% of patients achieving a complete response *(174)*. A similar study replaced cisplatin with carboplatin; 105 patients were treated with 135 mg/m^2 paclitaxel and AUC = 5 carboplatin on day 1 and 0.75 mg/m^2 topotecan on days 1–3. The regimen resulted in response rates of 88% and 93% in patients with extensive and limited disease, respectively *(175)*.

Topotecan (1.0–1.25 mg/m^2/day on days 1–5) and paclitaxel (135 mg/m^2 on day 5) were assessed in 28 patients able to be evaluated with untreated extensive disease with response rates of 60% *(176)*. Sequential paclitaxel-topotecan with G-CSF support had a similar overall response rate (56%) when 43 untreated patients with extensive-stage SCLC were treated with three cycles of paclitaxel (250 mg/m^2 over 3 hours every 2 weeks) followed by three cycles of topotecan (2.5 mg/m^2 for 5 days every 3 weeks). Despite the G-CSF support, significant hematological toxicity was observed with this regimen *(177)*. The response rates from these studies are comparable to those seen with standard front-line combination therapies (65–85%) *(178)*. Topotecan, in combination with cisplatin, has also been evaluated in SCLC patients as a second-line therapy. Topotecan (0.75 mg/m^2/d on days 1–5) in combination with cisplatin (60 mg/m^2 on day 1) resulted in response rates of 24% and 29% for resistant ($n = 42$) and sensitive ($n = 68$) patients, respectively *(179)*. These response rates are similar to those reported with topotecan monotherapy *(70,100,101,114)*.

5.3.2. Non-Small-Cell Lung Cancer

Clinical trials evaluating the efficacy of topotecan combination therapy in patients with NSCLC have found modest activity. Topotecan, in combination with etoposide, was administered to 19 patients with advanced NSCLC. Patients received topotecan as a continuous 72-hour infusion (0.85 mg/m^2/day) on days 1–3 of therapy. On days 7–9, patients were treated with oral etoposide (100 mg twice daily). Only one partial response (5%) was observed. This study sequenced the drugs to take advantage of elevated TOP-II levels seen after the administration of a TOP-I inhibitor *(160)*. However, this dosing schedule does not appear to be optimal because TOP-II levels may return to baseline levels within 24 hours of exposure to a TOP-I inhibitor *(180)*. The combination of gemcitabine and topotecan has been studied both as first-line therapy and in previously treated patients with advanced disease. As first-line therapy, patients (n = 53) treated with topotecan (1 mg/m^2 on days 1–5) and gemcitabine (1000 mg/m^2 (days 1 and 15) had a median survival of 7.6 months. One-year survival was 39% *(181)*. In previously treated patients with advanced NSCLC, the combination of topotecan and gemcitabine has resulted in response rates of 18–34%, indicating that further studies with this drug combination may be warranted *(182,183)*.

Preliminary data evaluating two other regimens also show promising results. A 42% response rate was observed when topotecan (0.5–1.0 mg/m^2/day on days 1–5) and vinorelbine (20–30 mg/m^2/day on days 1 and 5) were administered to 26 patients with recurrent or metastatic NSCLC *(184)*. After 47 patients with untreated, nonresectable, advanced NSCLC were treated with topotecan (0.5 mg/m^2/day on days 1–5) and carboplatin (AUC = 5 on day 1), response rates of 13% were observed. An additional 36% were deemed to have achieved some treatment benefit due to prolonged disease stabilization *(185)*.

5.4. Topotecan Combination Therapy and Hematological Malignancies

As a result of topotecan's single-agent activity in hematological malignancies, several studies have investigated the effectiveness of topotecan in combination with existing therapies. In one study, patients with MDS and chronic myelomonocytic leukemia were treated with topotecan (1.25 mg/m^2/day continuous iv infusion for 5 days) and cytarabine (ara-C) (1.0 g/m^2 daily for 5 days). Overall, 56% of the 86 patients had a complete remission; the median duration of remission was 34 weeks. Of the 59 patients with MDS, 61% had a complete remission. Notably, this regimen was effective in patients with both good-risk and poor-risk MDS (complete remission rates of 70% and 56%, respectively) *(186)*. The drug combination topotecan (1.0–2.5 mg/m^2/day) and etoposide (150 mg/m^2/day) was administered for 5 days to patients with recurrent or refractory non-Hodgkin's lymphoma. The overall response rate (n = 21) was 38%. Three patients (14%) achieved a complete remission *(187)*. Similarly, the combination of topotecan and paclitaxel was effective in treating patients with relapsed or refractory non-Hodgkin's lymphoma. Of the 66 patients able to be evaluated who received topotecan (1 mg/m^2/day on days 1–5) and paclitaxel (200 mg/m^2 on day 1), 48% responded to therapy *(188)*.

Clinical trials have evaluated the utility of topotecan combination therapy in patients with refractory or relapsed AML or acute lymphocytic leukemia. Many of these studies have evaluated three drug combinations in which topotecan and ara-C are combined with a third agent. When cyclophosphamide (500 mg/m^2 given every 12 hours on days 1 and 3) was combined with ara-C (2 g/m^2 daily on days 2–6) and topotecan (1.25 mg/m^2/day continuous infusion days 2–6), 17% of the 63 patients able to be evaluated had a complete remission. Subpopulation analysis showed that 23% of AML patients and 9% of acute lymphocytic leukemia patients responded to this therapy *(189)*. Higher response rates were observed in a three-drug study evaluating topotecan, ara-C, and idarubicin. Twenty-seven patients with refractory or relapse AML and high-risk MDS were treated with idarubicin (12 mg/m^2 days 1–3), ara-c (1 g/m^2 on days 1–5), and topotecan (1.25 mg/m^2/day on days 1–5). Overall, 52% achieved a complete remission (59% of AML and 40% of MDS patients) *(190)*. The response rates were not as impressive when Mylotarg (9 mg/m^2 on day 1) was added to topotecan (1.25 mg/m^2 on days 1–5) and ara-C (1 g/m^2 days 1–5) in patients with refractory AML or advanced MDS and significant toxicity was observed. Two of 17 patients (12%) had a complete response. Notably, 29% of patients had grade 3/4 hepatic transaminitis and one patient died of hepatic venoocclusive disease *(189)*.

A three-arm study has compared two drug combinations using topotecan and the TOP-II inhibitor, etoposide. AML patients were randomized to either topotecan and ara-C (n = 10), topotecan followed by etoposide (n = 15), or etoposide (n = 12) followed by topotecan. Of the 37 patients, only one complete remission was observed and that was in the topotecan and ara-C arm. As a result of the lack of activity, accrual into the treatment arms was terminated and it was concluded that none of the three treatment arms had antileukemic activity *(191)*. Similarly, minimal activity and significant toxicity was observed in non-Hodgkin's lymphoma patients treated with topotecan (1.25 mg/m^2 days 1–5) and etoposide (50 mg days 6–12) *(192)*. However, when topotecan treatment was followed by two TOP-II inhibitors, mitoxantrone and etoposide, significant response rates were observed in heavily pretreated patients with refractory acute leukemia. Seventeen patients received 1.5 mg/m^2 topotecan on days 1–3, 100 mg/m^2 etoposide, and 10 mg/m^2 mitoxantrone on days 4, 5, 9, and 10. Five patients (29%) had a complete or partial remission and an additional four patients (24%) had no evidence of disease, but had platelet counts of less than 100,000. Notably, topotecan resulted in increased TOP-II levels and the magnitude of TOP-II increase correlated with response to therapy *(193)*.

5.5. Topotecan High-Dose Chemotherapy and Transplant

Recent studies evaluating the efficacy of high-dose chemotherapy regimens containing topotecan followed by progenitor cell support have shown promising results *(194–196)*. Nineteen patients with previously untreated advanced-stage ovarian cancer received two cycles of carboplatin (AUC = 5) and paclitaxel (175 mg/m^2). Peripheral blood progenitor cells were collected before the induction of three cycles of high-dose therapy in which patients received topotecan (1.5–4.5 mg/m^2 daily for 5 days), paclitaxel (250 mg/m^2 over 24 hours), and carboplatin (AUC 12–16). Peripheral blood progenitor cell support permitted all three drugs to be administered with acceptable nonhematological toxicity. The overall clinical response rate was 95%, with 73% of patients achieving a complete clinical response *(196)*. Similarly, impressive response rates were found when previously treated advanced ovarian cancer patients were treated with cyclophosphamide (1 g/m^2/day on days –6, –5 and –4), melphalan (70 mg/m^2/day on days –3 and –2), and topotecan (1.25–4.0 mg/m^2/day on days –6 to –2), with stem cells infused on day 0. Of the 30 patients able to be evaluated, 93% had a response (50% complete response, 43% partial response) *(195)*. Although the response rates in these studies are promising, randomized studies are required to determine if these high-dose chemotherapy regimens are more effective than conventional therapy.

6. CLINICAL PERSPECTIVES AND FUTURE DIRECTIONS

Topotecan is approved as salvage therapy for patients with ovarian or SCLC. Clinical trials also have demonstrated promising antitumor activity in hematologic malignancies and squamous cell lung cancer. As a result of its unique mechanism of action and non–cross-resistance with standard therapies, combination regimens with topotecan should continue to be assessed to determine the role of topotecan as a component of first- or second-line drug combinations. Because previous studies have demonstrated that single-agent therapy may be just as effective as combination therapy in ovarian cancer, the addition of topotecan to front-line agents may not have a significant impact on survival rates *(197,198)*. The role of topotecan in combination therapy for lung cancer may be more promising because significant survival advantage has been demonstrated with combination therapy *(65)*. Similarly, high-dose chemotherapy regimens with topotecan may have utility in the bone marrow transplant setting. Myelosuppression is the dose-limiting toxicity; only at very high doses of topotecan is significant nonhematologic dose-limiting toxicity observed (i.e., mucositis, diarrhea, and erythema). As several studies have demonstrated, however, sequence and timing issues may be important in determining the efficacy of topotecan in combination regimens. Additional studies are warranted to characterize sequencing effects and maximize the therapeutic benefit of topotecan combination regimens.

Clinical trials continue to assess the optimal route of administration, dose, and schedule of topotecan. Clearly, the development of alternate routes of administration is a promising area of topotecan research that may impact the future potential of this drug. In ovarian cancer patients, high doses of topotecan can be effectively administered specifically to the peritoneal cavity using intraperitoneal administration of topotecan. Because the dose-limiting toxicity of intraperitoneal administration of topotecan is not myelosuppression, this is an attractive therapy to add to front-line systemic regimens that are myelosuppressive.

Clinical trials with oral topotecan demonstrate the activity of this therapy. It is likely, however, that because of physician reimbursement issues, the full potential of oral topotecan will be realized in combination regimens containing iv administration of other agents. The feasibility of administering oral topotecan with iv agents is currently being examined *(199)*. Preclinical results from liposomal formulations of topotecan indicate that this dosage form may provide a significant therapeutic advantage over free topotecan.

The currently approved dosing regimen (daily administration of topotecan for 5 consecutive days once every 3 weeks) can be quite inconvenient for patients, especially those who are elderly, frail, or have limited access to treatment facilities. The development of other agents, such as pegylated liposomal doxorubicin, which have comparable activity and a more convenient dosing schedule, emphasize the need to continue to investigate the optimal schedule of administration for topotecan. The CPT analog irinotecan is approved to be dosed on a more convenient weekly schedule. Because topotecan is combined with other agents, dosing schedules that maximize the clinical effectiveness of the drug while minimizing the inconvenience to the patient should be carefully considered.

Exciting new agents, such as monoclonal antibodies, tyrosine kinase inhibitors, and antiangiogenesis are being developed as novel treatments for cancer. Preclinical data suggest that topotecan may be effectively combined with some of these agents. Topotecan has antiangiogenic activity *(200–202)* and when combined with anti-VEGF therapy suppresses tumor growth in an animal model *(203,204)*. Changes in EGFR expression and/or function may influence sensitivity to topotecan and coadministration with a HER inhibitor has been shown to alter the accumulation and cytotoxic potential of topotecan *(205,206)*. This is an exciting frontier in topotecan research, which may translate into drug combinations that have broader and more effective clinical applications.

REFERENCES

1. Wall ME, Wani MC, Cook CE, Palmer KH, McPhail AT, Lim GA. 1966 Plant antitumor agents: I. The isolation and structure of camptothecin, a novel alkaloid leukemia and tumor inhibitor from *camptotheca accuminata.* J Am Chem Soc 88:3888–3890.
2. Kingsbury WD, Boehm JC, Jakas DR, et al. 1991 Synthesis of water-soluble (aminoalkyl)camptothecin analogues: inhibition of topoisomerase I and antitumor activity. J Med Chem 34:98–107.
3. Hertzberg RP, Caranfa MJ, Holden KG, et al. 1989 Modification of the hydroxy lactone ring of camptothecin: inhibition of mammalian topoisomerase I and biological activity. J Med Chem 32:715–720.
4. Hsiang YH, Liu LF. 1988 Identification of mammalian DNA topoisomerase I as an intracellular target of the anticancer drug camptothecin. Cancer Res 48:1722–1726.
5. D'Arpa P, Liu LF. 1989 Topoisomerase-targeting antitumor drugs. Biochim Biophys Acta 989:163–177.
6. Stewart L, Redinbo MR, Qiu X, Hol WG, Champoux JJ. 1998 A model for the mechanism of human topoisomerase I. Science 279:1534–1541.
7. Redinbo MR, Stewart L, Kuhn P, Champoux JJ, Hol WG. 1998 Crystal structures of human topoisomerase I in covalent and noncovalent complexes with DNA. Science 279:1504–1513.
8. Grochow LB, Rowinsky EK, Johnson R, et al. 1992 Pharmacokinetics and pharmacodynamics of topotecan in patients with advanced cancer. Drug Metab Dispos 20:706–713.
9. van Warmerdam LJ, ten Bokkel Huinink WW, Rodenhuis S, et al. 1995 Phase I clinical and pharmacokinetic study of topotecan administered by a 24-hour continuous infusion. J Clin Oncol 13:1768–1776.
10. Saylors RL, Stewart CF, Zamboni WC, et al. 1998 Phase I study of topotecan in combination with cyclophosphamide in pediatric patients with malignant solid tumors: a Pediatric Oncology Group Study. J Clin Oncol 16:945–952.
11. Rowinsky EK, Baker SD, Burks K, O'Reilly S, Donehower RC, Grochow LB. 1998 High-dose topotecan with granulocyte-colony stimulating factor in fluoropyrimidine-refractory colorectal cancer: a phase II and pharmacodynamic study. Ann Oncol 9:173–180.
12. Saltz L, Sirott M, Young C, et al. 1993 Phase I clinical and pharmacology study of topotecan given daily for 5 consecutive days to patients with advanced solid tumors, with attempt at dose intensification using recombinant granulocyte colony-stimulating factor. J Natl Cancer Inst 85:1499–1507.
13. Wall JG, Burris HA, Von Hoff DD, et al. 1992 A phase I clinical and pharmacokinetic study of the topoisomerase I inhibitor topotecan (SK&F 104864) given as an intravenous bolus every 21 days. Anticancer Drugs 3:337–345.
14. Haas NB, LaCreta FP, Walczak J, et al. 1994 Phase I/pharmacokinetic study of topotecan by 24-hour continuous infusion weekly. Cancer Res. 54:1220–1226.
15. Loos WJ, Gelderblom HJ, Verweij J, Brouwer E, de Jonge MJ, Sparreboom A. 2000 Gender-dependent pharmacokinetics of topotecan in adult patients. Anticancer Drugs 11:673–680.
16. Schellens JH, Creemers GJ, Beijnen JH, et al. 1996 Bioavailability and pharmacokinetics of oral topotecan: a new topoisomerase I inhibitor. Br J Cancer 73: 1268–1271.

17. Herben VM, Rosing H, ten Bokkel Huinink WW, et al. 1999 Oral topotecan: bioavailablity and effect of food co-administration. Br J Cancer 80:1380–1386.
18. Kuhn J, Rizzo J, Eckardt J, et al. 1995 Phase I bioavailability study of oral topotecan. Proc Am Soc Clin Oncol 14:474.
19. Zamboni WC, Bowman LC, Tan M, et al. 1999 Interpatient variability in bioavailability of the intravenous formulation of topotecan given orally to children with recurrent solid tumors. Cancer Chemother Pharmacol 43:454–460.
20. Gerrits CJ, Schellens JH, Burris H, et al. 1999 A comparison of clinical pharmacodynamics of different administration schedules of oral topotecan (Hycamtin). Clin Cancer Res 5:69–75.
21. Rowinsky EK, Grochow LB, Sartorius SE, et al. 1996 Phase I and pharmacologic study of high doses of the topoisomerase I inhibitor topotecan with granulocyte colony-stimulating factor in patients with solid tumors. J Clin Oncol 14:1224–1235.
22. Rowinsky EK, Grochow LB, Hendricks CB, et al. 1992 Phase I and pharmacologic study of topotecan: a novel topoisomerase I inhibitor. J Clin Oncol 10:647–656.
23. Tubergen DG, Stewart CF, Pratt CB, et al. 1996 Phase I trial and pharmacokinetic (PK) and pharmacodynamics (PD) study of topotecan using a five-day course in children with refractory solid tumors: a Pediatric Oncology Group Study. J Pediatr Hematol Oncol 18:352–361.
24. van Warmerdam LJ, Creemers GJ, Rodenhuis S, et al. 1996 Pharmacokinetics and pharmacodynamics of topotecan given on a daily-times-five schedule in phase II clinical trials using a limited-sampling procedure. Cancer Chemother Pharmacol 38:254–260.
25. Abbruzzese JL, Madden T, Sugarman SM, et al. 1996 Phase I clinical and plasma and cellular pharmacological study of topotecan without and with granulocyte colony-stimulating factor. Clin Cancer Res 2:1489–1497.
26. Furman WL, Baker SD, Pratt CB, Rivera GK, Evans WE, Stewart CF. 1996 Escalating systemic exposure of continuous infusion topotecan in children with recurrent acute leukemia. J Clin Oncol 14:1504–1511.
27. Herben VM, ten Bokkel Huinink WW, Beijnen JH. 1996 Clinical pharmacokinetics of topotecan. Clin Pharmacokinet 31:85–102.
28. Kaye SB, Workman P, Graham MA, Cassidy J, Jodrell D. 1993 Pharmacokinetics and early clinical studies of selected new drugs. Cancer Surv 17:371–396.
29. El-Gizawy SA, Hedaya MA. 1999 Comparative brain tissue distribution of camptothecin and topotecan in the rat. Cancer Chemother Pharmacol 43:364–370.
30. Blaney SM, Cole DE, Balis FM, Godwin K, Poplack DG. 1993 Plasma and cerebrospinal fluid pharmacokinetic study of topotecan in nonhuman primates. Cancer Res 53:725–727.
31. Baker SD, Heideman RL, Crom WR, Kuttesch JF, Gajjar A, Stewart CF. 1996 Cerebrospinal fluid pharmacokinetics and penetration of continuous infusion topotecan in children with central nervous system tumors. Cancer Chemother Pharmacol 37:195–202.
32. Rosing H, Herben VM, van Gortel-van Zomeren DM, et al. 1997 Isolation and structural confirmation of *N*-desmethyl topotecan, a metabolite of topotecan. Cancer Chemother Pharmacol 39:498–504.
33. Rosing H, van Zomeren DM, Doyle E, et al. 1999 Quantification of topotecan and its metabolite *N*-desmethyltopotecan in human plasma, urine and faeces by high-performance liquid chromatographic methods. J Chromatogr B Biomed Sci Appl 727:191–203.

34. Borkowski JM, Duerr M, Donehower RC, et al. 1994 Relation between age and clearance rate of nine investigational anticancer drugs from phase I pharmacokinetic data. Cancer Chemother Pharmacol 33:493–496.
35. O'Reilly S, Rowinsky E, Slichenmyer W, et al. 1996 Phase I and pharmacologic studies of topotecan in patients with impaired hepatic function. J Natl Cancer Inst 88:817–824.
36. Armstrong D, O'Reilly S. 1998 Clinical guidelines for managing topotecan-related hematologic toxicity. Oncologist 3:4–10.
37. Martin D, Hall DJ, Kincaid K. 2003 Phase II trial of weekly topotecan in advanced or recurrent endometrial adenocarcinoma [abstract]. Proc Am Soc Clin Oncol 22:491.
38. Morris R, Munkarah A. 2002 Alternate dosing schedules for topotecan in the treatment of recurrent ovarian cancer. Oncologist 7(Suppl. 5):29–35.
39. Homesley HD, Hall DJ, Martin DA, et al. 2001 A dose-escalating study of weekly bolus topotecan in previously treated ovarian cancer patients. Gynecol Oncol 83(2):394–399.
40. Rocondo G, Abbruzzese J, Newman B, et al. 1991 Phase I trial of topotecan administered by a 24-hour infusion. Proc Am Assoc Cancer Res 32:1229.
41. Sabiers J, Berger N, Berger S, Haaga JR, Hoppel CR, Wilson JKV. 1993 Phase I trial of topotecan administered as a 72 hour infusion. Proc Am Assoc Cancer Res 34:426.
42. Rowinsky EK, Adjei A, Donehower RC, et al. 1994 Phase I and pharmacodynamic study of the topoisomerase I-inhibitor topotecan in patients with refractory acute leukemia. J Clin Oncol 12:2193–2203.
43. Kantarjian HM, Beran M, Ellis A, et al. 1993 Phase I study of topotecan, a new topoisomerase I inhibitor, in patients with refractory or relapsed acute leukemia. Blood 81:1146–1151.
44. Burris HA, Awada A, Kuhn JG, et al. 1994 Phase I and pharmacokinetic studies of topotecan administered as a 72 or 120 h continuous infusion. Anticancer Drugs 5:394–402.
45. Hochster H, Liebes L, Speyer J, et al. 1994 Phase I trial of low-dose continuous topotecan infusion in patients with cancer: an active and well-tolerated regimen. J Clin Oncol 12:553–539.
46. Hochster H, Hibrahim J, Liebes L, O'Dwyer P, Benson A. 1997 Phase II study of 21-day topotecan continuous infusion for metastatic colorectal cancer (ECOG study 4293). Proc Am Soc Clin Oncol 16:1032.
47. Frangoul H, Ames MM, Mosher RB, et al. 1999 Phase I study of topotecan administered as a 21-day continous infusion in children with recurrent solid tumors: a report from the Children's Cancer Group. Clin Cancer Res 5:3956–3962.
48. von Pawel J, Gatzemeier U, Pujol JL, et al. 2001 Phase II comparator study of oral versus intravenous topotecan in patients with chemosensitive small-cell lung cancer. J Clin Oncol 19:1743–1749.
49. Clarke-Pearson DL, Van Le L, Iveson T, et al. 2001 Oral topotecan as single-agent second-line chemotherapy in patients with advanced ovarian cancer. J Clin Oncol 19:3967–3975.
50. Gore M, Oza A, Rustin G, et al. 2002 A randomised trial of oral versus intravenous topotecan in patients with relapsed epithelial ovarian cancer. Eur J Cancer 38:57–63.

51. Gerrits CJ, Burris H, Schellens JH, et al. 1998 Five days of oral topotecan (Hycamtin), a phase I and pharmacological study in adult patients with solid tumours. Eur J Cancer 34:1030–1035.
52. Gerrits CJ, Burris H, Schellens JH, et al. 1998 Oral topotecan given once or twice daily for ten days: a phase I pharmacology study in adult patients with solid tumors. Clin Cancer Res 4:1153–1158.
53. Creemers GJ, Gerrits CJ, Eckardt JR, et al. 1997 Phase I and pharmacologic study of oral topotecan administered twice daily for 21 days to adult patients with solid tumors. J Clin Oncol 15:1087–1093.
54. Hofstra LS, Bos AM, de Vries EG, et al. 2001 A phase I and pharmacokinetic study of intraperitoneal topotecan. Br J Cancer 85:1627–1633.
55. Plaxe SC, Christen RD, O'Quigley J, et al. 1998 Phase I and pharmacokinetic study of intraperitoneal topotecan. Invest New Drugs 16:147–153.
56. Burke TG, Gao X. 1994 Stabilization of topotecan in low pH liposomes composed of distearoylphosphatidylcholine. J Pharm Sci 83:967–969.
57. Subramanian D, Muller MT. 1995 Liposomal encapsulation increases the activity of the topoisomerase I inhibitor topotecan. Oncol Res 7:461–469.
58. Tardi P, Choice E, Masin D, Redelmeier T, Bally M, Madden TD. 2000 Liposomal encapsulation of topotecan enhances anticancer efficacy in murine and human xenograft models. Cancer Res 60:3389–3393.
59. Verschraegen CF, Jaeckle K, Giovanella B, Knight V, Gilbert BE. 2000 Alternative administration of camptothecin analogues. Ann NY Acad Sci 922:237–426.
60. Blaney SM, Cole DE, Godwin K, Sung C, Poplack DG, Balis FM. 1995 Intrathecal administration of topotecan in nonhuman primates. Cancer Chemother Pharmacol 36:121–124.
61. Dowlati A, Levitan N, Gordon NH, et al. 2001 Phase II and pharmacokinetic/pharmacodynamic trial of sequential topoisomerase I and II inhibition with topotecan and etoposide in advanced non-small-cell lung cancer. Cancer Chemother Pharmacol 47:141–148.
62. von Pawel J, Schiller JH, Shepherd FA, et al. 1999 Topotecan versus cyclophosphamide, doxorubicin, and vincristine for the treatment of recurrent small-cell lung cancer. J Clin Oncol 17:658–667.
63. Grochow L, Slichenmyer W, Rowinsky E, Donehower R, Forastier A, Chen T-L. 1994 Phase I clinical and pharmacologic study of topotecan in patients with hepatic or renal dysfunction. Ann Oncol 5(Suppl.):191.
64. McGuire WP, Hoskins WJ, Brady MF, et al. 1995 Assessment of dose-intensive therapy in suboptimally debulked ovarian cancer: a Gynecologic Oncology Group study. J Clin Oncol 13:1589–1599.
65. Schiller JH. 2001 Current standards of care in small-cell and non-small-cell lung cancer. Oncology 61(Suppl. 1):3–13.
66. Saltz L, Janik JE. 1997 Topotecan and the treatment of recurrent ovarian cancer: is there a role for granulocyte colony-stimulating factor? Semin Oncol 24(Suppl. 5):S5-26–S5-30.
67. ten Bokkel Huinink W, Gore M, Carmichael J, et al. 1997 Topotecan versus paclitaxel for the treatment of recurrent epithelial ovarian cancer. J Clin Oncol 15:2183–2193.
68. Creemers GJ, Bolis G, Gore M, et al. 1996 Topotecan, an active drug in the second-line treatment of epithelial ovarian cancer: results of a large European phase II study. J Clin Oncol 14:3056–3061.

69. Beran M, Kantarjian H, O'Brien S, et al. 1996 Topotecan, a topoisomerase I inhibitor, is active in the treatment of myelodysplastic syndrome and chronic myelomonocytic leukemia. Blood 88:2473–2479.
70. von Pawel J, Depierre A, Hans K, et al. 1997 Topotecan (Hycamptin) in small cell lung cancer (SCLC) after failure of first line therapy: multicentre phase II study. Eur J Cancer 33(Suppl. 8):229.
71. Hochster H, Speyer J, Wadler S, et al. 1996 Phase II study of topotecan (TPT) 21-day infusion in platinum-treated ovarian cancer: a highly active regimen (A NYGOG study). Proc Am Soc Clin Oncol 15:285.
72. McGuire WP, Blessing JA, Bookman MA, Lentz SS, Dunton CJ. 2000 Topotecan has substantial antitumor activity as first-line salvage therapy in platinum-sensitive epithelial ovarian carcinoma: a Gynecologic Oncology Group Study. J Clin Oncol 18:1062–1067.
73. Zamboni WC, Gajjar AJ, Heideman RL, et al. 1998 Phenytoin alters the disposition of topotecan and *N*-desmethyl topotecan in a patient with medulloblastoma. Clin Cancer Res 4:783–789.
74. Stewart CF, Baker SD, Heideman RL, Jones D, Crom WR, Pratt CB. 1994 Clinical pharmacodynamics of continuous infusion topotecan in children: systemic exposure predicts hematologic toxicity. J Clin Oncol 12:1946–1954.
75. Zamboni WC, Houghton PJ, Johnson RK, et al. 1998 Probenecid alters topotecan systemic and renal disposition by inhibiting renal tubular secretion. J Pharmacol Exp Ther 284:89–94.
76. Woessner RD, Eng WK, Hofmann GA, et al. 1992 Camptothecin hyper-resistant P388 cells: drug-dependent reduction in topoisomerase I content. Oncol Res 4:481–488.
77. Yang CH, Schneider E, Kuo ML, Volk EL, Rocchi E, Chen YC. 2000 BCRP/MXR/ABCP expression in topotecan-resistant human breast carcinoma cells. Biochem Pharmacol 60:831–837.
78. Fujimori A, Harker WG, Kohlhagen G, Hoki Y, Pommier Y. 1995 Mutation at the catalytic site of topoisomerase I in CEM/C2, a human leukemia cell line resistant to camptothecin. Cancer Res 55:1339–1346.
79. Sorensen M, Sehested M, Jensen PB. 1995 Characterisation of a human small-cell lung cancer cell line resistant to the DNA topoisomerase I-directed drug topotecan. Br J Cancer 72:399–404.
80. Danks MK, Garrett KE, Marion RC, Whipple DO. 1996 Subcellular redistribution of DNA topoisomerase I in anaplastic astrocytoma cells treated with topotecan. Cancer Res 56:1664–1673.
81. Buckwalter CA, Lin AH, Tanizawa A, Pommier YG, Cheng YC, Kaufmann SH. 1996 RNA synthesis inhibitors alter the subnuclear distribution of DNA topoisomerase I. Cancer Res 56:1674–1681.
82. Mo YY, Yu Y, Shen Z, Beck WT. 2002 Nucleolar delocalization of human topoisomerase I in response to topotecan correlates with sumoylation of the protein. J Biol Chem 277:2958–2964.
83. Chang AY, Garrow G, Boros L, Asbury R, Pandya K, Keng P. 1995 Clinical and laboratory studies of topotecan in breast cancer. Proc Am Soc Clin Oncol 13:118.
84. Ejendal KF, Hrycyna CA. 2002 Multidrug resistance and cancer: the role of the human ABC transporter ABCG2. Curr Protein Pept Sci 3:503–511.
85. Bates SE, Robey R, Miyake K, Rao K, Ross DD, Litman T. 2001 The role of half-transporters in multidrug resistance. J Bioenerg Biomembr 33:503–511.

86. Maliepaard M, Nooter K, Ma J, et al. 1996 Relationship between P-glycoprotein, multidrug resistance-associated protein, and cellular accumulation of topoisomerase I inhibitors. Proc am Assoc Cancer Res 37:313.
87. Chen AY, Yu C, Potmesil M, Wall ME, Wani MC, Liu LF. 1991 Camptothecin overcomes MDR1-mediated resistance in human KB carcinoma cells. Cancer Res 51:6039–6044.
88. Hoki Y, Fujimori A, Pommier Y. 1997 Differential cytotoxicity of clinically important camptothecin derivatives in P-glycoprotein-overexpressing cell lines. Cancer Chemother Pharmacol 40:433–438.
89. Hendricks CB, Rowinsky EK, Grochow LB, Donehower RC, Kaufmann SH. 1992 Effect of P-glycoprotein expression on the accumulation and cytotoxicity of topotecan (SK&F 104864), a new camptothecin analogue. Cancer Res 52: 2268–2278.
90. Mattern MR, Hofmann GA, Polsky RM, Funk LR, McCabe FL, Johnson RK. 1993 In vitro and in vivo effects of clinically important camptothecin analogues on multidrug-resistant cells. Oncol Res 5:467–474.
91. Hoskins P, Eisenhauer E, Beare S, et al. 1998 Randomized phase II study of two schedules of topotecan in previously treated patients with ovarian cancer: a National Cancer Institute of Canada Clinical Trials Group study. J Clin Oncol 16:2233–2337.
92. Kudelka AP, Tresukosol D, Edwards CL, et al. 1996 Phase II study of intravenous topotecan as a 5-day infusion for refractory epithelial ovarian carcinoma. J Clin Oncol 14:1552–1557.
93. Swisher EM, Mutch DG, Rader JS, Elbendary A, Herzog TJ. 1997 Topotecan in platinum- and paclitaxel-resistant ovarian cancer. Gynecol Oncol 66:480–486.
94. Bookman MA, Malmstrom H, Bolis G, et al. 1998 Topotecan for the treatment of advanced epithelial ovarian cancer: an open-label phase II study in patients treated after prior chemotherapy that contained cisplatin or carboplatin and paclitaxel. J Clin Oncol 16:3345–3352.
95. Gordon A, Carmichael J, Malfetano J, et al. 1998 Final analysis of a phase III, randomized study of topotecan (T) vs paclitaxel (P) in advanced epithelial ovarian carcinoma (OC): International Topotecan Study Group [abstract]. Proc Am Soc Clin Oncol 17:abstr 1374.
96. Gore M, ten Bokkel Huinink W, Carmichael J, et al. 2001 Clinical evidence for topotecan-paclitaxel non–cross-resistance in ovarian cancer. J Clin Oncol 19:1893–1900.
97. Gordon AN, Fleagle JT, Guthrie D, Parkin DE, Gore ME, Lacave AJ. 2001 Recurrent epithelial ovarian carcinoma: a randomized phase III study of pegylated liposomal doxorubicin versus topotecan. J Clin Oncol 19:3312–3322.
98. Brown JV 3rd, Peters WA 3rd, Rettenmaier MA, et al. 2003 Three-consecutive-day topotecan is an active regimen for recurrent epithelial ovarian cancer. Gynecol Oncol 88:136–140.
99. Gore M, Rustin G, Schuller J, et al. 2001 Topotecan given as a 21-day infusion in the treatment of advanced ovarian cancer. Br J Cancer 84:1043–1046.
100. Ardizzoni A, Hansen H, Dombernowsky P, et al. 1997 Topotecan, a new active drug in the second-line treatment of small-cell lung cancer: a phase II study in patients with refractory and sensitive disease. The European Organization for Research and Treatment of Cancer Early Clinical Studies Group and New Drug Development Office, and the Lung Cancer Cooperative Group. J Clin Oncol 15:2090–2096.

101. Eckhardt J, Gralla R, Palmer MC, et al. 1996 Topotecan as a second-line therapy in patients with small-cell-lung cancer: A phase II study [abstract]. Ann Oncol 7:107.
102. Perez-Soler R, Glisson BS, Lee JS, et al. 1996 Treatment of patients with small-cell lung cancer refractory to etoposide and cisplatin with the topoisomerase I poison topotecan. J Clin Oncol 14:2785–2790.
103. Schiller JH, Kim K, Hutson P, et al. 1996 Phase II study of topotecan in patients with extensive-stage small-cell carcinoma of the lung: an Eastern Cooperative Oncology Group Trial. J Clin Oncol 14:2345–2352.
104. Schiller JH, Adak S, Cella D, DeVore RF 3rd, Johnson DH. 2001 Topotecan versus observation after cisplatin plus etoposide in extensive-stage small-cell lung cancer: E7593—a phase III trial of the Eastern Cooperative Oncology Group. J Clin Oncol 19:2114–2122.
105. Kraut EH, Staubus A, Mayernick D, King G, Balcerzak SP. 1995 Phase II trial of topotecan in metastatic malignant melanoma. Proc Am Assoc Cancer Res 36:1420.
106. Beran M, Estey E, O'Brien SM, et al. 1998 Results of topotecan single-agent therapy in patients with myelodysplastic syndromes and chronic myelomonocytic leukemia. Leuk Lymphoma 31:521–531.
107. Blaney SM, Needle MN, Gillespie A, et al. 1998 Phase II trial of topotecan administered as 72-hour continuous infusion in children with refractory solid tumors: a collaborative Pediatric Branch, National Cancer Institute, and Children's Cancer Group Study. Clin Cancer Res 4:357–360.
108. Nitschke R, Parkhurst J, Sullivan J, Harris MB, Bernstein M, Pratt C. 1998 Topotecan in pediatric patients with recurrent and progressive solid tumors: a Pediatric Oncology Group phase II study. J Pediatr Hematol Oncol 20:315–318.
109. Kretschmar C, Kletzel M, Murray K, et al. 1995 Upfront phase II therapy with Taxol (Txl) and topotecan in untreated children (>365 days) with disseminated (INSS stage 4) neuroblastoma. Med Pediat Oncol 25:243.
110. Pinkerton CR, Blanc Vincent MP, Bergeron C, Fervers B, Philip T. 2000 Induction chemotherapy in metastatic neuroblastoma—does dose influence response? A critical review of published data standards, options and recommendations (SOR) project of the National Federation of French Cancer Centres (FNCLCC). Eur J Cancer 36:1808–1815.
111. Blaney SM, Phillips PC, Packer RJ, et al. 1996 Phase II evaluation of topotecan for pediatric central nervous system tumors. Cancer 78:527–531.
112. Kadota RP, Stewart CF, Horn M, et al. 1999 Topotecan for the treatment of recurrent or progressive central nervous system tumors—a Pediatric Oncology Group phase II study. J Neurooncol 43:43–47.
113. Lynch TJ, Kalish L, Strauss G, et al. 1994 Phase II study of topotecan in metastatic non-small-cell lung cancer. J Clin Oncol 12:347–352.
114. Perez-Soler R, Fossella FV, Glisson BS, et al. 1996 Phase II study of topotecan in patients with advanced non-small-cell lung cancer previously untreated with chemotherapy. J Clin Oncol 14:503–513.
115. Kindler HL, Kris MG, Smith IE, Slevin ML, Krebs JB. 1997 Continuous infusion topotecan as first-line therapy in patients with advanced non-small cell lung cancer (NSCLC): a Phase II study. Proc Am Soc Clin Oncol 16:472.
116. Weitz JJ, Marschke RF, Sloan JA, et al. 2000 A randomized phase II trial of two schedules of topotecan for the treatment of advanced stage non-small cell lung cancer. Lung Cancer 28:157–162.

117. Perez-Soler R, Khuri F, Pisters KM, et al. 1997 Phase II study of topotecan in patients with squamous carcinoma of the lung previously untreated with chemotherapy. Proc Am Soc Clin Oncol 16:450.
118. Mainwaring PN, Nicolson MC, Hickish T, et al. 1997 Continuous infusional topotecan in advanced breast and non-small-cell lung cancer: no evidence of increased efficacy. Br J Cancer 76:1636–1639.
119. White SC, Cheeseman S, Thatcher N, et al. 2000 Phase II study of oral topotecan in advanced non-small cell lung cancer. Clin Cancer Res 6:868–873.
120. Creemers GJ, Wanders J, Gamucci T, et al. 1995 Topotecan in colorectal cancer: a phase II study of the EORTC early clinical trials group. Ann Oncol 6:844–846.
121. Macdonald JS, Benedetti JK, Modiano M, Alberts DS. 1997 Phase II evaluation of topotecan in patients with advanced colorectal cancer. A Southwest Oncology Group trial (SWOG 9241). Invest New Drugs 15:357–359.
122. Saltz LB, Schwartz GK, Ilson DH, Quan V, Kelsen DP. 1997 A phase II study of topotecan administered five times daily in patients with advanced gastric cancer. Am J Clin Oncol 20:621–625.
123. Benedetti JK, Burris HA, 3rd, Balcerzak SP, Macdonald JS. 1997 Phase II trial of topotecan in advanced gastric cancer: a Southwest Oncology Group study. Invest New Drugs 15:261–264.
124. Scher RM, Kosierowski R, Lusch C, et al. 1996 Phase II trial of topotecan in advanced or metastatic adenocarcinoma of the pancreas. Invest New Drugs 13: 347–354.
125. O'Reilly S, Donehower RC, Rowinsky EK, Ord S, Grochow LB. 1996 A phase II trial of topotecan in patients with previously untreated pancreatic cancer. Anticancer Drugs 7:410–414.
126. Stevenson JP, Scher RM, Kosierowski R, et al. 1998 Phase II trial of topotecan as a 21-day continuous infusion in patients with advanced or metastatic adenocarcinoma of the pancreas. Eur J Cancer 34:1358–1362.
127. Asbury RF, Lipsitz S, Graham D, Falkson CI, Baez L, Benson AB 3rd. 2000 Treatment of squamous cell esophageal cancer with topotecan: an Eastern Cooperative Oncology Group Study (E2293). Am J Clin Oncol 23:45–46.
128. Macdonald JS, Jacobson JL, Ketchel SJ, et al. 2000 A phase II trial of topotecan in esophageal carcinoma: a Southwest Oncology Group study (SWOG 9339). Invest New Drugs 18:199–202.
129. Friedman HS, Kerby T, Fields S, et al. 1999 Topotecan treatment of adults with primary malignant glioma. The Brain Tumor Center at Duke. Cancer 85:1160–1165.
130. Macdonald D, Cairncross G, Stewart D, et al. 1996 Phase II study of topotecan in patients with recurrent malignant glioma. National Clinical Institute of Canada Clinical Trials Group. Ann Oncol 7:205–207.
131. Burch PA, Bernath AM, Cascino TL, et al. 2000 A North Central Cancer Treatment Group phase II trial of topotecan in relapsed gliomas. Invest New Drugs 18:275–280.
132. Rajkumar SV, Reid JM, Novotny PJ, et al. 2000 A randomized phase II and pharmacokinetic study of dacarbazine in patients with recurrent glioma. J Neurooncol 49:255–261.
133. Avgeropoulos NG, Batchelor TT. 1999 New treatment strategies for malignant gliomas. Oncologist 4:209–224.
134. Murphy BA, Leong T, Burkey B, Langer C, Forastiere A. 2001 Lack of efficacy of topotecan in the treatment of metastatic or recurrent squamous carcinoma of the

head and neck: an Eastern Cooperative Oncology Group Trial (E3393). Am J Clin Oncol 24:64–66.
135. Smith RE, Lew D, Rodriguez GI, Taylor SA, Schuller D, Ensley JF. 1996 Evaluation of topotecan in patients with recurrent for metastatic squamous cell carcinoma of the head and neck. A phase II Southwest Oncology Group study. Invest New Drugs 14:403–407.
136. Robert F, Soong SJ, Wheeler RH. 1997 A phase II study of topotecan in patients with recurrent head and neck cancer. Identification of an active new agent. Am J Clin Oncol 20:298–302.
137. Goldschmidt E, Bonneterre J, Fumoleau P, Oberling F, Cupissol D, Misset JL. 1997 A phase II study of topotecan on a daily x 5 schedule as second-line single agent therapy in patients with advanced breast cancer. Proc Am Soc Clin Oncol 16:598.
138. Levine EG, Cirrincione CT, Szatrowski TP, Canellos G, Norton L, Henderson IC. 1999 Phase II trial of topotecan in advanced breast cancer: a Cancer and Leukemia Group B study. Am J Clin Oncol 22:218–222.
139. Spaeth D, Bonneterre J, Marty M, Khayat D, Facchini T, Conroy T. 1997 Phase II studies of two trial regimens of topotecan as second-line single agent therapy in advanced breast cancer. Proc Am Soc Clin Oncol 16:675.
140. Oberhoff C, Kieback DG, Wurstlein R, et al. 2001 Topotecan chemotherapy in patients with breast cancer and brain metastases: results of a pilot study. Onkologie 24:256–260.
141. Holloway RW. 2003 Treatment options for endometrial cancer: experience with topotecan. Gynecol Oncol 90:S28–S33.
142. Wadler S, Levy DE, Lincoln ST, Soori GS, Schink JC, Goldberg G. 2003 Topotecan is an active agent in the first-line treatment of metastatic or recurrent endometrial carcinoma: Eastern Cooperative Oncology Group Study E3E93. J Clin Oncol 21:2110–2114.
143. Miller DS, Blessing JA, Lentz SS, Waggoner SE. 2002 A phase II trial of topotecan in patients with advanced, persistent, or recurrent endometrial carcinoma: a gynecologic oncology group study. Gynecol Oncol 87:247–251.
144. Noda K, Sasaki H, Yamamoto K, et al. 1996 Phase II trial of topotecan for cervical cancer of the uterus. Proc Am Soc Clin Oncol 15:754.
145. Bookman MA, Blessing JA, Hanjani P, Herzog TJ, Andersen WA. 2000 Topotecan in squamous cell carcinoma of the cervix: a phase II study of the Gynecologic Oncology Group. Gynecol Oncol 77:446–449.
146. Abu-Rustum NR, Lee S, Massad LS. 2000 Topotecan for recurrent cervical cancer after platinum-based therapy. Int J Gynecol Cancer 10:285–288.
147. Muderspach LI, Blessing JA, Levenback C, Moore JL Jr. 2001 A phase II study of topotecan in patients with squamous cell carcinoma of the cervix: a Gynecologic Oncology Group study. Gynecol Oncol 81:213–215.
148. Hudes GR, Kosierowski R, Greenberg R, et al. 1995 Phase II study of topotecan in metastatic hormone-refractory prostate cancer. Invest New Drugs. 13:235–240.
149. Klein CE, Tangen CM, Braun TJ, et al. 2002 SWOG-9510: evaluation of topotecan in hormone refractory prostate cancer: a Southwest Oncology Group study. Prostate 52:264–268.
150. Janik JE, Miller LL, Korn EL, et al. 2001 A prospective randomized phase II trial of GM-CSF priming to prevent topotecan-induced neutropenia in chemotherapy-naive patients with malignant melanoma or renal cell carcinoma. Blood 97:1942–1946.

151. Wall JG, Benedetti JK, O'Rourke MA, Natale RB, Macdonald JS. 1997 Phase II trial to topotecan in hepatocellular carcinoma: a Southwest Oncology Group study. Invest New Drugs 15:257–260.
152. Chou TC, Motzer RJ, Tong Y, Bosl GJ. 1994 Computerized quantitation of synergism and antagonism of taxol, topotecan, and cisplatin against human teratocarcinoma cell growth: a rational approach to clinical protocol design. J Natl Cancer Inst 86:1517–1524.
153. Cheng MF, Chatterjee S, Berger NA. 1994 Schedule-dependent cytotoxicity of topotecan alone and in combination chemotherapy regimens. Oncol Res 6:269–279.
154. Kaufmann SH, Gore SD, Letendre L, et al. 1996 Factors affecting topotecan sensitivity in human leukemia samples. Ann NY Acad Sci 803:128–142.
155. Kaufmann SH, Peereboom D, Buckwalter CA, et al. 1996 Cytotoxic effects of topotecan combined with various anticancer agents in human cancer cell lines. J Natl Cancer Inst 88:734–741.
156. Ma J, Maliepaard M, Nooter K, et al. 1998 Synergistic cytotoxicity of cisplatin and topotecan or SN-38 in a panel of eight solid-tumor cell lines. Cancer Chemother Pharmacol 41:307–316.
157. Romanelli S, Perego P, Pratesi G, Carenini N, Tortoreto M, Zunino F. 1998 In vitro and in vivo interaction between cisplatin and topotecan in ovarian carcinoma systems. Cancer Chemother Pharmacol 41:385–390.
158. Kim JH, Kim SH, Kolozsvary A, Khil MS. 1992 Potentiation of radiation response in human carcinoma cells in vitro and murine fibrosarcoma in vivo by topotecan, an inhibitor of DNA topoisomerase I. Int J Radiat Oncol Biol Phys 22:515–518.
159. Bonner JA, Kozelsky TF. 1996 The significance of the sequence of administration of topotecan and etoposide. Cancer Chemother Pharmacol 39:109–112.
160. Whitacre CM, Zborowska E, Gordon NH, Mackay W, Berger NA. 1997 Topotecan increases topoisomerase IIalpha levels and sensitivity to treatment with etoposide in schedule-dependent process. Cancer Res 57:1425–1428.
161. Rowinsky EK, Kaufmann SH, Baker SD, et al. 1996 Sequences of topotecan and cisplatin: phase I, pharmacologic, and in vitro studies to examine sequence dependence. J Clin Oncol 14:3074–3084.
162. Bolis G, Scarfone G, Villa A, Parazzini F. 2001 Phase II trial of topotecan, carboplatin, and paclitaxel as front-line therapy in suboptimal advanced epithelial ovarian cancer. Gynecol Oncol 81:331–333.
163. du Bois A, Luck HJ, Meier W, et al. 1997 Carboplatin/paclitaxel versus cisplatin/paclitaxel as first-line chemotherapy in advanced ovarian cancer: an interim analysis of a randomized phase III trial of the Arbeitsgemeinschaft Gynakologische Onkologie Ovarian Cancer Study Group. Semin Oncol 24(Suppl. 15):S15-44–S15-52.
164. Neijt JP, Engelholm SA, Tuxen MK, et al. 2000 Exploratory phase III study of paclitaxel and cisplatin versus paclitaxel and carboplatin in advanced ovarian cancer. J Clin Oncol 18:3084–3092.
165. Pignata S, Deplacido S, Scambia G, et al. 2003 Topotecan vs nihil after response to carboplatin and paclitaxel in advanced ovarian cancer. Early results of the MITO-1 (Multicenter Italian Trials in Ovarian Cancer) study [abstract]. Proc Am Soc Clin Oncol 22:1791.
166. Pfisterer J, Lortholary A, Kimmig R, et al. 2003 Paclitaxel/carboplatin (TC) vs. paclitaxel/carboplatin followed by topotecan (TC-Top) in first-line treatment of ovarian cancer FIGO stages IIb-IV. Interim results of a gynecologic cancer inter-

group phase III trial of the AGO Ovarian Cancer Study Group and GINECO [abstract]. Proc Am Soc Clin Oncol 22:1793.
167. McGuire WP, Hoskins WJ, Brady MF, et al. 1996 Cyclophosphamide and cisplatin compared with paclitaxel and cisplatin in patients with stage III and stage IV ovarian cancer. N Engl J Med 334:1–6.
168. Greggi S, Salerno MG, D'Agostino G, et al. 2001 Topotecan and gemcitabine in platinum/paclitaxel-resistant ovarian cancer. Oncology 60:19–23.
169. Sehouli J, Stengel D, Oskay G, et al. 2002 A phase II study of topotecan plus gemcitabine in the treatment of patients with relapsed ovarian cancer after failure of first-line chemotherapy. Ann Oncol 13:1749–1755.
170. Penson RT, Supko JG, Seiden MV, et al. 2001 A Phase I-II study of 96-hour infusional topotecan and paclitaxel for patients with recurrent Mullerian tumors. Cancer 92:1156–1167.
171. Hanjani P, Nolte S, Shahin MS. 2002 Phase II evaluation of 3-day topotecan with cyclophosphamide in the treatment of recurrent ovarian cancer. Gynecol Oncol 85:278–284.
172. Bookman MA. 2002 Developmental chemotherapy in advanced ovarian cancer: incorporation of newer cytotoxic agents in a phase III randomized trial of the Gynecologic Oncology Group (GOG-0182). Semin Oncol 29:20–31.
173. Copeland LJ, Bookman M, Trimble E. 2003 Clinical trials of newer regimens for treating ovarian cancer: the rationale for Gynecologic Oncology Group Protocol GOG 182-ICON5. Gynecol Oncol 90:S1–S7.
174. Frasci G, Nicolella G, Comella P, et al. 2001 A weekly regimen of cisplatin, paclitaxel and topotecan with granulocyte-colony stimulating factor support for patients with extensive disease small cell lung cancer: a phase II study. Br J Cancer 84:1166–1171.
175. Hainsworth JD, Morrissey LH, Scullin DC, Jr., et al. 2002 Paclitaxel, carboplatin, and topotecan in the treatment of patients with small cell lung cancer: a phase II trial of the Minnie Pearl Cancer Research Network. Cancer 94:2426–2433.
176. Jacobs S, Jett J, Belani C, et al. 1999 Topotecan and paclitaxel, an active couplet in untreated extensive disease in small cell lung cancer. Proc Am Soc Clin Oncol 18:470a.
177. Felip E, Rosell R, Domine M, et al. 2003 Sequential dose-dense paclitaxel followed by topotecan in untreated extensive-stage small-cell lung cancer: a Spanish Lung Cancer Group phase II study. Ann Oncol 14:1549–1554.
178. Kelly K. 2000 New chemotherapy agents for small cell lung cancer. Chest 117(Suppl. 1):156S–1562S.
179. Ardizzoni A, Manegold C, Debruyne C, et al. 2003 European organization for research and treatment of cancer (EORTC) 08957 phase II study of topotecan in combination with cisplatin as second-line treatment of refractory and sensitive small cell lung cancer. Clin Cancer Res 9:143–150.
180. Hammond LA, Eckardt JR, Ganapathi R, et al. 1998 A phase I and translational study of sequential administration of the topoisomerase I and II inhibitors topotecan and etoposide. Clin Cancer Res 4:1459–1467.
181. Joppert MG, Garfield DH, Gregurich MA, et al. 2003 A phase II multicenter study of combined topotecan and gemcitabine as first line chemotherapy for advanced non-small cell lung cancer. Lung Cancer 39:215–219.
182. Rinaldi D, Lormand N, Brierre J, et al. 2001 A phase I-II trial of topotecan and gemcitabine in patients with previously treated, advanced non-small cell lung cancer (LOA-3). Cancer Invest 19:467–474.

183. Rinaldi DA, Lormand NA, Brierre JE, et al. 2002 A Phase II trial of topotecan and gemcitabine in patients with previously treated, advanced nonsmall cell lung carcinoma. Cancer 95(6):1274–1278.
184. Stupp R, Bodmer A, Duvoisin B, et al. 2001 Is cisplatin required for the treatment of non-small-cell lung cancer? Experience and preliminary results of a phase I/II trial with topotecan and vinorelbine. Oncology 61(Suppl. 1):35–41.
185. Pujol JL, von Pawel J, Tumolo S, et al. 2001 Preliminary results of combined therapy with topotecan and carboplatin in advanced non-small-cell lung cancer. Oncology 61(Suppl. 1):47–54.
186. Beran M, Estey E, O'Brien S, et al. 1999 Topotecan and cytarabine is an active combination regimen in myelodysplastic syndromes and chronic myelomonocytic leukemia. J Clin Oncol 17:2819–2830.
187. Kancherla RR, Nair JS, Ahmed T, et al. 2001 Evaluation of topotecan and etoposide for non-Hodgkin lymphoma: correlation of topoisomerase-DNA complex formation with clinical response. Cancer 91:463–471.
188. Younes A, Preti HA, Hagemeister FB, et al. 2001 Paclitaxel plus topotecan treatment for patients with relapsed or refractory aggressive non-Hodgkin's lymphoma. Ann Oncol 12:923–927.
189. Cortes J, Estey E, Beran M, et al. 2000 Cyclophosphamide, ara-C and topotecan (CAT) for patients with refractory or relapsed acute leukemia. Leuk Lymph 36:479–484.
190. Lee ST, Jang JH, Suh HC, Hahn JS, Ko YW, Min YH. 2001 Idarubicin, cytarabine, and topotecan in patients with refractory or relapsed acute myelogenous leukemia and high-risk myelodysplastic syndrome. Am J Hematol 68:237–245.
191. Vey N, Kantarjian H, Beran M, et al. 1999 Combination of topotecan with cytarabine or etoposide in patients with refractory or relapsed acute myeloid leukemia: results of a randomized phase I/II study. Invest New Drugs 17:89–95.
192. Crump M, Couban S, Meyer R, et al. 2002 Phase II study of sequential topotecan and etoposide in patients with intermediate grade non-Hodgkin's lymphoma: a National Cancer Institute of Canada Clinical Trials Group study. Leuk Lymph 43158:1581–1587.
193. Mainwaring MG, Rimsza LM, Chen SF, et al. 2002 Treatment of refractory acute leukemia with timed sequential chemotherapy using topotecan followed by etoposide + mitoxantrone (T-EM) and correlation with topoisomerase II levels. Leuk Lymph 43:989–999.
194. Kushner BH, Cheung NK, Kramer K, Dunkel IJ, Calleja E, Boulad F. 2001 Topotecan combined with myeloablative doses of thiotepa and carboplatin for neuroblastoma, brain tumors, and other poor-risk solid tumors in children and young adults. Bone Marrow Transplant 28:551–556.
195. Donato ML, Gershenson DM, Wharton JT, et al. 2001 High-dose topotecan, melphalan, and cyclophosphamide (TMC) with stem cell support: a new regimen for the treatment of advanced ovarian cancer. Gynecol Oncol 82:420–426.
196. Prince HM, Rischin D, Quinn M, et al. 2001 Repetitive high-dose topotecan, carboplatin, and paclitaxel with peripheral blood progenitor cell support in previously untreated ovarian cancer: results of a Phase I study. Gynecol Oncol 81:216–224.
197. Colombo NobotIc. 2000 Randomised trial of paclitaxel (PTX) and carboplatin (CBDCA) versus a control arm of carboplatin or CAP (cyclophosphamide, doxorubicin, & cisplatin): The Third International Collaborative Ovarian Neoplasm Study (ICON3). Proc Am Soc Clin Oncol 19:1500.

198. Muggia FM, Braly PS, Brady MF, et al. 2000 Phase III randomized study of cisplatin versus paclitaxel versus cisplatin and paclitaxel in patients with suboptimal stage III or IV ovarian cancer: a Gynecologic Oncology Group study. J Clin Oncol 18:106–115.
199. Eckardt JR. 2001 Feasibility of oral topotecan plus intravenous paclitaxel in advanced non-small-cell lung cancer. Oncology 61(Suppl. 1):30–34.
200. O'Leary JJ, Shapiro RL, Ren CJ, Chuang N, Cohen HW, Potmesil M. 1999 Antiangiogenic effects of camptothecin analogues 9-amino-20(S)-camptothecin, topotecan, and CPT-11 studied in the mouse cornea model. Clin Cancer Res 5:181–187.
201. Nakashio A, Fujita N, Tsuruo T. 2002 Topotecan inhibits VEGF- and bFGF-induced vascular endothelial cell migration via downregulation of the PI3K-Akt signaling pathway. Int J Cancer 98:36–41.
202. McCrudden KW, Yokoi A, Thosani A, et al. 2002 Topotecan is anti-angiogenic in experimental hepatoblastoma. J Pediatr Surg 37:857–861.
203. Soffer SZ, Kim E, Moore JT, et al. 2001 Novel use of an established agent: Topotecan is anti-angiogenic in experimental Wilms tumor. J Pediatr Surg 36:1781–1784.
204. Soffer SZ, Moore JT, Kim E, et al. 2001 Combination antiangiogenic therapy: increased efficacy in a murine model of Wilms tumor. J Pediatr Surg 36:1177–1181.
205. Ling YH, Donato NJ, Perez-Soler R. 2001 Sensitivity to topoisomerase I inhibitors and cisplatin is associated with epidermal growth factor receptor expression in human cervical squamous carcinoma ME180 sublines. Cancer Chemother Pharmacol 47:473–480.
206. Erlichman C, Boerner SA, Hallgren CG, et al. 2001 The HER tyrosine kinase inhibitor CI1033 enhances cytotoxicity of 7-ethyl-10-hydroxycamptothecin and topotecan by inhibiting breast cancer resistance protein-mediated drug efflux. Cancer Res 61:739–748.

13 The Clinical Development of Lurtotecan

Experience With Water-Soluble and Liposomal Forms

Keith T. Flaherty, MD,
James P. Stevenson, MD,
Christopher J. Twelves, MD,
and Peter J. O'Dwyer, MD

CONTENTS

1. INTRODUCTION

Camptothecin (CPT) derivatives have become integral to the management of lung and colon cancer. They continue to be the subject of intense investigation. The parent compound, CPT, was extracted from the leaves of *Camptotheca acuminata* by Wall and Wani in 1957. The hydrophilic carboxylate salt entered clinical trials in the late 1960s. The lack of efficacy and unpredictable bone marrow and bladder toxicity halted its clinical development *(1)*. When topoisomerase I (TOP-I) was discovered as the target of CPT class of compounds 1985 *(2)*, there was a resurgence of interest in the compound.

Camptothecins in Cancer Therapy
Edited by: V. R. Adams and T. G. Burke © Humana Press Inc., Totowa, NJ

TOP-I is a non-energy–dependent enzyme that causes single-stranded breaks in DNA and allows relaxation of positively and negatively supercoiled DNA before transcription or replication *(3)*. The CPTs form covalently bound complexes with TOP-I and DNA. S-phase–specific cytotoxicity results from replication fork collision of DNA polymerase and the CPT/DNA adduct *(4)*. CPT-stabilized DNA cleavage complexes are not sufficient for cytotoxicity. The requirement for DNA replication has been shown by the protection against CPT-induced cytotoxicity by the DNA synthesis inhibitors hydroxyurea and aphidicolin *(5,6)*. Repair of TOP-I–mediated DNA damage is accomplished through ubiquitin/26S proteasome-mediated degradation of TOP-I *(7)*. Whereas normal tissues such as peripheral blood mononuclear cells downregulate TOP-I in response to incubation with CPT *(8)*, breast, colon, and leukemia cell lines do not *(9)*.

Subsequent to initial clinical trials, it was found that the structure of CPT derivatives is altered in plasma *(10)*. An equilibrium exists between the five-ring structure and the open E-ring (Fig. 1). The latter form of the drug has less than 10% of the activity of the closed-ring compound against topoisomerase in vitro and binds with high affinity to human serum albumin *(11)*. Although the active and inactive form of the drug exist in a 1:1 ratio in the plasma of mice, in humans the ratio shifts to 1:9 *(12)*. These findings led to the generation of CPT derivatives with a lower affinity for albumin. Substitutions at the 10 and 11 positions on the A-ring have been shown to increase in vitro activity, provided that there is no steric encroachment on the 12 position *(13)*. Alteration at the 20 position on the E-ring generally decreases activity *(14)*, with the exception of substitutions with CH2, Br, and Cl *(15,16)*. 10,11-ethylenedioxy-camptothecin is more water-soluble and more potently inhibits TOP-I compared with CPT by creating more stable TOP-I–DNA cleavage complexes *(17,18)*.

Two CPT derivatives have already shown remarkable antitumor activity in humans. Topotecan was generated by modifying the ninth and tenth position of the A-ring (Fig. 2). It was approved by the Food and Drug Administration for use in women with previously treated ovarian cancer based on the results of a Phase III trial comparing it with paclitaxel *(19)*. Irinotecan is a CPT analogue with modifications at the seventh and tenth position on the A-ring (*see* Fig. 2). It is approved for use in patients with colon cancer that have recurred or progressed after 5-Fluorouracil (5-FU)–based chemotherapy *(20,21)*.

2. WATER-SOLUBLE LURTOTECAN

2.1. Preclinical Studies

Lurtotecan (GI147211, GlaxoSmithKline) was created by the addition of an ethylenedioxy group bridging the tenth and eleventh position of the A-ring,

A

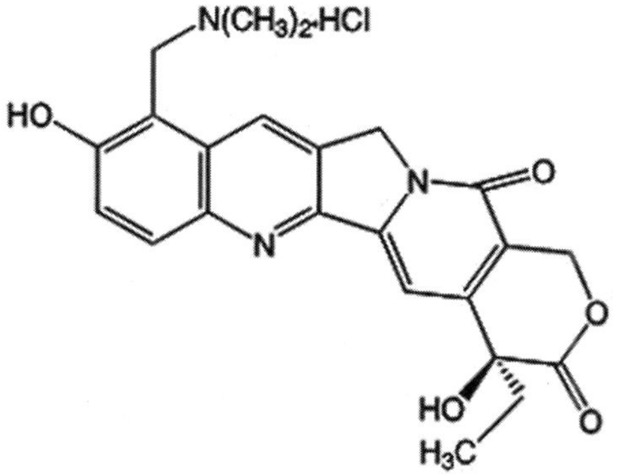

Topotecan hydrochloride

B

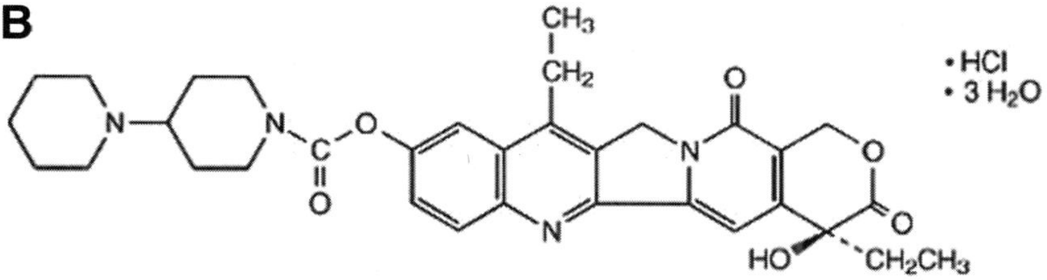

Irinotecan Hydrochloride

Fig. 1. Picture of camptothecin with rings lettered and positions numbered and picture of lurtotecan from GSK investigator brochure. (Adapted from Kohn & Pommier, Annal NY Acad Sci, 2001.)

as well as a 4- methylpiperazinomethylene moiety at the seventh position of the B ring yielding [7-(4-methylpiperazinomethylene)-10,11-ethylene-dioxy-20(S)-camptothecin] *(22)* (Fig. 3). It is more water-soluble than topotecan or CPT. Topoisomerase-mediated DNA strand breaks, a measure of topoisomerase activity, are inhibited with more than twofold greater potency by lurtotecan compared with topotecan. The IC_{50} for lurtotecan was significantly lower than topotecan in five human tumor cell lines. The efficacy was not reduced in the multidrug-resistant (MDR)–positive cell line, SKVLB. In two mouse xenograft models with implanted human colon cancer cell lines, lurtotecan showed dose-dependent reduction in tumor volume, whereas topotecan had only modest tumoristatic effect. Remarkable activity was also seen in a MX-1 breast cancer xenograft model. Toxicity in animal models resembled that of topotecan.

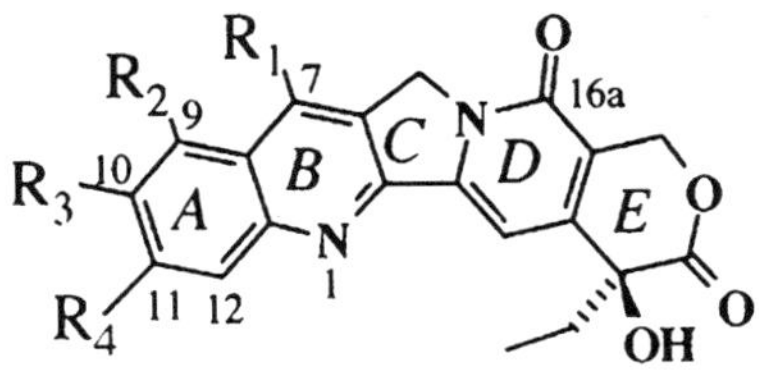

Fig. 2. Chemical structure of camptothecin. Topotecan contains substitutions at the ninth and tenth position of the A ring . Irinotecan has substitutions at the seventh and tenth position of the A ring.

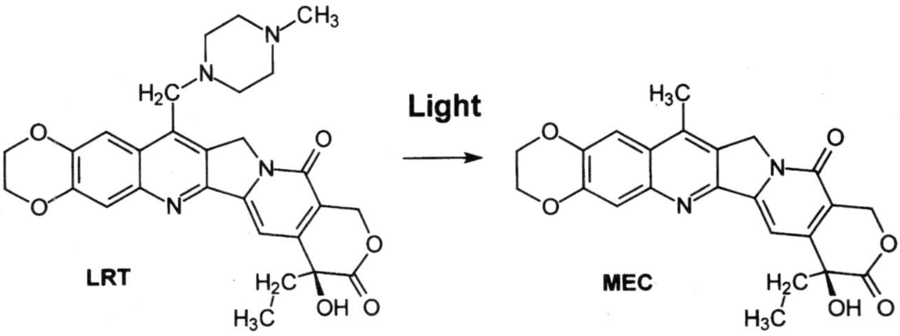

Fig 3. Chemical structure of lurtotecan.

2.2. Phase I Clinical Trials

A summary of the phase I clinical trials of water-soluble lurtotecan is presented in Table 1. In 1996, Gerrits et al. reported the results of a phase I trial of lurtotecan carried out at the Rotterdam Cancer Institute *(23)*. The drug was administered intravenously daily for 5 consecutive days every 3 weeks. Nineteen patients with advanced cancer were enrolled in the study; six had received prior chemotherapy, and nine had colorectal cancer. The dose was escalated from 0.3 to 1.5 mg/m^2/day. Neutropenia and thrombocytopenia were dose-limiting. The maximum tolerated dose (MTD) of 1.5 mg/m^2/day was determined by 11 instances of grade 4 neutropenia of 15 evaluable courses of treatment. Seven of 15 courses were complicated by grade 3 or 4 thrombocytopenia. There were no grade 3 or 4 nonhematologic toxicities, with mild nausea and vomiting being the most common adverse event. One patient with colon cancer had a short-lasting partial response and one patient with leiomyosarcoma had a minor response. Ten other patients had stable disease. Pharmacokinetic data were collected during the first 4 days of the first course on 18 patients. The area of the time-concentration curve (AUC) was linearly related to dose. The terminal half-life was 3.54 ± 0.99 hours.

Table 1
Clincal Trials of Water-soluble Lurtotecan

Phase I trials				
Investigator	*Schedule*	*Phase II dose*	*DLT*	*Responses*
Gerrits et al.	Days 1–5 q 3 weeks	1.5 mg/m^2/d × 5 days	Neutropenia	1 PR, 10 SD of 19 patients
Gerrits et al.	Day 1 PO, days 2–5 IV q 3 weeks	6.0 mg/m^2 PO, 1.5 mg/m^2/day × 4 days	Neutropenia and thrombocytopenia	7 SD of 27 patients
Eckhardt et al.	Days 1–5 q 3 weeks	1.5 mg/m^2/day × 5 days	Neutropenia	None
Paz-Ares et al.	72 hour CI q 4 weeks	1.2 mg/m^2/day × 3 days, heavily pretreated 1.75 mg/m^2/day × 3 days, minimally pretreated	Neutropenia and thrombocytopenia	3 PR, 2 MR of 44 patients
Stevenson et al.	7–21 day CI, 2 week break	0.4 mg/m^2/day × 21 days	Thrombocytopenia	2 PR, 2 SD of 38 patients

Phase II trials			
Investigator	*Regimen*	*Toxicity*	*Responses*
Sessa et al.	1.2 mg/m^2/day × 5 days q 3 weeks	25% grade 3 or 4 neutropenia 22% grade 3 or 4 thrombocytopenia	11 PR, 21 SD of 62 patients with SCLC
Gamucci et al.	1.2 mg/m^2/day × 5 days q 3 weeks	55% grade 3 or 4 neutropenia 20% grade 3 or 4 thrombocytopenia	3 PR, 9 SD of 20 patients with breast cancer 2 PR, 5 SD of 23 patients with NSCLC 7 SD of 19 patients with colorectal cancer

CI, continuous infusion; SCLC, small cell lung cancer; PR, partial response; NSCLC, non-small cell lung cancer; MR, minor response; SD, stable disease.

The following year, Gerrits et al. published the results of a phase I study using a single dose of oral lurtotecan on day 1, followed by 4 days of intravenous infusion *(24)*. The intravenous doses were fixed at 1.5 mg/m^2/day, based on the results of the all-intravenous phase I trial. Oral therapy was given on day 1 of the first two cycles only, because the goal of the study was to determine the bioavailability of the drug. The oral dose levels were 1.5, 3.0, and 6.0 mg/m^2. Nineteen patients were entered into the study. To determine the interaction between bioavailability and food intake, eight additional patients were added at the 6.0 mg/m^2 level. Grade 3 or 4 neutropenia or thrombocytopenia was observed in 5 of 30 and 4 of 30 treatments courses, respectively. Treatment delay secondary to persistent leukopenia occurred in 5 of 13 patients at the highest dose level. The AUC after a 6.0 mg/m^2 oral dose was 20.3 ng/mL/hour compared to 32.1 ng/mL/hour after an intravenous dose of 1.5 mg/m^2/day. The absolute bioavailability was 11.8 ± 4.5%. The half-life of the oral drug was 6.8 ± 3.1 hours. Seven patients, five of whom had colon cancer, experienced stable disease.

Another phase I study of intravenous lurtotecan was performed at the Institute for Drug Development in San Antonio and reported in 1998 *(25)*. Lurtotecan was administered daily for 5 days every 3 weeks. The dose was escalated from 0.3 to 1.75 mg/m^2/day and was guided by toxicity data available from the previous phase I trial. Twenty-four patients with advanced malignancies were enrolled, 11 of whom were minimally pretreated. Dose reduction for myelosuppression occurred in one patient at the 1.2 mg/m^2/day level and two patients at the 1.75 mg/m^2/day level. Although neutropenia was dose-limiting, it was not cumulative after repeated cycles. There were no dose limiting toxicities (DLTs) among six patients at 1.5 mg/m^2/day. However, at a dose of 1.75 mg/m^2/day, three of four patients experienced grade 4 neutropenia. Two of those patients required hospitalization for febrile neutropenia, one of whom died of respiratory failure secondary to pneumonia. Grade 4 thrombocytopenia occurred in one patient receiving 1 mg/m^2/day, two patients receiving 1.2 mg/m^2/day and two patients receiving 1.75 mg/m^2/day. Pharmacokinetic analyses revealed terminal half-lives of the lactone and total lurtotecan of 7.5 and 9.6 hours, respectively. The values from day 4 were not significantly higher than the day 1 values. There were no objective responses.

Paz-Ares et al. conducted a study at the Fox Chase Cancer Center and the University of Glasgow evaluating the tolerability, pharmacokinetics, and pharmacodynamics of lurtotecan given by 72-hour continuous infusion every 4 weeks *(26)*. Forty-four patients with solid tumors were enrolled and received 124 cycles with doses ranging from 0.25 to 2.5 mg/m^2/day. Neutropenia and thrombocytopenia were dose-limiting. Among four heavily pretreated patients at the 1.5 mg/m^2/day level, three experienced grade 4 thrombocytopenia in addition to grade 3 or 4 neutropenia. Thereafter, more heavily pretreated patients were enrolled at 1.2 mg/m^2/day, which was the recommended phase II dose for those patients. Among 10 minimally pretreated patients treated at 2.0 mg/m^2/day, 4 patients had dose-limiting hematologic toxicity. There were three instances of grade 4 neutropenia and four of grade 3 thrombocytopenia. Therefore, the recommended phase I or II dose for minimally pretreated patients was 1.75 mg/m^2/day. The first five patients received treatment through peripheral intravenous catheters; all of them developed phlebitis. The remainder of the patients in the study were treated through central venous catheters. The mean terminal elimination half-life was 7.5 ± 3.2 hours. A correlation was observed between steady-state concentration of lurtotecan and decline in neutrophils and platelets. Neutrophils were more sensitive with a half-maximal concentration of 0.75 ng/mL compared with 1.4 ng/mL for platelets. Two partial and two minor responses were observed at doses greater than or equal to 1.5 mg/m^2/day in patients with hepatoma, breast, and colorectal cancer; one partial response occurred in a woman with ovarian cancer treated with 0.5 mg/m^2/day.

In 1999, Stevenson et al. reported a multicenter pharmacokinetic study of lurtotecan given by prolonged continuous infusion to 38 patients with advanced malignancy *(27)*. All patients had a central venous catheter placed. Initially, the duration of infusion was escalated from 7 to 14 to 21 days at a fixed dose of 0.3 mg/m^2/day. For patients at each duration interval, treatment was repeated 2 weeks after the completion of the previous cycle, assuming that no DLTs were encountered. After five patients were treated at 0.3 mg/m^2/day for 21 days without defining an MTD, the dose of lurtotecan was escalated to 0.4 and 0.5 mg/m^2/day. Thrombocytopenia was the DLT at 0.5 mg/m^2/day. Four of eight patients at that level experienced grade 3 or 4 thrombocytopenia. Two of 14 patients treated with 0.4 mg/m^2/day for 21 days had grade 3 thrombocytopenia. Neutropenia was not dose-limiting, with one patient receiving 0.4 mg/m^2/day and two patients receiving 0.5 mg/m^2/day having had grade 3 neutropenia. Five patients developed grade 3 nausea and vomiting, which was controlled with antiemetics for most. Three patients experienced grade 3 fatigue and one patient had grade 3 diarrhea. A linear relationship between dose and AUC was observed ($r^2 = 0.76$). Two partial responses were observed in patients with breast and ovarian cancer. Two patients, with colorectal and ovarian cancer, had stable disease through eight cycles of therapy.

These trials provided evidence of predictable and dose-limiting hematologic toxicity. Altering the schedule of administration did not substantially alter this pharmacodynamic profile. Objective responses were observed in patients with previously refractory malignancies. Based on these results, phase II studies were undertaken to further delineate the toxicity and activity of this drug.

2.3. Phase II Clinical Trials

Four phase II clinical trials using lurtotecan by 30-minute infusion daily for 5 days every 3 weeks have been reported (Table 1). The first study was carried out by Sessa et al. at 16 European cancer centers. Sixty-seven patients with small-cell lung cancer that had progressed or recurred after first-line therapy were enrolled. Patients were treated with 1.2 mg/m²/day. Of the 62 patients who were evaluable for response, 34 had responded to their initial chemotherapy and relapsed more than 3 months after the completion of treatment. The others had initially responded, then relapsed within 3 months, had progressive disease after at least one cycle of chemotherapy or progressed after having stable disease for at least two cycles. Anemia was the most common toxicity, with 91% of patients having had at least grade 1. Neutropenia and thrombocytopenia were the most common moderate to severe toxicities. Grades 3 and 4 neutropenia occurred in 16.5% and 9% of cycles, respectively. Fifteen percent of cycles were complicated by grade 3 thrombocytopenia and 7% by grade 4 thrombocytopenia. The dose was reduced to 0.9 mg/m²/day in 16 patients (24%) who had grade 4 neutropenia or thrombocytopenia, and was increased to 1.5 mg/m²/day in five patients (7.5%) who had no hematologic or nonhematologic toxicity in the previous cycle. Three patients with refractory disease and eight patients with previously sensitive disease had partial responses (overall relative risk [RR] 16.6%, 95% confidence interval [CI] 8.5–27.5%). Twenty-one patients (32%) had stable disease. The median duration of responses was 133 days. The authors concluded that the toxicity and response data were no better than topotecan in the second-line treatment of small-cell lung cancer. In light of the greater expense of the drug, they felt that it did not warrant further investigation in the water-soluble form.

The three remaining phase II trials using 1.2 mg/m²/day of lurtotecan for 5 days every 3 weeks were carried out independently at several European cancer centers, but were reported together by Gamucci et al *(28)*. Twenty patients with pretreated breast cancer, 19 patients with no prior chemotherapy for advanced colorectal cancer and 23 patients with untreated non-small-cell lung cancer were eligible and enrolled in the study. Two hundred sixty-seven cycles were given and were evaluable for toxicity. Thirty-two percent of all patients experienced grade 3 neutropenia and 22% had grade 4. Thrombocytopenia was less common, with 20% of patients having either grade 3 or 4 toxicity. Neutropenic fever occurred in 10 patients (14.5%). Dose reductions for hematological toxicity occurred in 12% of patients, dose increases were made in 25% of patients, and treatment was delayed in 20% of patients because of hematological toxicity. Among 64 patients evaluable for response, 3 patients with breast cancer (RR 13%, 95% CI 0–26.7%) and 2 patients with non-small-cell lung cancer had partial responses

(RR 9.1%, 95% CI 0–19.3%). Nine patients with breast cancer, seven patients with colorectal cancer, and five patients with non-small-cell lung cancer had stable disease.

Although responses to single-agent lurtotecan were seen, the rates were not substantially greater than previously reported second- and third-line regimens. Although the tolerability of lurtotecan appeared to exceed that of CPT, there was not sufficient evidence of activity to warrant further investigation as a single agent. While these studies were carried out, attention turned to the development of a liposomal formulation of lurtotecan. Based on the application of this carrier to other chemotherapeutics, it was hoped that liposomal encapsulation of the drug would further increase the therapeutic index.

3.LIPOSOMAL LURTOTECAN

3.1. Preclinical Studies

It has been shown that cellular uptake of CPT requires energy-dependent transporters *(29)*. Resistance is mediated, in part, by overexpression of adenosine triphosphate-binding cassette proteins such as the mitoxantrone-resistance half-transporter *(30)* and MRP2 *(31)*. In an effort to enhance drug delivery to tumors, minimize exposure to normal tissues, and circumvent resistance mediated by extrusion of the drug from the intracellular compartment, lurtotecan was encapsulated in liposomes. This approach has been validated pharmacologically and clinically with doxorubicin and daunorubicin *(32)*. Liposomes stabilize the lactone form of the CPTs *(33)*. For the more hydrophilic CPT derivatives, the lactone form can be further stabilized by lowering the pH of the aqueous core of liposomes *(94)*. The opening of the lactone ring had been shown in vitro to account for at least a 90% loss of anti-TOP-I activity. The possibility of stabilizing the lactone form of lurtotecan in human plasma provided the mechanistic basis for optimism that this formulation would provide greater delivery of active drug to tumor cells than the water-soluble form.

The first preclinical report of the anticancer activity of liposomal lurtotecan was made by Colburn et al. in 1998 *(35)*. They were able to entrap more than 90% of the free drug in liposomes containing a pegylated lipid along with phosphatidylcholine, cholesterol, and another phospholipid. The average diameter of the particles was 100 nm. In rats, a 1250-fold increase in the AUC was seen with liposomal lurtotecan after a single intravenous bolus compared with a similar dose of the free drug. Toxicity and antitumor activity of liposomal lurtotecan was evaluated in a mouse xenograft model of implanted HT-29 colon cancer cells. The dose of liposomal lurtotecan was adjusted to match the toxicity profile of 20 mg/kg of free lurtotecan. The dose of free lurtotecan was determined based on a drug-related death in 1 of 10 animals treated at the higher dose level. There were 7 complete and 1 partial responses among the 10 mice treated with 3 mg/kg of liposomal lurtotecan compared to only 1 partial response out of 10 animals treated with 20 mg/kg of free lurtotecan. This formulation of liposomal lurtotecan has not been evaluated in humans.

Another formulation of liposome-encapsulated lurtotecan (NX 211, Gilead Sciences) was studied in animal models by Emerson et al. and reported in 2000 *(36)*. The liposomes used in this study were unilamellar particles averaging 100 nm in size and were composed of phosphatidylcholine and cholesterol in a 2:1 ratio. A 1435-fold increase in AUC was seen with liposomal lurtotecan compared with the free drug. The toxicity and efficacy of liposomal lurtotecan was compared with free lurtotecan and topotecan in two mouse xenograft models using ES-2 human ovarian carcinoma cells and KB human squamous cell carcinoma cells with and without the MDR phenotype. Using a wide range of doses of each drug, the lethal dose for 50% of the animals and the dose required for 60% or 80% tumor growth inhibition were determined. After separately determining the MTD for each drug in each xenograft model, the efficacy was compared. The therapeutic index of liposomal lurtotecan was 2.9 in the KB xenografts and 14.4 in the ES-2 xenografts. In the ES-2 xenografts, at a dose of 9 mg/kg of liposomal lurtotecan, three of eight animals had complete responses, with no toxic deaths occurring. The lurtotecan and topotecan treated groups had no complete responses and three toxic deaths each. The time to a fourfold increase in tumor size was four times longer in the liposomal lurtotecan-treated groups compared with untreated animals. The KB xenograft mice also demonstrated greater tumor sensitivity and growth delay when treated with liposomal lurtotecan compared with free lurtotecan. This result was seen in the MDR(+) and the MDR(–) KB xenografts. Using radiolabeled lurtotecan to measure concentration in tissue, tumor uptake of the drug was increased 9- to 67-fold with liposome encapsulation compared with the free drug.

Further pharmacokinetic studies in mice have been carried out in tumor-bearing mice treated with radiolabeled lurtotecan in the encapsulated or free form *(37)*. A 70-fold increase in concentration of lurtotecan in tumors was achieved with liposomal lurtotecan. The intratumoral AUC was 17-fold greater with liposomal lurtotecan compared with free lurtotecan. More than 95% of the radioactivity in tumors was the intact drug. Xenograft models have subsequently been employed to assess the efficacy of liposomal lurtotecan against implanted lung, breast, ovarian, renal, sarcoma, glioblastoma, and prostate cancer cell lines *(38)*. Response rates ranged from 6% to 43%. This formulation of liposomal lurtotecan has been taken to the clinic.

3.2. Phase I Clinical Trials

Three phase I clinical trials have been performed with liposomal lurtotecan and have been reported in abstract form (Table 2). At the 2000 American Society of Clinical Oncology (ASCO) annual meeting, Bos et al. reported on an ongoing phase I trial of liposomal lurtotecan given by 30-minute infusion once every 21 days *(39)*. At the time of publication, 15 patients had been enrolled and no dose-limiting toxicities had occurred. Three patients were treated with 0.4 mg/m^2, six with 0.8 mg/m^2, three with 1.6 mg/m^2, and three with 3.2 mg/m^2. The maximum plasma concentration of the drug increased across the first three dose levels, but the AUC did not. Accrual continued after this report was prepared. The results of this trial were updated at the 2001 ASCO meeting. Fourteen additional patients had been enrolled. An MTD of 4.3 mg/m^2 was defined by dose-limiting neutropenia and thrombocytopenia in three of five patients at that level. Therefore, the recommended Phase II dose was 3.8 mg/m^2. Objective response data were not provided in this report.

Rothenberg et al. reported on a multicenter phase I trial at the 2000 ASCO meeting *(40)*. Two schedules of liposomal lurtotecan were evaluated in concurrent studies. The first schedule consisted of liposomal lurtotecan given by 30-minute infusion on days 1 and 8 every 3 weeks; in the second, liposomal lurtotecan was given on days 1, 2, and 3 every 3 weeks. By the time of that report, eight patients had been treated using the first regimen at doses of 0.2, 0.4, 0.8, and 1.6 mg/kg/day. No DLTs had been encountered. Twenty patients were treated with the second schedule at doses of 0.15, 0.30, 0.6, 1.2, and 1.8 mg/m^2/day. Grade 3 thrombocytopenia was observed in two of four heavily pretreated patients at the highest dose level. Pharmacokinetic analysis from both studies showed a maximum AUC of 7.3 mcg/mL/hour in the 1.2 mg/m^2/day group using the second schedule. Taking all patients into account, the AUC for liposomal lurtotecan was 71-fold greater than the AUC for lurtotecan seen in prior studies. No objective responses were reported.

These results were also updated at the 2001 ASCO meeting *(41)*. The days 1 and 8 every 3 weeks schedule was evaluated in 18 further patients. An MTD of 3.2 mg/m^2/week was reached when two of six patients had dose-limiting neutropenia and thrombocytopenia. The recommended phase II dose was 2.4 mg/m^2/week for heavily pretreated patients and 2.8 mg/m^2/week for minimally pretreated patients. Based on the improved dose-intensity of this regimen compared with the once every 3 weeks schedule, it was chosen for further study. The schedule using liposomal lurtotecan on days 1, 2, and 3 every 3 weeks was evaluated in 17 additional patients. During dose escalation, patients were divided into minimally and heavily pretreated. An MTD of 1.8 mg/m^2/day for heavily pretreated patients was defined by

Table 2
Clinical Trials of Liposomal lurtotecan

Phase I trials				
Investigator	*Schedule*	*Phase II dose*	*DLT*	*Responses*
Bos et al.	Day 1 q 3 weeks	3.8 mg/m^2	Neutropenia and thrombocytopenia	None reported
Rothenberg et al.	Days 1 and 8 q 3 weeks	2.4 mg/m^2/day, heavily pretreated	Neutropenia and thrombocytopenia	PRs in unspecified
		2.8 mg/m^2/day, minimally pretreated	Neutropenia and thrombocytopenia	Number of patients with breast and ovarian cancer
	Days 1–3 q 3 weeks	1.5 mg/m^2/day, heavily pretreated	Thrombocytopenia	
		2.1 mg/m^2/day, minimally pretreated	Thrombocytopenia	
Felton et al.	Weekly for 4 weeks q 6 weeks	Not yet determined	Thrombocytopenia	None reported

PR, partial response; DLT, dose-limiting toxicity.

dose-limiting thrombocytopenia in two of four patients. The MTD for minimally pretreated patients was greater than 2.1 mg/m^2/day, based on dose-limiting thrombocytopenia in two of nine patients. The recommended Phase II doses for minimally and heavily pretreated patients was 1.5 mg/m^2/day and 2.1 mg/m^2/day. Partial responses were observed in patients with breast and ovarian cancer.

A fourth schedule was evaluated by Felton et al. at the San Antonio Institute for Drug Development and preliminary results were reported at the 2001 ASCO meeting. Liposomal lurtotecan was given by 30-minute infusion weekly for 4 weeks every 6 weeks. At the time of the report, nine patients had been treated with 0.4, 0.8, 1.6, and 2.4 mg/m^2/wk. One patient at the highest dose level experienced dose-limiting grade 4 thrombocytopenia. Although large interpatient variability was observed, pharmacokinetic studies from the first two dose levels yielded results that were consistent with earlier trials. No objective responses were reported.

4. SUMMARY

The development of novel TOP-I inhibitors continues to be of considerable interest. Lurtotecan represents a rationally developed CPT derivative with improved pharmacokinetics and pharmacodynamics compared with the parent compound. Early clinical trials of the water-soluble form of lurtotecan revealed a narrow therapeutic index based on dose-limiting myelosuppression. Liposome encapsulation has provided a mechanism for circumventing several of the pharmacokinetic limitations of the free drug. Animal models and phase I clinical trials have born out the hypothesis that more drug can be safely delivered with considerably increased tumor drug concentrations. Phase II clinical trials are under way in patients with refractory ovarian cancer, advanced head-and-neck cancer, recurrent small-cell lung cancer, and colorectal cancer. These studies will help to delineate the antitumor activity of this approach and seek to validate the efforts to engineer a more potent inhibitor of TOP-I.

REFERENCES

1. Muggia FM, Creaven PJ, Hansen HH, Cohen MH, Selawry OS. 1972 Phase I trial of weekly and daily treatment with camptothecin (NSC-100880): correlation with preclinical studies. Cancer Chemother Rep 56:515–521.
2. Hsiang YH, Hertzberg R, Hecht S, Liu LF. 1985 Camptothecin induces protein-linked DNA breaks via mammalian DNA topoisomerase I. J Biol Chem 260:14873–14878.
3. Liu LF. 1989 DNA topoisomerase poisons as anti-tumor drugs. Ann Rev Biochem 58:351–375.
4. Zhang H, D'Arpa P, Liu LF. 1990 A model for tumor cell killing by topoisomerase poisons. Cancer Cells 2:23–27.

5. Borovitskaya AE, D'Arpa P. 1998 Replication-dependent and -independent camptothecin cytotoxicity of seven human colon tumor cell lines. Oncol Res 10:271–276.
6. Holm C, Covey JM, Kerrigan D, Pommier Y. 1989 Differential requirement of DNA replication for the cytotoxicity of DNA topoisomerase I and II inhibitors in Chinese hamster DC3F cells. Cancer Res 49:6365–3638.
7. Desai SD, Liu LF, Vazquez-Abad D, D'Arpa P. 1997 Ubiquitin-dependent destruction of topoisomerase I is stimulated by the antitumor drug camptothecin. J Biol Chem 272:24159–24164.
8. Murren JR, Beidler DR, Cheng YC. 1996 Camptothecin resistance related to drug-induced down-regulation of topoisomerase I and to steps occurring after the formation of protein-linked DNA breaks. Ann NY Acad Sci 803:74–92.
9. Liu LF, Desai SD, Li TK, Mao Y, Sun M, Sim SP. 2000 Mechanism of action of camptothecin. Ann N Y Acad Sci 922:1–10.
10. Wall ME. 1998 Camptothecin and taxol: discovery to clinic. Med Res Rev 18:299–314.
11. Mi Z, Burke TG. 1994 Differential interactions of camptothecin lactone and carboxylate forms with human blood components. Biochemistry 33:10325–10336.
12. Mi Z, Burke TG. 1994 Marked interspecies variations concerning interactions of camptothecin with serum albumin. Biochemistry 33:12540–12545.
13. Jaxel C, Kohn KW, Wani MC, Wall ME, Pommier Y. 1989 Structure-activity study of the actions of camptothecin derivatives on mammalian topoisomerase I: evidence for a specific receptor site and a relation to antitumor activity. Cancer Res 49:1465–1469.
14. Hertzberg RP, Caranfa MJ, Holden KG, et al. 1989 Modifications of the hydroxy lactone ring of camptothecin: inhibition of mammalian topoisomerase I and biological activity. J Med Chem 32:715–720.
15. Lavergne O, Lesueur-Ginot L, Rodas F, et al. 1998 Homocamptothecins, synthesis and antitumor activity of novel E-ring-modified camptothecin analogues. J Med Chem 41:5410–5419.
16. Wang X, Zhou X, Hecht SM. 1999 Role of the 20-hydroxyl group in camptothecin binding by the topoisomerase I-DNA binary complex. Biochemistry 38:4374–4381.
17. Tanizawa A, Fujimori A, Fujimori Y, Pommier Y. 1994 Comparison of topoisomerase I inhibition, DNA damage, and cytotoxicity of camptothecin derivatives presently in clinical trials. J Natl Cancer Inst 86:836–82.
18. Tanizawa A, Kohn KW, Kohlhagen G, Leteurtre F, Pommier Y. 1995 Differential stabilization of eukaryotic DNA topoisomerase I cleavable complexes by camptothecin derivatives. Biochemistry 34:7200–7206.
19. ten Bokkel Huinink W, Gore M, Carmichael J, et al. 1997 Topotecan versus paclitaxel for the treatment of recurrent epithelial ovarian cancer. J Clin Oncol 15:2183–2193.
20. Rothenberg ML, Cox JV, DeVore RF, et al. 1999 A multicenter, phase II trial of weekly irinotecan (CPT-11) in patients with previously treated colorectal carcinoma. Cancer 85:786–795.
21. Rougier P, Bugat R, Douillard JY, et al. 1997 Phase II study of irinotecan in the treatment of advanced colorectal cancer in chemotherapy-naive patients and patients pretreated with fluorouracil-based chemotherapy. J Clin Oncol 15:251–260.
22. Emerson DL, Besterman JM, Brown HR, et al. 1995 In vivo antitumor activity of two new seven-substituted water-soluble camptothecin analogues. Cancer Res 55:603–609.

23. Gerrits CJ, Creemers GJ, Schellens JH, et al. 1996 Phase I and pharmacological study of the new topoisomerase I inhibitor GI147211, using a daily x 5 intravenous administration. Br J Cancer 73:744–750.
24. Gerrits CJ, Schellens JH, Creemers GJ, et al. 1997 The bioavailability of oral GI147211 (GG211), a new topoisomerase I inhibitor. Br J Cancer 76:946–951.
25. Eckhardt SG, Baker SD, Eckardt JR, et al. 1998 Phase I and pharmacokinetic study of GI147211, a water-soluble camptothecin analogue, administered for five consecutive days every three weeks. Clin Cancer Res 4:595–604.
26. Paz-Ares L, Kunka R, DeMaria D, et al. 1998 A phase I clinical and pharmacokinetic study of the new topoisomerase inhibitor GI147211 given as a 72-h continuous infusion. Br J Cancer 78:1329–1336.
27. Stevenson JP, DeMaria D, Sludden J, et al. 1999 Phase I/pharmacokinetic study of the topoisomerase I inhibitor GG211 administered as a 21-day continuous infusion. Ann Oncol 10:339–344.
28. Gamucci T, Paridaens R, Heinrich B, et al. 2000 Activity and toxicity of GI147211 in breast, colorectal and non-small-cell lung cancer patients: an EORTC-ECSG phase II clinical study. Ann Oncol 11:793–797.
29. Gupta E, Luo F, Lallo A, et al. 2000 The intestinal absorption of camptothecin, a highly lipophilic drug, across Caco-2 cells is mediated by active transporter(s). Anticancer Res 20:1013–1016.
30. Brangi M, Litman T, Ciotti M, et al. 1999 Camptothecin resistance: role of the ATP-binding cassette (ABC), mitoxantrone-resistance half-transporter (MXR), and potential for glucuronidation in MXR-expressing cells. Cancer Res 59:5938–5946.
31. Koike K, Kawabe T, Tanaka T, et al. 1997 A canalicular multispecific organic anion transporter (cMOAT) antisense cDNA enhances drug sensitivity in human hepatic cancer cells. Cancer Res 57:5475–5479.
32. Massing U, Fuxius S. 2000 Liposomal formulations of anticancer drugs: selectivity and effectiveness. Drug Resist Updat 3:171–177.
33. Burke TG, Staubus AE, Mishra AK. 1992 Liposomal stabilization of camptothecin's lactone ring. J Am Chem Soc 114:8318–8319.
34. Burke TG. Liposomal and micellar stabilization of camptothecin drugs. U.S. Patent 5,552,156. September 3, 1996.
35. Colbern GT, Dykes DJ, Engbers C, et al. 1998 Encapsulation of the topoisomerase I inhibitor GL147211C in pegylated (STEALTH) liposomes: pharmacokinetics and antitumor activity in HT29 colon tumor xenografts. Clin Cancer Res 4:3077–3082.
36. Emerson DL, Bendele R, Brown E, et al. 2000 Antitumor efficacy, pharmacokinetics, and biodistribution of NX 211: a low-clearance liposomal formulation of lurtotecan. Clin Cancer Res 6:2903–2912.
37. Desjardins JP, Abbott EA, Emerson DL, et al. 2001 Biodistribution of NX211, liposomal lurtotecan, in tumor-bearing mice. Anticancer Drugs 12:235–245.
38. Emerson DL, Bendele R, Brown E, et al. 2001 In vivo antitumor efficacy of liposomal lurtotecan (NX 211) in human xenografts. Proc Am Assoc Cancer Res 42:545.
39. Bos AM, Kehrer D, Sparreboom A, et al. 2000 Phase I study of NX 211 (liposomal lurtotecan) administered as a single dose every 3 weeks. Proc Am Soc Clin Oncol 19:768.
40. Rothenberg ML, Gelmon KA, Eisenhauer E, et al. 2000 Phase I evaluation of liposomal topoisomerase I inhibitor, NX 211, given on days 1,2,3 or days 1,8 every 3 weeks to patients with advanced solid tumors. Proc Am Soc Clin Oncol 19:769.

41. Eisenhauer EA, Verweij J, Rothenberg ML, et al. 2001 Phase I evaluation of liposomal topoisomerase I inhibitor, NX 211, administered by three schedules to patients with advanced solid tumors. Proc Am Soc Clin Oncol 19:409.

14 Preclinical and Clinical Development of Exatecan (DX-8951f)

A Hexacyclic Camptothecin Analog

Eric K. Rowinsky, MD

Contents

1. INTRODUCTION

The principal rationale for synthesizing exatecan (DX-8951f, Daiichi Pharmaceutical Co., Ltd, Japan) was to exploit physicochemical features of the camptothecins (CPTs) anticipated to yield an increased therapeutic advantage compared with currently available CPT analogs such as topotecan and irinotecan. The overall therapeutic profile sought in these efforts was greater and broader antitumor activity, decreased toxicity, and intrinsic activity without requiring metabolic activation, which may accentuate the fundamentally large interindividual variability in the pharmacologic behavior of the CPT analogs and consequently in their antitumor and toxicologic profiles. Exatecan has completed Phase I clinical development on a broad range of schedules and is currently undergoing more focused disease-directed Phase II and Phase III evaluations. Additionally, DE-310, a unique polymer prodrug of exatecan, which was developed to achieve protracted systemic exposure to the active drug after a single dose, is also undergoing early clinical development.

2. STRUCTURE

Exatecan (DX-8951f; (1*S*, 9*S*)-1-amino-9-ethyl-5-fluoro-1, 2, 3, 9, 12, 15-hexahydro-9-hydroxy-4-methyl-10*H*, 13*H*-benzo [*de*] pyrano [3', 4':6,7] indolizino[1,2-*b*]quinoline-10, 13-dione monomethane sulfonate (salt) dihydrate is a water-soluble, fluorinated, hexaphilic synthetic derivative of CPT that, in contrast to irinotecan, has intrinsic activity without undergoing metabolic activation. The chemical structure of the anhydrous base form of the drug, referred to as DX-8951, is shown in Fig. 1. The 20S stereoisomeric form is active, whereas the 20R form is inactive. The chemical structure of exatecan has been modified to render the molecule water-soluble by adding a ring structure between rings A (in position 9) and B (in position 7), and a fluorine in position 11. Similar to all CPT derivatives that inhibit topoisomerase I (TOP-I), the A-ring of the lactone form of the drug is hydrolyzed to form an open-ring hydroxy-acid species. The two species coexist in solution according to a reversible pH-dependent equilibrium, with an acidic pH favoring the formation of the closed-ring lactone form.

3. PRECLINICAL ACTIVITY

Interest in exatecan was first generated after the agent demonstrated 3 times greater potency than SN-38, the active metabolite of irinotecan, 10 times greater potency than topotecan, and 20 times greater potency than CPT at inhibiting TOP-I extracted from murine P388 leukemia; IC_{50} (concentration that inhibits 50%) values of 0.975, 2.71, 9.52, and 23.5 μg/mL were reported for exatecan1f, SN-38, topotecan, and CPT, respectively *(1)*. The inhibition of human TOP-I by the lactone was approximately 300-fold greater than that by the hydroxy-acid form. Exatecan was also approximately five times more potent than SN-38 at inhibiting DNA synthesis. Furthermore, in a study of the relative antitumor properties of the CPT analogs against a panel of 32 cell lines derived from human breast, gastric, colon, ovarian, cervical, lung, and hematopoietic neoplasms, the IC_{50} values of exatecan averaged 6- and 28-fold lower than SN-38 and topotecan, respectively *(1,2)*. A summary of the relative IC_{50} values of exatecan and the other CPT analogs according to tumor type is shown in Table 1. In the human tumor cloning assay, exatecan inhibited the growth of clonogenic

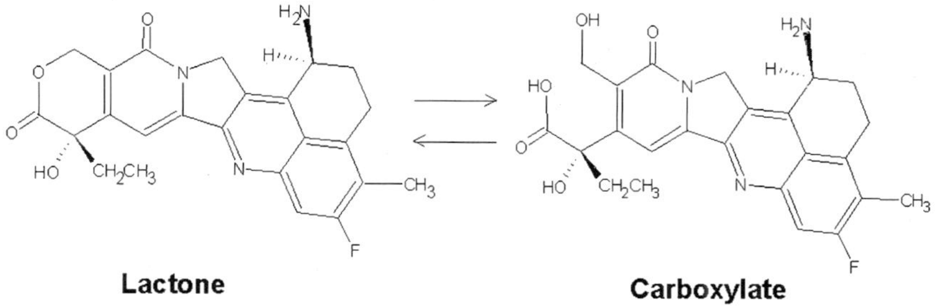

Fig. 1. Structure of the active exatecan lactone (left) undergoing reversible pH-dependent hydrolysis to its inactive open-ring form.

Table 1
In Vitro Cytotoxicity Against A Series of 32 Cancer Cell Lines: Summary According to Tumor Type

	IC_{50} (ng/mL)			
Tumor type	*Exatecan*	*SN-38*	*Topotecan*	*CPT*
Breaast	2.02	6.57	64.1	12.5
Colon	2.92	15.1	92.5	21.8
Stomach	1.53	15.1	30.6	13.0
Lung	0.87	7.37	35.3	9.99
Others	4.33	36.2	82.9	26.1
Summary	2.09	12.1	89.5	15.3

ID_{50}, drug concentration at which the growth is inhibited by 50%.

cells derived from patients with head and neck, non-small-cell lung, liver, lung, breast, colon, ovary, and prostate carcinomas in a dose-dependent manner, and exatecan and topotecan were not completely cross-resistant *(3)*.

Exatecan has shown activity against a wide range of human tumor xenografts in nude mice, including gastric, pancreatic, colon, breast, ovary, and lung cancers *(1,4,5)*. In addition, the agent demonstrated impressive antitumor activity against an intracranial xenograft of human RH30 rhabdomyosarcoma and various other pediatric solid neoplasms, murine lung and liver metastasis xenograft models, and both early and late stages of human acute myelogenous leukemia in a severe combined immunodeficient mouse model *(5–11)*. Exatecan also produced notable activity that was superior to gemcitabine in both orthotopic and traditional xenografts of human pancreatic cancer *(12)*. Although exatecan treatment resulted in impressive antitumor activity on both single and divided dosing administra-

Table 2
Comparison of the Antitumor Effects of Exatecan and CPT-11 Against Various Human Tumor Xenografts

		Exatecan total (75 mg/kg)		*Irinotecan (320 mg/kg)*	
Tumor type	*No. of tumors*	*>IR (80%)*	*>IR (58%)*	*>IR (80%)*	*>IR (58%)*
Gastric cancer	2	2 (100%)	2 (100%)	1 (50%)	2 (100%)
Colon cancer	6	6 (100%)	6 (100%)	4 (67%)	5 (83%)
Lung cancer	5	4 (80%)	5 (100%)	1 (20%)	2 (40%)
Breast cancer	2	2 (100%)	2 (100%)	2 (100%)	2 (100%)
Renal cancer	1	0 (0%)	0 (0%)	0 (0%)	0 (10%)
Total	16	14 (88%)	15 (94%)	8 (50%)	11 (69%)
p<0.05 p = 0.10					

IR, dose at which the specified percentage of tumor growth inhibition is produced by the drug as a single agent.

tion schedules, superior efficacy was generally noted against human tumor xenografts when the agent was administered on divided dosing schedules *(1,4)*. For example, in studies involving the in vivo homologous Meth A mouse fibrosarcoma model, a cyclical dosing pattern resulted in superior antitumor activity at lower doses of exatecan compared with a single dosing schedule. A comparison of the antitumor effects of exatecan and irinotecan at equitoxic doses against various human tumor xenografts is depicted in Table 2.

Several in vitro and in vivo investigations using human tumor cell lines and drug-resistant variants have demonstrated that exatecan, in contrast to topotecan and SN-38, is not affected by mechanisms of drug resistance conferred by overexpression of P-glycoprotein (Pgp) or breast cancer resistance protein, as well as decreased levels of TOP-I mRNA or protein *(9,12–18)*. In fact, exatecan is not a substrate for the Pgp multidrug transporter that confers multidrug resistance, whereas both topotecan and SN-38 are weak substrates for Pgp *(9,12–15)*. The impressive and distinctly different preclinical antitumor spectra of exatecan may, in part, be due to the fact that the agent is not a substrate for the Pgp multidrug transporter, in contrast to topotecan, 9-aminocamptothecin, and SN-38, which are weak substrates for the efflux pump *(13–16)*. The lack of cross-resistance of Pgp-overexpressing neoplasms to exatecan is indicated by the results of a study in which the agent exhibited similar antitumor activity against human lung cancer PC-6 and its multidrug resistance Pgp-overexpressing variant, PC-6/vincristine as shown in Table 3 *(9)*. Similarly, exatecan demonstrated roughly equiva-

Table 3
Comparison of the Antitumor Effects and Relative Resistance of Exatecan and Other Topoisomerase I-Targeting Agents Against Parental (PC-6) and Pgp Overexpressing (PC-6/Vincristine) Cancer Cell Lines

	IC_{50} *(ng/mL)*		
Agent	*PC*	*6 PC-6/Vincristine*	*Resistance ratio*
Exatecan	0.089	0.069	0.8
SN-38	0.655	0.751	1.1
Topotecan	1.73	4.36	2.5
Vincristine	0.284	107	380
Cisplatin	13.8	69	0.5

ID_{50}, dose associated with inhibition growth by 50%; Pgp, P-glycoprotein.

lent potencies against PC-6 and a SN-38–resistant subline characterized by impaired SN-38 accumulation without Pgp overexpression, and the antitumor activities of exatecan were similar against human pancreatic cancers SUIT-2 and KP-1N and their respective sublines that had acquired resistance to CPT-11 in vivo and SN-38 in vitro, presumably because of reduced levels of TOP-I mRNA and protein *(8)*. The magnitude of accumulation of drug within the cell was demonstrated to be a determinant of sensitivity to exatecan in vitro, and this phenomenon appears, in part, to be the basis for differential activity between CPT analogs *(8)*. Exatecan treatment has also been demonstrated to induce BRCP in vitro, but BRCP overexpression, which conferred resistance to 9-aminocamptothecin, SN-38, and irinotecan, was responsible for negligible to no resistance to exatecan *(17,18)*. Similarly, neither overexpression of Pgp, multidrug-resistance protein-1, or lung cancer–resistance protein conferred resistance to exatecan in a wide array of experimental human colon and ovarian cancers *(19)*. There is only one clear model of tumor resistance to exatecan, in which drug resistance relates to qualitative changes in the expression of TOP-I *(9,20)*. Evidence implicates "modifier" proteins such as ubiquitin, SUMO-1, and others, which bind to critical domains of TOP-I *(16,20)*. In addition, higher levels of the DNA repair protein O(6)-methylguanine-DNA methyltransferase have been demonstrated to be associated with resistance to exatecan and other CPT analogs, and treatment of drug resistance cells, presumptively because of increased O(6)-methylguanine-DNA methyltransferase activity, by a nontoxic O(6)-methylguanine-DNA methyltransferase inhibitor-augmented drug activity *(21)*.

4. PRECLINICAL PHARMACOLOGY

In preclinical pharmacology studies of exatecan in dogs and rodents using radiolabeled drug (^{14}C-exatecan) and high-performance liquid chromatography for differential quantification of lactone and total drug, the half-life ($t_{1/2}$) of the lactone ranged from approximately 20 to 30 minutes, and systemic exposure to the lactone was approximately 50% of total drug exposure *(22–28)*. In both species, the clearance rates of total drug and lactone were similar: lactone exposure accounted for approximately 50% of total exatecan exposure, and the pharmacokinetics of both total drug and lactone were dose-independent. Tissue distribution studies revealed exatecan uptake in all tissues; however, drug concentrations in brain were very low, suggesting that exatecan is not transported across an intact blood-brain barrier. Exatecan was also shown to be highly bound to plasma proteins in all species, and spectrometric studies indicated that the lactone is selectively stabilized by albumin under physiologic conditions. In vitro, plasma proteins were determined to be approximately 93, 86, 96, and 93% in rats, dogs, monkeys, and humans, respectively.

In rats treated with a single intravenous (iv) dose of ^{14}C-exatecan, urine and fecal recovery averaged 15% and 78% of the administered dose, respectively *(22–25)*. The majority of exatecan was metabolized to hydroxylated metabolites. The same hydroxylated metabolites have predominated after coincubation of exatecan and liver microsomes of multiple species, including humans, in vitro. These studies, and other in vitro and in vivo studies, have indicated that exatecan is highly metabolized to a 4-hydroxymethyl metabolite (UM-1) and a 3-hydroxy metabolite (UM-2), the structures of which are shown in Figure 2. The cytochrome P450 microsomal isoenzymes CYP3A4 and CYP1A2 are principally involved in metabolism of exatecan to UM-1 and UM-2, respectively *(22–28)*. The antitumor activities of both hydroxylated metabolites against P388 and PC-6 cancer cell lines were demonstrated to be substantially less than exatecan *(22,23,25,26,28)*. The hydroxylation of exatecan has been demonstrated to be inhibited in vitro by several known CYP3A substrates, including ketoconazole, nifedipine, erythromycin, and fentanyl *(22)*. There were no gender-related differences in exatecan metabolism, but an interindividual variation of hydroxylation, consisting of a 5.6-fold difference between the lowest and highest rates of hydroxylation in 29 human liver microsomal samples, was demonstrated *(22,23)*.

5. PRECLINICAL TOXICOLOGY

The toxicity profile of exatecan has been evaluated in mice, rats, and dogs before clinical trials *(22,25,26)*. The toxicity profile was consistent across all animal species. Rapidly proliferative tissues, including hematopoietic

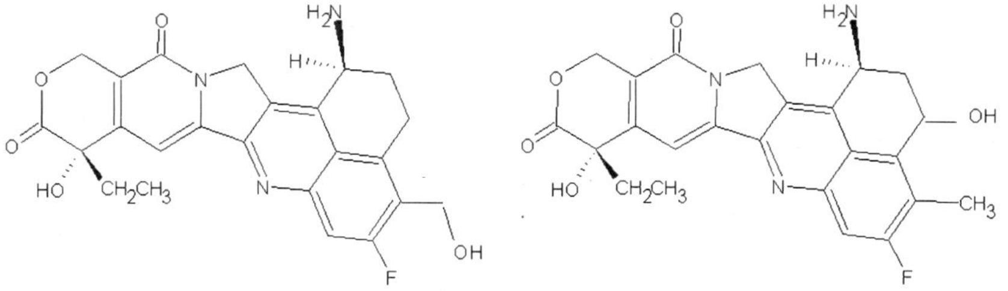

UM-1 **UM-2**

Fig. 2. Structures of the principal metabolites of exatecan 3-hydroxy metabolite (UM-1) (left) and a 3-hydroxy metabolite (UM-2) (right).

(neutropenia, thrombocytopenia, anemia, lymphopenia), gastrointestinal (vomiting diarrhea), lymph nodes, and reproductive tissues, have been most prone to the toxic effects of exatecan, and noncumulative myelosuppression, particularly neutropenia, was been the principal dose-limiting effect of exatecan on both single- and divided-dosing regimens in both rodents and dogs. In addition to being dose-dependent, hematologic toxicity appeared schedule-dependent, with more frequent (divided) dosing schedules associated with greater toxicity at equivalent doses. Similar to other CPT analogs, there has been considerable interspecies differences in drug tolerance, with dogs being more susceptible to toxicity than rodents. Therefore, the human equivalent of one-third of the low toxic dose in dogs was used to determine the starting dose for each corresponding schedule of administration in human clinical trials.

6. PHASE I DEVELOPMENT IN PATIENTS WITH ADVANCED MALIGNANCIES

6.1. Overall Clinical Scheme

The safety, dosing limits, and pharmacokinetics of multiple exatecan administration schedules were evaluated in phase I clinical evaluations according to a parallel and integrated development plan that linked studies in the United States, Europe, and Japan. The principal objective of this approach was to select an optimal dosing regimen for subsequent disease-directed clinical investigations. To achieve this goal, a core protocol was established to standardize clinical data evaluation including toxicity and efficacy criteria, definitions of unacceptable or dose-limiting toxicity (DLT) and maximum tolerated dose (MTD), inclusion and exclusion criteria, and supportive therapy paradigms. Another goal was to readily permit exchange of data in a timely manner among the three global regions so that all investigators had ready access to the data for decision making as dose escalation was in progress. Data were collected and processed in compliance with the International Committee on Harmonization guidelines.

Six phase I studies were initially conducted outside of Japan according to three schedules of administration and two durations of iv infusion *(25,26,29–36)*. Two studies were duplicated in Japan; however, these studies were directed to evaluate the pharmacokinetics of the exatecan lactone and total exatecan *(29,31)*, whereas the other studies were limited to measurements of total exatecan because of logistical considerations regarding the analysis of the exatecan lactone.

For each study, the starting dose was chosen as one-third of the toxic dose low for the corresponding schedule in the dog, which was the most sensitive species. There was no standardization of the method of dose escalation, because both modified Fibonacci and modified continual reassessment methods were employed. Interestingly, there were no significant differences between the methods in the number of dose escalation steps required to delineate and recommend phase II doses. However, MTDs were determined separately for heavily pretreated (HP) and minimally pretreated (MP) patients because the extent of prior treatment appeared to be a major determinant for the severity of the neutropenia, which was the principal toxicity. The definitions of HP and MP patients were derived prospectively, largely based on the results of prior Phase I studies of other TOP-I-targeting agents and chemotherapeutics in which neutropenia was the principal DLT *(37–39)*. HP patients were defined as those who had received more than six courses of alkylating-agent containing chemotherapy (or more than four courses of carboplatin), radiation therapy to more than 25% of hematopoietic reserves, and two or more courses of mitomycin C or nitrosourea. All toxic effects were graded according to the National Cancer Institute Common Toxicity Criteria, version 1.0. DLT was defined as grade 4 neutropenia (absolute neutrophil count [ANC] <500/μL) associated with fever (≥38.4°C) or lasting longer than 5 days), any grade 3 nonhematologic toxicity (excluding nausea and vomiting), grade 4 vomiting with maximum supportive care, any grade 3 or higher event requiring intensive care treatment, or the inability to start a second course after a 2-week treatment delay because of toxicity. The MTD was defined as the highest dose at which no more than 20% of patients experienced DLT during the first course.

6.2. Overall Pharmacokinetic Scheme

Initial analytical assays to measure plasma and urinary concentrations of exatecan and metabolites used high-performance liquid chromatography, but more sensitive liquid chromatographic/mass spectrometry/mass spectrophotometry assays were subsequently derived and validated *(23–28)*. The pharmacokinetics of exatecan were determined in all phase I studies using standard noncompartmental and compartmental pharmacokinetic methods. Compartmental analyses were performed to obtain more robust estimations of individual pharmacokinetic parameters. Initially, the individual data sets in each study were fit with either two- or three-compartment models using nonlinear least-squares regression *(40)*. The "goodness" of model fit (i.e. two- versus three-compartment model) was guided by inspection of the weighted sum of squares, dispersion of the residuals, standard errors of the fitted pharmacokinetic parameters, and the Akaike information criterion *(41)*. When the drug was administered on a 24-hour infusion schedule and concentrations were available for 24 hours posttreatment, the quality of the fit was as good using a two- or three-compartment model. Therefore, the two-compartment model was selected because of its simplicity. When exatecan was given as a 24-hour infusion and concentrations available for only 6 hours posttreatment, a single compartment model fit the data as well as the two- or three-compartment models, which is not surprising in view of the potential masking of the distribution phase by a 24-hour infusion schedule and the inability to adequately describe the terminal elimination phase because of the lack of plasma observations after 6 hours. In subjects treated with exatecan administered over 30 minutes and concentrations available for 24 hours posttreatment, a three-compartmental model was demonstrated to be systematically superior in fitting plasma concentrations based on the aforementioned criteria. Pharmacokinetic parameter estimates derived from these fits were then used as prior values for a population pharmacokinetic analysis, performed using an iterative two-stage methodology (IT2S) *(42–44)*. All concentrations were modeled using a weighting procedure of $Wj + 1/S_j^2$, where the variance of S_j^2 was calculated for each observation using the equation $S_j^2 = (a + b*Y)^2$, where a and b are the intercept and slope of each variance model. The slope is the residual variability associated with each concentration (i.e., sum of the intraindividual variability and the sum of all experimental errors), and the intercept is related to the limit of detection of the analytical assay. Variance parameter estimates were derived using maximum likelihood analysis (ADAPT-II Release 4; Biomedical Simulations Resource, University of Southern California, Los Angeles, CA) *(43)*. These estimates were used as beginning priors and were updated iteratively during the population pharmacokinetic analysis until a stable value was found *(43)*. The parameters derived were: the macro rate constants λ_1, λ_2, and λ_z associated with λ_1, λ_2, and λ_z (terminal) phases, respectively; λ_1–$t_{1/2}$, λ_2–$t_{1/2}$, λ_z–$t_{1/2}$, calculated as 0.693 divided by the respective macro constants; and V_{ss}, calculated as the sum of the central and peripheral volumes of distribution.

Urinary metabolites were detected using both high-performance liquid chromatography and liquid chromatographic/mass spectrometry/mass spectrophotometry methods and subsequently isolated, purified, and identified using nuclear magnetic resonance *(23,24,27)*. In the urine of rats and humans, both UM-1 and UM-2 were identified. Mass balance studies in humans are to precisely determine the extent of metabolite formation and excretion are ongoing (C. Takimoto, personal communication, September 2003). Furthermore, Phase I and pharmacokinetic studies in patients with various grades of hepatic or renal dysfunction are also being performed (C. Takimoto, personal communication, September 2003).

6.3. Clinical Results

6.3.1. Toxicity

The principal toxicity of exatecan was similar for all schedules of administration *(25,26,29–36)*. Myelosuppression, particularly neutropenia, was the principal DLT of exatecan. In HP patients, both neutropenia and thrombocytopenia were dose-limiting. On the daily × 5 every 3-week schedule, the ANC nadir was typically experienced between days 10 and 15, treatment delays resulting from unresolved neutropenia were uncommon, and there was no evidence of a cumulative effect of exatecan on the ANC nadirs in both MP and HP patients *(32)*. However, the relationship between exatecan dose and effect on neutrophils was steep in the dosing range evaluated. The steepness of this relationship is illustrated in Fig. 3, which shows that the percent decrements in ANC sharply increased to nearly 100% as the dose of exatecan was increased above 0.4 mg/m^2/day *(32)*. Severe thrombocytopenia and anemia occurred much less frequently than neutropenia, and were usually noted concomitant with severe neutropenia. These effects were also more severe in HP patients. Anemia related to exatecan was generally mild (grade 1) or moderate (grade 2) and cumulative in that it tended to progressively worsen with repetitive dosing.

Nonhematologics; effects consisted primarily of mild to moderate gastrointestinal toxicity. Nausea and vomiting were typically mild or moderate in severity, generally noted in the peritreatment period, and appeared to be dose-related. Nausea and vomiting were generally prevented or managed successfully with prochlorperazine or serotonin 5-hydroxytryptophan receptor antagonists, but routine premedication was not instituted because most events were nausea alone, mild in severity, and sporadic. Delayed emesis was not common. Mild to moderate diarrhea was also noted in patients, most of whom had been previously treated with fluoropyrimidine- or irinotecan-based regimens. Transient and reversible elevations of serum transaminases or alkaline phosphatase were also observed infrequently, and acute pancreatitis occurred in two patients (approximately 1%) in phase I trials. Alopecia that was dose-related, typically mild, and generally cumulative was also noted. Other toxicities included stomatitis, malaise, headache, anorexia, or alkaline phosphatase, altered taste sensation, and dizziness. These effects were noted across the entire exatecan dosing range and definite temporal

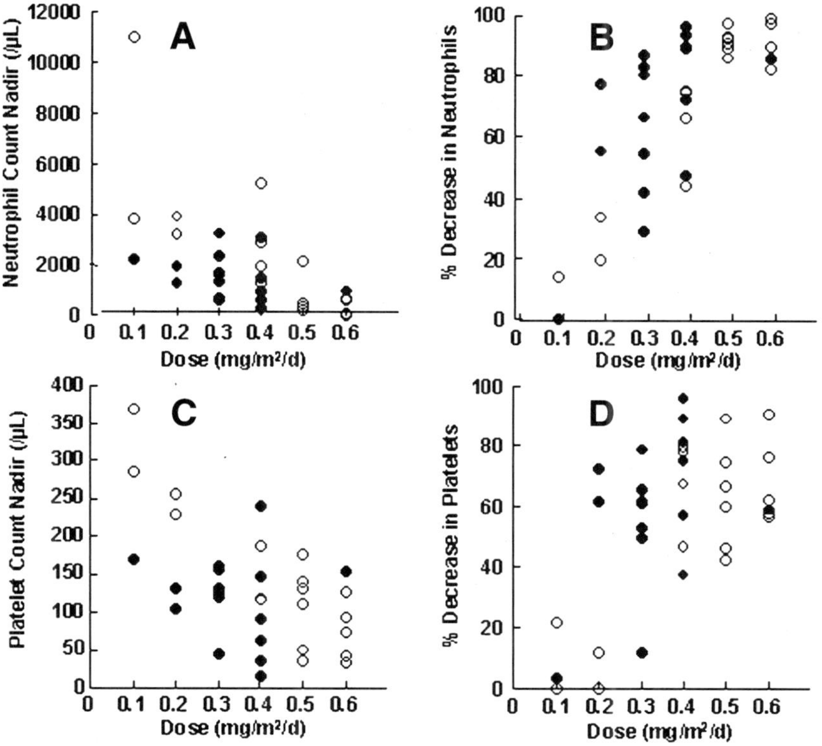

Fig. 3. Scatterplots depicting the effects of the dose of exatecan on **(A)** absolute neutrophil count (ANC) nadirs; **(B)** percentage change in the ANC; **(C)** platelet count nadirs; and **(D)** percentage change in platelet counts. The extent of prior treatment is also indicated. (●) heavily pretreated; (○) minimally pretreated.

relationships could not be discerned for any of these potential toxicities, indicating that the underlying malignant process may have contributed.

6.3.2. Maximum Tolerated Dose

The MTD and lowest doses associated with consistently intolerable toxicity (>MTD) are listed in Table 4. MP patients tolerated higher doses of exatecan than HP patients except for the single-dose, every-3-week regimen for which a single MTD was determined for HP and MP patients alike. However, this study involved only 12 patients, and the MTD was close to the starting dose. The MTDs for exatecan administered as a 30-minute iv infusion daily × 5 every 3 weeks were 0.5 and 0.3 mg/m²/day for MP and HP patients, respectively. Representative concentration versus time curves are shown in Fig. 4. The number of dose escalation steps in each study

Table 4
Pertinent Single-Agent Phase I Clinical Trials of Exatecan

Administration schedule	*Site (reference)*	*No. of patients*	*Prior treatment*	*MTD ($mg/m^2/day$)*	*>MTD ($mg/m^2/day$)*	*Principal DLT*	*Other toxicities*
30 minutes (day 1) every 3 weeks	IGR, France *(30)*	12	MP/HP	5.33	7.1	ANC	Nausea, vomiting, fever, alopecia, asthenia, anemia
	NCCE, Japan *(29)*	15	MP/HP	NR	NR	ANC	PLT
30 minutes daily × 5 every 3 weeks	IDD, USA *(32)*	36	MP	0.5	0.6	ANC	Nausea, vomiting, diarrhea, liver finctions, anemia
			HP	0.3	0.4	ANC, PLTs	
	NCH, Japan *(29)*	28	NR	0.4	0.45	ANC, PLTs	Nausea, vomiting, diarrhea, malaise
24-hour CI every 3 weeks	MDA (USA) *(33)*	22	MP	2.4	3.0	ANC	PLTs, anemia, nausea, vomiting, diarrhea
			HP	<2.4	3.0	ANC	
24-hour weekly × 3 every 4 weeks	MSKCC (USA) *(34)*	27	MP	1.0	1.2	ANC, PLTs	Nausea, vomiting, diarrhea, anorexia, asthenia, fever, stomatitis, alopecia, pancreatitis (with lipase elevation)
			HP	<0.8	0.8	ANC, PLTs	
30 minutes weekly × every 4 weeks	Oxford/Vrije (UK/Holland) *(35)*	35	MP	2.75	3.13	ANC	Diarrhea, alopecia, mucositis
			HP	2.06	2.35	ANC	
5- to 21-day CI every 4 weeks	IDD (USA) *(36)*	31	MP	0.15	0.23	ANC	Anemia, PLTs
			HP	0.15	0.23	ANC, PLTs	

ANC, absolute neutrophil pointl CI, continuous infusion; HP, heavily pretreated; IDD, Institute for Drug Development; IGR, Institute for Gustave Roussy; MDA, M. D. Anderson Cancer Center; MP, minimally pretreated; NCCE, National Cancer Institute East; NR, noot reported; PLTS, platelets.

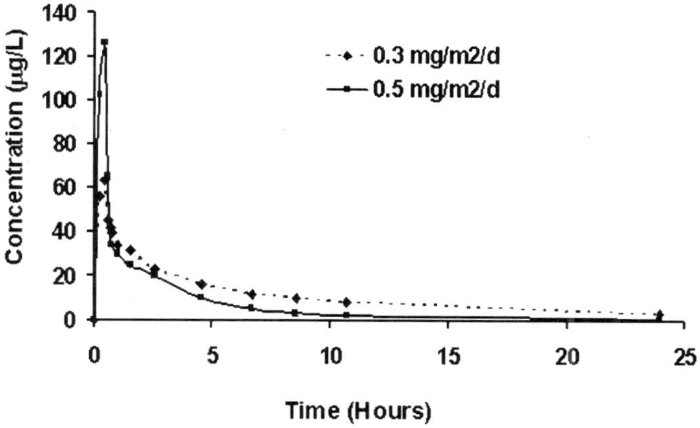

Fig. 4. Representative plasma total exatecan concentration-time profiles (day 1) in patients treated with DX-8951f at the 0.3 mg/m^2/day (◆) and 0.5 mg/m^2/day (■) dose levels.

reflected the MTD/starting dose ratios and was not related to the type of dose escalation scheme used. It was not possible to evaluate the impact of the modified continual reassessment method in these studies because of the small number of patients and early intervention of investigators in modifying the dose levels assigned by the modified continual reassessment scheme at toxic dose levels.

In a comparison of exatecan clinical and preclinical toxicokinetics, MTD/toxic dose low (TDL) ratio were similar (dog [2.0] and man [1.5–3.1]) *(45)*. On the other hand, human toxicokinetics appeared to be schedule-independent, whereas toxicokinetics in dogs were schedule-dependent, which might be explained by differences in metabolic rates between species.

6.3.3. Antitumor Activity

Major antineoplastic activity was observed in patients with several types of solid neoplasms in phase I investigations *(25,26,29–36)*. Partial responses (≥ 50% reduction in the sum of the bidimensional products of measurable tumors) were reported in previously treated patients with non–small-cell lung, extrapulmonary small cell, colorectal, and hepatocellular carcinomas and sarcoma. Disease stabilization, including minor responses (<50% reduction in the sum of the bidimensional products of measurable disease) was observed in patients with colorectal carcinoma, hepatocellular carcinoma, prostate carcinoma, and carcinoma of unknown primary type involving the peritoneum. Interestingly, antitumor activity was noted in cancers that were previously demonstrated to be resistant to other TOP-I-targeting therapeutics such as irinotecan and topotecan *(25,26,29–36)*. The 30-minute iv infusion daily × 5 every 3 week, 30-minute iv infusion weekly × 3 every 4 week,

Table 5
Mean Pharmacokinetic Parameters in Phase I Evaluations of Exatecan

Pharmacokinetic parameter	*Pharmacokinetic analytical method*	
	Noncompartmental	*Population compartmental*
Clearance (L/hour/m²)	1.87 (67%)	1.63 (64%)
Urinary excretion (%)	Not applicable	9.9 (60%)
Volume of distribution (central) (L/m²)	Not applicable	6.4 (28.7%)
Volume of distribution (steady-state) (L/m²)	17 (39%)	17.65 (28.9%)
Terminal half-life (hours)	9.1 (54%)	12.3 (60%)

Note: Represent mean value (coefficient of variation).

and the 5- to 21-day continuous iv infusion every 3–4 week regimens appeared to be associated with greater activity than the single-dose regimen or the 24-hour intermittent regimens, however, the phase I clinical trial is not the proper setting for generating comparative data regarding scheduling. There was no relationship between the number of patients demonstrating antitumor activity and the dose intensity of the regimens used in individual studies. The 30-minute daily × 5 every 3 week regimen, which appeared to be the most active in phase I evaluations, was selected as the principal regimen in phase II studies, whereas the corresponding MTDs for MP and HP patients, 0.3 and 0.5 mg/m²/day, were selected as phase II doses.

6.3.4. Clinical Pharmacology

The pharmacokinetics of exatecan were dose-independent within the dose range evaluated in phase I evaluations, with pharmacokinetic indices of exposure (e.g., AUC, C_{max}) proportionate to dose *(25,26,29–36)*. Similarly, both clearance and V_{ss} were dose-independent. There was no evidence of drug accumulation in the plasma over from day 1 to day 5 in most patients treated with exatecan as a 30-minute iv infusion on the daily for 5 days schedule *(32)*. Table 5 displays the mean pharmacokinetic parameters of exatecan in phase I evaluations, and plasma concentration curves for total exatecan in representative patients treated with 30-minute iv infusions are shown in Fig. 5. Both total exatecan and its lactone form were measured only in the 30-minute single iv dose every 3 week study conducted in Japan *(29)*. The AUC of the lactone was approximately 30% of the AUC of total exatecan, and the plasma AUC of UM-1 was 4% of the total exatecan AUC. Twenty-five percent of the administered dose of exatecan was recovered in the urine, and there was a 2:1 ratio between the UM-1 metabolite and unmetabolized exatecan *(25,29,31)*.

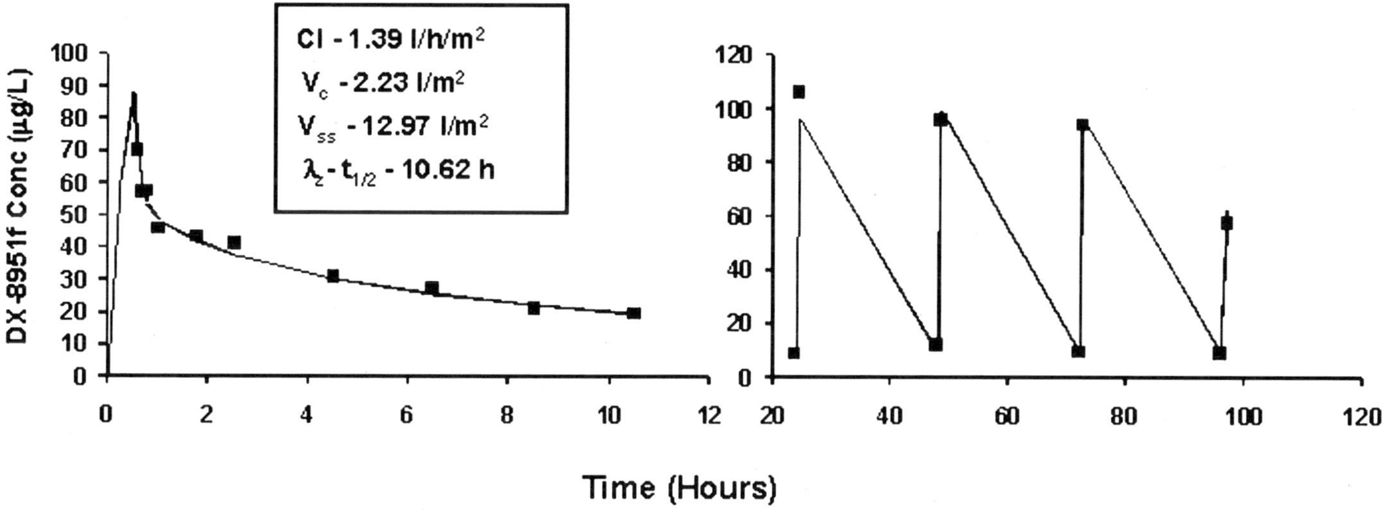

Fig. 5. Representative patient's plasma concentration data (■) fit to the population model using an IT2S approach. The patient was treated with exatecan at the 0.5 mg/m^2/day dose level. Pharmacokinetic parameter values derived from the population model are listed.

Because there was no evidence of nonlinear drug elimination, auto-induction, or inhibition of drug clearance based on visual inspection of individual plasma concentration-versus-time curves in the phase I studies, linear pharmacokinetic models were evaluated for quality of fit. The compartmental pharmacokinetic models developed in individual studies were very adequate in explaining the observed plasma concentrations and excreted urinary amounts of exatecan. In study PRT002, in which exatecan was administered as a 30-minute iv infusion on a daily × 5 every 3-week schedule, a two-compartment model consistently missed peak plasma concentrations and a three-compartment model was systematically superior in fitting all plasma concentration-time data sets for total exatecan on both days 1 and 5 *(25,32)*. Therefore, pharmacokinetic parameters derived from the triexponential model were used to develop a population pharmacokinetic model using an IT2S approach. A representative patient's plasma concentration data fit to this population model are shown in Fig. 5. Pertinent pharmacokinetic parameters for total exatecan derived from this model were nearly identical to those derived using noncompartmental methods, with mean (coefficient of variation) clearance, and terminal half-life values of 1.64 L/hour/m^2 *(57)* and 15.8 hours *(65)*, respectively. Mean values for the central and steady-state volumes of distribution, were 2.40 L/m^2 *(30)*, respectively *(25,32)*.

The relationships between the both the AUC and C_{max} values for total exatecan and the percentage decrements in neutrophils were consistently described by sigmoidal E_{max} models, as shown in Fig. 6A,B, which depicts scatterplots of individual data in study PRT002 and sigmoidal E_{max} models fitting the data *(32)*. With these models, the AUC and C_{max} values predicted to yield a 50% decrement in neutrophils (AUC_{50} and $C_{max\text{-}50}$) were 115 mg/hour/L and 31 mg/L, respectively. The relationships between pertinent pharmacokinetic parameters for total exatecan and platelet counts, as depicted in the scatterplots in Fig. 6C,D could be described adequately by neither linear nor nonlinear models. Within particular dose levels, pharmacokinetic parameters reflecting total exatecan exposure were generally greater in those patients who experienced dose-limiting myelosuppression during their first course, but the relatively small numbers of both dose-limiting events and patients at each dose level has limited the statistical power of such analyses. Such models may be very useful clinically as they may be able to predict which exatecan dosing regimens and doses would minimize decrements in blood cell counts.

7. DISEASE-DIRECTED (PHASE II–III) EVALUATIONS

Disease-directed evaluations of exatecan are currently being performed in both North America and Europe in patients with advanced carcinomas of the pancreas (first and second line), colon/rectum (second line, no prior CPT analog), ovary (relapsed after taxanes and platinum; no more than two prior

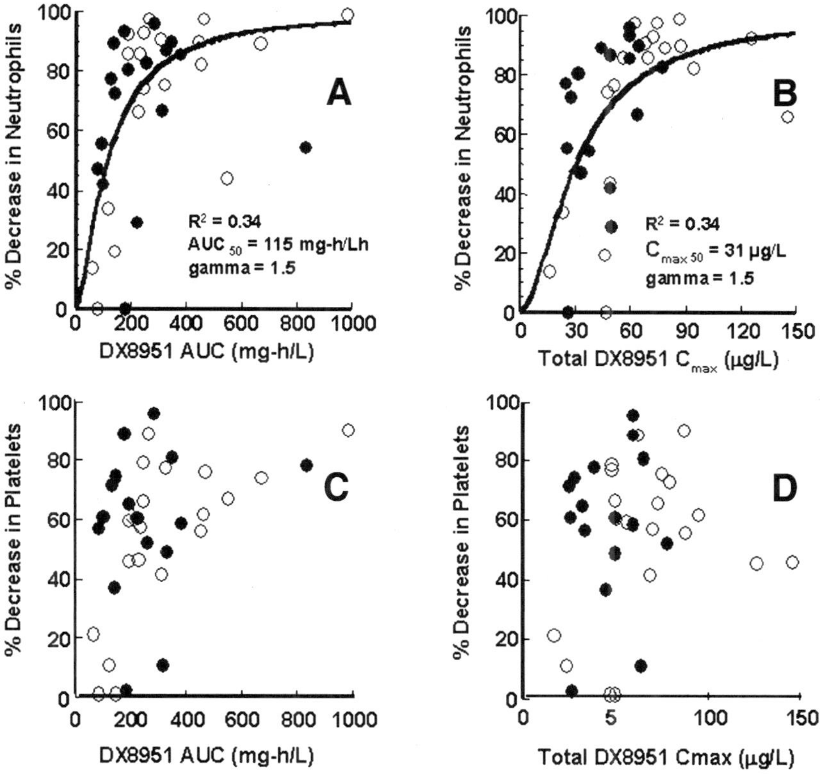

Fig. 6. Scatterplots depicting the relationships between percentage decrements in absolute neutrophil count during the first course of exatecan and total exatecan AUC (**A**) and C_{max} (**B**), and between percentage decrements in platelets during the first course and AUC (**C**) and C_{max} (**D**). The extent of prior treatment, as defined in the Patients and Methods section, is also indicated. (●) heavily pretreated; (?) minimally pretreated. The solid lines represent fits of sigmoidal E_{max} models to the data when appropriate.

regimens), uterine cervix (first or second line), lung (non-small cell; first line), liver (first or second line), biliary duct (first or second line), hormone-refractory prostate, head and neck (first line), and breast (relapsed after taxane and anthracycline; up to three prior regimens) *(25,46–56)*. In the majority of these trials, exatecan is being administered as a 30-minute iv infusion daily × 5 every 3 weeks. Starting doses for MP and HP patients have been 0.4–0.5 and 0.3 mg/m²/day, respectively. To ascertain information about the relative activity of various schedules of exatecan, patients with advanced ovarian cancer are being randomized to treatment with exatecan administered iv over 30 minutes on either a daily × 5 every 3 week schedule (starting dose, 0.3 mg/m^2/day) or weekly × 3 every 4 week schedule (starting dose, 2.1 mg/m^2/day) in a randomized phase II evaluation.

Perhaps the most intriguing and unique activity with exatecan to date has been noted in patients with advanced adenocarcinomas of the pancreas, biliary track, gallbladder, and liver *(49–53)*. At this juncture, the most advanced results are available from a Phase II study of exatecan in patients with advanced adenocarcinoma of the pancreas *(48–50)*. A single, multicenter trial of exatecan administered as a 30-minute infusion at a dose of 0.5 mg/m^2/day × 5 every 3 weeks was conducted in 39 patients with metastatic adenocarcinoma of the pancreas and a subset of 23 patients who had not received prior chemotherapy has been analyzed. Three patients (13%) had confirmed partial responses lasting 2.8, 4.3, and 10.1 months. The median survival time for the 23 previously untreated patients was 9.3 months. The 6-, 12-, and 24-month survival times were 70%, 39%, and 5%, respectively. Toxicity was primarily myelosuppression and fatigue. A phase I study of exatecan in combination with gemcitabine, conducted in patients with advanced solid malignancies, yielded phase II/III doses of exatecan of 2.0 mg/m^2 and gemcitabine 1000 mg/m^2 when both drugs were administered on a weekly × 3 every 3 week schedule *(51)*. The toxicity profile was similar to exatecan as a single-agent exatecan with the exception of apparently more severe thrombocytopenia. In the study, 7 of 31 patients with advanced pancreatic cancer who had received the regimen as additional therapy experienced major responses, including one complete and six partial responses. The median duration of response was 8 months and the median survival time was 8 months. The 6-, 12-, and 24-month survival times were 55%, 39%, and 19%, respectively. These results to two large-scale randomized trials in the North America and Europe, which have completed their accrual targets. In the North American study, a combination of exatecan and gemcitabine was compared with gemcitabine alone and in the European study, exatecan as a single-agent was compared with gemcitabine alone *(60,61)*. However, preliminary results from both studies indicate that no survival benefits were conferred.

A multicenter phase II study of exatecan 0.5 mg/m^2/day × 5 every 3 weeks has also been conducted in patients with advanced biliary and gallbladder carcinomas who received a maximum of one prior chemotherapy regimen *(52)*. Of 41 patients able to be evaluated for efficacy, 21 (50%) of whom had had prior chemotherapy, 2 (4.9%) had partial responses, 4 (9.8%) had minor responses, and 12 (29.3%) had stable disease as their best response. The median overall survival was 7.8 months and the 6- and 12-month survival rates were 61% and 32%, which will serve as the foundation for future combination studies in biliary and gallbladder carcinomas. In a phase II study involving 43 patients with hepatocellular carcinoma who had received a maximum of one prior chemotherapy regimen, exatecan was administered at a dose of 0.5 mg/m^2/day × 5 every 3 weeks *(53)*. Two patients had partial responses, whereas 6 had minor responses, and 14 had stable disease as their best response. The median time to progression was 3.3 months and median survival time was 7.4 months, with respective 6- and 12-month survival rates of 61% and 35%. Despite its modest activity as a single-agent activity, it was felt that the results provided a sufficient foundation for the development of relatively nontoxic exatecan-based multiagent regimens for hepatocellular carcinoma.

Exatecan administered as a 30-minute iv infusion at a dose of 0.5 mg/m^2/day × 5 every 3 weeks demonstrated no significant activity in a phase II study in patients with metastatic colorectal cancer who had received no prior treatment with CPT derivatives *(48)*. Similarly, negligible activity has been reported with exatecan 0.5 mg/m^2/day for 5 days every 3 weeks in previously untreated patients with advanced non–small-cell lung cancer (54). The major response rate was 5.1% and median times to progression and survival were 88 and 262 days, respectively. Moderate activity was observed in patients with advanced breast cancer who had experienced resistance or progressive disease after chemotherapy that included anthracyclines and taxanes *(55)*. Of 39 patients able to be evaluated, 3 (7.7%) experienced partial responses and 20 (51.3% had either a minor response or stable disease. Approximately 20% of patients had stable disease for at least 6 months. To characterize the activity of exatecan in patients with advanced ovarian cancer who were either refractory to or relapsed after both platinum agents and taxanes, patients were randomized to one of two dosing schedules: (Arm A) daily × 5 every 3 weeks, starting dose 0.3 mg/m^2/day, or (Arm B) weekly × 3 every 4 weeks, starting dose 2.1 mg/m^2 weekly *(47)*. In a preliminary report involving 47 patients (Arm A, $n = 31$; and arm B, $n = 16$) and including 23 patients who were able to be evaluated for response, two patients (both on Arm A) had partial responses and five subjects had stable disease as their best response. In a study of exatecan 0.5 mg/m^2/day × 5 every 3 weeks in previously untreated patients with non-small-cell lung cancer, partial responses were reported in 3 (18%) of 16 of patients who were able to be evaluated for response and 5 patients had stable disease as their best response *(51)*. Many other disease-directed studies in a wide array of adult solid malignancies are ongoing.

The potential utility of exatecan in pediatric malignancies is also being studied, beginning with a phase I study of exatecan as a 30-minute iv infusion daily × 5 every 3 weeks in pediatric patients with solid malignancies (starting dose, 0.25 mg/m^2/day). Furthermore, evaluations of exatecan in adult acute leukemias are also under way *(56)*. In a phase I study, doses of exatecan were escalated from 0.6 to 1.35 mg/m^2/day as a 30-minutes iv infusion daily × 5 every 3 weeks. Severe stomatitis was consistently noted at the 1.35 mg/m^2/day dose level. On the 30-minute infusion daily × 5 schedule, the 1.2 mg/m^2/day dose level appears tolerable, and increasing the duration of treatment from 5 to 7 days at the 0.9 mg/m^2/day dose level has not been associated with prohibitive toxicity. Antileukemic activity, primarily reductions in circulating blasts and bone marrow cellularity, has also been consistently noted across all dose levels in HP patients.

8. DE-310, A MACROMOLECULAR CARRIER OF DX-8951

DE-310 is a novel drug construct consisting of exatecan linked to a biodegradable carrier, carboxymethyldextran poly alcohol, via a peptide spacer. This macromolecular polymer drug deliver system was designed to enhance the antitumor efficacy of exatecan. The slow release of exatecan from the carrier in the tumor provides for a sustained level of localized active agent. The relatively greater acidic environment of malignant neoplasms compared with normal tissues may hypothetically favor the presence of the active lactone species in malignant neoplasms, potentially resulting in greater specificity. The supporting rationale for the development of DE-310 is that the molecule will accumulate and be retained preferentially in tumor tissue by the enhanced permeability and retention effect. The enhanced permeability into tumor tissue is due to leaky vascular architecture of the tumor blood vessels and pathophysiological mediators such as cytokines or vascular permeability factors. The retention effect is based on the lack of effective lymphatic clearance of macromolecules in tumor tissue. Thus macromolecules such as DE-310 may readily leak into tumor tissue through more permeable tumor blood vessels and may be retained in tumor tissue for a longer period. DE-310 is designed for iv administration. The macromolecular carrier used in the drug gradually depolymerizes within the body to be excreted in the urine. The peptide spacer serves as the DE-310 enzymatic cleavage site to give a low and sustained release of exatecan into tumor tissue, without prematurely releasing the drug into the systemic circulation. As a result, the number of required dosages may be reduced significantly when compared with other CPT derivatives in current use. Two phase I and pharmacokinetic studies of DE-310 administered as a single short infusion every 4 or 6 weeks have recently begun *(5,57)*. DLT on both schedules appear to be late myelosuppression, and transaminitis has been observed at doses above the MTD (6 and 7.5 mg/m^2 in HP and MP patients, respectively). Both conjugated exatecan and free exatecan concentrations increased linearly with dose and plasma drug concentrations were sustained for several weeks. The pharmacokinetic results from both studies were similar. In the every-4-week study, the mean (CV%) C_{max} for DE-310 in the form of conjugated exatecan was 4120 (21.2) ng/mL and the apparent terminal plasma half-life ($t_{1/2}$) was 208.8 (78.9) hours. The C_{max} of free exatecan was 5.8 (53.4) ng/mL and the $t_{1/2}$ was 175.1 (9.0) hours.

9. CONCLUSION

Exatecan was developed to exploit physicochemical properties that may result in superior antitumor activity, less toxicity and interindividual variability, and greater clinical feasibility than TOP-I–targeting agents in current clinical use. The agent was specifically selected for clinical development because of its relatively high potency and impressive activity against a broad range of human tumor cell lines and xenografts, including malignancies resistant to other CPT analogs and other classes of anticancer agents. Furthermore, unlike topotecan, 9-aminocamptothecin, and SN-38, exatecan is not a substrate for multidrug transporter Pgp, and retains activity against both tumor cell lines and xenografts with acquired multidrug resistance conferred by Pgp overexpression. Another hypothetical advantage of exatecan is that it is an intrinsically active compound and not a prodrug, which reduces concerns about interindividual variability in prodrug activation that could increase the fundamentally large interindividual variability in the toxicologic, pharmacokinetic, and antitumor profiles of the CPT analogs. Although schedule-dependence was not as prominent with exatecan in preclinical studies as with other CPT analogs, the cumulative results of these investigations indicate that maximal antitumor activity is achieved with divided dosing schedules, and these observations have served, in part, as the rationale for broad disease-directed evaluation of exatecan on a 30-minute infusion daily × 5 every 3 week schedule. In addition, exatecan demonstrated a safe and predictable toxicity profile when administered on the daily × 5 schedule, with manageable neutropenia being the principal DLT. Thrombocytopenia and anemia may be associated with neutropenia, particularly in HP patients treated at doses that approach the MTD. Nonhematologic toxicity has been less frequent and generally moderate. Exatecan also demonstrated dose-independent and predictable pharmacokinetics in the dose range evaluated and antitumor activity was consistently observed, including that against tumors that had been previously treated with topotecan or irinotecan. Although the ultimate clinical activity of exatecan will be defined only in appropriate phase II/III trials, exatecan's specific pattern of myelotoxicity, its relative paucity of nonhematologic toxicity, and its activity against a several types of neoplasms in early clinical evaluations, warranted broad disease-directed evaluations of exatecan on this administration schedule, which are nearing completion, as well as further developmental evaluations of DE-310, particularly in exatecan-sensitive tumor types, to maximize activity and optimize the therapeutic index.

REFERENCES

1. Mitsui I, Kumazawa E, Hirota Y, et al. 1995 A new water-soluble camptothecin derivative, DX-8951f, exhibits potent antitumor activity against human tumors in vitro and in vivo. Jpn J Cancer Res 86:776–782.

2. Okamoto R, Park JS, Hanaoka H, Nishiyama M. 1999 DX-8951f, a novel camptothecin derivative: critical determinants of the action and synergistic combination against gastrointestinal cancer cells [abstract]. Proc Am Assoc Cancer Res 40:712.
3. Lawrence RA, Izbicka E, DeJager R, et al. 1999 Comparison of DX-8951f and topotecan effects on tumor colony formation from freshly explanted adult and pediatric human tumor cells. Anti-Cancer Drugs 10:655–661.
4. Kumazawa E, Jimbo T, Ochi Y, Tohgo A. 1998 Potent and broad antitumor effects of DX-8951f, a water-soluble camptothecin derivative, against various human tumors xenografted in nude mice. Cancer Chemother Pharmacol 42:210–220.
5. Kumazawa E, Tohgo A. 1998 Antitumor activity of DX-8951f: a new camptothecin derivative. Exp Opin Invest Drugs 7:625–632.
6. Gonzales P, Marty J, Stringer SD, et al. 2000 In vivo antitumor activity of DX-8951f against an intracranial sarcoma tumor model [abstract]. Proc Am Assoc Cancer Res 41:1349.
7. Takiguchi S, Kumazawa E, Shimazoe T, Tohgo A, Kono A. 1997 Antitumor effect of DX-8951, a novel campotothecin analog, on human pancreatic tumor cells and their CPT-11-resistant variants cultured in vitro and xenografted into nude mice. Jpn J Cancer Res 88:760–769.
8. Joto N, Ishii M, Minami M, et al. 1997 DX-8951f, a water-soluble camptothecin analog, exhibits potent antitumor activity against a human lung cancer cell line and its SN-38-resistant variant. Int J Cancer 72:680–686.
9. Nomoto T, Nishio K, Ishidia T, Mori M, Saijo N. 1998 Characterization of a human small-cell lung cancer cell line resistant to a new water-soluble camptothecin derivative, DX-8951f. Jpn J Cancer Res 89:1179–1186.
10. Weitman S, DeJager R, Marty J, et al. 1999 Preclinical evaluation of DX-8951f against pediatric solid tumors [abstract]. Proc Am Soc Clin Oncol 18:762.
11. Vey N, Giles FJ, Kantarjian H, et al. 2000 The topoisomerase I inhibitor DX-8951f is active in a severe combined immunodeficient mouse model of human acute myelogenous leukemia. Clin Cancer Res 6:731–736.
12. Sun FX, Tohgo A, Bouvet M, et al. 2003 Efficacy of camptothecin analog DX8951f (exatecan mesylate) human pancreatic cancer in an orthotopic metastatic model. Cancer Res 63:80–85.
13. Hendricks CB, Rowinsky EK, Grochow LB, et al. 1992 Effect of P-glycoprotein expression on the accumulation and cytotoxicity of topotecan (SK &F 104864), a new campothecin analogue. Cancer Res 52:2268–2278.
14. Chen AY, Yu C, Potmesil M, et al. 1991 Camptothecin overcomes MDR1-mediated resistance in human KB carcinoma cells. Cancer Res 51:6039–6044.
15. Tsuruo T, Matsuzaki T, Matsushita M, et al. 1988 Antitumor effect of CPT-11, a new derivative of camptothecin, against pleotropic drug resistant tumors in vitro and in vivo. Cancer Chemother Pharmacol 21:71–74.
16. Mattern MR, Hofmann GA, Polsky RM, et al. 1993 In vitro and in vivo effects of clinically important camptothecin analogues in multi-drug resistant cells. Oncol Res 5:467–474.
17. van Hattum AH, Hoogsteen IJ, Schluper HM, et al. 2002 Induction of breast cancer resistance protein by the camptothecin derivative DX-8951f is associated with minor reduction of antitumour activity. Br J Cancer 87;665–672.
18. Ishii M, Iwahana M, Mitsui I, et al. 2000 Growth inhibitory effect of a new camptothecin analog, DX-8951 on various drug resistant sublines including BCRP-mediated camptothecin derative-resistant variants derived from the human lung cancer cell line PC-6. Anticancer Drugs 11:353–362.

19. van Hattum AH, Pinedo HM, Schluper HM, Erkelens CA, Tohgo A, Bov E. 2002 The activity profile of the hexacyclic camptothecin derivative DX-8951f in experimental human colon cancer and ovarian cancer. Biochem Pharm 64:1267–1277.
20. Liu L, Desai S, Sun M, et al. 2000 Mechanism of action of topoisomerase I and its inhibitors. Ann NY Acad Sci 922:1–10.
21. Okamoto R, Takano H, Okamura T, et al. 2002 O(6)-methylguanine-DNA methyltransferase (MGMT) as a determinant of resistance to camptothecan derivatives. Jpn J Cancer Res 93:93–102.
22. Daiichi Pharmaceutical Corporation. DX-8951f for injection. Investigators Brochure. Edition No. 2. Fort Lee, New Jersey, 1998.
23. Oguma T, Ohshima Y, Nakaoka M. 2000 Sensitive and high-performance liquid chromatographic method for the determination of the lactone plus hydroxy forms of the new camptothecin derivative DX-8951 in human plasma using fluorescence detection. J Chromatogr B Biomed Sci Appl 740:237–245.
24. Oguma T, Konno T, Inaba A, Nakaoka M. 2001 Validation study of assay method for DX-8951 and its metabolite in human plasma and urine by high-performance liquid chromatography/atmospheric pressure chemical ionization tandem mass spectrometry. Biomed Chromatogr 2:108–115.
25. DeJager R, Cheverton P, Tamanoi K, et al. 2000 DX-8951f: summary of phase I clinical trials. Ann NY Acad Sci 922:260–273.
26. Verschraegen CF, Royce M, Hammond L, Rowinsky EK. 2000 Exatecan. Curr Opin End Met Invest Drugs 2:1631–1638.
27. Oguma T, Konno T, Inaba A, Nakaoka M. 2001 Validation study of assay method for DX-8951 and its metabolite in human plasma and urine by high-performance liquid chromatography/atmospheric pressure chemical ionization tandem mass spectrometry. Biomed Chromatogr 15:108–115.
28. Oguma T, Yamada M, Konno T, Inukai K, Nakaoka M. 2001 High-performance liquid chromatographic analysis of lactone, an hydroxy acid of new antitumor drug, DX-8951 (exatecan), in mouse plasma. Biol Pharm Bull 24:176–180.
29. Minami H, Fujii H, Igarashi T, et al. 2001 Phase I study and clinical pharmacology of DX-8951f, a new camptothecin derivative, infused over 30 minutes every three weeks [abstract]. Clin Cancer Res 7:3056–3064.
30. Boige V, Raymond E, Faivre S, et al. 2000 Phase I and pharmacokinetic study of the camptothecin analog DX-8951f administered as a 30-minute infusion every 3 weeks in patients with advanced cancer. J Clin Oncol 18:3986–3992.
31. Kamiya Y, Yamamoto N, Yamada Y, et al. 1999 Phase I and pharmacokinetic (PK) study of DX-8951f, a novel camptothecin analog, given as a 30 minute infusion daily x 5 days [abstract]. AACR NCI EORTC Mol Targets Cancer Ther Suppl A:327.
32. Rowinsky EK, Johnson TR, Geyer CE Jr, et al. 2000 DX-8951f , a hexacyclic camptothecin analog, on a daily-times-five schedule: a phase I and pharmacokinetic study in patients with advanced solid malignancies. J Clin Oncol 18:3151–3163.
33. Royce ME, Hoff PM, Dumas P, et al. 2001 Phase I and pharmacokinetic study of exetacan mesylate (DX-8951f): a novel campothecin analog. J Clin Oncol 19:1493–1500.
34. Sharma S, Kemeny N, Schwartz GK, et al. 2001 A phase I study of topoisomerase I inhibitor exatecan mesylate (DX-8951f) given as weekly 24-hour continuous infusions three of every four weeks. Clin Cancer Res 7:3963–3970.
35. Braybrooke JP, Boven E, Bates NP, et al. 2003 Phase I and pharmacokinetic study of the topoisomerase I inhibitor, exatecan mesylate (DX-8951f), using a weekly

30-minute intravenous infusion, in patients with advanced solid malignancies. Ann Oncol 14;913–921.
36. Garrison MA, Hammond LA, Geyer CE, et al. 2003 A phase I and pharmokinetic study of the hexacyclic camptothecin analog exatecan mesylate (DX-8951F) administered as a protracted infusion in patients with advanced solid malignancies. Clin Cancer Res 9:2527–2537.
37. Rowinsky EK, Grochow LB, Sartorius SE, et al. 1996 Phase I and pharmacologic study of high doses of the topoisomerase I inhibitor topotecan with granulocyte colony-stimulating factor in patients with solid tumors. J Clin Oncol 14:1224–1235.
38. Rowinsky EK, Kaufman SH, Baker SD, et al. 1996 Sequences of topotecan and cisplatin: phase I, pharmacologic, and in vitro studies to examine sequence dependence. J Clin Oncol 14:3074–3084.
39. Rowinsky E, Grochow L, Hendricks C, et al. 1992 Phase I and pharmacologic study of topotecan : a novel topoisomerase I inhibitor. J Clin Oncol 10:647–656.
40. Metzler CM. 1987 Extended least squares (ELS) for pharmacokinetic models. J Pharm Sci 76:565–571.
41. Yamaoka K, Nakagawa T, Uno T. 1978 Application of Akaike's information criterion (AIC) in the evaluation of linear pharmacokinetic equations. J Pharmacokinet Biopharm 6:165–175.
42. Lalonde RL. Pharmacodynamics. In: Applied pharmacokinetics: principles of therapeutic drug monitoring. 3rd ed. Evans WE, Schentag JJ, Jusko WJ, eds. Applied Therapeutics, Washington, 1992, 4-1–4-33.
43. D'Argenio DZ, Schumitzky A. ADAPT-II users manual. Biomedical Simulation Resource, University of Southern California, 1997.
44. Collins DG, Forrest A. IT2s user's guide. State University of New York Buffalo, 1995.
45. Jager RD, Oguma T, Kajimura T, et al. 1999 Comparison of DX8951f clinical and preclinical toxicokinetics (TK) [abstract]. Proc Am Soc Clin Oncol 18:178A.
46. Kudelka A, Verschraegen CF, Vincent M, et al. 2000 Phase II study of intravenous DX-8951f in patients (Pts) with advanced ovarian, tubal, or peritoneal cancer refractory to platinum, taxane, and topotecan [abstract]. Proc Am Soc Clin Oncol 19:392A.
47. Calvert P, Jayson G, Atkinson R, et al. 2000 Phase II clinical and pharmacokinetic study of exatecan mesylate (DX-8951f) in patients with advanced ovarian cancer, refractory to, or relapsed after platinum and taxane [abstract]. Ann Oncol 11(Suppl. 4):84.
48. Royce, M, Saltz L, Rowinsky E, et al. 2003 A phase II study of intravenous exatecan mesylate (DX-8951f) administered daily for five days every three weeks to patients with advanced or metastatic adenocarcinoma of the colon or rectum. Invest. New Drugs. 22:53–61.
49. D'Adamo D, Hammond L, Donehower R, et al. 2001 Final results of a phase II study of DX-8951f (exatecan mesylate, DX) in advanced pancreatic cancer [abstract] Proc Am Soc Clin Oncol 37:134a.
50. O'Reilly EM, Hammond L, Sharma S, et al. 2000 A phase II study of exetecan mesylate (DX-8951f, DX) in advanced pancreatic cancer [abstract]. Proc Am Soc Clin Oncol 19:299a.
51. Talbot DC, White S, Jones P, et al. 2000 Phase II study of exatecan mesylate (DX-8951f) in advanced NSCLC [abstract]. Proc Am Soc Clin Oncol 19:549a.

52. O'Reilly EM, Lenzi R, Mani S, et al. 2002 Phase I study of DX-8951f (exatecan mesylate, DX) and gemcitabine (gem) in advanced solid malignancies [abstract]. Proc Am Soc Clin Oncol 21:99A.
53. Abou-Alfa GL, O'Reilly EM, Rowinsky EK, et al. 2002 Final results of a phase II study of DX-8951f (DX, exatecan mesylate) in biliary tree cancers. Proc Am Soc Clin Oncol 21:561.
54. Patt YZ, Rowinsky E, O'Reilly E, et al. 2002 Phase II trial of DX-8951f (exatecan mesylate) in hepatocellular carcinoma (HCC): a final analysis [abstract]. Proc Am Soc Clin Oncol 21:139a..
55. Braybrooke JP, Ranson M, Manegold C, et al. 2003 Phase II study of exatecan mesylate (DX-8951f) as first-line therapy for advanced non-small cell lung cancer. Lung Cancer 41:215–219.
56. Eteva FJ, Rivera E, Cristofanilli M, et al. 2003 A phase II study of intravenous exatecan mesylate (DX-8951f) administered daily for 5 days every 3 weeks to patients with metastatic breast cancer. Cancer 98:900–907.
57. Giles FJ, Cortes JE, Thomas DA, et al. 2002 Phase I and pharmacokinetic study of DX-8951f (exatecan mesylate), a hexacyclic campothecin, on a daily-time-five schedule in patients with advanced leukemia. Clin Cancer Res 8:2134–2141.
58. Takimoto CHM, Forero L, Schwartz GH, et al. 2003 A phase I and pharmacokinetic study of DE-310 administered as a 3 hour infusion every 4 weeks (wks) to patients (pts) with advanced solid tumors or lymphomas [abstract]. Proc Am Soc Clin Oncol 22:130.
59. De Jonge M, Sparreboom, A, De Bruijn P, et al. 2003 Phase I and PK study of DE-310 (D) given once every 2 or 6 wks (w) in pts with solid tumors [abstract]. Proc Am Soc Clin Oncol 22:130.
60. Cheverton P, Friess H, Andras C, et al. 2004 Phase III results of exatecan (DX-8951f) versus gemcitabine (Gem) in chemotherapy-naive patients with advanced pancreatic cancer (APC). Proc Am Soc Clin Oncol 23:314s.
61. O'Reilly EM, Abou-Alfa GK, Letourneau R, et al. 2004 A randomized phase III trial of DX-8951f (exatecan mesylate; DX) and gemcitabine (GEM) vs. gemcitabine alone in advanced pancreatic cancer (APC). Proc Am Soc Clin Oncol 23:315s.

15 Camptothecins in the Treatment of Primary Brain Tumors

Clinton F. Stewart, PharmD,
Markos Leggas, PhD,
and Henry S. Friedman, MD

CONTENTS

1. INTRODUCTION

The number of new cases of primary malignant brain tumors diagnosed in 2003 more than double the number of diagnosed cases of Hodgkin's disease, approximately 13,100 deaths were estimated to have occurred as a result of primary cancer of the central nervous system (CNS). Metastases to the brain from a systemic primary cancer are even more common. One estimate suggests that more than 100,000 patients per year die with symptomatic intracranial metastases. In addition, if benign cases are considered, approximately 36,000 brain tumors would have been diagnosed in 2002.

Camptothecins in Cancer Therapy
Edited by: V. R. Adams and T. G. Burke © Humana Press Inc., Totowa, NJ

The age- and sex-adjusted incidence of primary tumors of the CNS is estimated to be approximately 19 per 100,000 persons per year (11.8 per 100,000 for symptomatic tumors and 7.3 per 100,000 for asymptomatic tumors) *(1)*.

In adults, malignant astrocytomas, which include anaplastic astrocytoma and glioblastoma multiforme, are the most common glial tumors, with an annual incidence of 3 to 4 per 100,000 population *(1)*. Glioblastomas account for approximately 80% of all gliomas *(2)*. The peak age at onset for anaplastic astrocytomas is in the fourth or fifth decade, whereas glioblastomas usually present in the sixth or seventh decade.

The incidence of primary brain tumors is different in children, with astrocytoma still the most common type but followed by primitive neuroectodermal tumors (PNET). The astrocytomas may be divided into low grade, anaplastic, and glioblastoma multiforme, with the latter the most prevalent astrocytoma diagnosis. The second most common tumors are represented by the PNET, and medulloblastoma is the most common of this group; followed third by supratentorial PNET, and the newest category, atypical teratoid malignant rhabdoid. The remaining categories include ependymoma, oligodendroglioma, mixed glioma, and germ cell tumors. The peak incidence of malignant CNS disease is within the first decade of life, and thereafter the incidence trends downward.

In adults, the treatments for anaplastic astrocytoma and glioblastoma multiforme are the same. The initial intervention is gross total excision, where every effort is made to remove as much tumor as possible, followed by involved-field radiotherapy. The addition of radiotherapy doses up to of 60 Gy significantly prolongs survival *(1)*. Individual randomized, controlled studies of chemotherapy in addition to radiation therapy have demonstrated no significant improvement in median survival; however, meta-analysis of these data has noted a significant increase in survival. Although a controversy may exist regarding the use of chemotherapy, most agree that administration of chemotherapy will increase the proportion of long-term survivors. However, this increase in survival is modest, from less than 5% to less than 20%, leading some investigators to question the clinical relevance of chemotherapy when considering the permanent side effects associated with this treatment modality. Nevertheless, the potential for long-term survival in a population of these patients exceeds, in our belief, the anticipated toxicities, and we favor the use of adjuvant chemotherapy in adults with newly diagnosed malignant glioma.

Treatment of infants and children with CNS tumors presents a significant clinical challenge. As with adults, surgery and radiation are the two primary therapies, but for reasons unique to children, chemotherapy is often used. In both infants and children, chemotherapy plays a primary role in treatment because of the toxicities and late effects observed with radiotherapy. As indicated previously, medulloblastoma is the second most common pediatric CNS tumor type, and because it often disseminates throughout the neuraxis, chemotherapy and radiotherapy are the most appropriate therapy.

Despite aggressive therapy, the majority of patients—both adults and children—with brain tumors have poor prognosis and have brief survival periods. Thus, the development of new therapies for the treatment of primary and metastatic tumors of the CNS is needed. This review will focus on the results of preclinical studies and clinical trials that have evaluated camptothecin (CPT) analogs in the treatment of CNS tumors.

2. CAMPTOTHECIN ANALOGS ARE TOPOISOMERASE I-INTERACTIVE AGENTS

The antitumor activity of 20(S)-camptothecin, a naturally occurring alkaloid that was originally isolated from the Chinese tree *Camptotheca acuminata (Nyssaceae)*, has been recognized since the 1960s *(3,4)*. Results of clinical trials conducted in China that showed antitumor activity with CPT were not replicated in the United States, and, in fact, the US clinical trials were unfortunately associated with severe and unpredictable toxicities *(5–8)*, including primarily hemorrhagic cystitis. Figure 1 depicts the pentacyclic structure of CPT with a α-hydroxylactone system in the E-ring, which undergoes a reversible pH-dependent hydrolysis forming an anionic hydroxy-acid moiety. The major limitations of the natural alkaloid were its poor solubility in aqueous media and the rapid hydrolysis of the lactone ring at physiological pH.

The development of CPT analogs as clinical agents began in earnest after it was discovered that CPT exerted its antitumor activity via topoisomerase I (TOP-I) *(9)*. The approaches to improve on the parent CPT molecule have been to increase solubility and stabilize the labile lactone ring. Several CPT derivatives have been developed and evaluated in clinical and preclinical trials. These agents include 9-nitrocamptothecin (rubitecan) *(10–13)*, 9-amino-20(S)-camptothecin (9-AC) *(14–16)*, lurtotecan (GI 147211) *(17)*, 9-dimethylaminomethyl-10-hydroxycamptothecin (topo-tecan), and 7-ethyl-10-(4-[1-piperidino]-1-piperidino)-carbonyloxycampto-thecin (irinotecan) (*see* Fig. 1). However, only topotecan (Hycamptin) and irinotecan (Camptosar) have Food and Drug Administration approval for clinical use. The former is approved as second-line therapy for ovarian and small-cell lung cancer, and the latter for secondary or combination therapy for colon cancer.

CPT analogs are unique in their mode of action because they bind to and stabilize the normally transient DNA–TOP-I complex during the S-phase of the cell cycle *(18–20)*. After DNA ligation and unwinding, the drug-stabilized enzyme is unable to perform the religation step, resulting in a DNA single-strand break. Subsequently, collision of the replication "machinery"

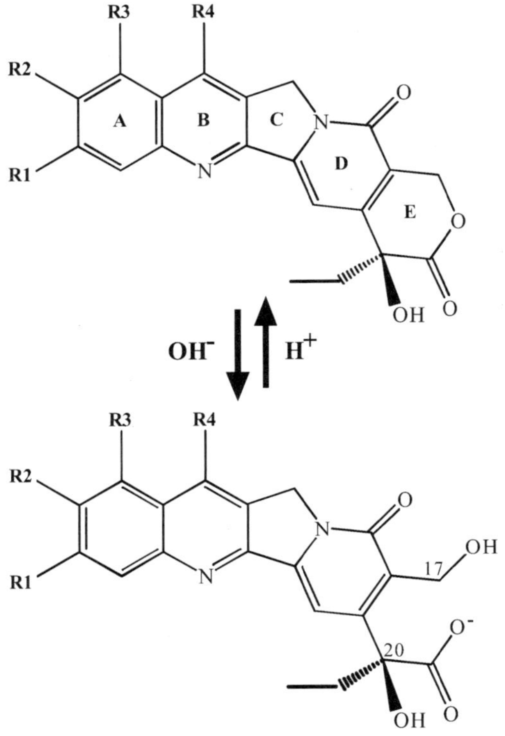

Compound	R1 (C-11)	R2 (C-10)	R3 (C-9)	R4 (C-7)
Camptothecin	H	H	H	H
Irinotecan	H	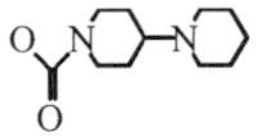	H	CH_2CH_2
Topotecan	H	OH	$CH_2N(CH_3)_2$	H
Lurtotecan	O	O	H	NCH_2NCH_3
9-Aminocamptothecin	H	H	NH_2	H
9-Nitrocamptothecin	H	H	$N0_2$	H

Fig. 1. As depicted in this figure, camptothecin analogs are pentacyclic structures, which vary by substitutions on the 7, 9, or 10 positions.

with this drug-stabilized complex can stall the replication fork and potentially result in the generation of DNA double-strand breaks, which may signal cells to initiate apoptosis. Consequently, considering CPTs' cell-cycle dependence, one can anticipate that their antitumor activity will depend both on drug concentration and duration of exposure. Results of preclinical studies show that the antitumor activity of the CPT analogs is clearly schedule- and systemic exposure–dependent *(21–24)*. This effect is consistent with the S-phase–specific cytotoxic action of these agents. Our preclinical xenograft data show that in many tumor models, the dose-response relationship for these agents is very steep. Below some minimal daily systemic exposure, virtually all antitumor activity is lost. Therefore, maximal efficacy requires that the duration of therapy be protracted while a crucial daily systemic exposure is maintained. In general, the relationship between systemic exposure and tumor response to the CPT analogs remains poorly defined for most human cancers. However, we have investigated these relationships for irinotecan and topotecan in several models of human pediatric and adult malignancies.

3. PRECLINICAL STUDIES OF CAMPTOTHECIN ANALOGS IN PRIMARY BRAIN TUMORS

3.1. Topotecan

In preclinical trials, the CPT analogs have shown considerable promise in the treatment of primary and metastatic CNS tumors, and a number of studies have addressed their distribution in brain tissue and cerebrospinal fluid (CSF). Rodent models have been used to determine the distribution of topotecan in the CNS. The brain extracellular fluid (ECF) distribution of CPT and topotecan lactone after a single intravenous (iv) bolus injection was studied in an awake, freely moving rat model using microdialysis techniques *(25)*. The CPT brain ECF to plasma ratio was greater than that for topotecan, but the topotecan lactone ECF concentrations were greater than the CPT concentrations. Straathof and colleagues studied the accumulation of topotecan in brain tumor tissue and adjacent normal tissue in rats bearing 9L glioma *(26)*. After an iv bolus of topotecan, the mean total topotecan concentration in brain tumor tissue was approximately 20-fold higher than in normal brain tissue. Moreover, dexamethasone pretreatment did not alter topotecan uptake into either tumor or normal brain tissue. In a study of intratumoral infusion of topotecan, Pollina and colleagues showed that topotecan significantly prolonged the survival of animals implanted with U87 glioma cells *(27)*. They also showed that after intratumoral topotecan infusions, cytotoxic topotecan concentrations could be measured up to 4.5 mm from the site of infusion.

Blaney and colleagues conducted a study in the nonhuman primate model of the pharmacokinetic behavior of topotecan in both plasma and CSF to measure the degree of CSF penetration *(28)*. Three nonhuman primates with indwelling Ommaya reservoirs received 10 mg/m^2 iv topotecan administered as a 10-minute infusion. Frequent plasma and CSF samples were assayed by reverse phase high-performance liquid chromatography (HPLC) to measure the concentration of topotecan lactone and total. Peak plasma topotecan concentrations ranged from 0.27 to 0.45 μ*M*, and peak CSF topotecan concentrations occurred 30 minutes after drug administration, ranging from 0.044 to 0.074 μ*M*. The mean ratio of the area under the CSF concentration-time curve to that in plasma was 0.32 (range 0.29–0.37). The mean CSF penetration of topotecan exceeds 30%, which is significantly greater than the penetration of most structurally similar chemotherapeutic agents.

Zamboni and colleagues used a nonhuman primate model to define the duration of topotecan iv infusion necessary to attain a cytotoxic exposure for medulloblastoma cells throughout the neuraxis *(29)*. Initially they used human medulloblastoma cell lines (Daoy, SJ-Med3) to estimate the length and extent of topotecan systemic exposure associated with inhibition of tumor cell growth or the exposure duration threshold. Results of the in vitro studies defined an exposure duration threshold as a topotecan lactone concentration of >1 ng/mL for 8 hours (IC_{99}) daily for 5 days. Topotecan systemic and CSF disposition was evaluated in rhesus monkeys that received topotecan 2.0 mg/m^2 as a 30-minute or 4-hour infusion. Plasma and CSF samples were assayed for topotecan lactone by HPLC, and the CSF exposures were compared with the estimated exposure duration threshold. Topotecan systemic clearance, penetration into fourth ventricle ($\%CSF_{4th}$), and lumbar space ($\%CSF_{LUM}$) were similar for the 30-minute and 4-hour infusion. At a topotecan lactone AUC_P of 140 ng/mL/hour, a 4-hour infusion achieved the desired topotecan exposure throughout the neuraxis (lateral and fourth ventricles and lumbar space), whereas a 30-minute infusion failed to achieve it in the lumbar space. In conclusion, prolonging topotecan infusion from 30 minutes to 4 hours at a targeted AUC_P achieves the exposure duration threshold throughout the neuraxis.

In preclinical trials, the CPT analogs have shown considerable promise in the treatment of primary and metastatic CNS tumors. However, preclinical studies have shown that the antitumor activity of topotecan is extremely schedule-dependent. Pawlik and colleagues examined the effect of various schedules of topotecan exposure in vitro on the production of TOP-I–DNA complexes. The schedule that maximized complex formation in vitro was then evaluated in a mouse xenograft assay; the results showed that an effective intermittent schedule of administration could be identified. However, the exact schedule may depend on the tumor type and the host sensitivity *(30,31)*.

3.2. Irinotecan

Blaney and colleagues evaluated the plasma and CSF disposition of the CPT analogs, irinotecan and its active metabolite SN-38, in a nonhuman primate model to determine their CSF penetration *(32)*. Irinotecan, 4.8 mg/kg (96 mg/m^2) or 11.6 mg/kg (225 mg/m^2), was infused over 30 minutes and plasma and CSF samples were obtained over 24 hours. Irinotecan and SN-38 lactone and total were measured by reverse-phase HPLC. For irinotecan, the AUC_{CSF}:AUC_P ratio was 14 ± 3%. CSF SN-38 lactone and carboxylate could not be measured (< 1.0 n*M*), thus the AUC_{CSF}:AUC_P ratio for SN-38 lactone was estimated to be ≤8%. Therefore, despite the structural similarity between topotecan and irinotecan, the CSF penetration of topotecan is substantially greater than that of irinotecan or SN-38.

Irinotecan was evaluated against a panel of human tumor xenografts derived from adult (high-grade glioma) and pediatric CNS malignancies (high-grade gliomas, medulloblastomas, ependymomas) *(33)*. Irinotecan was administered at 40 mg/kg intraperitoneally (ip) on days 1–5 and 8–12 and produced significant growth delays in all subcutaneous xenografts evaluated, including those sublines resistant to busulfan, cyclophosphamide, procarbazine, and melphalan. After treatment with irinotecan, statistically significant increases in survival were demonstrated in the two intracranial xenografts: D341 EP (73% increase) and D-456 MG (114% increase).

Vassal and colleagues conducted a study to evaluate the antitumor activity of irinotecan in five advanced stage subcutaneous medulloblastoma xenografts, using different schedules of administration *(34)*. With a 5-day schedule, the highest iv dose tested (40 mg/kg/day) induced complete regressions in four of five xenografts. Two xenografts, IGRM11 and IGRM33, were highly sensitive, and even at the lower dosage (27 mg/kg/day), animals survived tumor-free beyond 120 days after treatment. Irinotecan was significantly more active than cyclophosphamide, thiotepa, and etoposide against the three xenografts evaluated. To study the schedule dependency of its antitumor activity, CPT-11 was given iv at the same total doses over the same period (33 days) using either a protracted or a sequential schedule in IGRM34-bearing mice. With a dose of 10 mg kg/day given on days 0–4, days 7–11, days 21–25, and days 28–32 (total dose, 200 mg/kg), three of six animals were tumor-free on day 378. However, the same total dose given with a sequential schedule failed to induce complete regression.

Friedman and colleagues evaluated the combination of irinotecan and carmestine (BCNU) in a murine xenograft model of the glioma D-54 MG *(35)*. Previous studies showed this combination to have synergistic antitumor activity against D-54 MG, but the optimal schedule for the combination had not been determined. Athymic mice were transplanted with human glioma xenografts and were treated with two schedules of BCNU and irinotecan. The regimen in which BCNU (50 mg/m^2 ip on day 1) was administered 5 hours before irinotecan (30 mg/m^2 ip on days 1–5 and 8–12) demonstrated superior anticancer activity to regimens in which a single dose of BCNU was given after the irinotecan therapy. The investigators also reported that delaying irinotecan for 2 or 4 days after the initial BCNU dose reduces the activity of the combination. The mechanism of this schedule-dependent activity of BCNU and irinotecan remains to be elucidated, but it is hypothesized that O^6 adduct of guanine produced by BCNU is required for enhancement of irinotecan antitumor activity.

The combination of irinotecan with three different alkylating agents—1,3-bis(2-chloroethyl)-1-nitrosourea, busulfan, and cyclophosphamide—was evaluated against a panel of human tumor xenografts derived from CNS malignancies, including adult high-grade gliomas (D-54 MG, D-245 MG) and a childhood ependymoma (D-612 EP) *(36)*. In replicate experiments, the alkylating agents were given on day 1 in doses varying from 10% to 75% of the dose lethal to 10% of the animals, and irinotecan was given on days 1–5 and 8–12 in doses varying from 10% to 100% of the dose lethal to 10% of the animals. The antitumor effects of the various combinations ranged from less than additive (irinotecan and cyclophosphamide in D-54 MG) to statistically significant ($p < 0.001$) supra-additive effects (18.8 days above additive with 0.5 CPT-11 + 0.5 1,3-*bis*(2-chloroethyl)-1-nitrosourea in D-54 MG). These studies show that the combination of the topoisomerase inhibitor CPT-11 and alkylating agents may increase the antitumor effect and not increase host toxicity (0/10 deaths in both experiments cited previously).

The activity of temozolomide combined with irinotecan was evaluated against eight independent xenografts (four neuroblastoma, three rhabdomyosarcoma, and one glioblastoma) *(37)*. In all studies, temozolomide was administered orally daily for 5 consecutive days per cycle, because this was determined to be the optimal administration schedule during preliminary studies. Irinotecan was administered iv for 5 days for 2 consecutive weeks per cycle. Treatment cycles were repeated every 21 days for a total of three cycles over 8 weeks. In combination, temozolomide and irinotecan induced complete responses in four neuroblastomas, two rhabdomyosarcomas, and the glioblastoma line. The activity of the combination was significantly greater than the activity of either agent administered alone in four tumor lines. Of interest, the interaction appeared independent of tumor O^6-Methylguanine-DNA methyltransferase expression or mismatch repair phenotype, suggesting the mechanism of synergy may be independent of O^6-methylation by temozolomide. Pharmacokinetic studies indicated no detectable interaction between these two agents. Further, coadministration of irinotecan appeared to reduce the toxicity of temozolomide in tumor-bearing mice. However, results of a more recent study by Pommier and colleagues have shown that alkylating agents such as *N*-methyl-*N''*-nitro-*N*-nitrosoguanidine that covalently link alkyl groups at the 6 position of guanines in DNA lead to an 8-fold to 10-fold enhancement of Top1 cleavage complexes *(38)*. Presumably this will render the cell more sensitive to the effect of a TOP-I–interactive agent, accounting for the enhanced antitumor activity observed with the combination of temozolomide and irinotecan and with temozolomide and topotecan.

3.3. Other CPT Analogs

3.3.1. 9-Aminocamptothecin

The plasma and CSF pharmacokinetics of 9-AC were studied in a nonhuman primate model to determine CSF penetration. 9-AC, 0.2 mg/kg (4 mg/m^2) or 0.5 mg/kg (10 mg/m^2), was infused intravenously over 15 minutes *(32)*. Plasma and CSF samples were obtained over 24 hours, and lactone and total drug forms of 9-AC were measured by reverse-phase HPLC. 9-AC lactone CSF concentrations peaked 30–45 minutes after the dose (0.5 mg/kg dose) at 11–21 n*M*, and the ratio of the areas under the CSF and plasma concentration-time curves (AUC_{CSF}:AUC_P) was only 3.5 ± 2.1%. As with irinotecan and SN-38, 9-AC has much less CSF penetration than the structurally similar CPT analog topotecan.

3.3.2. Karenitecin

In a recent study the efficacy of Karenitecin, a novel highly lipophilic CPT derivative, was evaluated against a panel of human tumor xenografts derived from adult (high-grade glioma) and pediatric CNS malignancies (high-grade gliomas, medulloblastomas, ependymomas) *(39)*. Karenitecin was administered at 1.0 mg/kg via ip injection over 10 consecutive days; at this dosage, statistically significant growth delays were observed in all subcutaneous xenografts tested. This also included several sublines that were resistant to procarbazine and busulfan. Growth delays ranged from 12.1 days to more than 90 days. Karenitecin also had a favorable result in animals bearing intracranial xenografts, with a statistically significant increase observed in survival of animals bearing D-341 MED (69% increase) and D-456 MED (62% increase).

3.3.3. 20(S)-Camptothecin

The antitumor activity of 20(S)-camptothecin, a plant alkaloid isolated from *Camptotheca acuminata*, has been recognized for more than 20 years. A recent study reported the use of a microdialysis system coupled to a microbore HPLC assay to measure the disposition of unbound CPT in brain ECT after iv injection *(40)*. Within 10 minutes of injection, unbound CPT could be measured in brain ECF.

3.3.4. 7-Silylcamptothecins and Homocamptothecin

7-Silylcamptothecins, which represent a class referred to as silatecans, exhibit improved blood stability, potent inhibition of TOP-I, and sufficient lipophilicity to favor blood–brain barrier penetration *(41)*. Homocamptothecin contains an expanded seven-member β-hydroxylactone in place of the six-member α-hydroxylactone ring found in CPT *(42)*. Studies have shown that BN-80927, a novel homocamptothecin, is both a TOP-I- and TOP-II–interactive agent, and that the β-hydroxylactone ring stabilizes the TOP-I-DNA complexes retaining antitumor activity *(43–45)*.

4. CLINICAL TRIALS OF CAMPTOTHECIN ANALOGS IN PRIMARY BRAIN TUMORS

4.1. Topotecan

Topotecan has been evaluated in several Phase I studies to determine the dose-limiting toxicity (DLT) and maximum tolerated dose (MTD) at different administration schedules. A recent study evaluated topotecan administered as an ambulatory iv infusion for 21 days every 28 days, or after toxicity resolution, in 15 children with relapsed solid tumors *(46)*. The starting and maximum tolerated dose was 0.4 mg/m^2/day. At the MTD, equal number of patients (n = 3 each) experienced grade 4 neutropenia and grade 4 thrombocytopenia. Nonhematological toxicities were manageable. Objective responses were observed in two patients with ependymoma: one with rhabdomyosarcoma, and one with retinoblastoma metastatic to the brain.

In children with primary CNS tumors, we conducted a study of topotecan CSF disposition to describe the CSF penetration of topotecan lactone and hydroxy acid, to describe the effect of infusion length on CSF penetration, and to compare topotecan penetration into ventricular CSF and lumbar space *(47)*. Simultaneous plasma and CSF pharmacokinetic studies were performed on 24 patients enrolled in phase I or phase II trials of topotecan. The drug was administered as either a 30-minute infusion or a 24- or 72-hour continuous infusion. Serial plasma samples were collected and at selected times CSF samples were obtained from either a ventricular reservoir in patients with a ventricular-peritoneal shunt or from a lumbar puncture. Plasma and CSF samples were assayed for topotecan lactone and hydroxy acid by HPLC as described previously *(48,49)*. A three-compartment model was fit simultaneously to topotecan lactone and hydroxy-acid concentrations in the plasma and CSF. The AUC was numerically calculated from the final estimated parameters, and topotecan CSF penetration was defined as the CSF to plasma AUC ratio. In a small group of patients receiving topotecan by a 24-hour continuous infusion, the average CSF penetration was 44 ± 15% for topotecan lactone. We then compared the CSF penetration of topotecan lactone among three groups of children receiving topotecan by

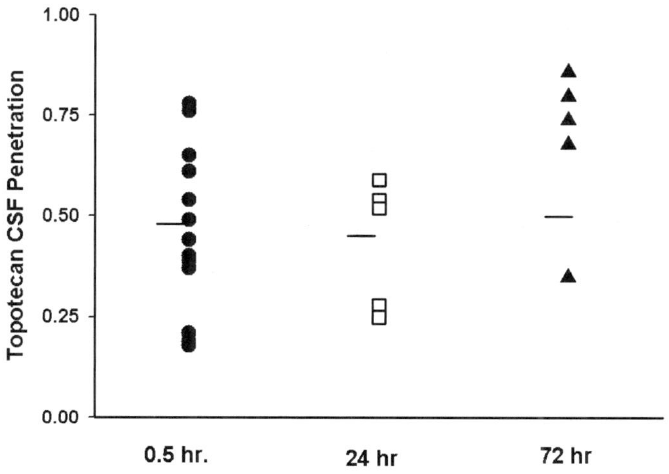

Fig. 2. CSF penetration of topotecan lactone was similar among three groups of children receiving topotecan by various length infusions (i.e., 30 minutess or 24 or 72 hours).

various length infusion (i.e., 30 minutes or 24 or 72 hours). The average CSF penetration was similar among the three groups (approximately 40%), and although slightly greater in the 72-hour group (approximately 58%) the difference was not statistically significant because of wide interpatient variability (Fig. 2). In a small number of patients, we were able to obtain simultaneous ventricular and lumbar CSF samples, and we found that topotecan CSF penetration in the lumbar space was approximately half that of the ventricular CSF, or approximately 20%.

Another recent phase I clinical trial in 40 children with refractory solid tumors was conducted to determine the MTD and DLT for topotecan administered by a 30-minute infusion for 5 consecutive days *(50)*. Among these patients, 9 were diagnosed with neuroblastoma and 10 with brain tumors. The starting and maximum tolerated dose was 1.4 mg/m^2/day. The DLT was thrombocytopenia and neutropenia. Grade 4 hematopoietic toxicity of brief duration was seen at all dose levels. Antitumor responses were seen in three patients with neuroblastoma and stable disease with continued therapy (>6 months) was seen in four patients, including one patient with anaplastic astrocytoma.

A phase I clinical trial was conducted of escalating topotecan dosages in association with a fixed systemic exposure of carboplatin with or without filgrastim in children *(51)*. Two separate cohorts of patients with solid tumors were studied: (1) patients with refractory or recurrent disease and (2) patients with no prior myelosuppressive therapy or newly diagnosed tumors for which there was no standard chemotherapy. Carboplatin was given on day 1 at an AUC of 6.5, followed by topotecan as a 72-hour continuous infusion; the starting topotecan dosage was 0.50 mg/m^2/day, and cycles were repeated every 21 days. Filgrastim was given at a dose of 5 μg/kg/day starting on day 4. Forty-eight of 51 patients were assessable for toxicity. In group 1, dose-limiting myelosuppression persisted despite de-escalation of topotecan to 0.3 mg/m^2/day and use of filgrastim. In group 2, the maximum-tolerated topotecan dosage was 0.5 mg/m^2/day for 3 days, and 0.6 mg/m^2/day for 3 days with filgrastim. No significant nonhematologic toxicities were observed. Among 46 patients assessable for response, 1 had complete response and 5 had a partial response, including 1 patient with an ependymoma and 1 patient with a PNET. Stable disease was observed in 18 patients, with 5 astrocytomas (range 1–195 days), 1 GBM (77+ days), 3 ependymomas (range 16–167 days), and 1 paraganglioma (113+ days). Although this combination possesses antineoplastic activity in pediatric solid tumors, hematologic toxicity precluded any meaningful dosage escalation, and filgrastim addition did not alter this. The potential for preservation of activity and diminution of toxicity with alternative sequences and schedules of administration (topoisomerase followed by alkylating or platinating agents) should be evaluated.

Kushner and colleagues studied a novel myeloablative regimen that consisted of topotecan, thiotepa, and carboplatin in 21 patients with poor-prognosis tumors *(52)*. The topotecan dosage was 2 mg/m^2 given iv on days –8, –7, –6, –5, –4; thiotepa 300 mg/m^2 by 3-hour iv infusion on days –8, –7, and –6; and carboplatin by 4-hour iv infusion on days –5, –4, and –3 targeted to an AUC of 7 mg/mL/minute (approximately 500 mg/m^2/day). Stem cell rescue was on day 0. Complete remissions were observed in 18 patients, and early toxicities included severe mucositis and erythema in all patients. Toxicities observed included a seizure, hypertension, and renal insufficiency followed by veno-occlusive disease. Posttransplant therapy included radiotherapy alone ($n = 4$) or biological agents for a subset of other patients. Event-free survivors include four of five patients with primary brain tumors (second partial recovery or complete recovery). These investigators suggest that this regimen results in favorable disease control with manageable toxicity.

Topotecan has been evaluated in numerous tumor types in phase II studies using different schedules as a single agent and in combination therapy. In a phase II clinical trial of 63 adult patients with malignant glioma, 25 were newly diagnosed and 38 had recurrent disease *(53)*. Topotecan was administered as a 2.6 mg/m^2 continuous infusion over 72 hours weekly. Toxicity was limited to infrequent grade 3 myelosuppression, with 17 of 38 patients requiring a dose reduction secondary to grade 3 thrombocytopenia. No other nonhematological toxicities were reported. In newly diagnosed patients, partial responses were noted in 2 of 14 evaluable patients with glioblastoma multiforme and in 1 of 8 evaluable patients with anaplastic astrocytoma. Three of 10 evaluable patients with recurrent anaplastic astrocytoma had a partial response. The authors noted that topotecan given in this schedule and dosage has modest activity, but they also noted that frequent use of anticonvulsants in their patients raises the possibility of subtherapeutic topotecan systemic exposure. This is based on a study by Zamboni and colleagues that showed the concomitant administration of phenytoin with topotecan increased the topotecan lactone clearance by approximately 45% *(54)*. Concomitant phenytoin also increased the plasma AUC of N-desmethyl topotecan approximately twofold. The other concern raised by Friedman and colleagues was that the schedule that was used (i.e., 72-hour infusion) may have been suboptimal, because preclinical studies have indicated that protracted exposure to the TOP-I-interactive agents is associated with greater antitumor effect.

The NCIC Clinical Trial Group conducted a phase II clinical trial of topotecan in patients with malignant glioma *(55)*. Adults with malignant glioma and recurrent contrast enhancing measurable disease were eligible. Topotecan 1.5 mg/m^2 iv was given daily for 5 days every 3 weeks. Response and toxic effects were assessed at the end of each cycle. Thirty-one patients were entered onto the study: 15 had glioblastoma, 16 had anaplastic astrocytoma, all had prior radiation, 15 had prior chemotherapy, and all were assessable for response and toxicity. Two patients (6%) responded: one had a complete radiographic response, but died with neutropenic sepsis, and the second had a prolonged partial response (>97 weeks). Twenty-one patients (68%) had stable disease for 5 to 86 + weeks (median 19) and eight (26%) had progressive disease after one cycle. Toxicity was primarily hematologic; 18 (58%) had grade 4 neutropenia ($<0.5 \times 10^9/1$), usually brief, and three (10%) grade 4 thrombocytopenia (<25,000/1). Twelve of 109 cycles (11%) were given at reduced dose. Topotecan in this dose and schedule has only modest activity in recurrent glioblastoma and anaplastic astrocytoma.

A recent phase II clinical trial of topotecan was conducted in 33 patients who developed evidence of progressive glioma after definitive radiation therapy *(56)*. Patients were treated with topotecan 1.5 mg/m^2 iv daily for 5 consecutive days repeated every 3 weeks or with 1.25 mg/m^2 if they had previously received nitrosourea-containing chemotherapy. However, the study showed that topotecan was not effective at this dose and schedule in patients with recurrent glioma. Hematological toxicities were observed in 16 patients. Grade 4 leukopenia in seven patients and grades 3 and 4 thrombocytopenia in nine patients. Two of the patients experiencing leukopenia did not survive infection-related complications. The majority of the patients experiencing toxicities were not on anticonvulsants (14 of 16). Only one patient experienced a partial response and the median survival time was approximately 20 weeks.

Nitschke and colleagues conducted a phase II clinical trial of a daily × 5 regimen of topotecan in 144 children with recurrent and progressive solid tumors *(57)*. Topotecan 2 mg/m^2/day was administered iv over 30 minutes for 5 days every 3 weeks. Three patients had complete responses (neuroblastoma *n* = 2; PNET), 2 patients had partial responses (Ewing's sarcoma; retinoblastoma), and 24 patients had minor responses or stable disease. The striking observation about the patients with stable disease was the duration of the resolution of the symptoms (median time on study for patients with stable disease was 8.5 months). Myelosuppression was the most prominent toxicity; however, only one patient died (on day 15 after the first course of therapy from sepsis). Nonhematological toxicities were mild and consisted primarily of nausea, vomiting, and rash.

In another phase II clinical trial, topotecan was administered as a 72-hour continuous infusion to 85 children with recurrent or refractory solid tumors *(58)*. Treatment was started at 1.0 mg/m^2/day and was escalated to 1.3 mg/m^2/day on subsequent cycles if the patient did not experience any dose-limiting toxicities on the first cycle. One patient with neuroblastoma had a complete response and one patient in the Ewing's sarcoma/PNET stratum had a partial response. Myelosuppression was the primary toxicity, and the primary nonhematological toxicity was mild nausea and vomiting. Despite the poor response rate the investigators suggested that, based on results of preclinical studies, consideration should be given to evaluating more prolonged schedules of topotecan administration in pediatric patients.

A phase II clinical trial of topotecan administered as a 24-hour infusion was performed to assess the activity of topotecan against childhood brain tumors *(59)*. Forty-five children with either a previously treated primary brain tumor that was refractory to standard therapy or an untreated brain stem glioma or glioblastoma multiforme received topotecan administered as a 24-hour iv infusion every 21 days. The initial dose was 5.5 mg/m^2 with escalation to 7.5 mg/m^2 on the second and subsequent doses in patients who did not experience dose-limiting toxicity. No complete or partial responses were observed in the patients with high-grade glioma (*n* = 9), medulloblastoma (*n* = 9), or brain stem glioma (*n* = 14). One of two patients with a low-grade glioma had a partial response lasting more than 17 months, three patients with a brain stem glioma had stable disease for 12 to 28 weeks, and one patient with a malignant neuroepithelial tumor and 1 patient with an optic glioma had stable disease for 41 weeks and 22 weeks, respectively. Dose escalation from 5.5 mg/m^2 to 7.5 mg/m^2 was well tolerated in the first 11 patients enrolled in this study who had not received prior craniospinal radiation therapy. The starting dose was subsequently increased to 7.5 mg/m^2 for patients without prior craniospinal radiation. Topotecan administered as a 24-hour infusion every 21 days is inactive in high-grade gliomas, medulloblastomas, and brain stem tumors.

A phase II clinical trial of topotecan given as a 72-hour continuous infusion in 88 children with recurrent or progressive CNS tumors was recently reported *(60)*. Treatment was begun at 1.0 mg/m^2/day and was escalated to 1.25 mg/m^2/day after the first six patients tolerated the initial dosage with minimal toxicities. No complete or partial responses were noted in these patients. The investigators expressed concern that topotecan efficacy might have been compromised by allowing patients to receive concomitant anticonvulsant therapy; however, a majority of patients (51/88) had one or more episodes of grade 3 or 4 neutropenia, suggesting that these patients received, at least, moderate dose intensity.

Topotecan has been evaluated in a phase II clinical trial in children with newly diagnosed high-risk medulloblastoma *(61)*. The hypothesis of the clinical trial was that pharmacokinetically guided topotecan dosing would attain a desired plasma AUC, yielding an appropriate CSF exposure as defined by preclinical models *(30)*. The objective of the study was to assess the antitumor efficacy of pharmacokinetically guided topotecan dosing in previously untreated patients with medulloblastoma and supratentorial PNETs. After maximal surgical resection, 44 children with high-risk medulloblastoma were enrolled, of which 36 were able to be evaluated for response. The topotecan window consisted of two cycles, administered initially as a 30-minute infusion daily × 5 days lasting 6 weeks. Pharmacokinetic studies were conducted on day 1 to attain a topotecan lactone AUC of 120–160 ng/mL/hour. After 10 patients were enrolled, the infusion was modified to 4 hours, but the dosage was still individualized. Of 36 patients able to be evaluated, 4 (11.1%) had a complete and 6 (16.6%) showed a partial response, and disease was stable in 17 patients (47.2%). Toxicity was mostly hematological with only one patient having treatment delay. The desired CSF topotecan exposure was achieved in seven of eight pharmacokinetic studies when the topotecan plasma AUC was within the target range. Topotecan, when pharmacokinetically guided to attain a target systemic exposure of 120–160 ng/mL/hr, is an effective agent against pediatric medulloblastoma in patients who have received no therapy other than surgery.

A phase I clinical trial was conducted by the Radiation Therapy Oncology Group to determine the maximum tolerated topotecan dosage that could be safely combined with standard cranial radiation for glioblastoma multiforme *(62)*. A secondary objective was to document the acute and late toxicities of this combination of chemotherapy and radiation. Forty-seven patients with histologically confirmed glioblastoma multiforme were entered into this phase I trial. Three cycles of topotecan were administered at 21-day intervals commencing at day 1 of cranial radiotherapy (60 Gy/30 fractions). Each cycle consisted of daily 30-minute iv infusions for 5 days. The topotecan dosage was escalated in three-dose increments from 0.5 mg/m^2/

day to 1.0 mg/m^2/day to 1.5 mg/m^2/day in different patient groups. The majority of patients were older than age 50. Three dose levels of topotecan were tested. Fifteen patients accrued to level 1 (topotecan dose 0.5 mg/m^2/day). No grade 4 toxicities were seen. Sixteen patients accrued to level 2 (topotecan dose 1.0 mg/m^2/day), five of whom had brief episodes of grade 4 neutropenia. Seventeen patients accrued to level 3 (1.5 mg/m^2/day). Six of these patients had brief episodes of grade 4 neutropenia and four developed grade 3 thrombocytopenia. No serious nonhematologic or late toxicities were seen. Median survival for all patients was 9.7 months. No apparent difference was noted in survival based on topotecan dose schedule. Toxicity was acceptable at an iv topotecan dose of 1.5 mg/m^2/day administered daily for 5 days every 21 days for three cycles. A phase II trial has been performed using this dose of topotecan.

In another study of topotecan added to radiation therapy, the change in quality of life and toxicity profiles was studied in a multicenter trial in patients that had histologically proven glioblastoma multiforme *(63)*. Including the pilot phase, 60 patients (41 male and 19 female; age range 26–76 years) were treated. Conventional fractionated conformal radiotherapy was performed with daily doses of 2.0 Gy to a total dose of 60 Gy. Topotecan (0.5 mg absolute dose) was administered intravenously 1 hour before irradiation for 30 doses or a cumulative dose of 15 mg. In addition to hematological and nonhematological toxicity, quality of life was assessed by the Karnofsky and Spitzer indices. Additionally, local control and survival time were recorded. Fifty-seven patients completed the combined therapy. Median administered dose of radiation was 60 Gy (16–76 Gy). Median cumulative topotecan dose was 15 mg (7.5–18.5 mg). Grade 3 toxicity was found in six cases (two hematological, two motoric disorder, one infection, one nausea) and grade 4 toxicity in three cases (one esophagitis, one motoric disorder, one mental disorder). Two patients died of septic disease most likely caused by steroid-induced immunosuppression. Mean Karnofsky index and Spitzer index initially, at the end of therapy, and 6 weeks after therapy showed values of 87%, 81%, and 80% and 19 points, 18 points, and 19 points, respectively. Median survival time was 15 months. This multimodal approach for patients with glioblastoma multiforme is well tolerated. Quality of life remains preserved and outpatient treatment is possible. The relatively long median survival time even for patients bearing macroscopic tumors is promising.

The Children's Cancer Study Group conducted a phase I clinical trial of daily topotecan administered as a 30-minute infusion along with fractionated radiotherapy for children with intrinsic pontine gliomas *(64)*. All patients received 50.4 Gy to the initial tumor volume with a 1.5 cm margin followed by a 9-Gy boost to the tumor volume plus a 1-cm margin. External beam radiotherapy was administered in a 1.8 Gy/fraction; patients were treated daily, 5 days per week. Topotecan was administered on the days of planned radiotherapy and was completed 30–60 minutes before initiation of radiotherapy. The starting topotecan dosage was 0.3 mg/m^2/day, and was escalated in standard fashion. Seventeen children were enrolled on this study; 16 completed protocol treatment (10 male and 6 female; age range <1–14 years). The DLT was hematological (neutropenia) and occurred at a topotecan dosage of 0.5 mg/m^2/day. No significant nonhematological toxicities were observed. The actuarial median survival time is 15 months (95% confidence interval [CI], 9.6–19 months) and the 1-year survival is 53%. The recommended safe MTD for daily topotecan for further Phase II studies is 0.4 mg/m^2 for 33 days, or a total dosage of 13.2 mg/m^2.

In a recently published study, 32 children with recurrent high-grade glioma received injectable formulation of topotecan administered orally once daily at a starting dosage of 0.4 mg/m^2 *(64a)*. In 19 evaluable patients, the maximum tolerated dosage was 0.9 mg/m^2/day, and the dose-limiting was hematological. Objective responses were observed in 2 of 13 evaluable patients that lasted for 2.5 and 9 months, respectively.

4.2. Irinotecan

Based on the highly promising preclinical activity of irinotecan in the xenograft model, several schedules and dosages of irinotecan have been evaluated in patients with primary CNS tumors. Friedman and colleagues conducted a phase II study of irinotecan in adults with recurrent or progressive malignant glioma to determine the antitumor activity, toxicity profile, and pharmacokinetics *(65)*. Patients with progressive or recurrent malignant gliomas were enrolled into this study and given irinotecan as a 90-minute iv infusion at a dose of 125 mg/m^2 once weekly for 4 weeks followed by a 2-week rest, which was considered one course. Plasma concentrations of irinotecan and its metabolites, SN-38 and SN-38 glucuronide, were determined in a subset of patients. All 60 patients who enrolled (36 males, 24 females) were treated with irinotecan and were evaluated for toxicity, response, and survival. Nine patients (15%; 95% CI, 6–24%) had a confirmed partial response, and 33 patients (55%) achieved stable disease lasting more than two courses (12 weeks). Toxicity observed during the study was limited to infrequent neutropenia, nausea, vomiting, and diarrhea. Pharmacokinetic data were available in 32 patients. Irinotecan, SN-38, and SN-38 glucuronide area under the plasma concentration-time curves through infinite time values in these patients were approximately 40%, 25%, and 25%, respectively, of those determined previously in patients with metastatic colorectal cancer not receiving enzyme-inducing anticonvulsants or chronic dexamethasone treatment. Response results document that irinotecan, given with a standard starting dosage and treatment schedule, has activity in patients with recurrent malignant glioma. However, the low incidence of severe toxicity and low systemic exposure of irinotecan and SN-38 achieved in this patient population suggest that concurrent treatment with anticonvulsants and dexamethasone enhances drug clearance.

The safety, tolerability, and efficacy of irinotecan given once every 3 weeks have been evaluated in the treatment of adults with malignant glioma *(66)*. These patients received irinotecan as a 90-minute iv infusion at a dose of 300 mg/m^2 once per week every 3 weeks. If after two courses the patient did not have grade 3/4 toxicity, the irinotecan dosage could be increased to 350 mg/m^2. Dose adjustments were made for toxicities. Fourteen patients were enrolled (11 males, 3 females) and were assessable for survival, response, and toxicity. The majority of patients (86%) had prior surgery. Two patients had a confirmed partial response and two patients (14%) had stable disease. Median survival was 24 weeks, and median time to tumor progression was 6 weeks. The primary hematological toxicity was grade 3/4 neutropenia, which was observed in 14% of patients. Infrequent grade 3/4 nonhematological toxicity was observed, possibly because of the concomitant use of enzyme-inducing anticonvulsants, which have been shown to alter irinotecan and SN-38 disposition by other investigators *(67)*. These investigators suggest that irinotecan has activity against recurrent malignant glioma using a dosing regimen of 300 mg/m^2 every 3 weeks, with limited toxicity.

In a phase I study, the MTDs and DLTs of a short course (daily × 5) of iv irinotecan was evaluated in children with refractory solid tumors *(68)*. Thirty-five children received 146 courses of irinotecan daily for 5 days every 21 days, in dosages ranging from 30 to 65 mg/m^2/day. Myelosuppression was the primary DLT in heavily pretreated patients (i.e., two prior chemotherapy regimens, no prior bone marrow transplantation, and no radiation to the spine, skull, ribs, or pelvic bones), and diarrhea was the DLT in less-heavily pretreated patients. The MTD in the heavily pretreated patient group was 39 mg/m^2, and the MTD in the less-heavily pretreated patients was 50 mg/m^2. A partial response was observed in one patient with neuroblastoma and in one patient with hepatocellular carcinoma. Stable disease (4–20 cycles) was observed in seven patients with a variety of malignancies including neuroblastoma, pineoblastoma, glioblastoma, brainstem glioma, osteosarcoma, hepatoblastoma, and a CNS rhabdoid tumor.

A phase II study of irinotecan (CPT-11) was conducted in children with high-risk malignant brain tumors *(69)*. A total of 22 children were enrolled in this study, including 13 with histologically verified recurrent malignant brain tumors (4 with glioblastoma multiforme [GBM], 1 anaplastic astrocytoma, 5 ependymoma, 3and medulloblastoma/PNET), 5 with recurrent diffuse pontine glioma, and 4 with newly diagnosed GBM. All patients with recurrent tumor had prior chemotherapy or irradiation. Each course of irinotecan consisted of 125 mg/m^2 per week given iv for 4 weeks followed by a 2-week rest period. Patients with recurrent tumors received therapy until disease progression or unacceptable toxicity. Patients with newly diagnosed tumors initially received three cycles of treatment to assess tumor response and then were allowed radiotherapy at physician's choice; patients who demonstrated a response to irinotecan before radiotherapy were allowed to continue the drug after radiation until disease progression or unacceptable toxicity. A 25–50% dose reduction was made for grade 3–4 toxicity. Responses were assessed after every course by gadolinium-enhanced magnetic resonance image of the brain and spine. Twenty-two patients received a median of two courses of CPT-11 (range 1–16). Responses were seen in four of nine patients with GBM or anaplastic astrocytoma (44%; 95% CI, 11–82%) (complete response in two patients with recurrent GBM lasting 9 months and 48+ months; partial response in one patient with a newly diagnosed midbrain GBM lasting 18 months before radiotherapy; and partial response lasting 11 months in one patient with recurrent anaplastic astrocytoma), one of five patients with recurrent ependymoma (partial response initially followed by stable disease lasting 11 months), and zero of five patients with recurrent diffuse pontine glioma. Two of three patients with medulloblastoma/PNET had stable disease for 9 and 13 months. Toxicity was mainly myelosuppression, with 12 of 22 patients (50%) suffering grade 3/4 neutropenia. Seven patients required dose reduction secondary to neutropenia. CPT-11, given in this schedule, appears to be active in children with malignant glioma, medulloblastoma, and ependymoma with acceptable toxicity. Ongoing studies will demonstrate if activity of CPT-11 can be enhanced when combined with alkylating agents, including carmustine and temozolomide.

In a multicenter phase II clinical trial, the antitumor efficacy of irinotecan was evaluated in chemotherapy-naive patients either before (Group A) or after (Group B) relapse following radiation therapy *(70)*. Fifty-two patients (25 in Group A and 27 in Group B) received a total of 191 cycles of irinotecan (350 mg/m^2 as a 90-minute infusion every 3 weeks). To minimize the potential for an interaction with enzyme-inducing anticonvulsant drugs, patients were recommended to use valproic acid or carbamazepine for 2 weeks before irinotecan. Of the 52 patients, 46 (22 in Group A and 24 in Group B) able to be evaluated for response, and of these one partial response (Group B), 7 minor responses (3 in Group A and 4 in Group B), and 12 patients with stable disease (7 in Group A and 5 in Group B) were noted. The median time to progression for Group A was 9 weeks compared with 14.4 weeks for Group B. The 6-month progression-free survival rates were 26% and 43% for Groups A and B, respectively. The primary toxicity was myelosuppression (neutropenia) occurring in 12.5% and 25.9% of the patients in Groups A and B, respectively. Grade 3/4 diarrhea occurred in less than 10% of the patients in either group. The investigators performed pharmacokinetic studies but because of limited numbers were unable to establish any statistical relation between SN-38 systemic exposure and outcome (e.g., toxicity, efficacy). Although they did note that the irinotecan clearance was lower in the two patients not receiving anticonvulsants than in patients receiving either valproic acid or enzyme-inducing anticonvulsants, the observation only confirms the earlier observations of Crews and colleagues *(67)*.

4.3. Other Camptothecin Analogs

In a phase II study, the antitumor activity of 9-AC was evaluated in a group of adults with high-grade astrocytomas *(71)*. 9-AC was administered as a 72-hour continuous infusion every 2 weeks to a total of 99 adults, 51 with newly diagnosed glioblastoma multiforme (before radiation therapy) and 48 patients with high-grade astrocytomas treated at time of tumor recurrence. The initial 9-AC dosage was 850 μg/m^2/day, but because of concomitant therapy with enzyme-inducing anticonvulsants, the dosage was escalated to a new MTD of 1776 μg/m^2/day for previously untreated patients and 1611 μg/m^2/day for previously treated patients. In the 38 assessable patients treated at the MTD, the overall response was 0 of 38. Furthermore, only one partial response was observed in the group of patients that received dosages less than the MTD, yielding an overall response rate of 2%. These data suggest that 9-AC lacks substantial antitumor activity in patients with newly diagnosed or recurrent high-grade astrocytoma.

5. SUMMARY

Treatment of patients with CNS tumors represents a significant clinical challenge because of the limited efficacy of traditional therapies and the potentially negative impact of available modalities. One factor that contributes to the ineffectiveness of current therapies is the unique physiology of the blood–brain barrier and the blood–CSF barrier that tightly regulates the transport of ions, nutrients, peptides, and drugs across these barriers and into the brain. The physiological regulation of these barriers and the specificity for controlling drug transport is not well understood. This likely contributes to the limited number of therapeutic agents that are effective in treating brain tumors. The CPT analogs topotecan and irinotecan are both used to treat patients with malignant brain tumors, but the distribution of these drugs into the brain is widely different. It was previously believed that drug distribution profiles in the CSF were controlled by passive diffusion and by physicochemical properties, but the discovery of P-glycoprotein (P-gp) and other ATP-binding cassette transport proteins in the brain has challenged that view. Thus it is highly likely that we have obtained the maximum therapeutic benefit from the CPTs using this empirical approach. Perhaps the only way to recognize the full antitumor potential promised from in vitro studies is to develop a more complete understanding of the regulation of the blood–brain barrier and the blood–CSF barrier and how CPT analogs are controlled with the CNS. Armed with this knowledge, the clinician could select the appropriate CPT, route, and dosage for the particular CNS malignancy to maximize the likelihood of an antitumor response.

REFERENCES

1. DeAngelis L. 2001 Brain tumors. N Engl J Med 344:114–123.
2. Radhakrishnan K, Mokri B, Parisi JE, et al. 1995 The trends in incidence of brain tumors in the population of Rochester, Minnesota. Ann Neurol 37:67–73.
3. Wall ME, Wani MC, Cook CE, Palmer KH. 1966 Plant antitumor agents. I. The isolation and structure of camptothecin, a novel alkaloidal leukemia and tumor inhibitor from Camptotheca acuminata. J Am Chem Soc 88:3888–3890.
4. Kepler JA, Wani MC, McNaull JN, Wall ME, Levine SG. 1969 Plant antitumor agents. IV. An approach toward the synthesis of camptothecin. J Org Chem 34:3853–3858.
5. Gottlieb JA, Guarino AM, Call JB, Oliverio VT, Block JB. 1970 Preliminary pharmacologic and clinical evaluation of camptothecin sodium (NSC-100880). Cancer Chemother Rep 54:461–470.
6. Muggia FM, Creaven PJ, Hansen HH, Cohen MH, Selawry OS. 1972 Phase I clinical trial of weekly and daily treatment with camptothecin (NSC-100880): correlation with preclinical studies. Cancer Chemother Rep 56:515–521.
7. Moertel CG, Schutt AJ, Reitemeier RJ, Hahn RG. 1972 Phase II study of camptothecin (NSC-100880) in the treatment of advanced gastrointestinal cancer. Cancer Chemother Rep 56:95–101.
8. Xu B. U.S./China Pharmacology Symposium. Burns JJ, Tsuchiatani PJ. 1980.
9. Hsiang YH, Hertzberg R, Hecht S, Liu LF. 1985 Camptothecin induces protein-linked DNA breaks via mammalian DNA topoisomerase I. J Biol Chem 260:14873–14878.
10. Konstadoulakis MM, Antonakis PT, Tsibloulis BG, et al. 2001 A phase II study of 9-nitrocamptothecin in patients with advanced pancreatic adenocarcinoma. Cancer Chemother Pharmacol 48:417–420.
11. Giovanella BC, Stehlin JS, Hinz HR, Kozielski AJ, Harris NJ, Vardeman DM. 2002 Preclinical evaluation of the anticancer activity and toxicity of 9-nitro-20(S)-camptothecin (Rubitecan). Int J Oncol 20:81–88.
12. Han Z, Wyche JH, Sands H, Pantazis P. 2001 9-Nitrocamptothecin is an effective drug for the treatment of human lung tumors: comparison of in vitro and in vivo studies. Anticancer Res 21:1823–1827.
13. Verschraegen CF, Vincent M, Abbruzzese JL, et al. 2000 Phase I study of 9-nitro-20(S)-camptothecin in combination with cisplatin for patients with advanced malignancies. Ann NY Acad Sci 922:345–348.
14. Hinz HR, Harris NJ, Natelson EA, Giovanella BC. 1994 Pharmacokinetics of the in vivo and in vitro conversion of 9-nitro-20(S)-camptothecin to 9-amino-20(S)-camptothecin in humans, dogs, and mice. Cancer Res 54:3096–3100.
15. Pantazis P, Kozielski AJ, Vardeman DM, Petry ER, Giovanella BC. 1993 Efficacy of camptothecin congeners in the treatment of human breast carcinoma xenografts. Oncol Res 5:273–281.

16. Takimoto CH, Thomas R. 2000 The clinical development of 9-aminocamptothecin. Ann NY Acad Sci 922:224–236.
17. Holthuis JJM, Postmus PE, van Oort WJ. 1986 Pharmacokinetics of high dose etoposide (VP16–213). Eur J Cancer Clin Oncol 22:1149–1155.
18. Liu LF, Desai SD, Li TK, Mao Y, Sun M, Sim SP. 2000 Mechanism of action of camptothecin. Ann NY Acad Sci 922:1–10.
19. Champoux JJ. 2001 DNA topoisomerases: structure, function, and mechanism. 2001 Annu Rev Biochem 70:369–413.
20. Stewart C. Topoisomerase I interactive agents. 2001 Cancer Chemother Biol Response Modif 19:85–128.
21. Houghton PJ, Chesire PJ, Myers L, Stewart CF, Synold TW, Houghton JA. 1992 Evaluation of 9-dimethylaminomethyl-10-hydroxycamptothecin against xenografts derived from adult and childhood solid tumors. Cancer Chemother Pharmacol 31:229–239.
22. Houghton PJ, Cheshire PJ, Hallman JD, et al. 1995 Efficacy of topoisomerase I inhibitors, topotecan and irinotecan, administered at low dose levels in protracted schedules to mice bearing xenografts of human tumors. Cancer Chemother Pharmacol 36:393–403.
23. Houghton PJ, Stewart CF, Zamboni WC, Thompson J, Danks MK, Houghton JA. 1996 Schedule dependent efficacy of camptothecins in models of human cancer. NY Acad Sci 803:188–201.
24. Zamboni WC, Stewart CF, Thompson J, et al. 1998 Relationship between topotecan systemic exposure and tumor response in human neuroblastoma xenografts. J Natl Cancer Inst 90:505–511.
25. El Gizawy SA, Hedaya MA. 1999 Comparative brain tissue distribution of camptothecin and topotecan in the rat. Cancer Chemother Pharmacol 43:364–370.
26. Straathof CS, van den Bent MJ, Loos WJ, Vecht CJ, Schellens JH. 1999 The accumulation of topotecan in 9L glioma and in brain parenchyma with and without dexamethasone administration. J Neurooncol 42:117–122.
27. Pollina J, Plunkett RJ, Ciesielski MJ, et al. 1998 Intratumoral infusion of topotecan prolongs survival in the nude rat intracranial U87 human glioma model. J Neurooncol 39:217–225.
28. Blaney SM, Cole DE, Balis FM, Godwin K, Poplack DG. 1993 Plasma and cerebrospinal fluid pharmacokinetic study of topotecan in nonhuman primates. Cancer Res 53:725–727.
29. Zamboni WC, Gajjar AJ, Mandrell TD, et al. 1998 A four-hour topotecan infusion achieves cytotoxic exposure throughout the neuraxis in the nonhuman primate model: implications for treatment of children with metastatic medulloblastoma. Clin Cancer Res 4:2537–2544.
30. Danks MK, Pawlik CA, Whipple DO, Wolverton JS. 1997 Intermittent exposure of medulloblastoma cells to topotecan produces growth inhibition equivalent to continuous exposure. Clin Cancer Res 3:1731–1738.
31 Pawlik CA, Houghton PJ, Stewart CF, Cheshire PJ, Richmond LB, Danks MK. 1998 Effective schedules of exposure of medulloblastoma and rhabdomyosarcoma xenografts to topotecan correlate with in vitro assays. Clin Cancer Res 4:1995–2002.
32. Blaney SM, Takimoto C, Murry DJ, et al. 1998 Plasma and cerebrospinal fluid pharmacokinetics of 9-aminocamptothecin (9-AC), irinotecan (CPT-11), and SN-38 in nonhuman primates. Cancer Chemother Pharmacol 41:464–468.

33. Hare CB, Elion GB, Houghton PJ, et al. 1997 Therapeutic efficacy of the topoisomerase I inhibitor 7-ethyl-10-(4-[1-piperidino]-1-piperidino)-carbonyl-oxy-camptothecin against pediatric and adult central nervous system tumor xenografts. Cancer Chemother Pharmacol 39:187–191.
34. Vassal G, Boland I, Santos A, et al. 1997 Potent therapeutic activity of irinotecan (CPT-11) and its schedule dependency in medulloblastoma xenografts in nude mice. Int J Cancer 73:156–163.
35. Friedman HS, Castellino RC, Elion GB, et al. 2000 Schedule-dependent activity of irinotecan plus BCNU against malignant glioma xenografts. Cancer Chemother Pharmacol 45:345–349.
36. Coggins CA, Elion GB, Houghton PJ, et al. 1998 Enhancement of irinotecan (CPT-11) activity against central nervous system tumor xenografts by alkylating agents. Cancer Chemother Pharmacol 41:485–490.
37. Houghton PJ, Stewart CF, Cheshire PJ, et al. 2000 Antitumor activity of temozolomide combined with irinotecan is partly independent of O6-methylguanine-DNA methyltransferase and mismatch repair phenotypes in xenograft models. Clin Cancer Res 6:4110–4118.
38. Pourquier P, Waltman JL, Urasaki Y, et al. 2001 Topoisomerase I-mediated cytotoxicity of *N*-methyl-*N*'-nitro-*N*-nitrosoguanidine: trapping of topoisomerase I by the O6-methylguanine. Cancer Res 61:53–58.
39. Keir ST, Hausheer F, Lawless AA, Bigner DD, Friedman HS. 2001 Therapeutic activity of 7-[(2-trimethylsilyl)ethyl)]-20 (S)-camptothecin against central nervous system tumor-derived xenografts in athymic mice. Cancer Chemother Pharmacol 48:83–87.
40. Tsai TH, Chen YF, Chou CJ, Chen CF. 2000 Measurement and pharmacokinetics of unbound 20(S)-camptothecin in rat blood and brain by microdialysis coupled to microbore liquid chromatography with fluorescence detection. J Chromatogr A 870:221–226.
41. Pollack IF, Erff M, Bom D, Burke TG, Strode JT, Curran DP. 1999 Potent topoisomerase I inhibition by novel silatecans eliminates glioma proliferation in vitro and in vivo. Cancer Res 59:4898–4905.
42. Lavergne O, Lesueur-Ginot L, Pla RF, et al. 1998 Homocamptothecins: synthesis and antitumor activity of novel E-ring- modified camptothecin analogues. J Med Chem 41:5410–5419.
43. Lavergne O, Harnett J, Rolland A, et al. 1999 BN 80927: a novel homocamptothecin with inhibitory activities on both topoisomerase I and topoisomerase II. Bioorg Med Chem Lett 9:2599–2602.
44. Lesueur-Ginot L, Demarquay D, Kiss R, et al. 1999 Homocamptothecin, an E-ring modified camptothecin with enhanced lactone stability, retains topoisomerase I-targeted activity and antitumor properties. Cancer Res. 59:2939–2943.
45. Bailly C, Lansiaux A, Dassonneville L, et al. 1999 Homocamptothecin, an E-ring-modified camptothecin analogue, generates new topoisomerase I-mediated DNA breaks. Biochemistry (Mosc) 38:15556–15563.
46. Frangoul H, Ames MM, Mosher RB, et al. 1999 Phase I study of topotecan administered as a 21-day continous infusion in children with recurrent solid tumors: a report from the Children's Cancer Group. Clin Cancer Res 5:3956–3962.
47. Stewart CF, Gajjar AJ, Heideman RL, Houghton PJ. 1998 Penetration of topotecan into cerebrospinal fluid after intravenous injection. Onkologie 21:22–24.

48. Stewart CF, Baker SD, Heideman RL, Jones D, Crom WR, Pratt CB. 1994 Clinical pharmacodynamics of continuous infusion topotecan in children: systemic exposure predicts hematologic toxicity. J Clin Oncol 12:1946–1954.
49. Zamboni WC, Stewart CF, Thompson J, et al. 1998 Relationship between topotecan systemic exposure and tumor response in human neuroblastoma xenografts. J Natl Cancer Inst 90:505–511.
50. Tubergen DG, Stewart CF, Pratt CB, et al. 1996 Phase I trial and pharmacokinetic (PK) and pharmacodynamics (PD) study of topotecan using a five-day course in children with refractory solid tumors: A Pediatric Oncology Group Study. J Ped Hematol Oncol 18:352–361.
51. Athale UH, Stewart C, Kuttesch JF, et al. 2002 Phase I study of combination topotecan and carboplatin in pediatric solid tumors. J Clin Oncol 20:88–95.
52. Kushner BH, Cheung NK, Kramer K, Dunkel IJ, Calleja E, Boulad F. 2001 Topotecan combined with myeloablative doses of thiotepa and carboplatin for neuroblastoma, brain tumors, and other poor-risk solid tumors in children and young adults. Bone Marrow Transplant 28:551–556.
53. Friedman HS, Kerby T, Fields S, et al. 1999 Topotecan treatment of adults with primary malignant glioma. The Brain Tumor Center at Duke. Cancer 85:1160–1165.
54. Zamboni WC, Gajjar AJ, Heideman RL, et al. 1998 Phenytoin alters the disposition of topotecan and *N*-desmethyl topotecan in a patient with medulloblastoma. Clin Cancer Res 4:783–789.
55. Macdonald D, Cairncross G, Stewart D, et al. 1996 Phase II study of topotecan in patients with recurrent malignant glioma. National Clinical Institute of Canada Clinical Trials Group. Ann Oncol 7:205–207.
56. Burch PA, Bernath AM, Cascino TL, et al. 2000 A North Central Cancer Treatment Group phase II trial of topotecan in relapsed gliomas. Invest New Drugs 18:275–280.
57. Nitschke R, Parkhurst J, Sullivan J, Harris MB, Bernstein M, Pratt C. 1998 Topotecan in pediatric patients with recurrent and progressive solid tumors: a Pediatric Oncology Group phase II study. J Pediatr Hematol Oncol 20:315–358.
58. Blaney SM, Needle MN, Gillespie A, et al. 1998 Phase II trial of topotecan administered as 72-hour continuous infusion in children with refractory solid tumors: a collaborative Pediatric Branch, National Cancer Institute, and Children's Cancer Group Study. Clin Cancer Res 4:357–360.
59. Blaney SM, Phillips PC, Packer RJ, et al. 1996 Phase II evaluation of topotecan for pediatric central nervous system tumors. Cancer 78:527–531.
60. Kadota RP, Stewart CF, Horn M, et al. 1999 Topotecan for the treatment of recurrent or progressive central nervous system tumors—a pediatric oncology group phase II study. J Neurooncol 43:43–47.
61. Stewart CF, Iacono LC, Chintagumpala M, Kellie SJ, Ashley D, Zamboni WE, et al. 2004 Results of a Phase II upfront window of pharmacokinetically guided topotecan in high-risk medulloblastoma and supratentorial primitive neuroectodermal tumor (PNET). J Clin Oncol 22:3357–3365.
62. Fisher BJ, Scott C, Macdonald DR, Coughlin C, Curran WJ. 2001 Phase I study of topotecan plus cranial radiation for glioblastoma multiforme: results of Radiation Therapy Oncology Group Trial 9507. J Clin Oncol 19:1111–1117.
63. Gross MW, Altscher R, Brandtner M, et al. 2001 Acute toxicity and changes in quality of life during a combined radio-chemotherapy of glioblastomas with topotecan (Hycamtin). Strahlenther Onkol 177:656–661.

64. Sanghavi SN, Needle MN, Krailo MD, Geyer JR, Ater J, Mehta MP. 2003 A phase I study of topotecan as a radiosensitizer for brainstem glioma of childhood: first report of the Children's Cancer Group-0952. Neurooncol 5:8–13.
64a. Wagner S, Erdlenbruch B, Langler A, et al. 2004 Oral topotecan in children with recurrent or progressive high-grade glioma: a Phase I/II study by the German Society for Pediatric Oncology and Hematology. Cancer 100:1750–1757.
65. Friedman HS, Petros WP, Friedman AH, et al. 1999 Irinotecan therapy in adults with recurrent or progressive malignant glioma. J Clin Oncol 17:1516–1525.
66. Cloughesy TF, Filka E, Nelson G, et al. 2002 Irinotecan treatment for recurrent malignant glioma using an every-3-week regimen. Am J Clin Oncol 25:204–208.
67. Crews K, Stewart CF, Jones-Wallace D, et al. 2002 Altered irinotecan pharmacokinetics in pediatric high-grade glioma patients receiving enzyme-inducing anticonvulsant therapy. Clin Cancer Res 8:2202–2209.
68. Blaney S, Berg SL, Pratt C, et al. 2001 A phase I study of irinotecan in pediatric patients: a pediatric oncology group study. Clin Cancer Res 7:32–37.
69. Turner CD, Gururangan S, Eastwood J, et al. 2002 Phase II study of irinotecan (CPT-11) in children with high-risk malignant brain tumors: the Duke experience. Neurooncol 4:102–108.
70. Raymond E, Fabbro M, Boige V, et al. 2003 Multicentre phase II study and pharmacokinetic analysis of irinotecan in chemotherapy-naive patients with glioblastoma. Ann Oncol 14:603–614.
71. Hochberg F, Grossman SA, Mikkelsen T, Glantz M, Fisher JD, Piantadosi S. 2000 Lack of efficacy of 9-aminocamptothecin in adults with newly diagnosed glioblastoma multiforme and recurrent high-grade astrocytoma. NABTT CNS Consortium. Neurooncol 2:29–33.

16 Camptothecins in the Treatment of Lung Cancer

Pankaj Kumar, MD,
Missak Haigentz, Jr., MD,
Jorge Gomez, MD,
and Roman Perez-Soler, MD

Contents

1. INTRODUCTION

Since 1987 lung cancer has been the leading cause of cancer death in both men and women. In 2003 an estimated 171,900 new cases of lung cancer were diagnosed in the United States, and an estimated 157,200 deaths occurred from the disease. The incidence rate of lung cancer is declining in men, from a high of 102.1 per 100,000 in 1984 to 81.1 per 100,000 in 1999. In the late 1990s the incidence of lung cancer seen in women, which had been steadily rising, leveled off to the current incidence rate of 52.4 per 100,000. Overall, the 1-year survival rates for lung cancer have increased from 34% in 1975 to 42% in 1998, mainly because of improvements in surgical techniques. However, the 5-year relative survival rate for all stages is only 15% *(1)*.

Camptothecins in Cancer Therapy
Edited by: V. R. Adams and T. G. Burke © Humana Press Inc., Totowa, NJ

Approximately 80% of lung cancer patients have non-small-cell lung cancer (NSCLC); small-cell lung cancer (SCLC) accounts for the remaining 20%. Most of the patients with NSCLC have advanced disease at onset, with 35% presenting with TNM stage III and 40% with stage IV disease. Unfortunately, less than 20% of these patients are candidates for curative surgery. Patients with unresectable disease have an extremely poor survival, with an average 5-year survival rate of less than 5%.

For SCLC a much simpler staging system is used, consisting of limited-stage disease (LD-SCLC) and extensive stage disease (ED-SCLC). Limited stage is defined as disease confined to one hemithorax that can be included in a single radiation field; patients with disease extending beyond one radiation portal are considered to have ED (approximately 60–70% of all SCLC cases). Patients with ED-SCLC are treated with systemic chemotherapy; those with LD-SCLC are treated with a combination of chemotherapy and radiation therapy. The median survival with the current chemotherapeutic regimens in extensive disease is only 7 to 12 months despite an overall response rate (ORR) of 60–80%. The dismal statistics are highlighted by the fact that more than 90% of patients with ED-SCLC will not survive beyond 2 years. The outcome is somewhat better in LD-SCLC, with a response rate of approximately 80–90% and a median survival of 12 to 16 months *(2)*. However, over the past 20 years, no major advances have been made in the treatment of SCLC *(3)*. Given such poor statistics, there is a pressing need to develop better systemic treatments for lung cancer.

Camptothecins, a new class of chemotherapeutic agents that act by inhibiting the topoisomerase I (Topo-I) enzyme, have shown activity in many cancers, including NSCLC and SCLC. In particular, two drugs from this class of agents, topotecan (Hycamtin, GlaxoSmithKline) and irinotecan (CPT-11; Camptosar, Pfizer) have been studied extensively and have shown promising results. Topotecan and irinotecan are the two camptothecins being used in the treatment of lung cancer in clinical practice, though several more agents are being evaluated in clinical and preclinical studies. Because of the current clinical utility of topotecan and irinotecan, in this chapter, we will address the use of these two agents in the treatment of lung cancer.

2. TOPOTECAN IN SMALL-CELL LUNG CANCER

Topotecan is approved by Food and Drug Administration (FDA) for use in patients with SCLC-sensitive disease after failure of first-line chemotherapy. Sensitive disease was defined as disease responding to chemotherapy but thereafter progressing at least 60 days (in the phase III study) or at least 90 days (in the phase II studies) after chemotherapy. The recommended dose of topotecan is 1.5 mg/m^2 by intravenous (iv) infusion over 30 minutes daily for 5 consecutive days, starting on day 1 of a 21-day course

(4). In the absence of tumor progression, a minimum of four cycles are recommended. It is also being studied as a first-line agent in SCLC. Several studies have been conducted in patients with SCLC using topotecan as a second-line therapy, both as a single agent and in combination with other drugs.

2.1. Topotecan as a Single Agent in the Second-Line Treatment of SCLC

Several studies have been performed to look at the efficacy of topotecan as a single agent in SCLC (Table 1). We have reviewed a few of these studies. The dose of topotecan in the majority of studies is 1.5 mg/m^2/day for 5 days every 3 weeks.

A study published by Perez-Soler et al. tested the efficacy of topotecan as a single agent in patients refractory to etoposide (defined as a lack of response or relapse within 3 months of last dose of etoposide and cisplatin). Topotecan was given at 1.25 mg/m^2/day during 30-minute infusions for 5 days every 21 days. Of 28 patients enrolled, partial responses (PRs) were observed in 11% (durable for 7, 8, and 19 weeks), minor response (MR) in 7%, stable disease (SD) in 17%, and progressive disease (PD) in 65%. The overall survival duration was 20 weeks. Grade 3/4 granulocytopenia and thrombocytopenia occurred in 70% and 31% of cycles, respectively. The study demonstrated that topotecan has modest activity against refractory SCLC, with myelosuppression being a common limiting toxicity. Notably, topotecan produced a response in these patients despite a prior exposure to etoposide; hence, the authors concluded that resistance to etoposide (a Topo-II inhibitor) does not confer resistance to topotecan *(5)*.

In a similar work, Depierre et al. studied patients with relapsed SCLC. This trial included refractory (progressed in <3 months of stopping treatment, $n = 48$) and sensitive (progressed >3 months after treatment, $n = 71$). Topotecan was given at 1.5 mg/m^2/day for 5 days over 30 minutes every 3 weeks. Ninety-eight patients were able to be evaluated. A response was seen in eight (8.1%) sensitive patients and one (1%) refractory patient. The median overall survival was 21.6 weeks (sensitive 25.7 weeks; refractory 16.3 weeks). Grade 3/4 neutropenia was seen in 88.7 and 69.6%, respectively. Nine patients in this study had central nervous system disease and there were four PR, three SD, and one CR (with radiation therapy) in this subgroup. Thus this study also reiterated that topotecan has modest activity in the relapsed patients with SCLC *(6)*.

Ardizzoni et al. performed a trial in patients with relapsed SCLC, including both refractory (relapsed in less than 3 months of chemotherapy) and sensitive patients (relapsed after 3 months of chemotherapy). Topotecan was given at the same dose as in the previous study, 1.5 mg/m^2/day for 5 days over 30 minutes every 3 weeks. Of the 92 patients enrolled, 47 were in the

Table 1
Single Agent Topotecan in SCLC as 2nd Line Agent

Author (Reference)	*Phase*	*Number*	*Prior Rx*	*Regimen*	*Response (%)*	*Median survival*
Perez Soler *(5)*	II	28	Yes	1.25 mg/m^2/day × 5 days q 3 weeks	PR 11, SD 17, MR 7	20 weeks
Depierre *(6)*	II	98	Yes	1.5 mg/m^2/day × 5 days q 3 weeks	OR 8.8	21.6 weeks
Ardizzoni *(7)*	II	92	Yes	1.5 mg/m^2/day × 5 days q 3 weeks	Sensitive 37.8 Refractory 6.4	21.6 weeks
von Powel *(8)*	III	106	Yes	Oral 2.3 mg/m^2/day × 5 days vs	OR 23	32 weeks
				Intravenous 1.5 mg/m^2/day × 5 days both q 21 days	OR 15	25 weeks

Rx, treatment; PR, partial response; SD, stable disease; OR, overall response; MR, minor response.

refractory arm and 45 in the sensitive arm. There were two PRs and one complete response (CR) reported in the refractory group, with an ORR of 6.4%. In this group, the median survival was 4.7 months versus 6.9 months in the sensitive group ($p = 0.002$). In the sensitive group there were 7 CRs and 13 PRs, with the regimen showing an ORR of 21.7%. The median survival of the responding patients was 12.5 months. The authors reported a high incidence of hematological toxicities, with grade 3/4 leukopenia seen in 28% and 46.8% of cycles, respectively, whereas nonhematological toxicities were mild *(7)*.

Topotecan is also investigationally available in an oral form, making it an attractive drug because of the ease of administration. von Powel et al. have recently studied this formulation in a phase II trial. They compared oral topotecan and iv topotecan in chemosensitive SCLC (relapsed at least 90 days after chemotherapy). Fifty-two patients were given oral topotecan 2.3 mg/m^2/day for 5 days every 21 days, and 54 were given iv topotecan at 1.5 mg/m^2/day for 5 days every 21 days. Data analysis demonstrated that oral topotecan had similar efficacy compared with the iv form. There were 1 CR and 11 PRs in the oral arm, with an ORR of 23.1%. In the iv arm, there were two CRs and six PRs, with the ORR being 14.8%. After accounting for all of the prognostic factors in a logistic regression model, the oral topotecan group was 1.6 times more likely to respond than the iv group (95% confidence interval [CI] for the odds ratio 0.50–5.15). The median duration of response was also higher in the oral group: 18 weeks versus 14 weeks in the iv group. The time to progression was 15 weeks in the oral and 13 weeks in the iv group, with the risk ratio being oral:iv of 0.98 (95% CI 0.63–1.54). Median survival was also higher in the oral group: 32 weeks in the oral arm and 25 weeks in the iv arm. After accounting for the prognostic factors the risk ratio oral:IV of survival was 0.90 (95% CI: 0.55–1.47). Both formulations of topotecan were well tolerated. The main reported toxicity was neutropenia though it was less common in the oral arm. Grade 4 neutropenia occurred in 35.3% patients in the oral group and 67.3% in the iv arm ($p = 0.001$). The incidence of fever and infections (grade ≥ 2) associated with grade 4 neutropenia was 5.1% in the oral arm and 3.3% in the iv topotecan arm. The incidence of severe thrombocytopenia and grade 3/4 anemia was similar in both groups. The main nonhematological toxicities seen were vomiting and nausea. Vomiting was observed in 36.5% of patients in the oral group and 31.5% in the iv group; the incidence of nausea was 26.9% and 40.7% in the oral and iv arms, respectively *(8)*. The results of this phase II study demonstrate that in this cohort of patients oral topotecan is as efficacious as the iv form. Gralla et al. recently presented the results of an international phase III study of oral versus iv topotecan administration in chemosensitive patients with SCLC *(9)*. The median survival of both groups was approximately 9 months, and quality of life outcomes were also similar.

Because the oral form is better tolerated than the iv formulation and does not require venipuncture, its usage is attractive in practice.

Another single-agent topotecan schedule with growing appeal is weekly scheduling. Greco et al. recently presented preliminary results of a Phase II trial of weekly topotecan in the second-line treatment of SCLC *(10)*. Of 17 patients enrolled to date, 9 of 11 patients with sensitive relapse had a PR, and 1 of 6 patients with resistant relapse also responded. The regimen was quite tolerable, with fatigue as the major nonhematologic toxicity.

2.1.1. Phase III Comparative Study of Topotecan With Cyclophosphamide, Doxorubicin, and Vincristine

The effects of topotecan in the relapsed patients were best illustrated in a phase III study conducted by von Powel et al. that compared topotecan to the then-standard cyclophosphamide, doxorubicin, and vincristine (CAV) in recurrent SCLC (Table 2). They treated 211 patients with SCLC who had relapsed 60 days after treatment with a first-line agent. Patients received 1.5 mg/m^2 of topotecan as a 30-minute infusion daily for 5 days every 21 days ($n = 107$) or CAV, which consisted of cyclophosphamide at 1000 mg/m^2, doxorubicin at 45 mg/m^2, and vincristine at the dose of 2 mg, all given on day 1 every 21 days ($n = 104$). In the topotecan group, 24.3% patients had a PR (none achieved a CR), and in the CAV group, 18.3% had an objective response (CR 1%, PR 17.3%; $p = 0.285$). The median survival in the topotecan group was 25 weeks and 24.7 weeks in the CAV group ($p = 0.795$). The median time to progression in the topotecan group was 13.3 weeks and 12.3 weeks in the CAV group. However, more patients in the topotecan group had an improvement of symptoms, in particular of dyspnea, fatigue, anorexia, hoarseness, and interference with daily activity. Grade 4 neutropenia was more common in the CAV group (51.4%) as compared with the topotecan group (37.8%); grade 4 thrombocytopenia and grade 3–4 anemia were more common in the topotecan arm *(11)*. The study concluded that topotecan is at least as effective as CAV in recurrent SCLC, thus establishing a definite role of topotecan in this group of patients.

2.2. Topotecan in Combination With Other Agents in Second-Line Treatment of SCLC

Most of the currently adopted regimens for the treatment of SCLC exploit the synergistic effects of a combination of drugs (Table 3). Using the same model, topotecan is being studied in combination with other drugs for SCLC.

Agelaki et al. reported phase I data of escalating doses of topotecan with epirubicin. The rationale behind this combination is to exploit the synergism between Topo-I and Topo-II inhibitors. Epirubicin is a semisynthetic derivative of doxorubicin with single-agent activity in SCLC that acts by stabilizing Topo-II–DNA complexes. Epirubicin has less hematologic,

Table 2
Topotecan Versus CAV—A Phase III Trial in SCLC as 2nd Line Agent.

Author (Reference)	*Phase*	*Number*	*Prior Rx*	*Regimen*	*Response (%)*	*Median survival*
von Powel *(11)*	III	211	Yes	Topotecan (n = 107) 1.5 mg/m^2/day × 5 days q 3 weeks	OR 24.3	25 weeks
				CAV regimen (n = 104) C-1000 mg/m^2 on day 1 A- 45 mg/m^2 on day 1 V- 2 mg on day 1 all q 3 weeks	OR 18.3	24.7 weeks

C, cyclophosphamide; A, doxorubicin; V, vincristine; OR, overalll response; Rx, treatment.

Table 3
Topotecan in Combination With Other Agents for 2nd Line Treatment of SCLC

Author (Reference)	Phase	Number	Prior Rx	Regimen (MTD)	Response (%)
Agelaki *(12)*	I	27	Yes	Topotecan 0.90 mg/m^2/day × 5 days Epirubicin 40 mg/m^2 on day 8, q 28 days	5
Frasci *(13)*	I	25	Yes ($n = 16$) No ($n = 9$)	Topotecan 2.25 mg/m^2, all q week Paclitaxel 85 mg/m^2 Cisplatin 40 mg/m^2 (+ GCSF days 3–5)	44
Thompson *(14)*	I	15	Yes	Topotecan 0.75 mg/m^2/day × days 1–3, q 21 days Paclitaxel 135 mg/m^2 day 1 Carboplatin AUC-5 day 1	53

MTD, maximum tolreable dose; Rx, treatment.

nonhema-tologic, and cardiac toxicity than doxorubicin. This study enrolled 27 patients with SCLC who had previously been treated with etoposide and cisplatin. Patient cohorts were given escalating doses of topotecan starting from 0.5 mg/m^2/day as a 30-minute infusion for 5 days, along with escalating doses of epirubicin starting from 40 mg/m^2 as a 10-minute infusion on day 8 given every 28 days. Seventy-three courses were given, and the reported MTD were 0.90 mg/m^2/day for topotecan and 40 mg/m^2 for epirubicin. Neutropenia was the DLT; grade 3/4 neutropenia was seen in 30% courses and grade 3–4 anemia in 10% courses. Seven courses were associated with fever, and there was one neutropenic septic death. There was some suggestion of response in this regimen—of the 20 patients able to be evaluated, 1 had complete response, 4 had disease stabilization, and 15 progressed. The median time to progression was 24 weeks; the median overall survival was 22 months *(12)*.

Frasci et al. reported results of a phase I trial encompassing a combination of topotecan, cisplatin, and paclitaxel with G-CSF (granulocyte-colony stimulating factor) in SCLC ($n = 25$) and ovarian cancer ($n = 19$). Of the 25 patients with SCLC, 9 were chemotherapy-naive and 16 had previously been treated. Topotecan was given along with cisplatin and paclitaxel in a weekly regimen along with G-CSF given from days 3 through 5 of each week. The MTDs were topotecan at 2.25 mg/m^2/week, cisplatin at 40 mg/m^2/week, and paclitaxel at 85 mg/m^2/week (as a 1-hour infusion). Grade 3–4 neutropenia, thrombocytopenia, and anemia were reported in 36 cycles, 15 cycles, and 5 cycles, respectively. Severe vomiting and diarrhea was seen in seven and four patients, respectively. Peripheral neuropathy was observed in 11 patients (42 cycles). An objective response was observed in 11 of 19 (58%) ovarian cancer and 11 of 25 (44%) SCLC patients; 3 patients in the SCLC group had a complete response. Of the 9 chemotherapy-naive patients with SCLC, 7 (78%) responded. This triplet combination appears tolerable and has activity in pretreated as well as chemotherapy-naive SCLC patients *(13)*.

Thompson et al. examined a combination of topotecan, paclitaxel, and carboplatin in a phase I study with or without growth factor support. The recommended doses for the phase II trial were topotecan at 0.75 mg/m^2 days 1–3, paclitaxel at 135 mg/m^2 on day 1, and carboplatin at AUC 5 (area under the curve) on day 1, all given every 21 days. They had 15 patients with SCLC; 8 of these 15 patients (53%) responded, including 1 CR. All of these patients had previously been treated with carboplatin and etoposide, and 2 had also been given paclitaxel. DLT was myelosuppression including grade 3/4 thrombocytopenia; however, only 2 of 100 courses were complicated by febrile neutropenia. A phase II trial is under way to evaluate the activity of this regimen *(14)*.

2.3. *Topotecan in SCLC as a First-Line Agent*

Many trials have been conducted studying topotecan as a single agent and in combination with other agents in the first-line setting.

2.4. *Single-Agent Topotecan in First-Line Treatment of SCLC*

Schiller et al. published a phase II Eastern Cooperative Oncology Group study of 48 previously untreated ED-SCLC patients treated with topotecan at 2.0 mg/m^2/day for 5 days (Table 4). The first 13 patients were treated without G-CSF, and the remaining 35 patients received G-CSF 5 mcg/m/kg for 10–14 days starting on day 6. Cycles were repeated every 3 weeks for a maximum of four cycles. Patients who had a PR after four cycles, SD after two cycles, or PD at any time received salvage chemotherapy with cisplatin and etoposide. Of the 48 patients, none had a CR and 19 had a PR, for an overall objective response rate of 39%. The median response duration was 4.8 months, the median survival was 10.0 months, and the 1-year survival was 39%. Eight of 34 patients (24%) who received salvage chemotherapy responded. Four of the 17 patients who did not respond to topotecan responded to salvage chemotherapy. Hematological toxicities were common: 92% of patients without G-CSF developed grade 3/4 neutropenia as compared with 29% in the G-CSF group *(15)*.

2.5. *Topotecan in Combination With Paclitaxel as First-Line Agent in SCLC*

Traditionally SCLC has been treated with drug combinations, and paclitaxel is emerging as one of the active agents in this disease (Table 5). Topotecan has been evaluated in combination with paclitaxel in many studies, and the data are summarized in the accompanying table. Of the five studies tabulated, four have demonstrated advantageous results.

2.5.1. Phase II Data

Jett et al. presented the preliminary report of a phase II trial of a combination of topotecan and paclitaxel with G-CSF in 1997. In this study, 12 patients able to be evaluated, previously untreated patients with ED-SCLC were treated with topotecan at a dose of 1 mg/m^2 over 30 minutes for 5 days along with paclitaxel 135 mg/m^2 iv over 24 hours on day 5, followed by G-CSF administration. In this study, the first three patients were given a higher dose of topotecan (1.25 mg/m^2/day); however, two patients developed life-threatening toxicity (grade 4), and one had a fatal infection at this dose. Accordingly, the dose of topotecan was decreased to 1 mg/m^2 for the rest of the group. They reported a CR in 2 (17%), PR in 9 (75%), and 1-yr survival of 50% (95% CI 20–74%) and 2-year survival of 25% (95% CI 4–55%). This early small trial showed that combination of topotecan and paclitaxel was

Table 4
Single Agent Topotecan in SCLC as First Line Therapy

Author (Reference)	*Phase*	*Number*	*Prior Rx*	*Regimen*	*Response (%)*	*Median survival*
Schiller *(15)*	II	48	None	Topotecan 2 mg/m^2/day × 5 days ± G-CSF q 3 weeks × 4 cycles maximum	PR 39	10 months

Rx, treatment; G-CSF, granulocyte colony-stimulating factor; PR, partial response.

Table 5
Topotecan in Combination With Paclitaxel as First Line Agent in ED-SCLC

Author (Reference)	*Phase*	*Number*	*Prior Rx*	*Regimen*	*Response (%)*	*Median survival*
Tweedy *(17)*	II	15	None	Topotecan 1 mg/m^2/day over 30 min days 1–5 Paclitaxel 135 mg/m^2 over 3 hours on day 5 G-CSF, q 28 days	CR 66 PR 33	
Jacobs *(18)*	II	29	None	Topotecan 1.25 mg/m^2/day over 30 min days 1–5 Paclitaxel 135 mg/m^2 over 24 hours on day 5 G-CSF, q 28 days	CR 21 PR 39	54 weeks
Lynch *(19)*	II	34	None	Topotecan 1 mg/m^2/day, days 1–5 Paclitaxel 175 mg/m^2 over 3 hours on day 1 G-CSF	CR 2 PR 61	9.44 months
Jett *(20)*	II	46	None	Alternating regimens q 21 day Etoposide 100 mg/m^2 + cisplatin 30mg/m^2 on days 1–3 of cycle 1, 3, 5, alternating with topotecan 1mg/m^2 day 1–5 + paclitaxel 200mg/m^2 day 5 with G-CSF starting day 6 of cycle 2, 4, 6	CR 8 PR 67	10.5 months
Schiller *(21)*	III	405	None	**Step 1** ($n = 405$) Cisplatin 60 mg/m^2 day 1 PR 30 Etoposide 120 mg/m^2 days 1–3, q 3 weeks Patients with stable or progressive disease randomized to either topotecan or observation	CR 2	9.5 months
				Step 2 Topotecan 1.5 mg/m^2/day × 5 days, q 3 week ($n = 115$) versus observation ($n = 115$)	CR 2 PR 5	8.7 months 9 months

ED-SCLC, extensive stage disease small-cell lung cancer; Rx, treatment; G-CSF, granulocyte colony-stimulating factor; CR, complete response; PR, partial response.

active against chemotherapy-naive SCLC patients exhibiting a response rate similar to other regimens used in SCLC *(16)*.

Tweedy et al. confirmed the results of Jett et al *(16)*; here, however, paclitaxel was administered over 3 hours as opposed to 24 hours. Of 15 chemotherapy-naive patients with ED-SCLC treated, high response rates were observed, with a CR in 10 (66%) and PR in 5 (33%). Although prophylactic cranial irradiation was not permitted, only 1 of 15 patients had developed brain metastasis at the time of reporting *(17)*.

Jacobs et al. presented their data in 1999 from a study that included 29 patients with no prior treatment for ED-SCLC. The starting doses were topotecan at 1.25 mg/m^2/day over 30 minutes for 5 days and paclitaxel at 135 mg/m^2 over 24 hours on day 5 followed by G-CSF. Cycles were repeated every 28 days. As reported by Jett et al. *(16)*, the dose of topotecan in this study required dose reduction to 1.0 mg/m^2/d after grade 4 myelosuppression was seen in the first three patients with one septic death. Seventeen patients (60%) in this study had a response, including 6 (21%) CR and PR in 11 (39%). The median survival was 54 weeks (95% CI, 39–72 weeks) with the 1- and 2-year survival probabilities of 50% and 15%, respectively *(18)*.

In 2000, Lynch et al. reported preliminary results of Cancer and Leukemia Group B 9430 trial. This trial began as a three-arm randomized phase II trial of novel doublets in untreated ED-SCLC to compare newer regimens to the standard combination of etoposide and cisplatin. One arm of the trial that used topotecan at 1.0 mg/m^2/day $\times$ 5 days and paclitaxel at the dose of 225 mg/m^2 on day 1 with G-CSF was closed early because of very high toxicity (3 toxic deaths among the first 13 patients). In its place, a fourth arm was opened with topotecan at 1.0 mg/m^2/day for 5 days and paclitaxel at 175 mg/m^2 over 3 hours on the first day of the cycle, along with G-CSF. Of the 34 ED-SCLC patients able to be evaluated, 1 (2%) had complete response and 22 (61%) had partial response, with the overall response of 68% (95% CI, 49–83%). The median overall survival was 9.44 months. Failure-free survival was 5.08 months and 1-year survival was estimated at 26.5%. These results were very comparable to the standard cisplatin and etoposide combination. As reported in previous studies, neutropenia was the most frequent toxicity: 24% had grade 3 and 29% had grade 4 neutropenia. This study did not demonstrate any advantages of topotecan and paclitaxel combination as compared with standard therapy with etoposide and cisplatin *(19)*.

Jett et al. recently published the results of a phase II trial of untreated patients with ED-SCLC. In this trial, a rather complicated schedule of etoposide and cisplatin (EC) alternating with topotecan and paclitaxel (TP) was used. Etoposide (100 mg/m^2 iv) and cisplatin (30 mg/m^2 iv) were administered on days 1, 2, and 3 of cycle 1, 3, and 5 topotecan (1.0 mg/m^2/day for

5 days) and paclitaxel (200 mg/m^2 iv day 5) with G-CSF starting on day 6 of cycles 2, 4, and 6. EC or TP was given every 21 days. The physicians were allowed to give radiation to the brain or chest at their discretion. Sixty-five patients received all six cycles and 78% received four cycles. Of 46 patients able to be evaluated, 4 (8%) patients had CR and 31 (67%) had PR. Median time to progression was 7 months (95% CI, 5.5–7.8) and the median survival was 10.5 months (95% CI, 7.8–11.7). The most frequently observed toxicity was myelosuppression: EC caused more grade 3–4 neutropenia than did TP (82% versus 64%), but less thrombocytopenia (13% versus 36%). This alternating schedule of EC and TP appears to have good activity against SCLC, with reasonable side effects *(20)*.

2.5.2. Phase III Data

The Eastern Cooperative Oncology Group conducted a phase III trial of 405 untreated ED-SCLC patients, the largest number of patients reviewed in any trial by us. This study consisted of two steps. In the first step, all patients were given four cycles of cisplatin at 60 mg/m^2 iv on day 1 and etoposide 120 mg/m^2 iv on days 1, 2, and 3 every 3 weeks. In the second step, patients who had stable disease or responding disease were then randomized to either observation or four cycles of topotecan 1.5 mg/m^2/day for 5 days every 3 weeks. The response rates of step one (induction etoposide and cisplatin) were CR 3% and PR 30%. With topotecan there were additional CR of 2% and PR of 5%. The median overall survival was 9.5 months. Progression-free survival in the topotecan group was 3.4 months compared with 2.3 months in the observation group ($p = 0.0001$). However, overall survival in the two arms was not significantly different: the observation group had a median survival of 8.7 versus 9.0 months in the topotecan arm ($p = 0.71$). Grade 4 neutropenia occurred in 50% of the step 1 group and 58% in the topotecan group in step 2. This study demonstrated that four cycles of cisplatin and etoposide followed by topotecan does not improve survival in ED-SCLC, but it does modestly improve the progression-free survival. The investigators concluded that four cycles of standard cisplatin and etoposide is an appropriate first-line treatment in good performance status (PS 0 to 2) ED-SCLC patients. This study showed that giving topotecan after a standard course of chemotherapy, in the hope that it would consolidate the gains of the prior treatment, has no impact on the overall survival. However, it could be argued that the model used in this study was not a suitable setting for maximizing the effects of topotecan *(21)*.

2.6. Topotecan in Combination With Other Agents as First-Line Regimens for the Treatment of SCLC

Work in this field is still in the early stages; several trials have been conducted to study the interaction between topotecan and other chemotherapeutic agents in SCLC (Table 6). Most of these studies are small and have been primarily for dose and schedule finding of drugs.

Murren et al. evaluated the combination of topotecan and cyclophosphamide with G-CSF in a phase II study in previously untreated ED-SCLC and SCLC patients in sensitive relapse (>3 months of progression-free survival). Prior treatment with cyclophosphamide or camptothecins was not permitted. Seventeen patients were able to be evaluated; the doses used were topotecan at 1 mg/m^2/day for 5 days and cyclophosphamide at 600 mg/m^2. The investigators reported an ORR of 29% with CR in two (11%) and PR in three (17%); stable disease was seen in four (23%) patients. Dose reduction was needed in three patients and one patient died from neutropenic sepsis. Myelosuppression was the most frequently observed toxicity *(22)*. This regimen appears to be active in SCLC though the data are quite early.

Smith et al. conducted a phase I trial to determine the MTD of topotecan in combination with a different alkylating agent, ifosfamide, in SCLC. This study was carried out in two steps: in the first step, all patients received topotecan and ifosfamide; thereafter chemotherapy-naive patients who had achieved an objective response after three cycles were treated with carboplatin at AUC of 6 and etoposide at 100 mg/m^2/day for 3 days. They enrolled 9 chemotherapy-naive patients and 4 patients who had previously received one prior chemotherapeutic regimen. Patients were initially given a fixed dose of ifosfamide at 2.5 mg/m^2 over 30 minutes on day 1 followed immediately by topotecan at different dose levels (0.68, 0.85, 1.05, and 1.3 mg/m^2/day for 3 days). The MTD of topotecan was determined to be 1.3 mg/m^2/day. Intravenous hydration and MESNA were given on day 1, and each cycle was repeated every 3 weeks. They reported one (7%) CR and four (28%) PR. Neutropenia was a common side effect in this study *(23)*. This Phase I study shows that topotecan can be combined with ifosfamide and the MTD of topotecan has been obtained. However, whether this model has significant clinical efficacy remains to be determined.

Preclinical studies show that combinations of Topo-I and Topo-II inhibitors might have an additive effect in tumor cells *(24)*. Cells that have acquired resistance to a certain class of drugs often develop hypersensitivity to another class of drugs; this phenomenon can be exploited by combining drugs from different classes *(25)*. With regard to camptothecins, it has been suggested that cells that have developed resistance to topotecan by downregulating Topo-I enzyme compensate for it by upregulating Topo-II, which could be an easy target for inhibitors of the Topo-II *(26)*. This rationale has been exploited in the studies reviewed in this section.

Etoposide, a Topo-II inhibitor, is commonly used in combination regimens in the treatment of SCLC. O'Neill et al. published results of a Phase I study of a 5-day schedule of iv topotecan and etoposide. They administered a 5-day course of topotecan as 30-minute infusions at dose levels of 0.5 and

Table 6

Topotecan in Combination With Other Agents in SCLC as First-Line Treatment

Author (Reference)	*Phase*	*Number*	*Prior Rx*	*Regimen*	*Response*
Murren *(22)*	II	17	Untreated and in sensitive relapse G-CSF, q 3 weeks	Topotecan 1 $mg/m^2/day \times 5$ days Cyclophosphamide 600 mg/m^2 on day 1	CR 11 PR 17
Smith *(23)*	I/II	14	Untreated ($n = 9$) Treated ($n = 4$)	Ifosfamide 2.5 gm/m^2 on day 1 and topotecan days 1–3 q 3 weeks	CR 7 PR 28
O'Neil *(27)*	I	12 LD-SCLC ($n = 3$) ED-SCLC ($n = 9$)	None	Topotecan MTD 1.3 $mg/m^2/day$ Topotecan at either 0.5 and 0.75 $mg/m^2/$ day with etoposide 60 $mg/m^2/day$, days 1–5, q 3 weeks Maximum six cycles	
Sorenson *(29)*	I	21 LD-SCLC ($n = 15$) ED-SCLC ($n = 6$)	None	Alternating cycle A and B Cycle A: Topotecan days 1–5 + cisplatin 50 mg/m^2 on day 5 Cycle B: Teniposide, carboplatin, vincristine Cisplatin MTD of topotecan: 1.5 $mg/m^2/day$	CR 33 PR 52
Dediu *(30)*	I/II	8 ED-SCLC	None	Topotecan 0.60 $mg/m^2/day$, days –4 Fractionated cisplatin 20 $mg/m^2/d$ on days 1–4 q 21 days	PR 88

Sensitive relapse, relapsing after 3 months of treatment; Rx, treatment; G-CSF, granulocyte colony-stimulating factor; CR, complete response; PR, partial response; MTD, maximum tolerable dose; LD, limited stage disease; ED, extensive stage disease.

0.75 mg/m^2/day followed by 1-hour infusions of fixed dose of etoposide at 60 mg/m^2/day. Of 19 patients enrolled with previously untreated SCLC, 18 (95%) patients responded (14 PRs and 4 CRs), and the median survival was 10 months. Neutropenia was commonly seen, although no toxic deaths were reported *(27)*.

The concept of combined Topo-I and Topo-II inhibition has been further explored in a trial of topotecan with etoposide in SCLC patients *(28)*. Using this approach, Reck et al. recently reported that of 28 patients able to be evaluated, a 50% response rate was observed (13 PRs and 1 CR). Furthermore, the regimen did not have any grade 4 hematological or nonhematological toxicity. Given that etoposide is a commonly used agent in SCLC, this combination of agents might have promise and needs to be explored further.

Sorenson et al. studied topotecan with cisplatin, another commonly used drug in SCLC. They enrolled previously untreated patients in a phase I study. Fifteen patients had LD-SCLC and six had ED-SCLC. This study consisted of giving two cycles alternately, cycle A and B, for a total of six cycles. Cycle A consisted of topotecan given on days 1–5 with cisplatin at the dose of 50 mg/m^2 on day 5. Cycle B included teniposide, carboplatin, vincristine, and cisplatin. The dose of topotecan was increased to dose levels of 0.75, 1.0, 1.25, and 1.5 mg/m^2/day. The MTD of topotecan in this study was determined as 1.5 mg/m^2/day with cisplatin 50 mg/m^2 on day 5 *(29)*.

The combination of topotecan and fractionated cisplatin without G-CSF was further reported by Dediu et al. in a phase I/II study. They administered topotecan at 0.60 mg/m^2 and cisplatin at 20 mg/m^2 both on days 1–4; this cycle was repeated every 21 days. Until the time of presentation of the abstract, they had enrolled eight patients, with a PR in seven (88%) patients. After a median follow-up of 5 months, there had been two relapses in the central nervous system. However, there were no reported cases of grade 3–4 myelotoxicity. The investigators concluded that the absence of CR and the high relapses along with the low toxicity observed suggest that a higher dose of drugs might be needed for optimum efficacy *(30)*.

2.7. Topotecan in Triplet Combinations for the First-Line Treatment of SCLC

Topotecan has been studied in triple combinations with other drugs that have demonstrated activity against SCLC (Table 7). The drugs that have been used include paclitaxel, etoposide, and carboplatin. All of these drugs have been found to have activity in SCLC either individually or in various combinations.

Faucette et al. presented the data of a phase I trial that studied a combination of carboplatin, topotecan, and etoposide. Specifically, the investigators examined the effect of sequencing of carboplatin with regard to its

Table 7
Topotecan in Triplet Combinations as First-Line Agent in SCLC

Author (Reference)	*Phase*	*Number*	*Prior Rx*	*Regimen*	*Response (%)*	*Median survival*
Faucette *(31)*	I	12 ED-SCLC	None	**Cohort 1** Carboplatin AUC-5 on day 1, followed by topotecan AUC-15 ±5 on days –5 Etoposide 100 mg/m^2/day po days 6–8 q 3 weeks for six cycles **Cohort 2** Topotecan AUC-15 ± 5 on days 1–5, followed by carboplatin AUC-5 on day 5 Etoposide 100 mg/m^2/day po days 6–8 q 3 weeks for six cycles		
Gillenwater *(32)*	I	28 ED-SCLC	None	Topotecan dose AUC-15 to 60 on days 1,–3 Carboplatin AUC-5 on day 3 Etoposide 100 mg/m^2/day po days 4– 6	OR 81 (CR 8)	10.9 months
Frasci *(33)*	II	37 ED-SCLC	None	Paclitaxel 85 mg/m^2 as 1 hour infusion plus cisplatin 40 mg/m^2 plus topoatecan 2.25 mg/m^2 over 30 minutes iv q week + GCSF on days 3–5	CR 22 PR 59	12.5 months
Hainsworth *(34)*	II	87 ED-SCLC and LD-SCLC	None	Topotecan 0.75 mg/m^2 IV, days 1–3 Carboplatin AUC-5 day 1 Paclitaxel 135 mg/m^2 iv over 1 hour on day 1 q 21 days q 21 days ×4 courses Responders given etoposide 50 mg alternating with 100 mg po days 1–10 Patients with LD given chest radiotherapy in third cycle	OR 90 (in ED 88) (in LD 93)	ED 8.2 months

Rx, treatment; ED, extensive disease; AUC, area under the curve; PO, by mouth; OR, overall response; LD, limited disease; IV, intravenous.

myelosuppressive effect. They enrolled 12 untreated ED-SCLC patients and divided the group in two cohorts. The first cohort received carboplatin on day 1 immediately before topotecan; in the second cohort, carboplatin was given on day 5, just after the fifth dose of topotecan. The doses used were carboplatin AUC 5 mg/min/mL on day 1 or 5, topotecan AUC 15 ± 5 ng/hr/mL days 1 to 5, and etoposide 100 mg/m^2/day orally days 6, 7, and 8. In the first cohort, 64% had grade 3/4 neutropenia and 71% had thrombocytopenia. The incidence of these toxicities was much lower in the second cohort, with only 41% experiencing neutropenia and 20% having thrombocytopenia. Surprisingly, the mean topotecan AUC in cohort 1 was actually lower than in cohort 2 (11.7 ± 2.4 versus 18.6 ± 1.8 ng/hr/mL, $p < 0.0001$). Thus giving carboplatin on day 1 before topotecan appears to be associated with a higher incidence of myelosuppression. The authors concluded that this disparity between the systemic dose of topotecan and the incidence of myelosuppression compels one to think that there are other mechanisms apart from mere sequencing of these three agents to account for this difference *(31)*.

Gillenwater et al. evaluated the maximum tolerated systemic exposure of topotecan with etoposide 100 mg/m^2 orally for 3 days and carboplatin AUC 5 in 28 untreated ED-SCLC patients. The maximum tolerated systemic exposure of topotecan was being determined at the time of reporting of this data, with AUC varying from 15 to 80. As expected in this study, the toxicity profile varies widely. The group with topotecan at AUC of 45 on days 1–3 had grades 3/4 neutropenia in 83%, thrombocytopenia in 50%, and anemia in 33%. On the other hand the group with a lower dose of topotecan, AUC 15 on days 1–3, had grades 3/4 neutropenia in 30%, thrombocytopenia in 15%, and anemia in 15%. The authors have thus recommended that this schedule of topotecan on days 1, 2, and 3; carboplatin on day 3; and etoposide on days 4, 5, and 6 be explored further *(32)*.

Frasci et al. published a phase II study of a weekly regimen consisting of cisplatin, paclitaxel, and topotecan in 37 chemotherapy-naive ED-SCLC patients. All patients received paclitaxel at 85 mg/m^2 as a 1-hour infusion followed by cisplatin at 40 mg/m^2 and topotecan at 2.25 mg/m^2 as a 30-minute infusion every week. G-CSF was administered on days 3, 4, and 5 of each week for at least six cycles. The patients that had clinical CR or PR received six more cycles. Those who did not have any response were instead given a combination of cyclophosphamide, doxorubicin, and etoposide. Thirty-three patients completed at least six cycles and were assessed for response. The authors reported 8 (22%) CR and 22 (59%) PR. Six of the complete responses were achieved after six cycles. In the two remaining patients with CR, tumor was present in liver and lung after six cycles that disappeared by the twelfth cycle. In five of eight patients who had a CR, the liver was the main site of disease. Twenty-six of 30 responders received 12 cycles. Seven of 10 patients with brain metastasis had a major response after six cycles, though these never completely regressed. At a 13-month median follow-up (range 4–26 months), the actuarial estimation of median failure-free survival was 8 months and the overall survival was 12.5 months. The projected 1-year and 2-year survivals in this study were 55% and 21%, respectively. Interestingly, patients with an increased serum lactate dehydrogenase (LDH) at the time of diagnosis had a median survival of only 7.5 months as compared with 14 months in the others. The patients with brain metastasis had median survival of 10 months as compared with 13 months seen in others. They did not report any toxic deaths. Grade 3 and 4 neutropenia was seen in 27% and 16% of patients, respectively. Only 17% had grade 3 thrombocytopenia, and none had grade 4 thrombocytopenia. Anemia was the most common toxicity seen in this study, with a drop in hemoglobin below 11 gm/L in all patients, with 19% of patients requiring transfusion. The response data in this study, as in many other studies, are modest, although this study does demonstrate a better survival outcome as compared with previous studies that have shown a survival of about 12 months in similar patients. From this study, it does appear that topotecan, paclitaxel, and cisplatin with G-CSF support can be given to ED-SCLC patients on a weekly basis with good safety data and that it results in good response and survival times *(33)*.

Hainsworth et al. published a phase II study of a combination of paclitaxel, carboplatin, and topotecan. One hundred and five previously untreated patients with LD-SCLC or ED-SCLC were enrolled in this trial. Patients were given paclitaxel at 135 mg/m^2 as a 1-hour infusion on day 1, carboplatin AUC 5 on day 1, and topotecan 0.75 mg/m^2 iv on days 1, 2, and 3. This cycle was repeated every 21 days for a total of four cycles. Those responding at the end of four cycles were then given three courses of etoposide 50 mg alternating with 100 mg orally from days 1 to 10 every 21 days. Patients with LD-SCLC received 45 Gy chest radiotherapy (1.8 Gy fractions/day), beginning concurrently with the third cycle of chemotherapy. Responses occurred in 88% of patients with extensive disease and in 93% of those with limited disease. ED-SCLC patients had a median survival of 8.2 months, and the median survival of patients with LD-SCLC was 17.2 months. Although toxicities were acceptable for patients with good performance status, toxicity was more pronounced in patients with Eastern Cooperative Oncology Group performance status of 2, with 5 of 12 patients (42%) having deaths from septic causes *(34)*. This study also demonstrated that the combination of paclitaxel, topotecan, and a platinum agent has activity against SCLC. Strictly speaking, the results of the these two studies cannot be compared, yet a noticeable point is the shorter median survival in the ED-SCLC patients in this study of 8.2 months compared with 10.9 months in the previous one.

3. TOPOTECAN IN NON-SMALL-CELL LUNG CANCER

NSCLC is a difficult disease to treat because the current options for this cancer fall far short, necessitating a search for more active drugs. Although topotecan is approved by the FDA for use in relapsed SCLC, it has been demonstrated to have activity against NSCLC. It is actively being studied both as a single agent and in combination with many other drugs.

3.1. TOPOTECAN IN NSCLC AS A SINGLE AGENT

Several studies have been conducted in stage IIIB and IV (unresectable stages) NSCLC using topotecan as a single agent (Table 8). In most of the studies, topotecan has been administered at 1.5 mg/m^2/day during 30-minute infusions for 5 days every 21 days, although it has also been studied as a continuous iv infusion over 21 days and in oral form as well.

Two phase II studies were published by Perez-Soler et al. studying topotecan in NSCLC. In the first study, 40 patients able to be evaluated with advanced NSCLC (stages IIIB and IV) were treated with topotecan at 1.5 mg/m^2/day during 30-minute infusions for 5 days every 21 days. Of the 40 patients, 19 had adenocarcinoma, 14 squamous carcinoma, and 7 had poorly differentiated carcinoma. Topotecan had modest activity in this group, as 6 of 40 patients (15%) had a PR with the duration being 8, 14, 18, 28, 56, and 61 weeks. Four had a minor response, 10 had stable disease, and 20 progressed. Interestingly, response was best seen in the squamous cell group with 5 of 14 patients (36%) having a PR. The overall survival in this study was 38 weeks, with a 1-year survival of 30%. Grade 3 and 4 granulocytopenia and thrombocytopenia were seen in 67% and 10% of courses, respectively *(35)*. Extending the results of the previous study, Perez-Soler et al. next studied topotecan in patients with untreated and unresectable stage IIIB and IV squamous-cell lung cancer. Of 29 assessable patients, 7 (24.1%) had a partial response, 2 (6.9%) had a minor response, 4 (13.8%) had stable disease, and 16 (55.2%) progressed. The overall survival of 40 weeks was similar to what was observed in the previous study *(36)*.

Lynch et al. had observed very different results in a phase II trial in untreated patients with stage IIIB and IV NSCLC in which topotecan was administered at a dose of 2 mg/m^2/day as 30-minute infusions for 5 days every 21 days. This trial ended prematurely because of a lack of observed response in the first 20 patients, despite marked myelosuppression. Grade 3 and 4 leukopenia was seen in 50% and 45% of patients, and Grade 3 and 4 thrombocytopenia was seen in 10% and 5%, respectively. Lethal febrile neutropenia was seen in one patient. The median overall survival was 7.6 months *(37)*. The lack of clinical responses to topotecan at 2.0 mg/m^2/day, a dose substantially higher than the that suggested by Rowinsky et al. in a previous Phase I study of 1.5 mg/m^2/day *(38)*, was surprising.

Table 8
Topotecan as a Single Agent in Non-Small-Cell Lung Cancer

Author (Reference)	*Phase*	*Number*	*Prior Rx*	*Regimen*	*Response (%)*	*Median survival (%)*	*1-Year survival (%)*	*TTP*
Perez Soler *(35)*	II	40	None	Topotecan 1.5 mg/m^2/day × 5 days q 21 days	PR 15 MR 10 SD 25	38 weeks	30	
Perez Soler *(36)*	II	35 sq cell	None	Topotecan 1.5 mg/m^2/day × 5 days q 21 days	PR 24 MR 6.9 SD 13.8	40 weeks		
Lynch*(37)*	II	20	None	Topotecan 2 mg/m^2/day × 5 days	OR 0 SD 55	30 weeks		
Kindler (39)	II	26	None	Topotecan by 21-day continuous infusion q 2–8 days 0.5 mg/m^2/day (n = 23) and 0.6 mg/m^2/day (n = 3)	PR 4 SD 31	36 weeks	39	2 months
Weitz *(40)*	II	75	None	**Arm A** Topotecan 1.5 mg/m^2/day × 5 days q 21 days	OR 16	257 days		101 days
				Arm B Topotecan 1.3 mg/m^2/day continuous infusion over 72 hours, q 4 weeks	OR 8	179 days		63 days
White *(41)*	II	29	None	Oral topotecan 2.3 mg/m^2/day × 5 days q 21 days	CR 0 PR 0 SD 43	39.9 weeks	33	12.3 weeks

Rx, treatment; TTP, time to progression; sq cell, squamous cell carcinoma; PR, partial response; MR, minor response; SD:, stable disease; OR, overall response.

Disappointing results were also obtained when topotecan was studied as a 21-day continuous iv infusion every 28 days. Kindler et al., in a phase II study of topotecan in patients with untreated stage IIIB and IV NSCLC, administered 86 cycles of continuous infusion topotecan to 26 patients. One patient had a PR, 6 had stable disease, and 19 patients had progressive disease. They reported a median survival of 9 months, time to progression of 2 months, and a 1-year survival of 39%. However, the study regimen seemed to have less myelosuppression than other studies with topotecan. Grade 4 neutropenia and thrombocytopenia were seen in only 4% and 8% of patients, respectively. Although no patients experienced febrile neutropenia, 16 of 86 courses of topotecan in this study were complicated by catheter related infections, a reflection of the prolonged handling of catheters *(39)*. Since the publication of this early work, few researchers have pursued this mode of delivery of topotecan because of the better responses seen with the 5-day course.

Another study looked at the mode of delivery of topotecan by comparing the 5-day course to a 72-hour infusion. In this trial, Weitz et al. studied 75 patients with untreated stage IIIB and IV NSCLC. Thirty-eight patients were given the traditional dose of topotecan at 1.5 $mg/m^2/day$ over 30 minutes for 5 days every 21 days (arm A) and 37 were given topotecan at 1.3 $mg/m^2/day$ by continuous iv infusion over 72 hours every 4 weeks (arm B). Although more responses were observed in arm A (16% in arm A as opposed to 8% in arm B), there was no statistically significant difference in time to progression and overall survival between the two arms. In arm A, the median time to progression was 101 days and the median survival time was 257 days; in arm B, the median time to progression was 63 days ($p = 0.83$) and the median survival time was 179 days ($p = 0.75$). There was more toxicity associated with the continuous infusion arm with grade 3 or 4 thrombocytopenia occurring in 37.8% versus 15.8% in arm A *(40)*.

Similar to the work using the oral formulation of topotecan in SCLC, oral topotecan has been investigated in NSCLC. In a phase II study, White et al. gave oral topotecan starting at the dose of 2.3 $mg/m^2/day$ for 5 days (first cycle) every 21 days for up to 6 cycles unless progression or unacceptable toxicity was seen. Dose modification was permitted from the second cycle onward based on drug tolerability. There were no CRs or PRs seen in this study. Of the 29 patients enrolled, 13 (43.3%) had stable disease; the median time to progression was 12.3 weeks, median survival was 39.9 weeks, and the 1-year survival was 33.3%. A total of 125 cycles were given, and 40% were associated with grade 3 or 4 neutropenia, 16.6% with grade 3 or 4 anemia, 1.6% with grade 3 or 4 thrombocytopenia, and 13% with grade 3 nausea and vomiting *(41)*. This study questions the utility of oral topotecan in NSCLC, although it would be imprudent to negate its use based on few studies.

3.2. Topotecan in Combination Regimens

NSCLC responds poorly to the commonly available chemotherapeutic agents (Table 9). As shown in the previous section, several studies have demonstrated modest activity of topotecan as a single agent in NSCLC, and it is conceivable that it might have a more efficacious response in combination with other drugs. Accordingly, topotecan is being studied in combination with other agents with demonstrated activity against NSCLC. Though work in this field is still preliminary, in this section we have reviewed a few studies.

Alkylating agents such as cisplatin have been used in various regimens in lung cancer. It has been suggested that topotecan might enhance the effects of these agents by inhibiting the repair of damaged DNA caused by alkylating agents. Using this rationale, Raymond et al. conducted a phase I study of topotecan with fixed dose of cisplatin in untreated NSCLC patients. Escalating doses of topotecan were given starting from 0.75 mg/m^2/day as 30-minute infusions for 5 days along with a fixed dose of cisplatin at 75 mg/m^2 on day 1 every 21 days. In this study, topotecan was given 90 minutes before cisplatin. Fourteen patients were assessable, and marked myelosuppression with severe thrombocytopenia and neutropenia were seen even at the lowest dose of topotecan and cisplatin planned in this study; as a result, this dose was not recommended for phase II studies *(42)*. In a very similar study, Bildat et al., in a phase I trial, gave escalating doses of topotecan at 0.5, 0.75, and 1.0 mg/m^2/day as 30-minute iv infusions on days 1–5 with a fixed dose of cisplatin at 25 mg/m^2 as a 30-minute iv infusion on days 1, 3, and 5, with cycles repeated every 22 days. Here topotecan was given 3 hours before cisplatin. The MTD of topotecan was reached at 0.75 mg/m^2/day; at this dose, the DLT was grade 4 neutropenia, observed in three of six (50%) patients. In this trial, four of nine patients achieved partial response *(43)*. This study demonstrated that a combination of topotecan and cisplatin is feasible at this dose level in advanced NSCLC, although with a very high degree of myelosuppression.

Wiesenfeld et al. conducted a randomized phase II trial which compared topotecan with cisplatin versus topotecan and paclitaxel; G-CSF support was used in both treatment arms. Arm A included topotecan at 1.25 mg/m^2 days 1–5 with cisplatin at 75 mg/m^2 on day 1; arm B consisted of topotecan at 1.0 mg/m^2 days 1–5 with paclitaxel at 190 mg/m^2 on day 1. G-CSF was given in both arms and the cycles were repeated every 28 days. Twenty-two patients were enrolled in arm A and 61 in arm B. Arm A was closed early because of a lack of response and severe toxicity—there was one septic death and another death from renal causes in this arm. The response rate was 14% in arm A and 24% in B with the Kaplan-Meier estimates of median time to progression of 115 days and 93 days in arms A and B, respectively. The median survival was 225 days in arm A and 184 days in arm B. As stated

Table 9
Topotecan in Combination With Other Agents in NSCLC

Author (Reference)	*Phase*	*Number*	*Prior Rx*	*Regimen*	*Response (%)*	*Median survival*
Raymond *(42)*	I	14	None	Topotecan 0.75 mg/m^2/day × 5 days q 21 days Cisplatin 75 mg/m^2 on day 1	PR 30.7	38 weeks
Bildat *(43)*	I	9	None	Topotecan 0.75 mg/m^2/day × 5 days q 22 days Cisplatin 25 mg/m^2 on days 1, 3, and 5	PR 44 SD 33	40 weeks
Wiesenfeld *(44)*	II	83	None	**Arm A** (n = 22) Topotecan 1.25 mg/m^2/day × 5 days Cisplatin 75 mg/m^2 day 1+ G-CSF	OR 14	225 days
				Arm B (n = 61) Topotecan 1.0 mg/m^2/day × 5 days Paclitaxel 190 mg/m^2 on day 1 + G-CSF	OR 24	184 days
Rinaldi *(47)*	I/II	18	Yes	Topotecan 0.75 mg/m^2/day × 5 days Gemcitabine 400 mg/m^2 days 1 and 5	PR 18 SD 32	40 weeks
Guarino *(48)*	I	25	None	Cisplatin 20 mg/m^2 days 1, 8, and 15 Gemcitabine 1000 mg/m^2 days 1 and 15 Topotecan 0.5–2 mg/m^2 days 1, 8, and 15 q 28 days	PR 24 SD 60	26 weeks

Rx, treatment; PR, partial response; SD, stable disease; G-CSF, granulocyte-colony stimulating factor; OR, overall response.

previously, the incidence of toxicity was higher in arm A: 62% had severe leukopenia and 76% had significant thrombocytopenia as opposed to 22% severe leukopenia and 1.6% significant thrombocytopenia in arm B. Arm A was also associated with a higher incidence of nonhematological toxicity. The authors concluded that neither arm was shown to have better results than the regimens available hitherto. Hence, neither arm was recommended for further studies *(44)*.

Topotecan has also been studied with gemcitabine. Gemcitabine is a pyrimidine analog that acts by inhibiting ribonucleotide reductase and by competing with deoxycytidine triphosphate for inclusion in the DNA molecule, resulting in premature chain termination. Gemcitabine has been approved for use in advanced pancreatic cancer and in advanced NSCLC. A phase II trial had demonstrated activity of gemcitabine as a single agent in NSCLC *(45)*, and a phase III trial has elucidated activity of gemcitabine with cisplatin in advanced NSCLC *(46)*. A phase I/II study was conducted by Rinaldi et al. to find the MTD and DLT of topotecan and gemcitabine. This study enrolled 17 patients with advanced NSCLC who had previously received chemotherapy. In this trial, both drugs were given iv over 30 minutes; topotecan was given for 5 consecutive days and gemcitabine was given on days 1 and 5 only. The MTD of these drugs were 0.75 mg/m^2 for topotecan and 400 mg/m^2 for gemcitabine. The DLTs were neutropenia and thrombocytopenia. At this dose level, 2 and 1 patients of a total of 10 had grade 3/4 neutropenia and thrombocytopenia, respectively. Partial response was seen in 3 of 17 patients (18%) and the median survival in this study was 10 months. This combination appears to be well-tolerated and appears to have activity against advanced NSCLC *(47)*.

Guarino et al. reported the results of an ongoing trial of weekly topotecan, cisplatin and gemcitabine in NSCLC. They enrolled 25 evaluable patients in this trial and gave fixed doses of cisplatin at 20 mg/m^2 over 30 minutes and gemcitabine at 1000 mg/m^2 over 30 minutes and escalating doses of topotecan over 30 minutes on days 1, 8, and 15 every 28 days. After the first cohort, gemcitabine was given on days 1 and 15 only because of marked thrombocytopenia. The MTD of topotecan was not reached but authors did not recommended a dose higher than 2 mg/m^2 of topotecan. After the change in the schedule of gemcitabine, 89% treatments were given as planned; grade 3 and 4 leukopenia was seen in two courses and one course, respectively; and none of the patients had febrile neutropenia. There were eight cases of grade 3 thrombocytopenia and no grade 4 thrombocytopenia *(48)*.

4. IRINOTECAN IN SMALL-CELL LUNG CANCER

Irinotecan is a Topo-I inhibitor that acts by forming a Topo-I–DNA-cleavable complex. Yakult Honsha Co., Ltd. in 1983 first synthesized Irinotecan, also known as CPT-11, in Japan. Thus it is not surprising that many pioneering studies of Irinotecan have been conducted in Japan. Irinotecan is actively being investigated for the treatment of both NSCLC and SCLC.

As mentioned previously, SCLC is a chemosensitive disease. Although current chemotherapy regimens in extensive stage disease produce an ORR of 60–80%, the median patient survival is only 7–12 months. In limited-stage disease, the response rate is approximately 80–90%, with a median survival of 12–16 months *(2)*. Despite initial high response rates, a great many of these patients relapse. In the past 20 years, no major advances have been made in the treatment of SCLC *(3)*. This leaves ample room for investigating new agents. A review of irinotecan in SCLC clearly demonstrates that it has substantial activity in this cancer.

4.1. Single-Agent Irinotecan in SCLC

In an early phase I study, it was found that irinotecan given once in 3 weeks at the dose of 200 to 250 mg/m^2 caused substantial side effects *(49)*, and it was observed that a weekly regimen of irinotecan was better tolerated *(50)* (Table 10). Accordingly, in most of the trials, it has been studied in a weekly dose.

Negoro et al. performed a phase II study of irinotecan in patients with previously untreated or previously treated non-small-cell carcinomas and small-cell carcinomas. In this study, irinotecan was given at a dose of 100 mg/m^2 iv infusion once per week for weeks or more. Among the patients with SCLC, the reported response rate was 37.1% (13 of 35 patients). Leukopenia and diarrhea were the DLTs *(51)*. Masuda et al. presented phase II data in refractory or relapsed patients, 5 had LD and 10 had ED. In this study, irinotecan was given at 100 mg/m^2 iv infusion once per week. Partial response was observed in 47% of patients (3 of 5 patients with LD and 4 of 10 patients with ED). The median duration of response was 58 days and the median survival was 187 days in the whole group. The main toxicities observed were leukopenia, anemia, diarrhea, nausea and vomiting, and pulmonary toxicity *(52)*.

Le Chevalier et al. studied irinotecan at the dose of 350 mg/m^2 given every 3 weeks. All patients had previously received an etoposide and cisplatin-based regimen. Five patients of 32 (16%) had an objective response, including one CR in a patient with brain metastasis. The median duration of response was 131 days and the overall survival was 125 days *(53)*.

DeVore et al. conducted a multicenter phase II trial in the United States and evaluated irinotecan in 44 patients with prior treatment. Irinotecan was given to SCLC patients with sensitive relapse ($n = 17$) and refractory relapse ($n = 27$). Patients who had previously achieved PR or CR and relapsed more than 3 months after completion of initial therapy were considered to have sensitive relapse. All other patients were considered refractory. The dose of

Table 10
Single Agent Irinotecan in SCLC

Author (Reference)	*Phase*	*Number*	*Prior Rx*	*Regimen*	*Response (%)*	*Median survival*	*Response duration*
Negoro *(51)*	II	35	Treated and untreated	Irinotecan 100 mg/m^2 q week × 3 wk or more	OR 37.1 CR 5		
Masuda *(52)*	II	15(LD 5 ED 10)	Yes	Irinotecan 100 mg/m^2/week	PR 47	187 days	58 days
Le Chevalier *(53)*	II	32	Yes	Irinotecan 350 mg/m^2 q 3 weeks	OR 16	125 days	131 days
DeVore *(54)*	II	44	Yes	Irinotecan 125 mg/m^2/week × 4 weeks then 2 weeks rest, repeated every 6 weeks	Sensitive: 35.3 Refractory: 3.7	5.9 months 2.8 months	4.6 months 2.9 months

Rx, treatment; LD, limited disease; ED, extensive disease; OR, overall response; sensitive and refractory relapse, patients who had previously achieved PR/CR and relapsed > 3 months after therapy, all others were considered to have refractory disease irinotecan was 125 mg/m^2 given over 90 minutes weekly for 4 weeks, followed by a rest period of 2 weeks; the cycle was repeated until disease progression. Their results were as follows: $n = 44$ patients, CR = 1 (2.3%), and PR = 6 (13.6%) for an overall intent-to-treat response rate of 15.9% (95% CI: 5.0–26.2). In this study, the median duration of response was 3 months, time to progression was 2.3 months, and the median survival was 4.8 months *(54)*.

4.2. Irinotecan-Based Combinations for the Treatment of SCLC

Irinotecan is being investigated in combination with other drugs in SCLC (Table 11). The combination of irinotecan and cisplatin in particular has been proven to be very effective, as demonstrated in the following section. It is also being studied with carboplatin, etoposide, and gemcitabine, among others.

4.2.1. Irinotecan and Cisplatin

Cisplatin is an integral component in the current chemotherapy regimens for SCLC. Preclinical models have suggested a synergistic interaction between irinotecan and cisplatin *(55)*.

4.2.1.1. Irinotecan and Cisplatin: Phase II Trials

Kudoh et al. conducted a phase II trial in 75 untreated patients with SCLC, 40 (53%) of whom had LD and 35 (47%) had ED. Irinotecan was given at 60 mg/m^2 as a 90-minute iv infusion on days 1, 8, and 15. After the irinotecan infusion, cisplatin 60 mg/m^2 was given on day 1 only, and cycles were repeated every 28 days. Patients with LD received four cycles followed by thoracic radiation, whereas patients with ED were given six cycles of chemotherapy. Among patients with LD ($n = 40$), CR was achieved in 12 (30%) and PR in 21 (53%) for an ORR of 83%. The median response duration was 8 months, median survival was 14.3 months, and 2-year survival was 17.5%. Among patients with ED ($n = 35$), CR was achieved in 10 (29%) and PR in 20 (57%) for an ORR of 86%. The median response duration was 6.6 months, median survival was 13 months, and 2-year survival was reported as 21.7%. Observed grade 3–4 toxicities were neutropenia in 77%, diarrhea in 19%, and anemia in 39% of patients *(56)*.

Okishio et al., in a phase II trial, studied 16 previously treated SCLC patients using a combination of irinotecan and cisplatin. In this trial, irinotecan, 60 mg/m^2 was given on days 1, 8, and 15, and cisplatin 60 mg/m^2 was given on day 1 only every 28 days. As might be expected in this trial, the response seen was much subdued as compared with the untreated population in the previous study. This trial reported an objective response in 3 (19%) patients and the median survival was reported to be 5.7 months *(57)*.

Table 11
Irinotecan in Combination Regimens in SCLC Irinotecan and Cisplatin

Author (Reference)	*Phase*	*Number*	*Prior Rx*	*Regimen*	*Response (%)*	*Median survival*	*Response duration*
Phase II data							
Kudoh *(56)*	II	LD ($n = 40$)	No	Irinotecan 60 mg/m^2 days 1, 8, and 15 Cisplatin 60 mg/m^2 day 1 q weeks × 4 cycles then radiotherapy	CR 30 PR 53	14.3 months	8 months
		ED ($n = 35$)	No	Irinotecan 60 mg/m^2 days 1, 8, and 15 Cisplatin 60 mg/m^2 day 1 q 4 weeks × 6 cycles	CR 29 PR 57	13 months	6.6 months
Okishio *(57)*	II	ED 16	Yes	Irinotecan 60 mg/m^2 days 1, 8, and 15 Cisplatin 60 mg/m^2 day 1 q 4 weeks		19	5.7 months
Phase III data							
Noda *(58)*	III	ED 154 ($n = 77$)	No	Irinotecan 60 mg/m^2 days 1, 8, and 15 Cisplatin 60 mg/m^2 days 1 q 4 weeks × 4 cycles	OR 65 CR 2 PR 63	12.8 months (PFS 6.9 months)	
		($n = 77$)	No	Cisplatin 80 mg/m^2 day 1 Etoposide 100 mg/m^2 days 1–3 q 3 weeks × 4 cycles	OR 52 CR 7 PR 45	9.4 months (PFS 4.8 months)	
Irinotecan and carboplatin							
Suguira *(60)*	II	16 LD = 13 ED = 3	No	Irinotecan 50 mg/m^2 days 1, 8, and 15 Carboplatin 300 mg/m^2 day 1 q 4 weeks	LD 77 ED 67		

Hirose *(61)*	II	22 Refractory and relapsed patients		Carboplatin AUC-5 day 1 Irinotecan 50 mg/m^2 days 1 and 8 q 3 weeks	68.2	194 days	
Naka *(62)*	II	29 Refractory and relapsed patients		Irinotecan 50 mg/m^2 days 1, 8, and 15 Carboplatin AUC-2 days 1, 8, and 15 q 4 weeks	31	6.1 months	(TTP 3.5 months)
Irinotecan and Etoposide							
Masuda *(63)*	II	24	Yes	Irinotecan 70 mg/m^2 days 1, 8, and 15 Etoposide 80 mg/m^2 days 1–3 (rhGCSF days 4–21)	CR 12.5 PR 58	271 days	4.6 months
Nakamura *(64)*	II	50 ED	No	Irinotecan 60 mg/m^2 days 1, 8, and 15 Etoposide 80 mg/m^2 days 2–4	OR 66 CR 10	12 months	

Rx, treatment; LD, limited disease; CR, complete response; PR, partial response; ED, extensive disease; OR, overall response; PFS, progression free survival.

4.2.1.2 Irinotecan and Cisplatin: Phase III Trials

Noda et al. recently published the results of a multicenter randomized phase III study in ED-SCLC patients conducted in Japan that compared irinotecan plus cisplatin with cisplatin and etoposide, an established regimen for SCLC. The original planned size of this study was 230, but accrual was stopped at 154 because of significantly better results in the irinotecan arm. Each arm had 77 patients, and the patient characteristics were comparable in the two arms. The patients in the irinotecan plus cisplatin arm were given 60 mg/m^2 irinotecan on days 1, 8, and 15, along with 60 mg/m^2 of cisplatin on day 1 only every 4 weeks. The patients in the other arm were given etoposide at the dose of 100 mg/m^2 on days 1, 2, and 3, and cisplatin 80 mg/m^2 on day 1 every 3 weeks. A total of four chemotherapy cycles was given. ORRs were 65.6% in the irinotecan plus cisplatin arm, as compared with 54.1% in the cisplatin and etoposide arm. The overall survival was significantly greater in the irinotecan plus cisplatin arm: 12.8 months versus 9.4 months in the cisplatin and etoposide arm ($p = 0.002$). The progression-free survival was also higher in the irinotecan arm, 6.9 months versus 4.8 months ($p = 0.003$). Myelosuppression was greater in the etoposide arm (92.2% versus 65.3%, $p < 0.001$), whereas diarrhea was more frequent in irinotecan arm (16% versus 0%, $p < 0.001$). Though the CR rate appeared to be somewhat higher in the cisplatin and etoposide arm, the higher survival rates of the irinotecan plus cisplatin are attractive and perhaps offer a new approach in the management of metastatic SCLC patients *(58)*. These are indeed impressive results; to confirm the findings, an intergroup phase III study in the United States is ongoing.

4.2.2. Irinotecan and Carboplatin

Carboplatin is better tolerated than cisplatin and has been studied in a phase I trial in combination with irinotecan by Fukuda et al. In this trial, the authors recommended that in future phase II trials. irinotecan be administered at 50 mg/m^2 on days 1, 8, and 15, with carboplatin AUC of 5. Neutropenia, thrombocytopenia, and diarrhea were the DLTs *(59)*.

Suguira et al., in a phase II study of irinotecan and carboplatin, concluded that carboplatin at 300 mg/m^2 on day 1 and irinotecan at 50 mg/m^2 on days 1, 8, and 15 given every 4 weeks is an effective combination in SCLC. They studied 16 previously untreated patients with SCLC and reported two CRs and eight PRs (RR 77%) in patients with limited disease, and two PRs (67%) in patients with extensive disease. The hematological toxicities were grade 4 leukopenia (in one course) and grade 3 thrombocytopenia (in two); the nonhematological toxicities were grade 3 diarrhea (in one course) and grade 3 nausea and vomiting (in one course) *(60)*.

The safety and efficacy of irinotecan plus carboplatin in refractory or relapsed SCLC patients was studied by Hirose et al. *(61)* and Naka et al. *(62)*.

Hirose et al. employed a regimen of carboplatin at AUC of 5 on day 1 plus irinotecan administered as 50mg/m^2 infusions only on days 1 and 8 of a 3-week cycle. Responses in this population of 22 patients were seen in 68.2%, mostly in patients with sensitive relapses. Grade 3/4 hematological toxicities included neutropenia in 63% of patients, thrombocytopenia in 58%, and anemia in 67%. Grade 3 diarrhea developed in 21% of patients and grade 3/4 infection in 13% *(61)*. Naka et al. evaluated a regimen in which patients were treated at 4-week intervals with a combination of irinotecan at 50 mg/m^2 and carboplatin AUC of 2 on each of days 1, 8, and 15. The observed ORR for this regimen was 31%, although the median time off of chemotherapy before study entry was 3.5 months. Again, the major toxicity was myelosuppression. Here, however, grade 3/4 neutropenia and thrombocytopenia occurred in 52% and 21% of patients, respectively. Grade 3/4 diarrhea was seen in only 7% *(62)*. These combination regimens appear to be active in the second-line setting with acceptable toxicity.

4.2.3. Irinotecan and Etoposide

Phase II trials have looked at the combination of irinotecan and etoposide, and it has been demonstrated to have efficacy in previously treated as well as untreated patients. Masuda et al. treated 24 patients with refractory or relapsed disease in a phase II trial of irinotecan and etoposide. All of these patients had previously received cisplatin and etoposide or an anthracycline-based regimen. Irinotecan at 70 mg/m^2 was given on days 1, 8, and 15 and etoposide was at 80 mg/m^2 on days 1, 2, and 3; G-CSF was given days 4–21 and this cycle was repeated every 4 weeks. Fourteen patients had a PR and three had CR, for an ORR of 71%. The median response duration was 4.6 months, and median survival was 271 days *(63)*. Nakamura et al. studied this combination in previously untreated ED-SCLC patients. In this study, 50 patients were given irinotecan at 60 mg/m^2 on days 1, 8, and 15, and etoposide was given at 80 mg/m^2 iv on days 2, 3, and 4. The reported ORR in this trial was 66% with a CR of 10%. The observed median survival was 12 months. Grade 3/4 toxicities were as follows: neutropenia (72%), leukopenia (28%), and anemia (4%). In this trial, grade 3/4 diarrhea was observed in only 2% of patients *(64)*.

4.2.4. Irinotecan, Cisplatin, and Etoposide Combination

Given the proven first-line activity of the three agents, Sekine et al. have recently published the results of a Japanese Clinical Oncology Group randomized phase II trial of irinotecan, cisplatin, and etoposide combinations administered weekly or every 4 weeks for patients with untreated ED-SCLC *(65)*. Sixty patients were randomized to be treated with weekly therapy (consisting of cisplatin at 25 mg/m^2 weekly × 9; irinotecan 90 mg/m^2 once on weeks 1, 3, 5, 7, and 9; and etoposide 60 mg/m^2 days 1–3 of week 2) or with every-4-week therapy (cisplatin at 60 mg/m^2 on day 1; irinotecan at 60 mg/m^2 on days 1, 8, and 15; and etoposide days 1–3 every 4 weeks for four cycles. Prophylactic G-CSF support was provided in both arms. Although the toxicity profile and the response rates were similar between the two arms, the median survival of the every-4-week arm was 12.9 months as opposed to 8.9 months in the weekly arm.

4.2.5. Irinotecan and Paclitaxel

Rushing et al. conducted a phase I study of a combination of irinotecan and paclitaxel in previously treated patients with SCLC. Paclitaxel was given in escalating doses, as a 30-minute infusion followed by a 45-minute infusion of irinotecan given at a fixed dose of 60 mg/m^2 on days 1, 8, and 15 every 28 days. In this study, two cycles of treatment were given. The DLT could not be identified at the time of reporting because of the unpredictability of toxicity. Of the 15 patients treated, 6 patients had grade 2 and 1 patient had grade 3 diarrhea, and 1 patient died of sudden unexplained death without other known toxicity. Three patients had pneumonia at different dose levels, one died with absolute neutrophil count of 1400, another patient with an absolute neutrophil count of <500, and yet another patient had an absolute neutrophil count of 3400. Three had grade 3 leukopenia without neutropenia. One had pulmonary embolus at the earliest dose level. Of the 11 patients able to be evaluated for response, 4 had achieved a CR and 1 a partial remission. The predictable toxicities in this trial were diarrhea and anemia; at the time of reporting, the DLT had not been reached (66).

4.3. Irinotecan in Multimodality Regimens for the Treatment of SCLC

Several studies are being conducted to define the role of irinotecan along with radiation therapy for the treatment of limited-stage SCLC. Kudoh et al. conducted a phase II study of irinotecan combined with cisplatin in previously untreated SCLC. Irinotecan 60 mg/m^2 was given on days 1, 8, and 15 along with cisplatin 60 mg/m^2 on day 1 every 28 days. Four cycles of chemotherapy were followed by thoracic irradiation to patients with LD and six courses were given to patients with ED. The reported results were an ORR of 83% in LD with a CR rate of 30%. The median response duration was 8.0 months in this group with a median survival of 14.3 months. The grade 3 or 4 toxicities were neutropenia (77%), leukopenia (45%), diarrhea (19%), and anemia (39%). Two patients died from neutropenia associated with diarrhea *(67)*.

5. IRINOTECAN IN NON-SMALL-CELL LUNG CANCER

In this section, we highlight some of the important studies in this field.

Table12
Irinotecan as a Single Agent in Advanced NSCLC

Author (Reference)	*Phase*	*Number*	*Regimen*	*Response (%)*	*Median survival*
Fukuoka *(68)*	II	73	100 mg/m²/week	31.9	42 weeks
Negoro *(69)*	II	128	100 mg/m²/week × 3 or more weeks	34 (untreated) 0 (treated)	
Baker *(70)*	II	48	100 mg/m²/week × 4 weeks, then 2-week rest	15	6.2 months

5.1. Single-Agent Irinotecan in NSCLC

Several phase II trials have been conducted using irinotecan as a single agent for advanced NSCLC; these have established a role of irinotecan in this cancer (Table 12).

In 1992, Fukuoka et al. published a phase II study of irinotecan in patients with untreated and inoperable NSCLC. Of the 72 assessable patients, 3 had stage I or II disease, 30 had stage III, and 40 had stage IV. CPT-11 was given at a dose of 100 mg/m²/day by an iv infusion over 90 minutes once per week; this was continued if the patient responded and if the toxicities were acceptable. A median of six doses were given to patients. In this study, a response was seen in 23 patients (31.9%), including a response rate of 31.3% in stages I–III and 32.5% in stage IV patients. No CRs were observed. The median survival was 42 weeks, and the median duration of response in patients with PR was 15 weeks. The main toxicities were leukopenia and diarrhea. Grade 3–4 leukopenia was seen in 18 patients (25%), and 15 patients (21%) had grade 3–4 diarrhea. Other common toxicities were nausea and vomiting (22%), anemia (15%), and alopecia (4%) *(68)*.

In 1991, Negoro et al. studied irinotecan in patients with lung cancer and reported significant results with this drug. This was a three-arm study: group A included previously untreated NSCLC patients (n = 67); group B had previously treated NSCLC patients (n = 26); and group C included patients with SCLC (n = 35). Patients were treated with irinotecan at a dose of 100 mg/m² by an iv infusion once per week for 3 or more weeks. The study reported a single-agent response rate of 34.3% in group A, 0% in B, and 37.1% in C. The DLTs of this study were leukopenia and diarrhea *(69)*.

Baker et al. conducted a multicenter trial of irinotecan in patients with advanced (stage IIIB and IV) NSCLC. Irinotecan cycles were given at 100 mg/m² every week for 4 weeks, followed by a 2-week rest. Forty-eight patients were enrolled and 41 were assessable. Results demonstrated a partial response in six patients (15%), median response duration of 4.7 months, time to progression of 2.8 months, and median survival of 6.2 months. Late diarrhea was a common toxicity seen in this trial—grade 3 and 4 diarrhea was seen in 6.3% and 10.4%, respectively. None had grade 4 neutropenia, although grade 3 neutropenia was seen in 14.6% of patients *(70)*.

5.2. Irinotecan and Cisplatin Combinations

Cisplatin is a commonly used drug in the treatment of advanced lung cancer, and cisplatin-based regimens have been found to confer survival benefits in NSCLC as compared with best supportive care *(71)* (Table 13). Preclinical models have suggested synergy between irinotecan and cisplatin. Accordingly, several studies have been conducted studying irinotecan and cisplatin combinations in NSCLC.

5.2.1. Phase II Trials

DeVore reported a phase II study of irinotecan and cisplatin in advanced (stage IIIB and IV) NSCLC. In this trial, irinotecan was given at 60 mg/m^2 on days 1, 8, and 15 and a single dose of cisplatin at 80 mg/m^2 was given on day 1 after irinotecan. The study enrolled 11 stage IIIB and 41 stage IV patients. Objective responses were seen in 28.8% patients, including 2 CRs and 13 PRs. The median duration of response was 5.9 months, and time to progression was 5.1 months. The median survival was 9.9 months, and the 1-year survival rate was 37%. The toxicity profile included late diarrhea (17.3%), neutropenia (46.1%), and nausea (32.7%). In 60% of patients in this trial the dose of CPT-11 had to be decreased to ≤40 mg/m^2, primarily because the protocol did not allow dose adjustment of cisplatin *(72)*.

Jagasia et al. studied a different dose and schedule of irinotecan and cisplatin. In this study, 30 mg/m^2 of cisplatin was given as a 30-minute infusion and irinotecan 65 mg/m^2 was given just after cisplatin as a 30-minute infusion. Both the drugs were given weekly for 4 weeks followed by a rest period of 2 weeks; this cycle was continued for a maximum of six cycles. Seven patients had stage IIIB and 43 had stage IV disease. The study reported an objective response rate of 36%, median survival of 11.6 months, and a 1-year survival of 46%. Grade 3/4 toxicities were diarrhea (26%), neutropenia (26%), anemia (14%), and thrombocytopenia (14%). This particular regimen was well tolerated and had significant efficacy *(73)*.

Mori et al. studied yet another regimen—a combination of cisplatin at 20 mg/m^2/day for 5 days as a continuous iv infusion and irinotecan 160 mg/m^2/day as a bolus on day 1 with G-CSF. They reported an objective response in 24 of 41 patients (58.5%) with a 1-year survival of 44%. Grade 3/4 diarrhea was reported in 23%, granulocytopenia in 15%, and anemia in 15% of patients *(74)*. In a study by Ueoka et al., cisplatin was administered at 60 mg/m^2 on days 1 and 8 and irinotecan was given at 50 mg/m^2 also on days

Table 13
Irinotecan and Cisplatin in Combination in Advanced NSCLC

Author (Reference)	*Phase*	*Number*	*Regimen*	*Response (%)*	*Median survival*	*1-year survival (%)*
DeVore *(72)*	II	52	Irinotecan 60 mg/m^2 days 1, 8, and 15 Cisplatin 80 mg/m^2 day 1	28.8	9.9 months	37
Jagasia *(73)*	II	50	Irinotecan 65 mg/m^2/day Cisplatin 30 mg/m^2/day q week × 4 weeks then 2 week rest	36	11.6 months	46
Mori *(74)*	II	41	Irinotecan 160 mg/m^2 day 1 bolus Cisplatin 20 mg/m^2/day × 5 day continuous iv	58.5	44.8 weeks	44
Ueoka *(75)*	II	41	Irinotecan 50 mg/m^2 days 1 and 8 Cisplatin 60 mg/m^2 days 1 and 8 q 4 weeks	41	13 months	58
Masuda *(76)*	III	133	**Arm A:** Cisplatin 80 mg/m^2 on day 1 Irinotecan 60 mg/m^2 days 1, 8, and 15	43	50.3 weeks	47.5
		132	**Arm B:** Irinotecan 100 mg/m^2 days 1, 8, and 15	21	46.1 weeks	40.7
		133	**Arm C:** Cisplatin 80 mg/m^2 on day 1 Vindesine 3 mg/m^2 on days 1, 8, and 15	31	47.4 weeks	37.9
Niho *(77)*	III	98	**Arm A:** Irinotecan 60 mg/m^2 on days 1, 8, and 15 Cisplatin 80 mg/m^2 on day 1	29	45.4 weeks	45.4
		101	**Arm B:** Cisplatin 80 mg/m^2 on day 1 Vindesine 3 mg/m^2 on days 1, 8, and 15	22	49.6 weeks	49.6

1 and 8, with cycles repeated every 4 weeks. They reported a response rate of 41% (17 of 41 patients), a median survival of 13 months, 1-year survival of 58%, and 2-year survival of 20%. Grade 3 and 4 toxicities were leukopenia (40%), thrombocytopenia (43%), anemia (42%), diarrhea (27%), and nausea and vomiting (26%). There was one death *(75)*.

5.2.2. Phase III Trials

Masuda et al. conducted a randomized multicenter phase III trial. This trial enrolled 398 patients with stage IIIB and IV disease. The patients were assigned to three arms. Arm A had 130 evaluable patients and consisted of cisplatin at 80 mg/m^2 on day 1 and irinotecan 60 mg/m^2 on days 1, 8, and 15. Arm B had 126 assessable patients, and these patients were given cisplatin at 80 mg/m^2 on day 1 and vindesine 3 mg/m^2 on days 1, 8, and 15. Arm C had 129 patients; these patients were treated with irinotecan alone at 100 mg/m^2 on days 1, 8, and 15. Response was seen in 55 (43%), 38 (31%), and 26 (21%) patients in arms A, B, and C, respectively. The median survival was 50.3 weeks, 47.4 weeks, and 46.1 weeks in the three arms, and the 1-year survival rate was 47.5%, 37.9%, and 40.7% in arms A, B, and C, respectively. Grade 4 neutropenia was highest in arm B (53.2%) and least in arm C (7.9%). Irinotecan arms were associated with a higher incidence of diarrhea: 12.6% in arm A, at least 4% in arm B, and 15% in arm C. This study showed a survival advantage with the combination of irinotecan and cisplatin *(76)*.

Niho et al. also presented a randomized phase III trial in patients with untreated stage IIIB or IV NSCLC comparing irinotecan and cisplatin versus vindesine and cisplatin. The two treatment arms of this trial were the same as arm A and B in the previous trial, with cycles repeated every 4 weeks. There was no difference between the two arms in terms of survival. Median survival was 45.4 weeks and 49.6 weeks in regimen A and B, respectively. There was a higher incidence of neutropenia in the vindesine arm (83% versus 63%) in this study *(77)*.

Fukuoka et al. evaluated the survival outcome in metastatic NSCLC (stage IV) patients in the two previously mentioned studies. Taken together, these studies had a total of 358 patients with stage IV NSCLC. A total of 139 had been assigned to the irinotecan and cisplatin arm, 134 to the vindesine and cisplatin arm, and 85 were treated with irinotecan alone. Cox regression analysis of the data showed that the irinotecan and cisplatin arm was associated with a significantly improved survival as compared with vindesine and cisplatin arm (hazard ratio 0.697; 95% CI 0.525–0.925, $p = 0.012$) *(78)*.

5.3. Irinotecan and Carboplatin

Many trials have shown that carboplatin-based regimens are as efficacious as cisplatin-based regimens and that these are associated with significantly less toxicity than cisplatin-based regimens *(79,80)* (Table 14). Thus studies have explored the efficacy and tolerability of irinotecan and carboplatin combinations.

Several Phase I studies have demonstrated that this is a feasible combination. Takeda et al. conducted a phase I study in advanced NSCLC patients. In this trial, a fixed dose of carboplatin was given at an AUC of 5 mg/mL/minute (using Calvert formula) on day 1 and irinotecan was given iv over 90 minutes on days 1, 8, and 15. This cycle was repeated every 28 days. Based on this work, the MTD of irinotecan was determined to be 60 mg/m^2; however, the authors recommended 50 mg/m^2 for phase II trials. Three of five patients given irinotecan at 60 mg/m^2 developed grade 4 neutropenia and thrombocytopenia. This study reported an ORR of 35.3%, median survival of 10.5 months, and a 1-year survival of 35.3% *(81)*. Fukuda et al. used irinotecan in a similar model in NSCLC (n = 11) and SCLC (n = 13) (and one case of colon cancer) and determined that the MTD of irinotecan was 60 mg/m^2 given on days 1, 8, and 15 with carboplatin AUC of 5 on day 1. The DLTs were neutropenia, thrombocytopenia, and diarrhea *(82)*. Okamoto et al. also recommended that irinotecan be administered at 60 mg/m^2 on days 1, 8, and 15 with carboplatin AUC of 5 on day 1 with G-CSF support *(83)*.

In a phase II study involving 36 advanced NSCLC patients, Mukohara et al. administered irinotecan at 50 mg/m^2 iv over 90 minutes on days 1, 8, and 15 with carboplatin AUC 5 mg/mL/minute (Calvert formula) on day 1. This cycle was given every 28 days for at least two cycles. They reported an ORR of 25%, a median survival of 10.8 months, and a 1-year survival rate of 38.9%. The following toxicities were reported using Japanese Clinical Oncology Group criteria: grade 3/4 neutropenia in 76.5%, grade 3 anemia in 26.5%, grade 3/4 thrombocytopenia in 47.1%, grade 3 nausea/vomiting in 36.1%, and grade 3/4 diarrhea in 5.9% *(84)*.

5.4. Irinotecan and Taxanes

Few studies have evaluated the combination of irinotecan and taxanes in NSCLC (Table 15). Taxanes have been shown to have significant activity in lung cancer. In a randomized trial, docetaxel was demonstrated to have activity in patients with NSCLC who had previously been treated with a platinum-containing chemotherapy drug *(85)*. Preclinical studies have looked at the combination of camptothecins and taxanes and have reported a degree of synergism in these two classes *(86)*.

Murren et al. administered paclitaxel at a fixed dose of 75 mg/m^2 weekly and gave escalating doses of irinotecan every week and determined that the MTD of weekly irinotecan in this combination was 50 mg/m^2. In this trial irinotecan was given as a 90-minute infusion followed immediately by paclitaxel over 1 hour every week for 4 weeks, followed by a 2-week rest. The DLT was neutropenia; mild diarrhea and fatigue were reported as the common nonhematological toxicities *(87)*.

Table 14
Irinotecan and Carboplatin in NSCLC

Author (Reference)	*Phase*	*Number*	*Regimen*	*Response (%)*	*Median survival*	*1-year survival (%)*
Fukuda *(82)*	I	NSCLC (n = 11) SCLC (n = 13)	MTD: Irinotecan 60 mg/m^2 on days 1, 8, and 15 Carboplatin AUC 5	NSCLC 36 SCLC 80		
Okamoto *(83)*	I	20	Recommended dose: Irinotecan 60 mg/m2 days 1, 8, and 15 Carboplatin AUC 5 G-CSF on all days except 1, 8, and15			
Mukohara *(84)*	II	36	Irinotecan 50 mg/m^2 days 1, 8, and 15 Carboplatin AUC 5 day 1	OR 25	10.8 months	39

MTD, maximum tolerable doses; AUC, area under the curve; G-CSF, granulocyte colony-stimulating factor.

Table 15
Irinotecan and Taxanes in Combination for NSCLC

Author (Reference)	*Phase*	*Number*	*Regimen*	*Response (%)*
Irinotecan and paclitxel				
Murren *(87)*	I	21	Irinotecan 50 mg/m^2 Paclitaxel 75 mg/m^2 q week	
Rosen *(88)*	I	17	Irinotecan 225 mg/m^2 Paclitaxel 100 mg/m^2 q 3 weeks	
Irinotecan and docetaxel				
Masuda *(90)*	I	32	Irinotecan 50 mg/m^2 days 1, 8, and 15 Docetaxel 50 mg/m^2 day 2 q 28 days	37
Adjei *(91)*	I	18	Irinotecan 160 mg/m^2 Docetaxel 65 mg/m^2 q 3 weeks	
Takeda *(92)*	II	112	DC arm (n = 53) Docetaxel 60 mg/m^2 day 1 Cispaltin 80 mg/m^2 day 1	40.9
			DI arm (n = 59) Docetaxel 60 mg/m^2 day 8 Irinotecan 60 mg/m^2 days 1 and 8	35.2

DC, docetaxel plus cisplatin; DI, docetaxel plus irinotecan.

Rosen et al. studied a regimen of these two drugs given every 3 weeks in a phase I trial in 17 patients with solid tumors. However, they could not escalate these drugs above their starting dose. The starting doses were paclitaxel at 100 mg/m^2 and irinotecan at 225 mg/m^2 given every 3 weeks. The main DLTs were neutropenic fever and grade 3 or higher diarrhea, seen in 5 of 17 (29%) patients. No pharmacokinetic differences were observed in either irinotecan or its metabolite SN-38 in the presence of paclitaxel *(88)*. Asai et al., on the other hand, had reported significant pharmacokinetic interaction between irinotecan and paclitaxel. They treated patients with an irinotecan infusion (over 90 minutes) on days 1 and 8 and paclitaxel (as a 3-hour infusion) on day 8 90 minutes after the end of irinotecan infusion, every 4 weeks. They reported that at level 2 of the dosing schedule (consisting of paclitaxel at 135 mg/m^2 and irinotecan at 50 mg/m^2), the AUC of irinotecan and its metabolites on day 8 were significantly higher than on day 1 *(89)*. This is a markedly different result than the previous trial, implying that there are important drug-to-drug interactions that need to be further elucidated.

Other combinations of docetaxel and irinotecan have also been evaluated in phase I and II studies. Masuda et al. presented the result of a phase I study in 32 patients with stage IIIB and IV NSCLC. Their recommended phase II dose was 50 mg/m^2 for irinotecan given on days 1, 8, and 15 and 50 mg/m^2 for docetaxel given on day 2 only, with cycles repeated every 28 days. The DLTs in this study were neutropenia and diarrhea. They reported a partial response in 11 of 30 (37%) patients with a median survival of 48 weeks and a 1-year survival rate of 44.9%. Importantly, pharmacokinetic analysis showed that irinotecan did not affect the pharmacokinetics of docetaxel *(90)*.

Adjei et al. have studied a different regimen of these drugs and have given these drugs in a three weekly regimen. In a phase I study in advanced cancers, they treated 18 patients with irinotecan iv over 90 minutes followed by docetaxel iv over 60 minutes every 3 weeks. The proposed phase II doses as per this trial are irinotecan at 160 mg/m^2 and docetaxel at 65 mg/m^2. The most common DLT in this report was myelosuppression, with grade 4 neutropenia observed in 11 of 18 (61%) patients. They reported dose-dependent diarrhea in this group with severe diarrhea in four patients who did not take adequate antidiarrheal treatment *(91)*.

Takeda et al. presented the result of a randomized phase II trial that compared docetaxel plus cisplatin (DC) versus docetaxel plus irinotecan (DI) in patients with advanced NSCLC. Fifty-three (44 who were able to be evaluated) patients were randomized to the DC arm and received docetaxel 60 mg/m^2 on day 1 and cisplatin 80 mg/m^2 on day 1. A total of 59 (54 who were able to be evaluated) patients were randomized to the DI arm to receive 60 mg/m^2 docetaxel on day 8 and irinotecan 60 mg/m^2 on days 1 and 8. Both regimens were repeated every 3 weeks. The response rates and myelosuppression were similar in both arms. In the DC arm, the response rate was 40.9%, whereas in the DI arm, response rate was 35.2%. The median time to progression was 19.9 weeks in the DC arm and 20.7 weeks in the DI arm. Median survival was 33.9 weeks in the DC and 39.1 weeks in the DI arm. The toxicity profile in the DC and DI arms was as follows: grade 3–4 anemia 16.7%/12.1%; grade 3–4 neutropenia 74.5%/74.6%; grade 3–4 thrombocytopenia 2.0%/1.7%; grade 2–4 serum creatinine 17.7%/13.6%, grade 2–4 vomiting 85.1%/53.5%, and grade 2–4 diarrhea 21.3%/41.3% (incidence of vomiting was higher in the DC arm whereas incidence of diarrhea was higher in the DI arm) *(92)*.

5.5. Irinotecan in Other Combinations

Studies have shown that combinations of paclitaxel and carboplatin have activity in advanced lung cancer and are well tolerated *(79)* (Table 16). This

Table 16
Irinotecan in Triplet Combinations in NSCLC

Author (Reference)	*Phase*	*Number*	*Regimen*	*Response (%)*	*Median survival*
Socinski *(93)*	I	32	Paclitaxel 175 mg/m^2 + Carboplatin AUC 5 Irinotecan 100 mg/m^2 day 1 q 3 weeks	39	11 months
Fujita *(94)*	I	22	Irinotecan 50 mg/m^2 Docetaxel 60 mg/m^2 Carboplatin AUC-5 (+ GCSF)	38.1	278 days

AUC, area under the curve; G-CSF, granulocyte colony-stimulating factor.

combination causes mild myelosuppression and a cumulative sensory neuropathy. Accordingly, it has been argued that the combination of an active third agent, such as irinotecan, to this combination is feasible and possibly beneficial.

Socinski et al. conducted a phase I trial in 33 patients with stage IIIB and IV NSCLC using a combination of irinotecan, paclitaxel, and carboplatin. The recommended dose was irinotecan at 100 mg/m^2, paclitaxel at 175 mg/m^2, and carboplatin at AUC 5 every 3 weeks. With this combination, they reported an objective tumor response in 39%, median survival of 11 months, time to tumor progression of 6.8 months, and a 1-year survival probability of 0.46. The DLTs were neutropenia and diarrhea. Grade 3/4 neutropenia was observed in 50% of patients, and six (19%) of these patients developed neutropenic fever and diarrhea *(93)*.

Fujita et al. studied a combination of irinotecan, docetaxel, and carboplatin with G-CSF support given every 3 weeks in 22 patients with stage IIIB and IV NSCLC. The dose that they arrived at was irinotecan 50 mg/m^2 plus docetaxel 60 mg/m^2 and carboplatin AUC 5, all administered on day 1 with G-CSF on days 5–15. The DLT in this study was diarrhea. The response rate was 38.1%, and the median survival was 278 days *(94)*.

Irinotecan has also been studied with gemcitabine with the recommended dose from a phase I analysis being gemcitabine 1000 mg/m^2 and irinotecan 100 mg/m^2 given on days 1 and 8 every 3 weeks, with no grade 4 hematological or any major nonhematological toxicity observed at this dose level *(95)*.

5.6. Irinotecan in Multimodality Therapy of NSCLC

Irinotecan has been studied concurrently with radiation therapy as a single agent and in combinations with other agents that have activity in lung cancer.

Takeda et al. used a combination of irinotecan given weekly with concurrent radiotherapy (60 Gy in 30, 2.0 Gy fractions over 6 weeks) in stage III NSCLC. The recommended phase II dose of irinotecan from this study was 45 mg/m^2. Three of five patients given 60 mg/m^2 developed grade 3/4 esophagitis and pneumonitis. One patient died of pneumonitis at 45 mg/m^2. In this study, the ORR was 76.9%, with a 1-year survival of 61.5% *(96)*.

A combination of irinotecan and cisplatin or carboplatin with radiation therapy has also been studied. Fukuda et al., in a phase I study, recommended irinotecan at 60 mg/m^2 on days 1, 8, and 15 with cisplatin at 80 mg/m^2 on day 1 with concurrent radiotherapy in patients with locally advanced NSCLC and reported a response rate of 65% with esophagitis, neutropenia, and thrombocytopenia being common toxicities *(97)*. Chakravarthy et al., in a phase I trial, have used escalating doses of weekly irinotecan (starting from 30 mg/m^2) and carboplatin AUC of 2 with concurrent radiation therapy. Nausea, vomiting, and esophagitis were the main DLTs in this study *(98)*.

6. CONCLUSIONS

The treatment of lung cancer is a Herculean task; the agents available to oncologists have not changed the perspective of this disease over the past several years. However, the introduction of camptothecins as a class of anticancer agents has definitely strengthened our therapeutic armamentarium.

We have focused our attention on the two agents in this class that are in widespread clinical use currently: topotecan and irinotecan. Topotecan is approved by the FDA for the treatment of patients with SCLC-sensitive disease after failure of first-line chemotherapy. Topotecan has also been demonstrated to have activity as a first-line agent in SCLC. Moreover, it is being studied in NSCLC patients with encouraging results. Interesting work is being carried out by combining topotecan with other agents to maximize its potential. Irinotecan is also an attractive agent to treat both SCLC and NSCLC patients. In particular, the combination of irinotecan with cisplatin in SCLC is very active and may even have better results than the currently used regimens, potentially changing the standard of care for the treatment of patients with this disease.

In this chapter, we have tried to present the published data in concise form. Interest in these drugs has stimulated numerous ongoing investigations, potentially expanding their role in cancer therapy, which have not been covered. Furthermore, many novel camptothecins in development have not been presented in this chapter. With continued research and new options, we are hopeful for the future of camptothecins in the treatment of patients with lung cancer.

REFERENCES

1. American Cancer Society. Cancer facts and figures 2003. Available at: http://www.cancer.org/docroot/STT/stt_0_2003.asp?sitearea=STT&level=1. Accessed June 28, 2004.
2. Ginsberg RJ, Vokes EE, Rosenzweig K. Non-small cell lung cancer. In: Cancer principles and practice of oncology, 6th ed. DeVita VT, Hellman S, Rosenberg SA, eds. Lippincott Williams & Wilkins, Pennsylvania, 2001, pp. 925–983.
3. Chute JP, Chen T, Feigal E, et al. 1999 Twenty years of phase III trials for patient with extensive stage SCLC: perceptive progress. J Clin Oncol 17:1794–1801.
4. Prescribing information for Hycamtin-Topotecan. Smith-Kline Beecham Pharmaceuticals, Philadelphia, Pennsylvania.
5. Perez-Soler R, Glisson BS, Lee JS, et al. 1996 Treatment of patients with small cell lung cancer refractory to etoposide and cisplatin with the topoisomerase I poison topotecan. J Clin Oncol 14:2785–2790.
6. Depierre A, von Powel J, Hans K, et al. 1997 Evaluation of topotecan (Hycamtin) in relapsed small cell lung cancer (SCLC). A multicenter phase II study. Lung Cancer Suppl abstract # 1267.

7. Ardizzoni A, Hansen H, Dombernowsky P, et al. 1997 Topotecan, a new active drug in the second line treatment of small cell lung cancer: a phase II study in patients with refractory and sensitive disease. J Clin Oncol 15:2090–2096.
8. von Powel J, Gatzemeier U, Pujol JL, et al. 2001 Phase II comparator study of oral versus intravenous topotecan in patients with chemosensitive small cell lung cancer. J Clin Oncol 19:1743–1749.
9. Gralla R, Eckardt J, von Pawel J, et al. 2003 Quality of life with single agent oral topotecan vs intravenous topotecan in patients with chemosensitive small cell lung cancer (SCLC). An international phase III study [abstract]. Lung Cancer.41(Suppl. 2):20.
10. Greco F, Burris H, Yardley D, et al. 2003 Phase II trial of weekly topotecan in the second-line treatment of small cell lung cancer. Lung Cancer 41 (Suppl. 2):237.
11. von Powel J, Schiller JH, Shepard FA, et al. 1999 Topotecan versus cyclophosphamide, doxorubicin and vincristine for the treatment of recurrent SCLC. J Clin Oncol 17:658–667.
12. Agelaki S, Kakolyris S, Palamidas P, et al. 2001 A dose escalation study of topotecan in combination with epirubicin in pretreated patients with small cell lung cancer. Lung Cancer 34:133–139.
13. Frasci G, Panza N, Comella P, et al. 1999 Cisplatin-topotecan-paclitaxel weekly administration with G-CSF support for ovarian and small cell lung cancer patients: a dose finding study. Ann Oncol 10:355–358.
14. Thompson D, Hainsworth JD, Burris HA, et al. 1999 A phase I trial of topotecan, paclitaxel and carboplatin with or without growth factor support. Proc Am Soc Clin Oncol 18:230a.
15. Schiller JH, KyungMann K, Hutson P, et al. 1996 Phase II study of topotecan in patients with extensive stage small-call carcinoma of lung: an Eastern cooperative oncology group trial. J Clin Oncol 14:2345–2352.
16. Jett JR, Day R, Levitt G, et al. 1997 Topotecan and paclitaxel in extensive stage small cell lung cancer (ED-SCLC) patients without prior therapy. Lung Cancer 18(Suppl 1).
17. Tweedy CR, Andrews DF, Ball T. 1999 Topotecan and paclitaxel in extensive stage small cell lung cancer as initial therapy. Proc Am Soc Clin Oncol 18:525a.
18. Jacobs SA, Jett JR, Belani CP, et al. 1999 Topotecan and paclitaxel, an active couplet, in untreated extensive disease small cell lung cancer. Proc Am Soc Clin Oncol (abstract 1814).
19. Lynch TJ, Herndon JE, Lyss AP, et al. 2000 Paclitaxel + topotecan + GCSF for previously untreated extensive small cell lung cancer: preliminary analysis of Cancer and Leukemia Group B (CALGB) 9430. Proc Am Soc Clin Oncol 18:470a.
20. Jett JR, Hatfield AK, Hillman S, et al. 2003 Alternating chemotherapy with etoposide plus cisplatin and topotecan plus paclitaxel in patients with untreated, extensive-stage small cell lung carcinoma: a phase II trial of the North Central Cancer Treatment Group. Cancer 97:2498–2503.
21. Schiller JH, Adak S, Cella D, et al. 2001 Topotecan versus observation after cisplatin plus etoposide in extensive-stage small-cell lung cancer: E7593—a phase III trial of the Eastern Cooperative Oncology Group. J Clin Oncol 19:2114–2212.
22. Murren J, Kraut E, Balcerzak S, et al. 1998 Phase II trial of topotecan and cyclophosphamide with G-CSF in high risk small cell lung cancer. Proc Am Soc Clin Oncol 17:495a.
23. Smith MJ, Spenser R, Zhang R, et al. 1998 Phase I/II a study of sequential ifosfamide and topotecan in patients with Small cell lung cancer. Proc Am Soc Clin Oncol 17:500a.

24. Johnson RK, McCabe FL, Tu Y, et al. 1992 Combination regimens with topotecan in animal tumor models. Ann Oncol 3(Suppl. 1) (abstract 107).
25. Whitacre CM, Zborowska E, Gordon NH, et al. 1997 Topotecan increases topoisomerase II alpha levels and sensitivity to treatment with etoposide in schedule dependent process. Cancer Res 57:1425–1428.
26. Sugimoto Y, Tsukahara S, Oh-hara T, et al. 1990 Elevated expression of DNA topoisomerase II in camptothecin resistant human tumor cell lines. Cancer Res 50:7962–7965.
27. O'Neill P, Clark PI, Smith D, et al. 2001 A phase I trial of a 5-day schedule of intravenous topotecan and etoposide in previously untreated patients with small-cell lung cancer. Oncology 61(Suppl. 1):25–29.
28. Reck M, Buchholz E, Groth G, et al. 2003 Phase-II trial of topotecan and etoposide in extensive disease small cell lung cancer. Lung Cancer 41:(Suppl. 2) 232.
29. Sorenson M, Jensen PB, Herrstedt J, et al. 2000 A dose escalating study of topotecan preceding cisplatin in previously untreated patients with small cell lung cancer. Ann Oncol 11:829–835.
30. Dediu M, Radut M, Crisan E, et al. 2000 Topotecan and fractionated cisplatin as first line chemotherapy for extensive small cell lung cancer (E-SCLC): a phase I/II study. Proc Am Soc Clin Oncol 19:533a.
31. Faucette SR, McCune JS, Donahue AE, et al. 1999 Impact of carboplatin sequence on myelosuppression and systemic exposure of topotecan in small cell lung cancer. Proc Am Soc Clin Oncol 18:210a.
32. Gillenwater HH, McCune, Donahue AE, et al. 2000 Phase I trial of topotecan, carboplatin, and etoposide for extensive stage small cell lung cancer (ES-SCLC). Proc Am Soc Clin Oncol 19:533a.
33. Frasci G, Nicolella G, Comella P, et al. 2001 A weekly regimen of cisplatin, paclitaxel and topotecan with granulocyte-colony stimulating factor support for patients with extensive disease small cell lung cancer a phase II study. Br J Cancer 84:1166–1171.
34. Hainsworth JD, Morrissey LH, Scullin DC Jr, et al. 2002 Paclitaxel, carboplatin and topotecan in the treatment of small cell lung cancer: a phase II trial of the Minnie Pearl Cancer Research Network. Cancer 94:2426–2433.
35. Perez-Soler R, Fossella FV, Glisson BS, et al. 1996 Phase II study of topotecan in patients with advanced non-small cell cancer previously untreated with chemotherapy. J Clin Oncol 14:503–513.
36. Perez-Soler R, Khuri F, Pisters KM, et al. 1997 Phase II study of topotecan in patients with squamous carcinoma of the lung previously untreated with chemotherapy. Proc Am Soc Clin Oncol 16:450a.
37. Lynch TJ, Kalish L, Strauss G, et al. 1994 Phase II study of topotecan in metastatic non small cell lung cancer. J Clin Oncol 12:347–352.
38. Rowinsky E, Growchow L, Hendricks C, et al. 1992 Phase I and pharmacologic study of topotecan: a novel topoisomerase I inhibitor. J Clin Oncol 10:647–656.
39. Kindler HL, Kris MG, Smith IE et al. 1997 Continuous infusion topotecan as first line therapy in patients with non-small cell lung cancer: a phase II study. Proc Am Soc Clin Oncol 16:472a.
40. Weitz JJ, Marschke Jr. R, Sloan JA, et al. 2000 A randomized phase II trial of two schedules of topotecan for the treatment of advanced stage non-small cell lung cancer. Lung Cancer 28:157–162.
41. White SC, Cheeseman Sue, Thatcher N, et al. 2000 Phase II study of oral topotecan in advanced non-small cell lung cancer. Clin Cancer Res 6:868–873.

42. Raymond E, Burris HA, Rowinsky EK, et al. 1997 Phase I study of daily times five topotecan and single injection of cisplatin in patients with previously untreated non small cell lung carcinoma. Ann Oncol 8:1003–1008.
43. Bildat S, Eberhardt W, Song HQ, et al. 2000 A phase I trial of topotecan (T) in combination with cisplatin (P) in patients with non-small cell lung cancer (NSCLC) Stage IV. Proc Am Soc Clin Oncol 19:228a.
44. Wiesenfeld M, Marks R, Grill J et al: 1997 A randomized phase II study of topotecan and cisplatin with filgrastim (GCSF) versus topotecan and paclitaxel (Taxol) with filgrastim in patients with advanced non small cell lung cancer. Proc Am Soc Clin Oncol (abstract 1755).
45. Hansen HH, Sorensen JB, et al. 1997 Efficacy of single agent Gemcitabine in advanced NSCLC: a review. Semin Oncol 24:38–41.
46. Rosell R, Tonato M, Sandler A, et al. 1998 The activity of Gemcitabine plus cisplatin in randomized trials in untreated patients with advanced non small cell lung cancer. Semin Oncol 25:27–34.
47. Rinaldi D, Lormand N, Brierre J, et al. 2001 A phase I-II trial of topotecan and gemcitabine in patients with previously treated, advanced non small cell lung cancer (LOA-3). Cancer Invest 19:467–4784.
48. Guarino M, Schneider C, Grubbs S, et al. 2000 Dose escalation study of weekly topotecan, cisplatin and gemcitabine in inoperable or recurrent NSCLC. Proc Am Soc Clin Oncol 19:541a.
49. Taguchi T, Wakui A, Hasegawa T, et al. 1990 Phase I study of CPT-11.Research group of CPT-11. Gan To Kagaku Ryoho 17:115–120.
50. Negoro S, Fukuoka M, Masuda N, et al. 1991 Phase I study of weekly intravenous infusion of CPT-11, a new derivative of camptothecin, in the treatment of advanced non small cell lung cancer. J Natl Cancer Inst 83:1164–1168.
51. Negoro S, Fukuoka M, Niitani H, et al. 1991 A phase II study of CPT-11, a camptothecin derivative, in patients with primary lung cancer. CPT-11 Cooperative Study Group. Gan To Kagaku Ryoho 18:1013–1019.
52. Masuda N, Fukuoka M, Kusunoki Y, et al. 1992 CPT-11: a new derivative of camptothecin for the treatment of refractory and relapsed small cell lung cancer. J Clin Oncol 10:1225–1229.
53. Le Chevalier T, Ibrahim N, Chomy P, et al. 1997 A phase II study of irinotecan (CPT-11) in patients with small cell lung cancer progressing after initial response to first line chemotherapy. Proc Am Soc Clin Oncol 16:450a.
54. DeVore RF, Blanke CD, Denham CA, et al. 1998 Phase II study of Irinotecan (CPT-11) in patients with previously treated SCLC. Proc Am Soc Clin Oncol 17:457a.
55. Kudoh S, Takada M, Masuda N, et al. 1993 Enhanced antitumor efficacy of a combination of CPT-11, a new derivative of camptothecin and cisplatin against human tumor xenografts. Jpn J Cancer Res 84:203–207.
56. Kudoh S, Fujiwara Y, Takada Y, et al. 1998 Phase II study of irinotecan combined with cisplatin in patients with previously untreated SCLC. J Clin Oncol 6:1068–1074.
57. Okishio K, Furuse K, Kawahara M. 1998 A phase II study of irinotecan (CPT-11) and cisplatin in previously treated SCLC. Proc Am Soc Clin Oncol 17:497a.
58. Noda K, Nishiwaski Y, Kawahara M, et al. 2002 Irinotecan plus cisplatin compared with etoposide plus cisplatin for extensive small cell lung cancer. N Engl J Med 346:85–91.

59. Fukuda M, Fukuda M, Oka M, et al. 1999 Phase I study of irinotecan combined with carboplatin in previously untreated solid cancers. Clin Cancer Res 5:3963–3969.
60. Suguira S, Saka H, Ando M, et al. 1998 Phase II and pharmacokinetic/pharmacodynamic study of carboplatin and irinotecan in patients with SCLC. Proc Am Soc Clin Oncol 17:502a.
61. Hirose T, Horichi N, Ohmori T, et al. 2003 Phase II study of irinotecan and carboplatin in patients with the refractory or relapsed small cell lung cancer. Lung Cancer 40:333–338.
62. Naka N, Kawahara M, Okishio K, et al. 2002 Phase II study of weekly irinotecan and carboplatin for refractory or relapsed small-cell lung cancer. Lung Cancer 37:319–323.
63. Masuda N, Matsui K, Negoro S, et al. 1998 Combination of irinotecan and etoposide for treatment of refractory and relapsed SCLC. J Clin Oncol 16:3329–3334.
64. Nakamura S, Kudoh S, Komuta K, et al. 1999 Phase II study of irinotecan combined with etoposide for previously untreated extensive disease SCLC. Proc Am Soc Clin Oncol 18:470a.
65. Sekine I, Nishiwaki Y, Noda K, et al. 2003 Randomized phase II study of cisplatin, irinotecan and etoposide combinations administered weekly or every 4 weeks for extensive small-cell lung cancer (JCOG9902-DI). Ann Oncol 14:709–714.
66. Rushing DA, Tipping SJ, Clouse LH, et al. 1999 Phase I study of the combination of irinotecan (CPT-11) and paclitaxel (taxol) in previously treated patients (pts) with small cell carcinoma of the lung (SCCL). Proc Am Soc Clin Oncol 18:484a.
67. Kudoh S, Fujiwara Y, Takada Y, et al. 1998 Phase II study of irinotecan combined with cisplatin in patients with previously untreated small-cell lung cancer. West Japan Lung Cancer Group. J Clin Oncol 16:1068–1074.
68. Fukuoka M, Niitani H, Suzuki A, et al. 1992 A phase II study of CPT-11, a new derivative of camptothecin, for previously untreated non-small cell lung caner. J Clin Oncol 10:16–20.
69. Negoro S, Fukuoka M, Niitani H, et al. 1991 A phase II study of CPT-11, a camptothecin derivative, in patients with primary lung cancer. CPT-11 cooperative study group. Gan To Kagaku Ryoho 18:1013–1019.
70. Baker L, Khan R, Lynch T, et al. 1997 Phase II study of irinotecan (CPT-11) in advanced non small cell lung cancer. Proc Am Soc Clin Oncol 16:461a.
71. Non-small cell lung cancer collaborative group; chemotherapy in non-small cell lung cancer: a meta-analysis using updated data on individual patients from 52 randomized clinical trials. 1995 BMJ. 311:899–909.
72. DeVore RF, Johnson DH, Crawford J, et al. 1999 Phase II study of irinotecan plus cisplatin in patients with advanced non small cell lung cancer. J Clin Oncol. 17:2710–2720.
73. Jagasia MH, Langer CJ, Johnson DH, et al. 2001 Weekly irinotecan and cisplatin in advanced non small cell lung cancer: a multicenter phase II study. Clin Cancer Res. 7:68–73.
74. Mori K, Machida S, Yoshida T, et al. 1999 A phase II study of irinotecan and infusional cisplatin with recombinant human granulocyte colony stimulating factor support for advanced non small cell lung cancer. Cancer Chemother Pharmacol 43:467–470.

75. Ueoka H, Kiura K, Hiraki S et al. 1999 Fractionated administration of cisplatin (CDDP) and irinotecan (CPT-11) in patients with stage IIIB and IV non small cell lung cancer: a phase II study. Proc Am Soc Clin Oncol 18:525a.
76. Masuda N, Fukuoka M, Negoro S, et al. 1999 Randomized trial comparing cisplatin (CDDP) and irinotecan (CPT-11) versus CDDP and vindesine (VDS) versus CPT-11 alone in non small cell lung cancer, a multicenter phase III study. Proc Am Soc Clin Oncol 18:459a.
77. Niho S, Nagao K, Nishiwaki Y, et al. 1999 Randomized multicenter phase III trial of irinotecan (CPT-11) and cisplatin (CDDP) versus CDDP and vindesine (VDS) in patients with advanced NSCLC. Proc Am Soc Clin Oncol18:492a.
78. Fukuoka M, Nagao K, Ohashi Y, et al. 2000 Impact of irinotecan (CPT-11) and cisplatin (CDDP) on survival in previously untreated metastatic non small cell lung cancer. Proc Am Soc Clin Oncol 19:495a.
79. Kelly K, Crowley J, Bunn PA Jr, et al. 2000 Randomized phase III trial of paclitaxel plus carboplatin versus vinorelbine plus cisplatin in the treatment of patients with advanced non small cell lung cancer: a southwest oncology group trial. J Clin Oncol 19:3210–3218.
80. Schiller JH, Harrignton D, Belani CP, et al. 2002 Comparison of four chemotherapy regimens for advanced non-small-cell lung cancer. N Engl J Med 346:92–98.
81. Takeda K, Negoro S, Takifuji N, et al. 2001 Dose escalation study of irinotecan combined with carboplatin for advanced non small cell lung cancer. Cancer Chemother Pharmacol 48:104–108.
82. Fukuda M, Oka M, Soda H, et al. 1999 Phase I study of Irinotecan combined with carboplatin in previously untreated solid cancers. Clin Cancer Res 5:3963–3969.
83. Okamoto H, Nagamoto A, Kunitoh H, et al. 1998 A phase I clinical and pharmacologic study of carboplatin and irinotecan regimen with recombinant human granulocyte–colony stimulation factor in the treatment of patients with advanced NSCLC. Cancer 82:2166–2172.
84. Mukohara T, Takeda K, Miyazaki M, et al. 2000 Phase II study of irinotecan (CPT-11) and carboplatin (CBDCA) in advanced non-small-cell lung cancer (NSCLC). Proc Am Soc Clin Oncol 19:534a.
85. Fossella V, Devore R, Kerr RN, et al. 2000 Randomized phase III trial of docetaxel versus vinorelbine or ifosfamide in patients with advanced NSCLC previously treated with platinum containing chemotherapy regimens. The TAX 320 NSCLC study group. J Clin Oncol 18:2095–2103.
86. Chou TC, Motzer RJ, Tong Y, et al. 1994 Computerized quantitation of synergism and antagonism of taxol, topotecan and cisplatin against human teratocarcinoma cell growth: a rational approach to clinical protocol design. J Natl Cancer Inst 86:1517–1524.
87. Murren JR, Peccerillo K, DiStasio SA, et al. 2000 Dose escalation and pharmacokinetic study of irinotecan in combination with paclitaxel in patients with advanced cancer. Cancer Chemother Pharmacol 46:43–50.
88. Rosen P, Schaaf LJ, Knuth DW, et al. 1999 Phase I and pharmacokinetic trial of CPT-11 and paclitaxel in patients with advanced cancer. Proc Am Soc Clin Oncol 18:177a.
89. Asai G, Yamamoto N, Sakai S, et al. 2000 Paclitaxel affects pharmacokinetics of irinotecan and its metabolites. Proc Am Soc Clin Oncol 19:199a.
90. Masuda N, Negoro S, Kudoh S, et al. 2000 Phase I and pharmacologic study of docetaxel and irinotecan in advanced NSCLC. J Clin Oncol 18:2996–3003.

91. Adjei AA, Klein CE, Kastrissios H, et al. 2000 Phase I and pharmacokinetics study of irinotecan and docetaxel in patients with advanced solid tumors: preliminary evidence of clinical activity. J Clin Oncol 18:1116–1123.
92. Takeda K, Yamamoto N, Negoro S, et al. 2000 Randomized phase II study of docetaxel (DOC) plus cisplatin (CDDP) versus DOC plus irinotecan in advanced non-small-cell lung cancer (NSCLC); a West Japan Thoracic Oncology Group (WJTOG) Study. Proc Am Soc Clin Oncol 19:497a.
93. Socinski MA, Sandler AB, Miller LL, et al. 2001 Phase I trial of the combination of irinotecan, paclitaxel and carboplatin in patients with NSCLC. J Clin Oncol 19:1078–1087.
94. Fujita A, Takabatake H, Tagaki S, et al. 2000 Phase I study of carboplatin, docetaxel and irinotecan with recombinant human granulocyte colony stimulating factor support in patients with advanced NSCLC. Anticancer Drugs 11:821–824.
95. Rocha Lima CM, Eckardt JR, Leong SS, et al. 1999 Single agent gemcitabine and gemcitabine/irinotecan combination (irinogem) in NSCLC. Semin Oncol 26(5 Suppl. 16):43–50.
96. Takeda K, Negoro S, Kudoh S, et al. 1999 Phase I/II study of weekly irinotecan and concurrent radiation therapy for locally advanced NSCLC. Br J Cancer 79:1462–1467.
97. Fukuda M, Fukuda M, Soda H, et al. 1999 Phase I study of irinotecan and cisplatin with concurrent thoracic radiotherapy in locally advanced NSCLC. Proc Am Soc Clin Oncol (abstract 1796).
98. Chakravarthy A, Choy H, DeVore RD, et al. 2000 Phase I trial of outpatient weekly irinotecan and carboplatin with concurrent radiation therapy for stage III unresectable NSCLC: a Vanderbilt Cancer Center Affiliate Network (VCCAN) trial. Proc Am Soc Clin Oncol 19:520a.

17 Use of Camptothecins in the Treatment of Leukemia and Related Disorders

Benjamin M. F. Mow, MD, *and Scott H. Kaufmann,* MD, PhD

CONTENTS

1. INTRODUCTION

Even though current therapy is capable of inducing remissions in 60–80% of adults with acute leukemia *(1,2)*, the vast majority of patients are not cured *(3–5)*. This is particularly true for the elderly, who account for the majority of cases of acute myelogenous leukemia (AML) *(6,7)*. Because of unrelated medical problems, as well as a higher incidence of certain resistance mechanisms (e.g., overexpression of the mdr1 multidrug transporter), eradicating AML in these patients has been particularly problematic *(8,9)*. These clinical observations highlight the need for new agents to treat AML.

Better treatments are also needed for patients with myelodysplastic syndrome (MDS), a group of clonal bone marrow disorders characterized by

Camptothecins in Cancer Therapy
Edited by: V. R. Adams and T. G. Burke © Humana Press Inc., Totowa, NJ

dysplastic hematopoiesis, excessive apoptosis, and a propensity to develop into AML *(10,11)*. This group of disorders includes chronic myelomonocytic leukemia (CMML), a pathogenetically and morphologically distinct entity that has a median survival of 8–30 months *(12)*, and the disorders refractory anemia, refractory anemia with ringed sideroblasts, refractory anemia with excess blasts (RAEB), and refractory anemia with excess blasts in transformation (RAEB-T). Of particular interest for the present review are RAEB and RAEB-T: patients with these disorders have median survivals of 6–12 months and <6 months, respectively *(13–15)*. Because the results of treatment using chemotherapy, growth factors, or hematopoietic stem cell transplantation have been disappointing in these high-grade categories of MDS *(16)*, new therapeutic agents are needed.

As reviewed elsewhere in this book (*see* Chapter 1), the camptothecins (CPTs) are a group of anticancer agents that target the nuclear enzyme topoisomerase I (TOP-I). According to current models, these agents primarily affect the relegation step of this enzyme, thereby transiently stabilizing covalent TOP-I–DNA complexes. An interaction of these covalent TOP-I–DNA complexes with advancing replication forks (reviewed in ref. *17*) or, under some circumstances, transcription complexes *(18)* results in the formation of DNA double-strand breaks, which then set into motion biochemical events leading to cell-cycle arrest or apoptosis (*see* Chapter 4).

Based on this unique mechanism of action, one can make several predictions about the cellular features that would render cells more or less resistant to this class of agents. First, cells expressing elevated levels of certain drug exporters (e.g., mdr1 [reviewed in ref. *19*] or the more recently cloned transporter BCRP *[20–22]*) could potentially exhibit resistance as a consequence of diminished drug accumulation. Second, cells with decreased TOP-I levels would stabilize fewer covalent TOP-I–DNA complexes and sustain less toxicity during drug treatment (reviewed in refs. *19* and *23*). Third, because the interaction of TOP-I complexes with advancing replication complexes is particularly effective at generating DNA double-strand breaks, cells that are not traversing S-phase would be more resistant to this class of agents *(24,25)*. Finally, because CPTs kill cells by inducing apoptosis *(26–30)*, cellular changes that alter the coupling between DNA damage and activation of the apoptotic machinery would be expected to affect sensitivity to this class of agents.

In the sections that follow, we will review clinical trials in which CPTs have been administered to patients with leukemias or MDS. In addition, because these diseases are ideally suited for the evaluation of potential mechanisms of resistance that might occur in the clinical setting, we will describe some of the assays performed to evaluate the actions of CPT analogs in clinical leukemia isolates from patients receiving these drugs.

2. ANTILEUKEMIC ACTIVITY OF CAMPTOTHECIN

One of the two original phase I trials of CPT included a patient with relapsed AML *(31)*. This patient experienced clearance of blasts from his peripheral circulation, a decrease in his marrow blasts from 80 to 20%, and resolution of splenomegaly. In the face of negative phase II trials of CPT for colon carcinoma and metastatic melanoma, as well as unpredictable and unmanageable toxicity *(32,33)*, this potential antileukemic activity of CPT was ignored.

3. ANTILEUKEMIC ACTIVITY OF SINGLE-AGENT TOPOTECAN

3.1. Phase I Studies

The demonstration that CPT is active in murine P388 leukemia isolates that are resistant to a variety of other agents *(34,35)* prompted renewed interest in CPT in the 1980s. Based on subsequent studies, two water-soluble CPT derivatives, topotecan and irinotecan, have been licensed for the treatment of patients with various solid tumors (*see* Chapters 11 and 12). Both of these, as well as other derivatives, have been tested in patients with various leukemias.

Phase I trials in solid-tumor patients demonstrated that neutropenia was the principal dose-limiting toxicity (DLT) of topotecan on all schedules tested *(19,36)*. The observation that this myelosuppression was brief and noncumulative suggested that topotecan spares the hematopoietic stem cell compartment. Furthermore, nonhematological side effects such as nausea, vomiting, diarrhea, rash, fever, and fatigue were mild and infrequent at the maximum tolerated dose (MTD) *(19,36,37)*.

Based on the observation that CPTs are particularly toxic to cells in S phase *(25,38)* and the realization that only a small percentage of blasts pass through S phase during a 24-hour exposure period *(39–41)*, initial phase I studies of topotecan in patients with hematological malignancies (Table 1) used a continuous infusion regimen. Kantarjian et al. administered escalating doses of topotecan by 5-day continuous infusion (CI) to 27 heavily pretreated acute leukemia patients, 70% of whom were receiving topotecan as their second or subsequent salvage regimen *(42)*. The DLT was mucositis, which was observed in two of five patients who received 11.8 mg/m^2 topotecan per course. Another patient treated at this dose level developed prolonged myelosuppression. At the MTD of 2 mg/m^2/day, these toxicities were not observed. Other nonhematological side effects, including nausea, vomiting, and diarrhea, were also uncommon. An 11% complete response (CR) rate was observed, with a higher response rate in patients receiving

Table 1
Leukemia Trials of Topotecan Administered as a Single Agent

Reference	*Disease type*	*No. of patients/ median age*	*Dosing schedule*	*Response rates*	*DLT*	*Comments*
42	AML, ALL, AUL, CML-B	27/51	CI × 5 days with MTD at 2 $mg/m^2/day$	11% CR 7% PR 4% HI	Mucositis	Response did not correlate with in vitro covalent complex assay
43	AML, ALL, CML-B	17/40	CI × 5 days with MTD at 2.1/$mg/m^2/day$	1 CR in CML-B 1 PR in AML	Mucositis	Response rates showed no correlation to in vitro studies
45	T-cell ALL, B-progenito ALL, B-cell ALL, AML	13/11	CI × 5 days with individualized dosing based on MTSE at 4 ng/mL	1 CR 1 PR	Mucositis	
49	AML, ALL, CML-B	14/50	30 minute daily infusion × 5 days with MTD at 4.5 $mg/m^2/day$	0% CR	High fever, rigors, hemolytic anemia, hyperbilirubinemia	
47	AML, ALL	49/9	30 minute daily infsion × 9 days with MTD at 2.4 $mg/m^2/day$	2 CR, 6 PR	Typhlitis, diarrhea, mucositis	
50	High-risk ALL	13/45	CI × 5 days with MTD at 2.1 $mg/m^2/day$ followed by standard ALL therapy	1/13 CR 6/13 HI	Mucositis, diarrhea	Terminated prematurely, 2 deaths. Bcl-2 levels were lower in responders

58	CMML, MDS	60/66	CI × 5 days with MTD at 2 mg/m²/day	31% CR 8/11 cyto-genetic	Mucositis	Mortality 20%, median survival 10.5 months
59	CLL	12/63	30 minute daily infusion × 5 days with MTD at 4.5 mg/m²/day	0% CR		No activity

AML, acute myeloid leukemia; ALL, acute lymphocytic leukemia; AUL, acute undifferentiated leukemia; CI, continuous infusion, CML-B, blast crisis of chronic myelogenous leukemia; CR, complete remission; HI, hematological improvement; MTD, maximum tolerated dose; MTSE, maximum tolerated systemic exposure; NR, not reported; PR, partial remission.

topotecan as their first salvage regimen. Although the report of Kantarjian et al. did not contain any pharmacokinetic analysis, a filter binding assay was used to examine levels of topotecan-stabilized covalent TOP-I–DNA complexes. These complexes were below the limit of detection when blasts were isolated directly from drug-treated patients.

The same 5-day CI schedule was used in a National Cancer Institute–sponsored phase I trial in acute leukemia patients performed by Rowinsky and coworkers *(43)* (*see* Table 1). The MTD was determined to be 2.1 mg/m^2/day, with mucositis again being the DLT. Although transient clearance of peripheral blasts was observed in the majority of patients, the CR rate was 12%. Pharmacokinetic analysis revealed that steady-state topotecan concentrations (lactone + carboxylate) were 26 ± 7 n*M* at the MTD. Evaluation of the response of blasts to topotecan ex vivo revealed that the concentrations required to inhibit leukemic colony formation by 90% ranged from 6 to 22 n*M*. Further examination revealed a wide range of TOP-I expression among the various pretreatment leukemia samples, with many specimens containing elevated levels of TOP-I relative to normal marrow. Unfortunately, differences in pretreatment cell cycle distribution, P-glycoprotein–mediated drug efflux, and pretreatment TOP-I levels did not appear to explain the variations in sensitivity to topotecan in vitro or in vivo *(43,44)*. The observed decrease in circulating blasts was, however, positively correlated with topotecan dosage.

In an attempt to individualize treatment, Furman and coworkers performed a pharmacokinetically guided phase I trial of topotecan administered as a 5-day CI to pediatric patients with relapsed and refractory leukemias *(45)*. Consistent with this type of trial design, the dose was adjusted based on pharmacokinetic data to achieve a target area under the concentration-vs-time curve; and the target area under the curve was increased in a predefined manner with each successive cohort until the maximum tolerated systemic exposure (MTSE) was achieved. To perform this trial, Furman and coworkers measured steady-state topotecan lactone concentrations by high-performance liquid chromatography and adjusted the infusion rate if the actual concentration differed from the target concentration by >20%. The MTSE was determined to be 4 ng/mL (9.5 n*M*) × 5 days. Mucositis was the DLT. Responses were observed in 2 of 13 (15%) children treated (*see* Table 1). Although peripheral blasts cleared completely after seven courses in six additional patients, progressive disease was noted before or soon after the scheduled time of retreatment. The authors argued that this approach adjusted for interpatient pharmacokinetic variability, thereby permitting more rapid and precise determination of a MTSE that can be used in subsequent phase II trials. Interestingly, the MTSE determined in this fashion was in remarkable agreement with the calculated lactone concentration of 3.8 ng/mL (8.6 n*M*) at the MTD in the more traditional phase I study of Rowinsky et al. *(43)*. Moreover, the pharm-acokinetically guided trial did not provide any new insight into the optimal dose for treating acute leukemia, because responses were still seen at targeted exposures as low as 1.5 ng/mL (3.6 n*M*) topotecan lactone.

To build on xenograft data showing that increasing the topotecan dose beyond a certain threshold offered no advantage, whereas prolonging the exposure time above that threshold resulted in increased efficacy *(46)*, Furman et al. examined a schedule involving continuous topotecan infusion for up to 12 consecutive days every 3 weeks in children with acute leukemia *(47)*. In this Phase I study, the DLTs were typhlitis, diarrhea, and mucositis; and the MTD was 2.4 mg/m^2/day for 9 days. Among the 49 patients (24 AML, 25 ALL) treated on this trial, there were 2 CRs and 6 PRs.

An alternative approach for achieving prolonged drug exposure would be daily or almost daily oral dosing. With this in mind, Beran and colleagues conducted a phase I trial of oral topotecan administered on days 1–5, 8–12, and 15–19 of cycles lasting 5 to 7 weeks in patients with AML and high-risk MDS *(48)*. The DLT was grade 3/4 diarrhea, nausea, and vomiting; the MTD was 1.4 mg/m^2/day. Drug levels in blood or bone marrow were not reported. Among 26 patients entered on study, there were 4 CRs (15%).

Because administration of topotecan on multiple consecutive days has proven more effective than continuous drug infusion in solid tumor patients (reviewed in Chapter 12), Rowinsky and coworkers *(49)* also evaluated the feasibility of a 30-minute daily topotecan infusion for 5 consecutive days in patients with refractory or relapsed acute leukemia (*see* Table 1). Mucositis was not observed on this schedule. Instead, the DLT was an unusual constellation of side effects that included high fever, rigors, precipitous anemia, and hyperbilirubinemia. These effects were observed at a dose level of 5.75 mg/m^2/day but not at the MTD of 4.5 mg/m^2/day. No CRs were observed on this schedule. Pharmacokinetic analysis revealed that topotecan lactone concentrations peaked at 90–140 n*M* at the MTD and decreased with a terminal half-life of 2–4 hours. Additional studies revealed that pretreatment TOP-I content of leukemic blasts varied widely but did not correlate with clinical response. In contrast to studies reported in tissue culture cell lines, these was no evidence in the leukemia samples that levels of the related enzyme topoisomerase II (TOP-II) were inversely related to TOP-I levels. This observation has implications for the use of topotecan in combination with TOP-II poisons, as will be discussed in the section 4.1.

3.2. Phase II Trials

Gore et al. performed a phase II study of topotecan in high-risk untreated ALL patients *(50)*. The observation that TOP-I levels were particularly high in ALL blasts *(43)*, coupled with the demonstration that topotecan exhibited significant antileukemic activity in a severe combined immunodeficiency

(SCID) mouse model of human B-lineage ALL *(30)*, provided the rationale for studying topotecan in ALL. Based on evidence that the activity of investigational agents is much higher in untreated patients than in relapsed or refractory cases *(51–56)*, Gore and coworkers chose to study untreated ALL patients using a so-called "window" trial design. After topotecan was administered as a 2.1 mg/m^2/day CI for 5 days, patients were observed until day 21 to assess response. If there was a CR or no response, patients were then treated with aggressive conventional chemotherapy to avoid compromising their chances of remission. If a partial or minimal response was observed, a second cycle of topotecan was given before standard treatment. In this trial, the primary nonhematological toxicities attributable to topotecan were mucositis and diarrhea. Although topotecan induced marked cytolytic responses in all 14 ALL patients, evidence of residual leukemia was universally observed in day 14 bone marrow samples. Two patients expired during induction therapy. The one patient who achieved a CR remained in remission for 17 months before expiring from central nervous system relapse. Ancillary studies again showed no relationship between steady-state plasma topotecan concentrations and hematological response or toxicity. Although the low response rate and small sample size made it difficult to draw firm conclusions about factors that might have affected topotecan sensitivity during this trial, it was observed that the CR and two partial responses occurred in patients whose blasts had the lowest levels of the anti-apoptotic protein Bcl-2.

The activity of topotecan in refractory/relapsed AML was evaluated in a still unpublished phase II trial performed at the M.D. Anderson Cancer Center *(57)*. No CRs were seen among the 14 patients enrolled. However, the possibility of false negative results is very real when new drugs are evaluated in relapsed/refractory patients whose prior therapy might have selected for blasts harboring a variety of mechanisms of drug resistance.

Another phase II study evaluated the activity of single-agent topotecan in 60 patients with MDS *(58)*. The median age of these patients was 66 years, with 83% being older than 60 years of age. Topotecan was administered as a CI of 2 mg/m^2/day for 5 days. An overall response rate of 31% was seen in this study, with a higher response rate for MDS (37%) than for CMML (27%). Responses were more frequent in chemotherapy-naive patients and in those whose clones lacked Ras mutations. These responses were, however, obtained at the cost of considerable morbidity and mortality. Febrile neutropenia occurred in 85%, grade 3/4 mucositis in 23%, grade 3/4 diarrhea in 17%, and nausea and vomiting in 28%. Moreover, there was a 20% mortality during the first 4 weeks of topotecan treatment. With a median follow-up of 31 months, the median survival was only 10.5 months. Although encouraging activity was seen in some patients with poor prognosis karyotypes, it is unclear whether this treatment altered the dismal prognosis associated with this group of disorders.

O'Brien and coworkers completed a phase II trial of topotecan in chronic lymphocytic leukemia (CLL) patients *(59)*. When 12 patients were treated with daily infusions of 4.5 mg/m^2/day for 5 days, no responses were observed. Based on earlier observations that continuous exposure to 1.6 μ*M* topotecan for 72 hours was required to kill 50% of a population of CLL cells in vitro *(60)*, as well as the pharmacokinetic parameters described previously *(43,49)*, the negative results of the CLL trial were perhaps predictable. Several factors might have contributed to this lack of activity, including the low percentage of S-phase cells and the almost universal expression of the antiapoptotic protein Bcl-2 in CLL.

In summary, the most widely studied schedule of topotecan in hematological malignancies is a 5-day CI. On this schedule, the MTD of 2.1 mg/m^2/day is approximately threefold higher than the MTD achieved in solid tumor patients *(43)*. At this dose, topotecan has shown modest activity in clonal myeloid hematological disorders. The principal nonhematological toxicity observed is mucositis. Although the myelosuppression observed with topotecan is reversible and noncumulative, it is sufficiently prolonged at the leukemic MTD that there is a significant risk of neutropenic infections and death. Moreover, the ancillary studies performed to date have generally failed to predict clinical responsiveness, thereby preventing the individualization of treatment. Because of the toxicity, limited efficacy, and inability to prospectively identify patients who might benefit from this agent, treatment of MDS and leukemia patients with single-agent topotecan is strongly discouraged outside the context of clinical trials.

4. TOPOTECAN-CONTAINING COMBINATIONS

The results cited previously have led to the conclusion that administration of topotecan alone is unlikely to significantly benefit patients with leukemia. Because this drug has some activity, albeit limited, against hematological malignancies, there has been interest in examining the effect of combining it with other agents. The rationale for these combinations has been extensively reviewed *(61)*. In the paragraphs that follow, we briefly describe the preclinical results that support the testing of these combinations and then review the results observed in the clinical setting.

4.1. Sequential Topotecan and Etoposide

When the early clinical studies of TOP-I poisons were being planned, there was considerable enthusiasm for combining these agents with TOP-II poisons such as etoposide or daunorubicin. The original basis for these studies was the observation that tissue culture cells selected in vitro for resistance to TOP-I poisons sometimes contained elevated TOP-II levels and displayed hypersensitivity to etoposide *(62,63)*. On the other hand, simultaneous administration of TOP-I and TOP-II poisons to unselected tissue culture cells resulted in antagonistic effects, in part because the TOP-I poisons inhibited the ongoing RNA synthesis that was required to convert etoposide-stabilized TOP-II–DNA complexes into cytotoxic DNA double-strand breaks *(64,65)*. When the agents were administered sequentially, however, the cytotoxic effects of the combination could be at least additive and sometimes synergistic *(66,67)*. Similar schedule dependence was observed in vivo using murine L1210 leukemia model *(68)*.

A phase I study of topotecan and etoposide in leukemia patients was performed by the National Cancer Institute of Canada (Table 2) *(69)*. In light of the preclinical data cited previously, topotecan was administered as a 5-day CI followed by bolus etoposide on days 6–8. Eleven patients with refractory acute leukemia (median age 46) were entered on study. Mucositis was observed at a topotecan dose of 1.5 mg/m^2/day combined with etoposide 100 mg/m^2/day. Grade 4 neutropenia and thrombocytopenia were also noted in all courses; and one patient died of neutropenic sepsis. These toxicities were sufficiently severe that no further dose escalation was attempted. A hematological and cytogenetic CR was seen in a CML patient in blast crisis (response rate 9%). Ancillary studies failed to confirm the reciprocal regulation of TOP-I and TOP-II levels observed in tissue culture cells. Although TOP-II levels increased in peripheral blasts within 72 hours of starting topotecan, they returned to near baseline by day 5 despite continued topotecan administration. In bone marrow blasts, TOP-II levels actually appeared to decrease by day 5. The expected increase in TOP-II levels at the time of etoposide treatment was not observed.

A second phase I study of sequential topotecan and etoposide was performed by Cooper and coworkers *(70)*. In this study, patients with refractory or relapsed acute leukemia were treated with escalating doses of topotecan administered as a CI over 72 hours followed by daily infusions of 100 mg/m^2/day etoposide on days 4–8. Grade 3/4 neutropenia and thrombocytopenia were noted in all courses. Toxicities at 1.10–1.35 mg/m^2/day topotecan included two deaths resulting from neutropenic sepsis, as well as grade 3/4 hyperbilirubinemia (two patients) and mucositis, diarrhea, and peripheral neuropathy (one patient each). The most common grade 3/4 nonhematological toxicities—mucositis, diarrhea, and reversible hepatic dysfunction—correlated with plasma topotecan concentrations. CRs were observed in 2 of 29 patients. Ancillary studies again failed to confirm the expected reciprocal regulation of TOP-I and TOP-II. In particular, TOP-I and TOP-II both decreased during the topotecan infusion in all except one patient and did not correlate with response. This topotecan-induced decrease in TOP-II levels might be explained, in part, by the induction of p53 and resulting downregulation of TOP-IIα gene transcription observed in leukemic cell lines *(71)*.

4.2. Simultaneous Topotecan and Liposomal Daunorubicin

In an attempt to identify a non–cytarabine-containing regimen, investigators at the M.D. Anderson Cancer Center examined the effect of administering topotecan 1.25 mg/m^2/day by continuous infusion for 3 days and liposomal daunorubicin 100 mg/m^2/day by brief infusion on days 1–3. In a phase I trial in patients with refractory and relapsed leukemias, this combination demonstrated a 19% response rate (cited in ref. *72*). In contrast, when administered to patients with newly diagnosed AML or high-grade MDS without or with thalidomide, this same regimen yielded a CR rate of 0/17 and was dropped from a multiarm phase II trial *(72)*. This disappointing result is consistent with earlier preclinical data indicating that topotecan and daunorubicin are antagonistic when administered simultaneously *(44)*.

4.3. Topotecan and Mitoxantrone

In a limited phase II study, the combination of topotecan 1.5 mg/m^2/day by continuous infusion for 5 days accompanied by mitoxantrone 12 mg/m^2/day on days 1–3 was studied in patients with MDS or with chronic myelogenous leukemia (CML) in accelerated phase or blast crisis *(73)*. Morphological CRs lasting 45–400 days were observed in four of seven patients with accelerated phase CML, two of four with CML in lymphoid blast crisis, and two of six with MDS. Ancillary studies were not reported. These results, however, are more promising than seen with some of the other combinations and might warrant further investigation.

4.4. Sequential Topotecan and Etoposide/Mitoxantrone

In a further extension of this approach, Mainwaring et al. performed a phase I/II study of topotecan 1.5 mg/m^2/day by continuous infusion for 3 days followed on days 4, 5, 9, and 10 with etoposide 100 mg/m^2/day and mitoxantrone 10 mg/m^2/day *(74)*. Grade 3 mucositis was observed in 29% of patients. In this heavily pretreated group of patients, 4 of 17 achieved a CR, and another 4 of 17 met the criteria of a CR except for inadequate platelet counts (CR_p). Interestingly, examination of paired marrow samples collected before treatment and on day 4 revealed that a $\geq$ 40% increase in TOP-IIα signal on day 4 correlated with response to therapy. Again, the high response rate in this small group of patients suggests that this regimen might merit further investigation.

4.5. Sequential Topotecan and Cytarabine

As indicated elsewhere in this volume (*see* Chapter 4), the interaction between advancing replication forks and drug-stabilized covalent TOP-I–DNA complexes generates the bulk of the cytotoxic DNA double-strand breaks. Consistent with this model, agents that inhibit DNA replication have

Table 2
Leukemia Trials of Topotecan-Containing Combinations

Reference	*Disease type*	*No. of patients/ median age*	*Drug combination*	*Dosage*	*Response rates*	*Side effects*
69	AML, CML-B	11/46	Topotecan (CI)/ etoposide	T: MTD 1.5 $mg/m^2/day \times 5$ days before etoposide E: bolus 100 $mg/m^2/day \times 3$ days	1 CR in CML-B	Mucositis was DLT
70	AML, ALL, CML-B	29/63	Topotecan (CI)/ etoposide	T: 72 h infusion followed in 24 hours by E: 100 $mg/m^2/day \times 5$ days	1 CR in relapsed AML, 1 CR in relapsed ALL	Grade 4 neutropenia and thrombocytopenia in all
76	AML, ALL, CML-B	53/50	Topotecan (30 min infusion)/ cytarabine	C: 1 $g/m^2/day \times 5$ days before T MTD for T 4.75 $mg/m^2/day \times 5$ days in high risk patients MTD T 7 $mg/m^2/day \times 5$ day in low risk patients	AML 10% CR ALL 50% CR CML-B 13% CR	Mucositis was DLT All developed neutropenic fever
77	AML	37/58	Topotecan (CI)/ etoposide or cytarabine	T then C (d1-5) T then E (d6-7) T then E (d1-2) *See* text for detail	1 CR	Mucositis was DLT
79	MDS, CMML	86/64	Topotecan/ cytarabine	T: 1.25 $mg/m^2/day \times 5$ days C: 1 $g/m^2 \times 5$ days	CR 56%	Grade 3/4 mucositis or diarrhea 2% Neutropenic fever 63% Mortality 7% during induction
78	AML	12/61	Topotecan/ cytarabine	T: 1.25 $mg/m^2/day \times 5$ days C: 1 $g/m^2 \times 5$ days	2 CR	Trial closed early because of poor efficacy

72	AML	11/NA	Topotecan/ liposomal daunorubicin	T: 1.25 mg/m^2/day × 3 days LD: 100 mg/m^2/day, days 1–3	0 CR	Arm closed because of poor efficacy
73	MDS, CML-B	24/38	Topotecan/ mitoxantrone	T: 1.5 mg/m^2/day × 5 days M: 12 mg/m^2/day, days 1–3	8 CR	Mucositis 69% Diarrhea 67%
74	AML, ALL	17/NA	Topotecan, mitoxantrone, etoposide	T: 1.5 mg/m^2/day, days 1–3 M: 10 mg/m^2/day, days 4, 5, 9 and 10 E: 100 mg/m^2/day, days 4, 5, 9 and 10	4 CR, 4 CR_p	Mucositis 29% Neutropenic fever 65%
100	AML, MDS	17/55	Topotecan Cytarabine Mylotarg	T: 1.25 mg/m^2/day × 5 days C: 1 g/m^2 × 5 days OG: 9 mg/m^2, day 1	2 CR	Grade 3/4 transaminase elevation 29% Hepatin veno-occlusive disease 7%
82	AML, ALL, CML-B	14/NA	Topotecan/ cyclophos-phamide	Cy: 40 mg/kg × day 1 T: 1.5-1.8 mg/m^2/day × 5 days	3 CR	MTD not reached
86	AML, ALL, CML-B	11/64	Topotecan/ carboplatin (Cb)	T: 0.5 mg/m^2/day × 5 days Cb: 150 mg/m^2/day × 5 days	3 CR	Prolonged myelo-suppression in all
96	AML, MDS	27/42	Topotecan, idarubicn, cytarabine	T: 1.25 mg/m^2/day × 5 days I: 12 mg/m^2 × 3 days C: 2 g/m^2 × 5 days	52% CR	Myelosuppression 100%, neutropenic fever 89%
94	AML, ALL	63/57	Topotecan (CI)/ cytara-bine / cyclophosphamide	Cy: 500 mg/m^2 every 12 h, days 1–3 T: 1.25 mg/m^2/day, days 2–6 C: 2 g/m^2, days 2–6	17% CR	Myelosuppression 100%, neutropenic fever 24%, nonhematologic toxicity mainly GI

AML, acute myeloid leukemia; ALL, acute lymphocytic leukemia; CML-B, chronic myeloid leukemia in blast phase; CMML, chronic myelomonocytic leukemia; C, cytarabine; CI, continuous infusion; CR, complete response; Cy, cyclophosphamide; DLT, dose limiting toxicity; GI, gastrointestinal; LD, liposomal daunorubicin; Mi, mitoxantrone; MDS, myelodysplastic syndrome; OG, gemtuzumab ozogamicin (Mylotarg); T, topotecan; min, minute; MTD, maximum tolerated dose.

been observed to antagonize the cytotoxic effects of TOP-I poisons. These results provide a potential explanation for the less than additive effects observed in vitro *(44)* when topotecan was combined with cytarabine, a known inhibitor of DNA synthesis *(75)*.

To avoid this potential antagonism between cytarabine and topotecan, Seiter et al. performed a phase I trial (*see* Table 2) in which cytarabine and topotecan were administered sequentially to 53 patients with refractory acute leukemia *(76)*. This trial was preceded by experiments to determine the effects of sequentially administering the two agents in vitro. These investigators found that treatment of HL-60 human leukemia cells with cytarabine followed by drug removal and then treatment with topotecan induced apoptosis in more cells than treatment with topotecan alone. In light of this result, cytarabine 1 g/m^2/day was administered as a 2-hour infusion daily for 5 days. Twelve hours after each cytarabine dose (i.e., when the remaining plasma concentrations of cytarabine would be expected to be minimal), topotecan was infused over 30 minutes. Mucositis was the DLT. In addition, all patients developed neutropenic fever and three patients died from sepsis. The MTD of topotecan was 4.75 mg/m^2/day for 5 days in high-risk patients (≥2 prior chemotherapy regimens) and 7 mg/m^2/day for 5 days in low-risk patients (<2 prior regimens and Eastern Cooperative Oncology Group performance status of <2). CR rates of 10% in AML, 50% in ALL, and 13% in blast crisis CML were observed. Remissions were, however, short-lived. Flow cytometry performed on peripheral blood and bone marrow samples revealed that those leukemias with higher S-phase fractions were more likely to achieve bone marrow aplasia with this regimen.

4.6. Alternative Approaches to Combining Topotecan With Cytarabine or Etoposide

Vey et al. *(77)* used a pre-phase II Bayesian selection design to examine three different patient groups and three different regimens in poor-risk AML (*see* Table 2). Patients were divided into three different risk groups based on karyotype, duration of first CR, number of prior salvage treatments, and response to last salvage therapy. An expected CR rate was then calculated for each group based on historical data. Within each stratum, patients were then randomized to one of three different treatments containing escalating doses of topotecan (starting dose 1 mg/m^2/day) administered as a CI for 5 days. The treatments were: topotecan CI on days 1–5 and cytarabine 1 g/m^2, days 1–5 as a 2-hour infusion; topotecan CI on days 1–5 followed by etoposide 250 mg/m^2 twice daily over 3 hours on days 6–7; or etoposide 250 mg/m^2 twice daily on days 1–2 followed by topotecan CI on days 3–7. A dose-finding phase was conducted in the poorest stratum of each arm. The Bayesian design was then used to assess whether the CR rate with each regimen was sufficient to merit investigation in a Phase II trial. The treatment arms were terminated after enrolling 37 patients because only one CR was observed. The principal cause of failure was insufficient antileukemic activity rather than toxicity. The authors concluded that the agents administered on these schedules did not warrant a phase II evaluation in poor prognosis AML patients.

The disappointing results with topotecan CI on days 1–5 + cytarabine on days 1–5 have been duplicated elsewhere *(78)*. A phase II trial of this combination produced no major extrahematological toxicities, but also only 2 CRs in 12 patients with refractory or relapsed AML. The results so disappointed the authors that they terminated the study early.

4.7. Phase II Trial of Concomitant Topotecan and Cytarabine in MDS

In view of the single-agent activity of topotecan in MDS, the M.D. Anderson group performed a phase II trial of topotecan + cytarabine in patients with this group of clonal hematological disorders. As indicated in Table 2, patients received topotecan 1.25 mg/m^2/day as a 5-day CI with brief infusions of cytarabine 1 gm/m^2/day on days 1–5 *(79)*. The median number of courses administered was two. At a median follow-up of 7 months, all 86 patients (median age 64) were assessable for toxicity and response. The therapy was relatively well tolerated, with 5% of patients developing grade 3–4 mucositis or diarrhea and 7% dying during induction therapy. The CR rates were reportedly 61% in patients with MDS and 44% in CMML, yielding an overall CR rate of 56%. The median duration of response was 34 weeks. These response rates were higher than observed after administration of single-agent topotecan (*see* Section 3.2.). Moreover, there was no statistically significant difference in the CR rates between the International Prognostic Scoring System risk groups (intermediate-1, intermediate-2, and high-risk). Impressively, 71% of MDS patients with a poor-prognosis karyotype achieved a CR with this regimen.

In a subsequent report, the same investigators described a cohort of 357 patients with newly diagnosed AML or high-grade MDS (presumably including the same original 82 MDS patients) who were treated with the same topotecan/cytarabine regimen *(80)*. Other patient cohorts were treated with idarubicin + cytarabine or fludarabine + cytarabine. Post hoc statistical analysis of this nonrandomized group of patients revealed a CR rate of 59%, median event-free survival of 36 weeks and median overall survival of 41 weeks for patients receiving topotecan/cytarabine. The authors found no evidence that topotecan + cytarabine was superior to idarubicin + cytarabine, which had a CR rate of 77% in a nonequivalent population.

It appears that the same MDS patients were described a third time by Beran and coworkers *(81)*, who reported an overall CR rate of 58% in 394 patients with newly diagnosed high-grade MDS treated in a nonrandomized fashion with one of five regimens, including topotecan + cytarabine. Although multivariate analysis failed to demonstrate a difference in remission rate among the regimens, topotecan + cytarabine had the lowest treatment-related mortality (5.4%).

In summary, it appears that the combination of topotecan + cytarabine administered according to the schedule described previously induces remissions in a substantial fraction of patients with high-grade MDS. This is in contrast to its lack of activity in relapsed and refractory acute leukemia *(77,78)* and its inferiority to standard induction regimens in newly diagnosed AML *(80)*. In MDS, a heterogeneous disorder in which patients live a variable length of time after diagnosis, properly controlled studies are required to determine whether the high CR rates seen with topotecan + cytarabine translate into altered survival.

4.8. Phase I Trials of Topotecan With DNA-Damaging Agents

Miller and coworkers performed a phase I trial of topotecan + cyclophosphamide in patients with relapsed and refractory leukemia *(82)*. This study was based on preclinical data suggesting that topotecan + cyclophosphamide exhibit additive or synergistic cytotoxic effects on tissue culture cells in vitro *(44,83,84)*, as well as clinical data indicating that myelosuppression is the DLT when topotecan and cyclophosphamide are administered to solid-tumor patients *(85)*. In the phase I leukemia trial (*see* Table 2), cyclophosphamide was administered at a dose of 40 mg/kg on day 1, followed by escalating doses of topotecan by 5-day CI on days 2–6. At the time of the most recent update, the MTD had not been reached. Of the 14 patients entered on study, 3 with AML achieved a CR. The final results of this trial, along with the ancillary studies examining potential mechanisms of resistance to this combination, remain to be reported.

Kaufmann et al. *(86)* performed a phase I trial of topotecan + carboplatin in patients with relapsed/refractory leukemia (*see* Table 2). The rationale for this study was the observation that the cytotoxic effects of topotecan and cisplatin are additive or synergistic in a variety of tissue culture cells *(83,87)* and in animal leukemia models *(88)*, possibly because CPT analogs inhibit the removal of platinum-associated DNA interstrand cross-links *(89)*. Carboplatin was chosen for the human leukemia trial because of its lower renal toxicity and its demonstrated single-agent activity in relapsed and refractory leukemia *(90–92)*. In the combination trial *(86)*, topotecan and carboplatin were administered to patients by 5-day CI starting with doses of 0.5 mg/m^2/day and 150 mg/m^2/day, respectively. At the time this study was last updated, 11 patients had received 19 cycles of therapy at two dose levels. Prolonged myelosuppression was observed in all patients, but other DLT were not observed. A total of three CRs (27%) was observed.

4.9. Three-Drug Combinations for Relapsed/Refractory Leukemia

In view of the additive or synergistic effects observed with topotecan and DNA-damaging agents in vitro *(83,87)* and in murine leukemia models *(88)*, as well as the admittedly modest single-agent antileukemic activity of cyclophosphamide in the clinical setting *(93)*, the M.D. Anderson group added cyclophosphamide to the topotecan + cytarabine regimen described previously (*see* Table 2) *(94)*. Sixty-three patients (median age 57 years) received cyclophosphamide 500 mg/m^2 administered as a brief infusion every 12 hours on days 1–3, accompanied by topotecan 1.25 mg/m^2/day by CI on days 2–6 and cytarabine 2 g/m^2 by 4-hour daily infusion on days 2–6. With this regimen, myelosuppression was universal, and a median of 29 days was required for neutrophil counts to reach 1000/mm^3. Five patients died during the first 28 days after therapy. Fever and weight loss, the most common nonhematological toxicities, were within the range expected with other induction regimens. Gastrointestinal side effects were also mild in most patients (mucositis grade 3 in 5%). Although a preliminary report indicated that the response rate with this regimen was 60% in AML *(95)*, prompting the Eastern Cooperative Oncology Group to initiate a confirmatory Phase II study (M. Litzow and M. Tallman, personal communication), a more complete report *(94)* indicated an overall CR rate of 17% in the 63 patients enrolled in this study, with CR rates of 23% in both AML and ALL patients.

Rather than building a regimen around the presumed mechanistic consequences of combining topotecan with various agents, an alternative has been to empirically combine topotecan with a "standard" cytarabine + anthracycline induction regimen. Using this approach, Lee et al. explored a regimen consisting of cytarabine 1 g/m^2 over 2 hours every 12 hours on days 1–5, idarubicin 12 mg/m^2 on days 1–3, and topotecan 1.25 mg/m^2/day by CI over days 1–5 in 27 patients with refractory/relapsed AML and high-grade MDS *(96)*. In addition to severe myelosuppression in all patients and documented infections in 89%, reversible grade 3–4 mucositis and diarrhea were observed in 26% and 7%, respectively. There was an 11% early death rate with this combination. Nonetheless, the CR rate was 52% and was somewhat higher in relapsed/refractory AML (59%) than MDS (40%). The median remission duration and median survival were 6 and 12 months, respectively, in this pretreated patient population. Four MDS patients who achieved CR maintained continuous CR with a median follow-up of 11 months. These results require confirmation in a further study.

Other investigators have attempted to build on the fludarabine and cytarabine combination that is used to treat high-risk and elderly AML patients *(97,98)*. A pilot study indicated that administration of fludarabine 15 mg/m^2/day on days 1–4 followed 4 hours later by cytarabine 2 gm/m^2/day over 4 hours and topotecan 1.25 mg/m^2/day over 4 hours is well tolerated and has a CR rate of 60% in newly diagnosed AML *(99)*. The reported activity of this regimen in elderly patients and those with secondary AML needs to be confirmed in a larger phase II or phase III study.

Other empiric approaches appear less promising. Cortes et al. reported that addition of the immunotoxin conjugate gemtuzumab ozogamicin (Mylotarg) 9 mg/m^2 iv over 2 hours on day 1 to the cytarabine/topotecan regimen described in Sections 4.6 and 4.7 resulted in grade 3/4 elevations in serum transaminase levels in 29% of patients, with 6% mortality resulting from hepatic veno-occlusive disease, but had only a 12% CR rate in 17 patients with relapsed or primary refractory AML *(100)*.

5. ANTILEUKEMIC STUDIES OF IRINOTECAN

Irinotecan is water-soluble, semisynthetic CPT analog that is converted by carboxylesterases into the more potent derivative 7-ethyl-10-hydroxy-camptothecin (SN-38). As indicated in Chapter 11, SN-38 stabilizes TOP-I–DNA complexes, thereby setting into motion biochemical changes that result in replication fork-associated DNA double-strand breaks, cell cycle arrest, and apoptosis. Compared to topotecan, which has a terminal serum half-life of 3 hours *(101)*, the pharmacokinetic profile of irinotecan is characterized by a long elimination half-life for both the parent compound (6 hours) and SN-38 (11–13 hours) *(102,103)*.

When irinotecan was administered to solid-tumor patients as a brief infusion every 3–4 weeks, an early phase I study revealed dose-limiting leukopenia at 350 mg/m^2 *(104)*. Grade 3/4 diarrhea was also frequently observed. Based on concerns about the combination of leukopenia and diarrhea at doses ≥250 mg/m^2, a phase II dose of 200 mg/m^2 was recommended in solid-tumor patients *(104)*.

Because of the presence of a potentially dose-limiting nonhematological toxicity, formal phase I testing of irinotecan in patients with hematological disorders was not performed. Instead, a multi-institution phase II study of irinotecan *(105)* was completed in 62 heavily pretreated leukemia and lymphoma patients (median age 46) based on the results of the phase I solid-tumor trial. Two administration schedules were planned for the initial phase of the study: on schedule A, irinotecan was administered as a single 60-minute infusion at 200 mg/m^2 on day 1 of every 3- to 4-week cycle; on schedule B, irinotecan was given as a 60-minute infusion at 40 mg/m^2/day on days 1–5 of each cycle. When an interim analysis showed no responses of leukemia or lymphoma patients to schedule A and no responses of acute leukemia patients to schedule B, these schedules were replaced by two new schedules: on schedule C, irinotecan was given as a 60-minute infusion of 40 mg/m^2 for 3 days every week; on schedule D, irinotecan was administered as a 60-minute infusion at 20 mg/m^2 twice per day on days 1–7 of a planned 3- to 4-week cycle. As seen in the earlier phase I study in solid-tumor patients, leukopenia was more marked than thrombocytopenia, with reversible grade 3/4 leukopenia occurring in 71% of the lymphoma patients enrolled in this study. Diarrhea was also noted in 71% of patients. Among the 26 patients with acute leukemia enrolled in this trial, the response rate was 0/14 in patients treated on schedules A–C and 3 out of 12 (25%) in patients treated on schedule D. Although the number of patients was small, subset analysis revealed that relapsed patients and patients with primary refractory disease each had a 33% response rate (1 CR/3 patients in each category), but patients with relapses that were unresponsive to other salvage regimens had only a 5% response rate (1 CR/20 patients).

A follow-up report summarized results obtained from 50 patients with acute leukemia or blast crisis CML treated with irinotecan at a dose of 15–20 mg/m^2 twice daily for 7 days every 2–4 weeks *(106)*. Of 17 patients with ALL, 2 showed a partial response (12%). No responses were seen in the 24 patients with AML.

Because of these disappointing results, irinotecan has not received much further study as a single agent in AML. In acute lymphoid leukemias, the only single-agent Phase II trial reported is a multi-institution trial examining the effect of irinotecan 40 mg/m^2/day on days 1–3 of each week in patients with relapsed/refractory acute T-cell leukemia/lymphoma *(107)*. Although 1 CR and 4 PRs were observed in 13 assessable patients, the median CR duration of 31 days was disappointing.

More recently, a small phase II study of single-agent irinotecan administered at 200 mg/m^2 every 2 weeks in MDS patients who were not candidates for cytarabine + anthracycline therapy was reported *(108)*. Because this irinotecan-treated group showed faster hematologic recovery than is usually seen in topotecan-treated MDS patients, there were fewer hospitalizations. In 26 previously untreated MDS patients, 1 CR and 4 PRs were observed. Because the median duration of these responses, however, was only 4 months, it is not clear whether further study of this agent in MDS is justified.

Combinations involving irinotecan have not been extensively studied in leukemia patients. Based on the promising activity of gemcitabine + irinotecan in solid tumor patients, 11 patients with relapsed or refractory acute leukemia were treated with 40 mg/m^2 daily for 3 days followed by infusional gemcitabine at 10 mg/m^2/minute for increasing lengths of time *(109)*. The DLTs were reversible stomatitis and esophagitis, and the MTD was gemcitabine 7200 mg/m^2 (12-hour infusion). One CR (9%) and one PR (9%) were observed.

In summary, irinotecan has little activity against the acute leukemias. These disappointing results might reflect the expression of the transporter BCRP (ABC G2) in a majority of acute leukemia specimens *(110,111)* and the high sensitivity of SN-38 accumulation to this transporter *(20,22)*. The activity of irinotecan as a single agent in MDS is also modest, and it remains to be determined whether combinations containing irinotecan have any role in the treatment of hematological malignancies.

6. TRIALS OF OTHER CAPMTOTHECINS IN LEUKEMIA

9-Aminocamptothecin (9-AC, *see* Chapter 9) has also been evaluated in leukemia patients. Preclinical studies demonstrated dramatic activity of a lipid formulation of this agent in an animal model of colon cancer *(112)*. Activity against human leukemia in a SCID mouse model was also demonstrated *(113)*. Phase I clinical trials in solid-tumor patients revealed that the DLT was myelosuppression *(114,115)*. Two groups have performed phase I trials of 9-AC in relapsed/refractory acute leukemia patients *(116,117)*. Results of these studies have demonstrated that the 9-AC dose can be increased threefold to fourfold in leukemia patients (1.4 mg/m^2/day by 7-day CI) before dose-limiting mucositis is encountered *(117)*. Even though 9-AC was capable of inducing marrow hypoplasia, it appeared to lack sufficient activity on this schedule to induce any objective responses *(116,117)*. Phase I trials of 9-AC in combination with other antileukemic agents are in progress (J. P. Eder, personal communication).

More recently, exatecan (DX-8951f) was also evaluated in patients with acute leukemia. Preclinical studies demonstrated that the activity of this agent in SCID mice inoculated with the KBM3 human leukemia line was both dose- and schedule-dependent, with protracted schedules giving improved survival *(118)*. Based on these results, and the observation that hematological toxicity was dose-limiting in phase I trials of exatecan in solid-tumor patients, a phase I trial investigating daily × 5 and daily × 7 intravenous infusion schedules was performed in patients with relapsed/refractory acute leukemias and MDS *(119)*. As is the case with topotecan, stomatitis was dose-limiting. The recommended phase II dose was 0.9 mg/m^2/day × 5 days. Among 24 patients, only 1 PR (4%) was observed.

7. CONCLUSIONS

Although TOP-I poisons have been in clinical trials for more than a decade, the studies summarized in this chapter provide only limited information regarding the efficacy of TOP-I poisons in patients with hematological malignancies. Most of the studies reported to date were phase I clinical trials. It is important to keep in mind that the primary goals of a phase I study are to define the toxicities and determine the MTD of a treatment. By its very nature, a phase I trial involves administration of agents at multiple dose levels, including dose levels that might be inadequate to produce an antineoplastic response. Moreover, only 6 to 10 patients are treated at the MTD in the typical Phase I trial. Accordingly, these trials provide little information about the antineoplastic activity of the treatments under study. In addition, Phase I trials are typically performed on patients whose disease has recurred after treatment with conventional agents. It is likely that the previous treatment has selected for neoplastic cells that are resistant to subsequent therapy.

Even with these caveats in mind, the results suggest that the activity of TOP-I poisons in acute leukemia is modest. The phase II window trial of topotecan in high-risk ALL revealed a CR rate of 7% *(50)*. The activity of single-agent topotecan in AML was likewise limited *(57)*.

Some of the phase I trials of topotecan-containing two-drug regimens have appeared more promising. In particular, the topotecan + cyclophosphamide and topotecan + carboplatin trials have demonstrated response rates of 20–30% in patients with relapsed/refractory acute leukemia and blast crisis CML (*see* Table 2). These regimens are also appealing because preclinical studies have demonstrated additive or greater than additive effects of the combinations in vitro and in vivo. In both trials, CRs were observed at a wide range of dose levels, providing a hint that the regimens might be active. Based on the responses observed in the phase I topotecan + cyclophosphamide trial, a phase II trial of this combination is currently in progress (C. Miller, personal communication). If this combination continues to show promise, it might be reasonable to assess its true antileukemic potential by performing a phase II window trial in previously untreated patients.

Results of the Bayesian phase I trial of topotecan + cytarabine versus sequential topotecan/etoposide did not provide evidence of sufficient activity to warrant a phase II trial of these combinations in relapsed/refractory leukemia. Although it might be argued that the patients enrolled in this study were heavily pretreated and, therefore, were unlikely to respond to any subsequent regimen, it is precisely these patients who need additional effective antileukemic treatments. Accordingly, most hematologists would have little enthusiasm for testing regimens such as these in untreated patients if the same regimens display little or no activity in patients with recurrent AML.

In contrast to its limited activity in relapsed or refractory acute leukemia, the topotecan + cytarabine combination has been reported to display remarkable activity in MDS and CMML. Studies to confirm these results and determine whether this regimen alters the natural history of these disorders appear to be warranted. Given the high frequency of MDS and the extremely poor prognosis of patients with RAEB and RAEB-T, it should be possible to address these questions rapidly.

Additional studies to evaluate the antileukemic potential of other CPT derivatives also appear to be reasonable. Given the limited effectiveness of current therapy in elderly (age >60 years) patients with AML, new therapeutic options are clearly needed. Oral topotecan has been shown to have different pharmacokinetic characteristics that might translate into a superior therapeutic index with a different toxicity profile from that of the iv formulation. Oral dosing also avoids the potential complications of central vein catheters, facilitates multiday dosing, and enhances convenience *(120–122)*. In view of the dramatic activity of the irinotecan/cisplatin combination in lung cancer *(123,124)*, it also might be reasonable to consider trials of irinotecan/carboplatin in relapsed/refractory leukemia. It will also be interesting to see whether myelosuppression is the DLT of the silatecans (*see* Chapter 8) in solid tumor patients. If so, additional studies in leukemia patients might be warranted for these CPT derivatives as well.

The current paucity of single-agent activity in acute leukemia might prompt some hematologists to abandon this entire class of agents. The anthracyclines, however, provide a nice example of a class of compounds in which some analogs (e.g., daunorubicin, idarubicin) appear to have preferential activity in acute leukemia, whereas others (e.g., doxorubicin, epirubicin) appear to be more active in solid tumors. Accordingly, we would argue that limited testing of new CPT derivatives in patients with hematological malignancies remains reasonable.

As these trials go forward, it will be important to include ancillary studies that attempt to identify the mechanisms of resistance to TOP-I poisons that play an important role in the clinical setting. Over the past several years, a number of additional factors that can affect CPT sensitivity have emerged. First, Brangi et al. *(20)* identified the ATP-binding cassette transporter BCRP/ABCG2 as a determinant of cellular SN-38 and topotecan accumulation. Several groups subsequently reported expression of BCRP mRNA in clinical leukemia specimens *(110,111)*, raising the question of whether BCRP plays a role in the response of human leukemias to topotecan or irinotecan. Second, Bjornsti and coworkers reported that cdc45 and dpb11, two proteins involved in processing of Okazaki fragments during DNA replication, play a role in determining whether the collision of replication forks with TOP-I–DNA complexes generates cytotoxic lesions *(125)*. Relatively little is known about the expression of these polypeptides in human leukemia. Finally, studies in mammalian tissue culture cells have implicated the DNA damage-responsive kinase ATM (mutated in ataxia telangiectasia) and the downstream kinase Chk2 (checkpoint kinase 2) in topotecan-induced cell-cycle perturbations *(126)*. Additional studies have also implicated the related kinases ATR (ATM- and Rad3-related) and Chk1 in CPT sensitivity *(127)*. Relatively little is known about the function of these pathways in clinical leukemia cells in vivo. If the TOP-I-directed agents continue to be tested in leukemia patients, it would be informative to know whether the presence or absence of these resistance mechanisms correlates in some way with the responses that are observed in the clinic.

ACKNOWLEDGMENTS

The authors gratefully acknowledge support from the National Cancer Institute (R01 CA73709) and secretarial assistance of Deb Strauss.

REFERENCES

1. Lowenberg B, Downing JR, Burnett A. 1999 Acute myeloid leukemia. N Engl J Med 341:1051–1062.
2. Pui CH, Evans WE. 1998 Acute lymphoblastic leukemia. N Engl J Med 339:605–615.
3. Appelbaum FR, Kopecky KJ. 1997 Long-term survival after chemotherapy for acute myeloid leukemia: the experience of the Southwest Oncology Group. Cancer 80:2199–2204.
4. Bennett JM, Young ML, Andersen JW, et al. 1997 Long-term survival in acute myeloid leukemia: the Eastern Cooperative Oncology Group experience. Cancer 80:2205–2209.
5. Bloomfield CD, Lawrence D, Byrd JC, et al. 1998 Frequency of prolonged remission duration after high-dose cytarabine intensification in acute myeloid leukemia varies by cytogenetic subtype. Cancer Res 58:4173–4179.
6. Rowe JM. 2000 Treatment of acute myelogenous leukemia in older adults. Leukemia 14:480–487.
7. Stone RM, Mayer RJ. 1993 The approach to the elderly patient with acute myeloid leukemia. Hematol Oncol Clin North Am 7:65–79.
8. Advani R, Saba HI, Tallman MS, et al. 1999 Treatment of refractory and relapsed acute myelogenous leukemia with combination chemotherapy plus the multidrug resistance modulator PSC 833 (Valspodar). Blood 93:787–795.
9. Hoelzer D, Gokbuget N. 2000 New approaches to acute lymphoblastic leukemia in adults: where do we go? Semin Oncol 27:540–559.
10. Rosenfeld C, List A. 2000 A hypothesis for the pathogenesis of myelodysplastic syndromes: implications for new therapies. Leukemia 14:2–8.
11. Bennett JM, Catovsky D, Daniel MT, et al. 1982 Proposals for the classification of the myelodysplastic syndromes. Br J Haematol 51:189–199.
12. Fenaux P, Beuscart R, Lai JL, Jouet JP, Bauters F. 1988 Prognostic factors in adult chronic myelomonocytic leukemia: an analysis of 107 cases. J Clin Oncol 6:1417–1424.
13. Hoagland HC. 1995 Myelodysplastic (preleukemia) syndromes: the bone marrow factory failure problem. Mayo Clinic Proc 70:673–676.
14. Parker JE, Mufti GJ. 1998 Ineffective haemopoiesis and apoptosis in myelodysplastic syndromes. Br J Haematol 101:220–230.
15. Heaney ML, Golde DW. 1999 Myelodysplasia. N Engl J Med. 340:1649–1660.
16. Dansey R. Myelodysplasia. 2000 Curr Opin Oncol 12:13–21.
17. Kaufmann SH. 1998 Cell death induced by topoisomerase-targeted drugs: more questions than answers. Biochim Biophys Acta 1400:195–211.
18. Wu J, Liu LF. 1997 Processing of topoisomerase I cleavable complexes into DNA damage by transcription. Nucleic Acids Res 25:4181–4186.
19. Slichenmyer WJ, Rowinsky EK, Donehower RC, Kaufmann SH. 1993 The current status of camptothecin analogues as antitumor agents. J Natl Cancer Inst 85:271–291.

20. Brangi M, Litman T, Ciotti M, et al. 1999 Camptothecin resistance: role of the ATP-binding cassette (ABC), mitoxantrone-resistance half-transporter (MXR), and potential for glucuronidation in MXR-expressing cells. Cancer Res 59:5938–5946.
21. Schellens JH, Maliepaard M, Scheper RJ, et al. 2000 Transport of topoisomerase I inhibitors by the breast cancer resistance protein. Potential clinical implications. Ann NY Acad Sci 922:188–194.
22. Erlichman C, Boerner SA, Hallgren CG, et al. 2001 The HER tyrosine kinase inhibitor CI1033 enhances cytotoxicity of 7-ethyl-10-hydroxycamptothecin and topotecan by inhibiting breast cancer resistance protein-mediated drug efflux. Cancer Res 61:739–748.
23. Nitiss JL, Wang JC. 1996 Mechanisms of cell killing by drugs that trap covalent complexes between DNA topoisomerases and DNA. Mol Pharmacol 50:1095–1102.
24. Li LH, Fraser TJ, Olin EJ, Bhuyan BK. 1972 Action of camptothecin on mammalian cells in culture. Cancer Res 32:2643–2650.
25. Horwitz SB, Horwitz MS. 1973 Effects of camptothecin on the breakage and repair of DNA during the cell cycle. Cancer Res 33:2834–2846.
26. Kaufmann SH. 1989 Induction of endonucleolytic DNA cleavage in human acute myelogenous leukemia cells by etoposide, camptothecin, and other cytotoxic anticancer drugs: a cautionary note. Cancer Res 49:5870–5878.
27. Del Bino G, Darzynkiewicz Z. 1991 Camptothecin, teniposide, 4′-(9-acridinylamino)-3-methanesulfon-*m*-anisidide, but not mitoxantrone or doxorubicin, induced degradation of nuclear DNA in the S phase of HL-60 cells. Cancer Res 51:1165–1169.
28. Kharbanda S, Rubin E, Gunji H, et al. 1991 Camptothecin and its derivatives induce expression of the c-*jun* protooncogene in human myeloid leukemia cells. Cancer Res 51:6636–6642.
29. Solary E, Bertrand R, Kohn KW, Pommier Y. 1993 Differential induction of apoptosis in undifferentiated and differentiated HL-60 cells by DNA topoisomerase I and II inhibitors. Blood 81:1359–1368.
30. Uckun FM, Stewart CF, Reaman G, et al. 1995 In Vitro and in vivo activity of topotecan against human B-lineage acute lymphoblastic leukemia cells. Blood 85:2817–2828.
31. Gottlieb JA, Guarino AM, Call JB, Oliverio VT, Block JB. 1970 Preliminary pharmacologic and clinical evaluation of camptothecin sodium (NSC-100880). Cancer Chemother Rpt 54:461–470.
32. Moertel CG, Schutt AJ, Reitemeier RJ, Hahn RG. 1972 Phase II study of camptothecin (NSC-100880) in the treatment of advanced gastrointestinal cancer. Cancer Chemother Rpt 56:95–101.
33. Gottlieb JA, Luce JK. 1972 Treatment of malignant melanoma with camptothecin (NSC-10088). Cancer Chemother Rpt 56:103–105.
34. Johnson RK, Chitnis MP, Embrey WM, Gregory EB. 1978 In vivo characteristics of resistance and cross-resistance of an adriamycin-resistant subline of P388 leukemia. Cancer Treat Rep 62:1535–1547.
35. Johnson RK, Howard WS. 1982 Development and cross-resistance characteristics of a subline of P388 leukemia resistant to 4′-(9-acridinylamino)-methanesulfon-m-anisidide. Eur J Cancer Clin Oncol 18:479–487.
36. Potmesil M. 1994 Camptothecins: from bench research to hospital wards. Cancer Res 54:1431–1439.

37. O'Leary J, Muggia FM. 1998 Camptothecins: a review of their development and schedules of administration. Eur J Cancer 34:1500–1508.
38. D'Arpa P, Beardmore C, Liu LF. 1990 Involvement of nucleic acid synthesis in cell killing mechanisms of topoisomerase poisons. Cancer Res 50:6919–6924.
39. Mauer AM, Fisher V. 1962 Comparison of the proliferative capacity of acute leukaemia cells in bone marrow and blood. Nature 193:1085–1086.
40. Killmann S-A. 1965 Proliferative activity of blast cells in leukemia and myelofibrosis. Acta Med Scan 178:263–280.
41. Mauer AM, Fisher V. 1966 Characteristics of cell proliferation in four patients with untreated acute leukemia. Blood 28:428–445.
42. Kantarjian HM, Beran M, Ellis A, et al. 1993 Phase I study of topotecan, a new topoisomerase I inhibitor, in patients with refractory or relapsed acute leukemia. Blood 81:1146–1151.
43. Rowinsky EK, Adjei AA, Donehower RC, et al. 1994 Phase I and pharmacodynamic study of the topoisomerase I-inhibitor topotecan in patients with refractory acute leukemia. J Clin Oncol 12:2193–2203.
44. Kaufmann SH, Gore SD, Letendre L, et al. 1996 Factors affecting topotecan sensitivity in human leukemia samples. Ann NY Acad Sci 803:128–142.
45. Furman WL, Baker SD, Pratt CB, Rivera GK, Evans WE, Stewart CF. 1996 Escalating systemic exposure of continuous infusion topotecan in children with recurrent acute leukemia. J Clin Oncol 14:1504–1511.
46. Houghton PJ, Cheshire PJ, Hallman JD, et al. 1995 Efficacy of topoisomerase I inhibitors, topotecan, and irinotecan, administered at low dose levels in protracted schedules to mice bearing xenografts of human tumors. Cancer Chemother Pharmacol 36:393–403.
47. Furman WL, Stewart CF, Kirstein M, et al. 2002 Protracted intermittent schedule of topotecan in children with refractory acute leukemia: a pediatric oncology group study. J Clin Oncol 20:1617–1624.
48. Beran M, O'Brien S, Thomas DA, et al. 2003 Phase I study of oral topotecan in hematological malignancies. Clin Cancer Res 9:4084–4091.
49. Rowinsky EK, Kaufmann SH, Baker S, et al. 1996 A phase I and pharmacologic study of topotecan on a 30 minute infusion daily for five day schedule in patients with refractory acute leukemia. Clin Cancer Res 2:1921–1930.
50. Gore SD, Rowinsky EK, Miller CB, et al. 1998 A phase II "window" study of topotecan in untreated patients with high risk adult acute lymphocytic leukemia. Clin Cancer Res 4:2677–2689.
51. Ettinger DS. 1990 Evaluation of new drugs in untreated patients with small-cell lung cancer: its time has come. J Clin Oncol 8:374–377.
52. Castleberry RP, Cantor AB, Green AA, et al. 1994 Phase II investigational window using carboplatin, iproplatin, ifosfamide, and epirubicin in children with untreated disseminated neuroblastoma: a Pediatric Oncology Group study. J Clin Oncol 12:1616–1620.
53. Kearns CM, Blakley RL, Santana VM, Crom WR. 1994 Pharmacokinetics of cladribine (2-chlorodeoxyadenosine) in children with acute leukemia. Cancer Res 54:1235–1239.
54. Harris MB, Cantor AB, Goorin AM, et al. 1995 Treatment of osteosarcoma with ifosfamide: comparison of response in pediatric patients with recurrent disease versus patients previously untreated: a Pediatric Oncology Group study. Med Pediatr Oncol 24:87–92.

55. Schiller JH, Kim K, Hutson P, et al. 1996 Phase II study of topotecan in patients with extensive-stage small-cell carcinoma of the lung: an Eastern Cooperative Oncology Group Trial. J Clin Oncol 14:2345–2352.
56. Perez-Soler R, Fossella FV, Glisson BS, et al. 1996 Phase II study of topotecan in patients with advanced non-small-cell lung cancer previously untreated with chemotherapy. J Clin Oncol 14:503–513.
57. Cortes J, Kantarjian HM. 2000 Promising approaches in acute leukemia. Invest New Drugs 18:57–82.
58. Beran M, Estey E, O'Brien SM, et al. 1998 Results of topotecan single-agent therapy in patients with myelodysplastic syndromes and chronic myelomonocytic leukemia. Leuk Lymph 31:521–531.
59. O'Brien S, Kantarjian H, Ellis A, Zwelling L, Estey E, Keating M. 1995 Topotecan in chronic lymphocytic leukemia. Cancer 75:1104–1108.
60. Silber R, Degar B, Costin D, et al. 1994 Chemosensitivity of lymphocytes from patients with B-cell chronic lymphocytic leukemia to chlorambucil, fludarabine, and camptothecin analogs. Blood 84:3440–3446.
61. Rowinsky EK, Kaufmann SH. 1997 Topotecan in combination chemotherapy. Semin Oncol 24:S11–S26.
62. Gupta RS, Gupta R, Eng B, et al. 1988 Camptothecin-resistant mutants of Chinese hamster ovary cells containing a resistant form of topoisomerase I. Cancer Res 48:6404–6410.
63. Sugimoto Y, Tsukahara S, Oh-hara T, Liu LF, Tsuruo T. 1990 Elevated expression of DNA topoisomerase II in camptothecin-resistant human tumor cell lines. Cancer Res 50:7962–7965.
64. D'Arpa P, Beardmore C, Liu LF. 1990 Involvement of nucleic acid synthesis in cell killing mechanisms of topoisomerase poisons. Cancer Res 50:6919–6924.
65. Kaufmann SH. 1991 Antagonism between camptothecin and topoisomerase II-directed chemotherapeutic agents in a human leukemia cell line. Cancer Res 51:1129–1136.
66. Bertrand R, O'Connor PM, Kerrigan D, Pommier Y. 1992 Sequential administration of camptothecin and etoposide circumvents the antagonistic cytotoxicity of simultaneous drug administration in slowly growing human colon carcinoma HT-29 cells. Eur J Cancer 28A:743–748.
67. Chen S, Gomez SP, McCarley D, Mainwaring MG. 2002 Topotecan-induced topoisomerase IIalpha expression increases the sensitivity of the CML cell line K562 to subsequent etoposide plus mitoxantrone treatment. Cancer Chemother Pharmacol 49:347–355.
68. Johnson RK, McCabe FL, Yu Y. 1992 Combination regimens with topotecan in animal tumor models. Ann Oncol 3:85.
69. Crump M, Lipton J, Hedley D, et al. 1999 Phase I trial of sequential topotecan followed by etoposide in adults with myeloid leukemia: a National Cancer Institute of Canada Clinical Trials Group Study. Leukemia 13:343–347.
70. Cooper BW, Donaher E, Lazarus HM, et al. 2003 A phase I and pharmacodynamic study of sequential topotecan and etoposide in patients with relapsed or refractory acute myelogenous and lymphoblastic leukemia. Leuk Res 27:35–44.
71. Nair JS, Kancherla R, Seiter K, Traganos F, Tse-Dinh YC. 2000 Action of topoisomerase targeting drugs on non-Hodgkin's lymphoma and leukemia. Correlation of clinical and cell culture studies. Ann NY Acad Sci 922:326–329.
72. Cortes J, Kantarjian H, Albitar M, et al. 2003 A randomized trial of liposomal daunorubicin and cytarabine versus liposomal daunorubicin and topotecan with or

without thalidomide as initial therapy for patients with poor prognosis acute myelogenous leukemia or myelodysplastic syndrome. Cancer 97:1234–1241.
73. Park SJ, Kim DW, Kim HJ, et al. 2000 Topotecan-based combination chemotherapy in patients with transformed chronic myelogenous leukemia and advanced myelodysplastic syndrome. Korean J Intern Med 15:122–126.
74. Mainwaring MG, Rimsza LM, Chen SF, et al. 2002 Treatment of refractory acute leukemia with timed sequential chemotherapy using topotecan followed by etoposide + mitoxantrone (T-EM) and correlation with topoisomerase II levels. Leuk Lymph 43:989–999.
75. Chabner BA. Cytidine analogues. In: Cancer chemotherapy and biotherapy. Chabner BA, Longo DL, eds. Lippincott-Raven, Pennsylvania, 1996, 213–233.
76. Seiter K, Feldman EJ, Halicka HD, et al. 1997 Phase I clinical and laboratory evaluation of topotecan and cytarabine in patients with acute leukemia. J Clin Oncol 15:44–51.
77. Vey N, Kantarjian H, Beran M, et al. 1999 Combination of topotecan with cytarabine or etoposide in patients with refractory or relapsed acute myeloid leukemia: results of a randomized phase I/II study. Invest New Drugs 17:89–95.
78. Pagano L, Mele L, Voso MT, et al. 2001 The association of topotecan and cytarabine in the treatment of secondary or relapsed acute myeloid leukemia. Haematologica 86:440–441.
79. Beran M, Estey E, O'Brien S, et al. 1999 Topotecan and cytarabine is an active combination regimen in myelodysplastic syndromes and chronic myelomonocytic leukemia. J Clin Oncol 17:2819–2830.
80. Estey EH, Thall PF, Cortes JE, et al. 2001 Comparison of idarubicin + ara-C-, fludarabine + ara-C-, and topotecan + ara-C-based regimens in treatment of newly diagnosed acute myeloid leukemia, refractory anemia with excess blasts in transformation, or refractory anemia with excess blasts. Blood 98:3575–3583.
81. Beran M, Shen Y, Kantarjian H, et al. 2001 High-dose chemotherapy in high-risk myelodysplastic syndrome: covariate-adjusted comparison of five regimens. Cancer 92:1999–2015.
82. Miller CB, O'Reilly S, Sartorius S, et al. 1997 A phase I and pharmacologic study of a combination of cyclophosphamide (CY) and topotecan (TOPO) in patients (Pts) with refractory leukemia. Proc Am Soc Clin Oncol 16:203a.
83. Kaufmann SH, Peereboom D, Buckwalter CA, Svingen PA, Donehower RC, Rowinsky EK. 1996 Cytotoxic effects of topotecan combined with various anticancer agents in human cancer cell lines. J Natl Cancer Inst 88:734–741.
84. Janss AJ, Cnaan A, Zhao H, Shpilsky A, Levow C, Sutton L, et al. 1998 Synergistic cytotoxicity of topoisomerase I inhibitors with alkylating agents in human brain tumor cell lines. Anticancer Drugs 9:641–652.
85. Murren JR, Anderson S, Fedele J, et al. 1997 Dose-escalation and pharmacodynamic study of topotecan in combination with cyclophosphamide in patients with refractory cancer. J Clin Oncol 15:148–157.
86. Kaufmann SH, Letendre L, Litzow M, et al. 1998 Phase I study of continuous infusion (CI) topotecan (TPT) and carboplatin (CBDCA) for relapsed or refractory acute leukemia. Proc Am Soc Clin Oncol 17:28a.
87. Cheng MF, Chatterjee S, Berger NA. 1994 Schedule-dependent cytotoxicity of topotecan alone and in combination chemotherapy regimens. Oncol Res 6:269–279.
88. Johnson RK, McCabe FL, Gallagher G. 1992 Comparative efficacy of topotecan, irinotecan, camptothecin and 9-aminocamptothecin in preclinical tumor models. Ann Oncol 3:85.

89. Fukuda M, Nishio K, Kanzawa F, et al. 1996 Synergism between cisplatin and topoisomerase I inhibitors, NB-506 and SN-38, in human small cell lung cancer cells. Cancer Res 56:789–793.
90. Meyers FJ, Welborn J, Lewis JP, Flynn N. 1989 Infusion carboplatin treatment of relapsed and refractory acute leukemia: evidence of efficacy with minimal extramedullary toxicity at intermediate doses. J Clin Oncol 7:173–178.
91. Martinez JA, Martin G, Sanz GF, Sempere A, Jarque I, de la Rubia J. 1991 A phase II clinical trial of carboplatin infusion in high-risk acute nonlymphocytic leukemia. J Clin Oncol 9:39–43.
92. Vogler WR. 1993 High-dose carboplatin in the treatment of hematologic malignancies. Oncology 50(Suppl. 2):42–46.
93. Pierce M, Shore N, Sitarz A, Murphy ML, Louis J, Severo N. 1966 Cyclophosphamide therapy in acute leukemia of childhood. Cooperative study conducted by members of Children's Cancer Cooperative Group A. Cancer 19:1551–1560.
94. Cortes J, Estey E, Beran M, et al. 2000 Cyclophosphamide, ara-C and topotecan (CAT) for patients with refractory or relapsed acute leukemia. Leuk Lymph 36:479–484.
95. Kantarjian H. New developments in the treatment of acute myeloid leukemia: focus on topotecan. Sem Hematol 36:16–25.
96. Lee ST, Jang JH, Suh HC, Hahn JS, Ko YW, Min YH. 2001 Idarubicin, cytarabine, and topotecan in patients with refractory or relapsed acute myelogenous leukemia and high-risk myelodysplastic syndrome. Am J Hematol 68:237–245.
97. Keating MJ, Estey E, O'Brien S, Kantarjian H, Robertson LE, Plunkett W. 1994 Clinical experience with fludarabine in leukaemia. Drugs 47(Suppl 6):39–49.
98. Visani G, Tosi P, Zinzani PL, et al. 1994 FLAG (fludarabine + high-dose cytarabine + G-CSF): an effective and tolerable protocol for the treatment of 'poor risk' acute myeloid leukemias. Leukemia 8:1842–1846.
99. Leoni F, Ciolli S, Nozzoli C, Santini V, Fanci R, Rossi Ferrini P. 2001 Fludarabine, cytarabine and topotecan (FLAT) as induction therapy for acute myeloid leukemia in the elderly: a preliminary report. Haematologica 86:104.
100. Cortes J, Tsimberidou AM, Alvarez R, et al. 2002 Mylotarg combined with topotecan and cytarabine in patients with refractory acute myelogenous leukemia. Cancer Chemother Pharmacol 50:497–500.
101. Rowinsky EK, Grochow LB, Hendricks CB, et al. 1992 Phase I and pharmacologic study of topotecan: a novel topoisomerase I inhibitor. J Clin Oncol 10:647–656.
102. Rowinsky EK, Grochow LB, Ettinger DS, et al. 1994 Phase I and pharmacological study of the novel topoisomerase I inhibitor 7-ethyl-10-[4-(1-piperidino)-1-piperidino] carbonyloxycamptothecin (CPT-11) administered as a ninety-minute infusion every 3 weeks. Cancer Res 54:427–436.
103. Chabot GG. 1997 Clinical pharmacokinetics of irinotecan. Clin Pharmacokinet 33:245–259.
104. Taguchi T, Wakui A, Hasegawa K, et al. 1990 Phase I clinical study of CPT-11. Research group of CPT-11. Gan To Kagaku Ryoho 17:115–120.
105. Ohno R, Okada K, Masaoka T, et al. 1990 An early phase II study of CPT-11: a new derivative of camptothecin, for the treatment of leukemia and lymphoma. J Clin Oncol 8:1907–1912.
106 Ota K, Ohno R, Shirakawa S, et al. 1994 Late phase II clinical study of irinotecan hydrochloride (CPT-11) in the treatment of malignant lymphoma and acute leukemia. The CPT-11 Research Group for Hematological Malignancies. Gan To Kagaku Ryoho 21:1047–1055.

107. Tsuda H, Takatsuki K, Ohno R, et al. 1994 Treatment of adult T-cell leukaemia-lymphoma with irinotecan hydrochloride (CPT-11). CPT-11 Study Group on Hematological Malignancy. Br J Cancer 70:771–774.
108. Ribrag V, Suzan F, Ravoet C, et al. 2003 Phase II trial of CPT-11 in myelodysplastic syndromes with excess of marrow blasts. Leukemia 17:319–322.
109. Bass AJ, Gockerman JP, Hammett E, et al. 2002 Phase I evaluation of prolonged-infusion gemcitabine with irinotecan for relapsed or refractory leukemia or lymphoma. J Clin Oncol 20:2995–3000.
110. Ross DD, Karp JE, Chen TT, Doyle LA. 2000 Expression of breast cancer resistance protein in blast cells from patients with acute leukemia. Blood 96:365–368.
111. Abbott BL, Colapietro AM, Barnes Y, Marini F, Andreeff M, Sorrentino BP. 2002 Low levels of ABCG2 expression in adult AML blast samples. Blood 100: 4594–4601.
112. Giovanella BC, Stehlin JS, Wall ME, et al. 1989 DNA topoisomerase I–targeted chemotherapy of human colon cancer in xenografts. Science 246:1046–1048.
113. Jeha S, Kantarjian H, O'Brien S, Vitek L, Beran M. 1998 Activity of oral and intravenous 9-aminocamptothecin in SCID mice engrafted with human leukemia. Leuk Lymph 32:159–164.
114. Rubin E, Wood V, Bharti A, et al. 1995 A phase I and pharmacokinetic study of a new camptothecin derivative, 9-aminocamptothecin. Clin Cancer Re 1:269–276.
115. Takimoto CH, Dahut W, Marino MT, et al. 1997 Pharmacodynamics and pharmacokinetics of a 72-hour infusion of 9-aminocamptothecin in adult cancer patients. J Clin Oncol 15:1492–1501.
116. Eder JP, Rubin E, Stone R, et al. 1996 Trials of 9-amino-20(S)-camptothecin in Boston. Ann NY Acad Sci 803:247–255.
117. Vey N, Kantarjian H, Tran H, et al. 1999 Phase I and pharmacologic study of 9-aminocamptothecin colloidal dispersion formulation in patients with refractory or relapsed acute leukemia. Ann Oncol 10:577–583.
118. Vey N, Giles FJ, Kantarjian H, Smith TL, Beran M, Jeha S. 2000 The topoisomerase I inhibitor DX-8951f is active in a severe combined immunodeficient mouse model of human acute myelogenous leukemia. Clin Cancer Res 6:731–736.
119. Giles FJ, Cortes JE, Thomas DA, et al. 2002 Phase I and pharmacokinetic study of DX-8951f (exatecan mesylate), a hexacyclic camptothecin, on a daily-times-five schedule in patients with advanced leukemia. Clin Cancer Res 8:2134–2141.
120. Burris HA. 1999 The evolving role of oral topotecan. Semin Hematol 36:26–32.
121. de Jonge MJ, Loos WJ, Gelderblom H, et al. 2000 Phase I pharmacologic study of oral topotecan and intravenous cisplatin: sequence-dependent hematologic side effects. J Clin Oncol 18:2104–2115.
122. Gerrits CJ, Schellens JH, Burris H, et al. 1999 A comparison of clinical pharmacodynamics of different administration schedules of oral topotecan (Hycamtin). Clin Cancer Res 5:69–75.
123. Masuda N, Fukuoka M, Takada M, et al. 1992 CPT-11 in combination with cisplatin for advanced non-small-cell lung cancer. J Clin Oncol 10:1775–1780.
124. Kudoh S, Fujiwara Y, Takada Y, et al. 1998 Phase II Study of Irinotecan Combined with Cisplatin in Patients with Previously Untreated Small-Cell Lung Cancer. West Japan Lung Cancer Group. J Clin Oncol 16:1068–1074.
125. Reid RJD, Fiorani P, Sugawara M, Bjornsti M-A. 1999 CDC45 and DPB11 are required for processive DNA replication and resistance to DNA topoisomerase I-mediated DNA damage. Proc Natl Acad Sci USA 96:11440–11445.

126. Chaturvedi P, Eng WK, Zhu Y, et al. 1999 Mammalian Chk2 is a downstream effector of the ATM-dependent DNA damage checkpoint pathway. Oncogene 18:4047–4054.
127. Cliby WA, Lewis KA, Lilly KK, Kaufmann SH. 2002 S phase and G_2 arrests induced by topoisomerase I poisons are dependent on ATR kinase function. J Biol Chem 277:1599–1606.

Index

D

E

R

S

Y